Atlas of Liver Pathology

A Pattern-Based Approach

MICHAEL TORBENSON, MD
Department of Laboratory Medicine and Pathology
Mayo Clinic
Rochester, MN

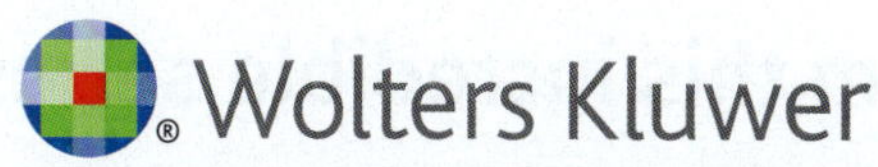

Philadelphia • Baltimore • New York • London
Buenos Aires • Hong Kong • Sydney • Tokyo

Acquisitions Editor: Ryan Shaw
Product Development Editor: Ariel S. Winter
Marketing Manager: Tyrone Williams
Production Project Manager: Bridgett Dougherty
Design Coordinator: Holly McLaughlin
Senior Manufacturing Coordinator: Beth Welsh
Prepress Vendor: TNQ Technologies

9 8 7 6 5 4 3 2 1

Printed in China

Library of Congress Cataloging-in-Publication Data

Names: Torbenson, Michael S., author.
Title: Atlas of liver pathology: a pattern-based approach / Michael Torbenson.
Description: Philadelphia: Wolters Kluwer, [2020] | Includes bibliographical references and index.
Identifiers: LCCN 2018061560 | ISBN 9781496396976 (hardback)
Subjects: | MESH: Liver—pathology | Liver Diseasest
Classification: LCC RC846.9 | NLM WI 700 | DDC 616.3/6207—dc23
LC record available at https://lccn.loc.gov/2018061560

shop.lww.com

CCS0219

PREFACE

The *Pattern-Based Approach* series is dedicated to providing pathology textbooks that more closely reflect the challenges of daily sign-out than conventional texts do. In other words, the focus is on practical clinical and histological findings that you actually need to know. This stands in contrast to books dedicated to comprehensive coverage, for which the goal is to provide all information about an entity, much of which is interesting, much of which is not, and most of which is not that important in getting your case signed out properly. That is not to mean that this book covers only common entities because it does not neglect the rare entities either. Instead, the focus is always on practical findings that are good to know, including clinical, histological, and molecular findings, but with an emphasis on histology. For this reason, there are lots of images (~790), succinct text, and organizational tools as outlined below that make the book even easier to navigate.

- Chapters begin with a "Chapter Checklist" that outlines the chapter for ease of reference. Similar "Checklists" are found throughout the chapter to help reinforce important aspects of complicated topics.
- The "Pearls & Pitfalls" sections include real lessons from the best of all instructors: experience. These sections highlight diagnostic clues, mimics, and pitfalls.
- The "Frequently Asked Questions" sections focus on important and recurrent clinical and histological questions.
- Approaches to reporting particularly challenging cases are illustrated in "Sample Note" sections.
- Each chapter ends with a "Near Misses Section," which uses a case-based approach to illustrate key diagnostic pitfalls.
- Each chapter also has a corresponding "Quiz" section online to reinforce important teaching points and provide a tool for self-assessment.

Liver pathology can be very challenging and a pattern-based approach is the perfect starting point for providing excellent patient care. This book is not perfect, as few books are, but I hope you like it and find it useful, especially when you are working on actual clinical material. In the end, I believe that there is no greater calling for a textbook than to be considered practical and useful by those who have it in their offices.

ACKNOWLEDGMENTS

I thank Drs Arnold, Lam-Himlin, and Montgomery for the invitation to write this book: three outstanding gastrointestinal (GI) pathologists and three wonderful people. I also thank the Acquisition Editor, Ryan Shaw, who has always been a pleasure to work with.

At Mayo Clinic, I am fortunate to work with Alison Smarzyk-Carlson, who does a fantastic job helping find case material for images, pulling obscure articles from the library, and helping with all of the other logistical aspects of writing this book.

Many thanks are also extended to all of the pathologists who have sent cases in consultation—I have learned a great deal from you and the difficult cases you have encountered. Thank you! And of course, I also thank you for reading this front material, which does not happen very often.

CONTENTS

1 BASIC PATTERNS IN LIVER PATHOLOGY

CHAPTER OUTLINE

INTRODUCTION

Liver pathology can be daunting, especially medical liver biopsy specimens. Sometimes it helps to remember that you do not need to be all-knowing. Instead, the patients and the clinicians are asking you to look at the liver biopsy and determine three principal things: (1) the major pattern of injury and its differential; (2) the degree of active injury; (3) and the amount of fibrosis. You are most likely to do an excellent job with these tasks if you start off by correctly recognizing the basic histological pattern of liver injury, a task usually performed best by using your low-power lenses. The need for this first step of identifying the major pattern of injury will be obvious to most readers, yet you might be surprised at how many times this step is skipped, and the pathologists jump right ahead to grading injury and staging fibrosis, which tends to make the pathology report less useful. Thus, this chapter will focus on the most common patterns of liver injury and lists the top three most common causes in the differential. Longer differentials for each pattern are found in their respective chapters.

ACUTE HEPATITIS VERSUS CHRONIC HEPATITIS VERSUS ACUTE-ON-CHRONIC HEPATITIS

As noted above, in most cases, the clinicians and patients are asking you to look at the liver biopsy and determine the major pattern of injury and its differential. In some cases, the histological findings can also provide insight into whether the injury is acute or chronic. Cases with definite fibrosis must have an element of chronicity (Fig. 1.1), as do cases with other structural abnormalities such as bile duct duplication, ductopenia, or periductal fibrosis.

When evaluating fibrosis as evidence for chronicity, do not be tricked by portal expansion due to either marked portal inflammation or ductular proliferation, both of which can mimic portal fibrosis. Also, do not be tricked by bridging necrosis, which can mimic bridging fibrosis. As another interpretative pitfall, finding more portal inflammation than lobular inflammation is sometimes mistaken as evidence for chronic hepatitis, but this is not true.

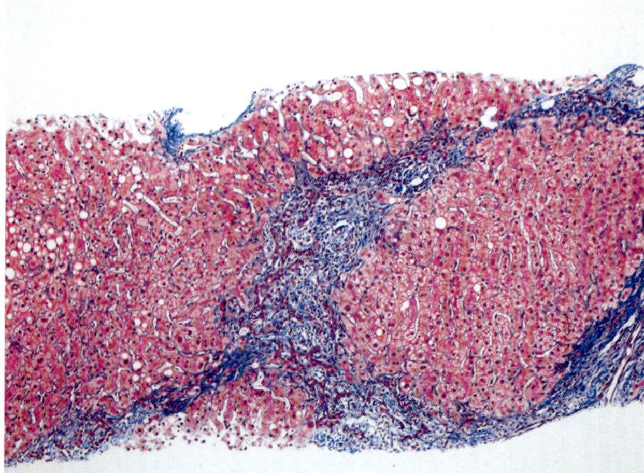

Figure 1.1. **Chronic hepatitis.** This case shows advanced fibrosis, with bridging fibrosis and focal parenchymal nodularity, indicating a chronic hepatitis.

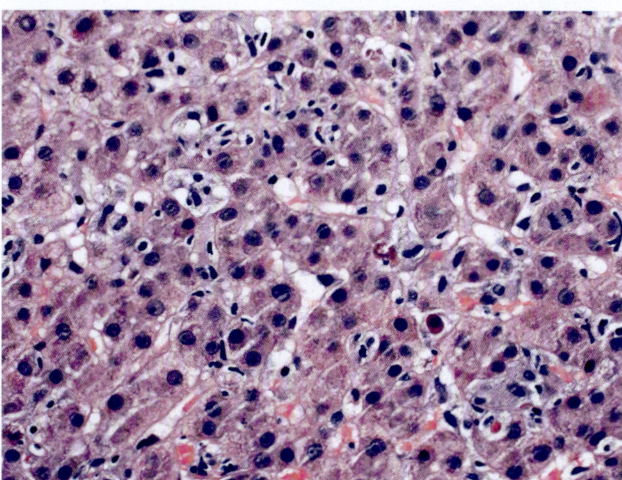

Figure 1.2. **Acute hepatitis.** In this case, the patient presented clinically with acute hepatitis and the biopsy shows moderate diffuse lobular hepatitis, a pattern that strongly suggests either acute hepatitis or acute-on-chronic hepatitis. In this case, there was no histological or clinical evidence for underlying chronic liver disease.

Histological changes that indicate the injury pattern is acute include finding marked lobular inflammation (Fig. 1.2) and or significant necrosis, as both are too injurious to the liver to be a chronic injury pattern. Of note, many biopsies will show patterns that could fit for either acute or chronic injury, so pathology is not always informative on this point. However, if there are histological features of both, then the findings are most commonly a chronic hepatitis with either a flare of the underlying liver disease, or a superimposed acute liver injury. Autoimmune hepatitis and hepatitis B are the two chronic livers diseases most likely to have clinically evident flares, which sometimes lead to liver biopsies, which can show an acute-on-chronic injury pattern.

ACUTE LIVER FAILURE

CHECKLIST: Causes of Acute Liver Failure

- ☐ Acetaminophen (40% to 50%)
  - ○ This percent is from the United States, Canada, and Europe but is less common elsewhere
- ☐ Idiosyncratic drug reactions (10% to 20%)
- ☐ Acute viral hepatitis (10% to 20%)
  - ○ Hepatitis A or B most common
- ☐ Idiopathic (20% to 30%)
- ☐ Rare causes
  - ○ Wilson disease
  - ○ Autoimmune hepatitis
  - ○ Alcoholic liver disease
  - ○ Budd–Chiari syndrome
  - ○ Nonhepatotropic viruses such as adenovirus and herpes simplex virus

The term acute hepatitis should not be confused with acute liver failure. From the clinical prospective, acute hepatitis simply means new onset elevations in liver enzymes within the last 6 months. In contrast, acute liver failure means an abrupt onset of severe liver disease that leads to encephalopathy and coagulopathy soon after clinical presentation. Although its not very relevant to surgical pathology, clinical studies further divide acute liver failure into hyperacute liver failure (<1 week from clinical presentation to encephalopathy or coagulopathy), acute liver failure (1 to 4 weeks), and subacute liver failure (4 to 13 weeks).[1]

The histological pattern of injury will depend on the etiology and can range from bland necrosis to vascular disease to marked hepatitis. Overall, most cases tend to fall into patterns of either extensive bland necrosis or marked hepatitis. Evidence for underlying liver disease in the form of fibrosis can be present when there is acute-on chronic injury.

The necrosis can also be described using the terms *zonal*, when a clear zonal pattern of necrosis is evident, and *panacinar*, when the necrosis involves multiple acini. In cases of panacinar necrosis, zonal patterns may still be evident in some areas of the specimen. *Massive necrosis* is just like it sounds and typically shows only a small rim of surviving hepatocytes around the zone 1 region. *Submassive necrosis* is not used entirely consistently in the literature. Sometimes this term is used to describe cases that fall in between pancacinar necrosis and massive necrosis, and in other cases, the term is used when a liver with massive necrosis also shows regenerative nodules, indicating the initial injury occurred long enough ago to allow significant liver regeneration.

Advanced fibrosis and the percent necrosis in liver biopsies both have prognostic information. Advanced fibrosis, which is defined as bridging fibrosis or cirrhosis, indicates a worse prognosis. For necrosis, the risk of death is low when there is less than 25% necrosis on biopsy but increased with 75% or more necrosis.[2-4]

ALMOST-NORMAL LIVER

CHECKLIST: Differential Diagnosis for an Almost-Normal Liver Biopsy in the Setting of Elevated Liver Enzymes

- ☐ Systemic autoimmune conditions
- ☐ Vascular outflow disease
- ☐ Low-grade or intermittent ischemic injury
- ☐ Metabolic syndrome (even if there is no fat on the biopsy)
- ☐ Drug effects

CHECKLIST: Differential Diagnosis for an Almost-Normal Liver Biopsy in the Setting of Portal Hypertension or Ascites

- ☐ Hepatoportal sclerosis
- ☐ Portal venopathy
- ☐ Peritoneal serositis without liver disease

The almost-normal liver pattern can be very challenging because you have to look very carefully not to miss subtle diagnoses (Fig. 1.3). Biopsies are usually prompted by either unexplained liver enzyme elevations or by unexplained portal hypertension/ascites. The differential in these two settings are different. However, in both cases, the histological findings are minimal, and by definition, there should be no significant inflammation, fatty change, cholestasis, biliary tract disease, fibrosis, or other evidence of active or chronic liver disease. In some biopsies with an almost-normal liver pattern, the liver injury is likely very mild and patchy and was missed on the biopsy. In other cases, the liver injury does not lead to microscopic changes. The etiology for elevated liver enzymes in 25% of cases with an almost-normal liver biopsy remains idiopathic despite full clinical and histological evaluation.

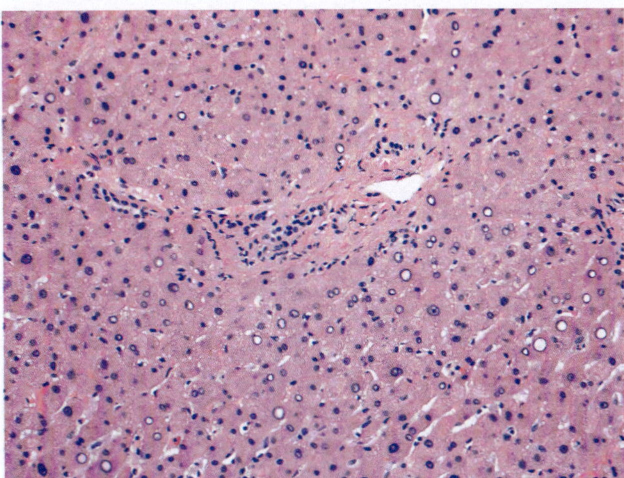

Figure 1.3. **Almost-normal liver.** This biopsy was performed for mildly elevated liver enzymes. There is no significant inflammation, fatty change, biliary tract disease, or fibrosis. Clinical follow-up studies did not identify the cause and the enzymes eventually normalized.

CHECKLIST: Differential for an Almost-Normal Liver Biopsy

These findings are subtle and can mimic an almost-normal biopsy

Abnormal Hepatocytes

- □ Hepatic glycogenosis
- □ Glycogen pseudo–ground glass change
- □ Alpha-1-antitrypsin deficiency

Structural Changes

- □ Nodular regenerative hyperplasia
- □ Hepatoportal sclerosis
- □ Early bile duct loss

Other

- □ Amyloid
- □ Stellate cell hyperplasia

RESOLVING HEPATITIS PATTERN

CHECKLIST: Resolving Hepatitis Pattern

- □ Acute self-limited viral infection
- □ Idiosyncratic drug reaction

The resolving hepatitis pattern of injury can also look like an almost-normal liver biopsy when the changes are mild. The biopsy shows no or minimal portal chronic inflammation and minimal or absent lobular hepatitis but does show scattered clusters of pigmented macrophages in the lobules (Fig. 1.4). The PASD stain will also highlight these clusters, which represent "clean-up" efforts in a site of prior mild lobular injury (Fig. 1.5). The most common cause is an acute self-limited viral infection or an idiosyncratic drug reaction, where the drug was stopped before the liver biopsy was performed. In most cases, the cause is suggested more by the clinical findings and clinical history than by the histological changes. However, the biopsy findings are important because they help rule out more significant liver disease.

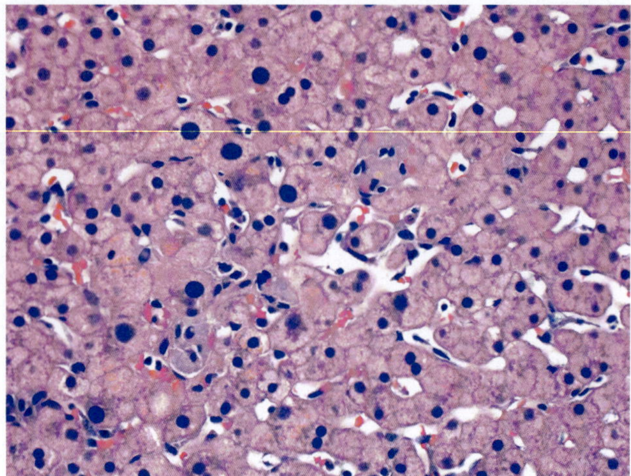

Figure 1.4. **Resolving hepatitis pattern.** This biopsy was performed 5 weeks after presentation of an acute hepatitis. By the time of the biopsy, the liver enzymes had decreased considerably. The biopsy shows scattered clusters of pigmented macrophages, but little active hepatitis or evidence for other forms of ongoing liver injury.

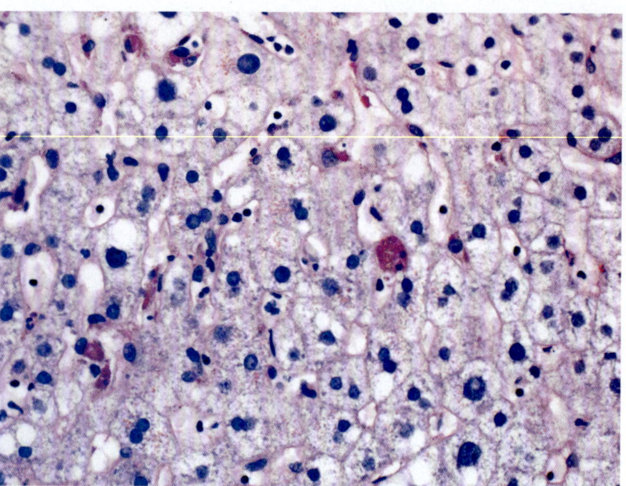

Figure 1.5. **Resolving hepatitis pattern, PASD stain.** The macrophages are easy to see because of their strong granular cytoplasmic staining on PASD stain.

CYTOPLASMIC CHANGES

Most cytoplasmic changes affect hepatocytes and lead to either diffuse cytoplasmic clearing or to distinct cytoplasmic inclusions. Diffuse cytoplasmic clearing usually results from glycogen accumulation in the setting of poorly controlled diabetes (Fig. 1.6). In infants and children, the differential also can include glycogen storage disease and urea cycle defects.

Distinct inclusions are further subdivided based on morphology. Large, single, pale inclusions that fill up most of the cytoplasm are called ground glass change in the setting of chronic hepatitis B and pseudo–ground glass change outside the setting of chronic hepatitis B (Fig. 1.7). The cytoplasmic ground glass changes can look exactly alike whether caused by chronic hepatitis B or by drug effects, so immunostains for hepatitis B surface antigen are important to perform. Most cases of pseudo–ground glass change are drug related.[5] A single drug or class of drug has not been identified, but most cases are found in association with immunosuppression and multiple medications.[5] Rarely, cases of glycogen pseudo–ground glass are idiopathic, and no cause is identified after routine clinical, laboratory, and histological evaluation. Other very rare genetic diseases can lead to similar inclusions, including type IV glycogen storage disease, fibrinogen storage disease, and LaFora disease.

Smaller more eosinophilic inclusions are found in zone 1 hepatocytes in alpha-1-antitrypsin deficiency (Fig. 1.8) and other genetic conditions that are very rare, such as antithrombin 3 deficiency and antichymotrypsin deficiency. The globules in alpha-1-antitrypsin deficiency are nicely highlighted by PASD stains (Fig. 1.9). Rarely, smaller eosinophilic inclusions have been reported in zone 3 hepatocytes in cases of chronic passive congestion of the liver.

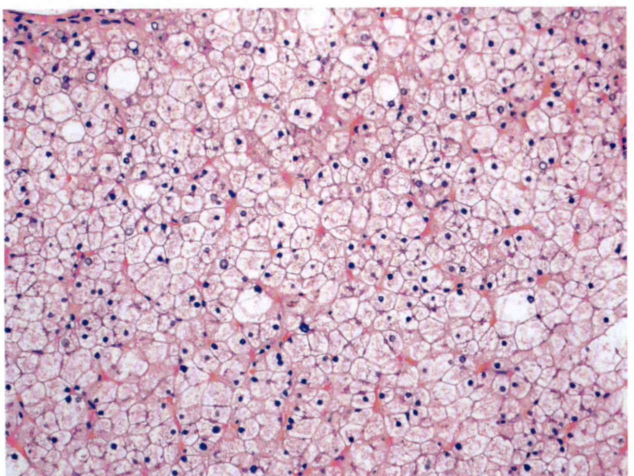

Figure 1.6. **Glycogenic hepatopathy.** The hepatocytes are mildly enlarged and show pale cytoplasm in this biopsy from a young man with poorly controlled type 1 diabetes mellitus.

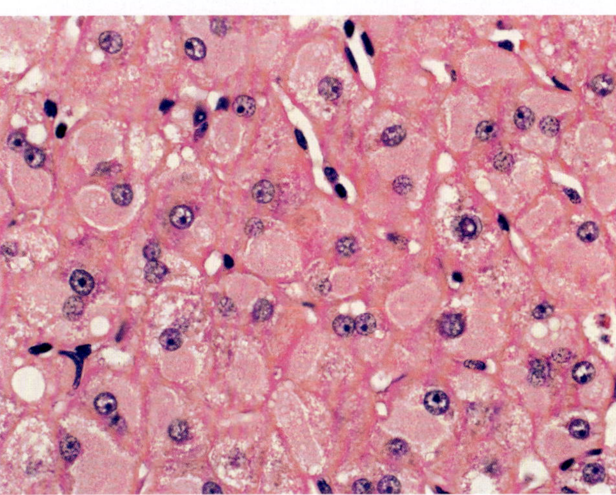

Figure 1.7. **Ground glass change in chronic hepatitis B.** Many of the hepatocytes contain a single large pale inclusion. These inclusions develop only in long-standing chronic hepatitis B infection and only in a subset of these cases. The changes of glycogen pseudo–ground glass change (usually a drug effect) can look exactly alike, so correlation with clinical and serological findings is important.

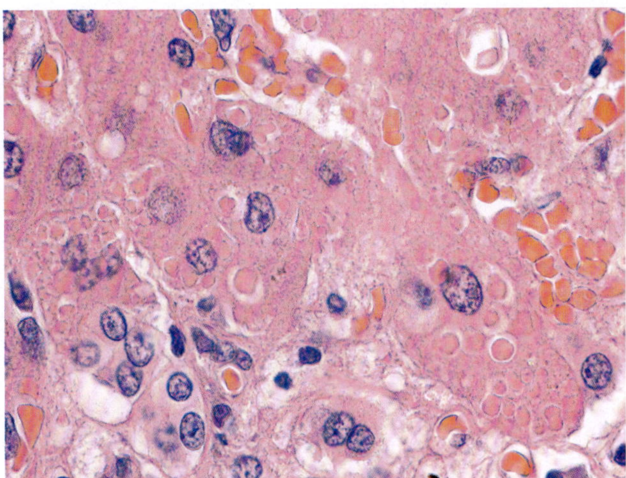

Figure 1.8. **Hepatocyte inclusions, alpha-1-antitrypsin deficiency.** The periportal hepatocytes show multiple round, pink globules.

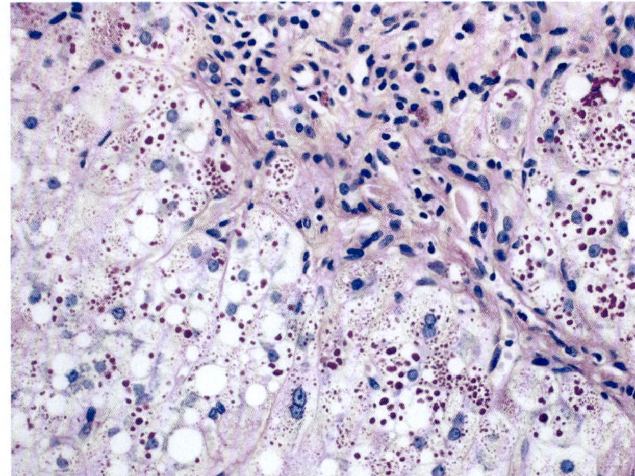

Figure 1.9. **Hepatocyte inclusions, alpha-1-antitrypsin deficiency, PASD stain.** The globules are highlighted by a PASD stain.

BLAND LOBULAR NECROSIS

CHECKLIST: Zone 1 Pattern of Necrosis

- ☐ Halothane toxicity (zone 3 necrosis more typical)
- ☐ Ferrous iron toxicity
- ☐ White phosphorous toxicity
- ☐ Endotoxin release from *Proteus vulgaris*
- ☐ Industrial chemicals such as allyl alcohol
- ☐ Hepatitis A

CHECKLIST: Zone 2 Pattern of Necrosis

- ☐ Poisons
- ☐ Heavy metals such as berrylium
- ☐ Yellow fever virus

CHECKLIST: Zone 3 Pattern of Necrosis

- ☐ Drug reaction including acetaminophen
- ☐ Various toxins
- ☐ Ischemia

CHECKLIST: Punched-out Azonal Pattern of Necrosis

- ☐ HSV
- ☐ VZV
- ☐ Adenovirus

Bland lobular necrosis results from direct liver injury that is not caused by the immune system. Thus, there is hepatocyte necrosis with relatively little or no inflammation (Fig. 1.10). Marked lobular inflammation from viral hepatitis, autoimmune hepatitis, or drug effect is also commonly associated with zone 3 necrosis or with bridging necrosis, but this pattern of necrosis is classified with the hepatitic pattern of injury.

In the bland lobular necrosis pattern of injury, the surviving hepatocytes commonly show cholestasis, and there often is mild small droplet steatosis (Fig. 1.11). If there has been sufficient time between the injury and the biopsy, the portal tracts can show a bile ductular reaction, and there may be mild lymphohistiocytic inflammation. Over time, the ductular reaction can extend out into the lobules in areas of parenchymal loss (Fig. 1.12). These areas will also show mild lymphohistiocytic inflammation. The proliferating bile ductules are often positive on iron stain (Fig. 1.13), but this does not indicate hemochromatosis and does not have any etiological significance.

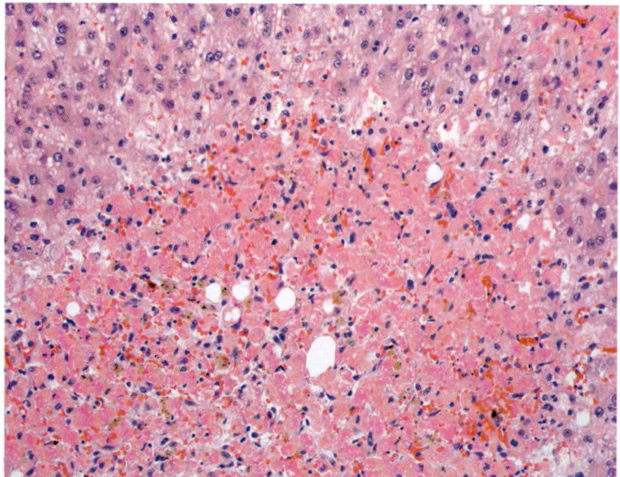

Figure 1.10. **Bland lobular necrosis.** There is extensive liver necrosis with relatively little inflammation in this case of acetaminophen toxicity. There is marked hepatocyte necrosis and hemorrhage surrounding the central vein (zone 3).

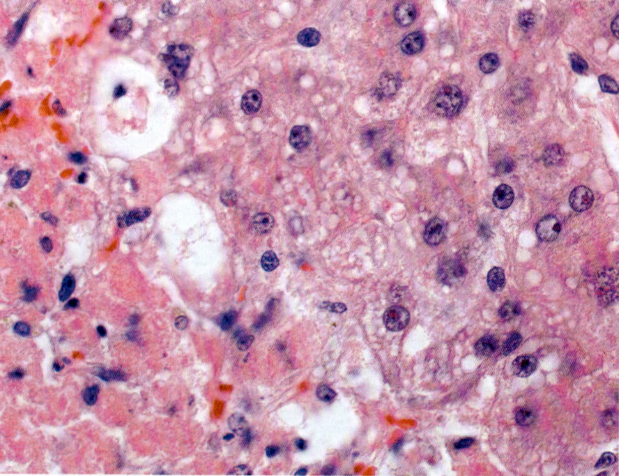

Figure 1.11. **Bland lobular necrosis, additional changes.** The surviving hepatocytes (same case as Fig. 1.10) show small droplets of fat in their cytoplasm. Necrotic hepatocytes are present in the lower left of the image.

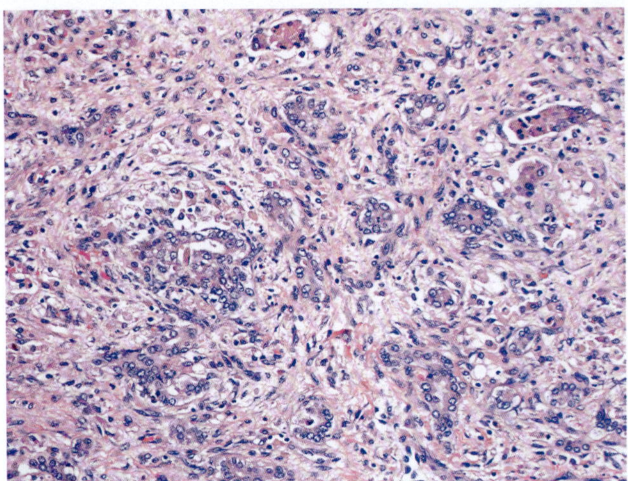

Figure 1.12. **Bland lobular necrosis, later stage.** The liver now shows a brisk reactive/reparative bile ductular response in the areas of parenchymal collapse. There also was mild nonspecific inflammation in the lobules and the portal tracts.

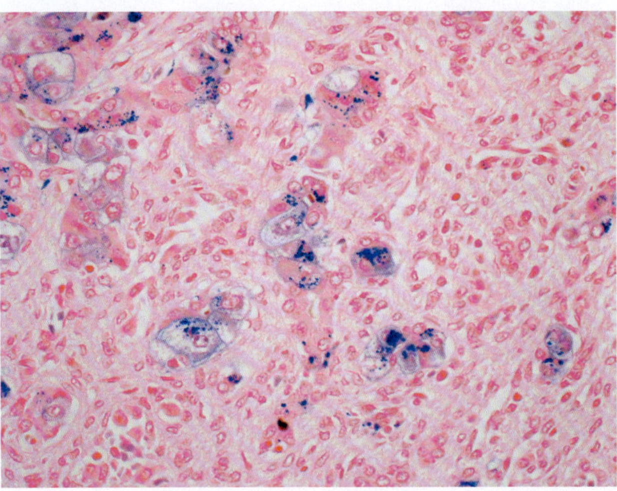

Figure 1.13. **Bland lobular necrosis, later stage, iron stain.** The proliferating bile ductules show mild nonspecific iron deposition. Sometimes the iron deposits can be moderate, but this finding is reactive in nature and does not indicate hemochromatosis.

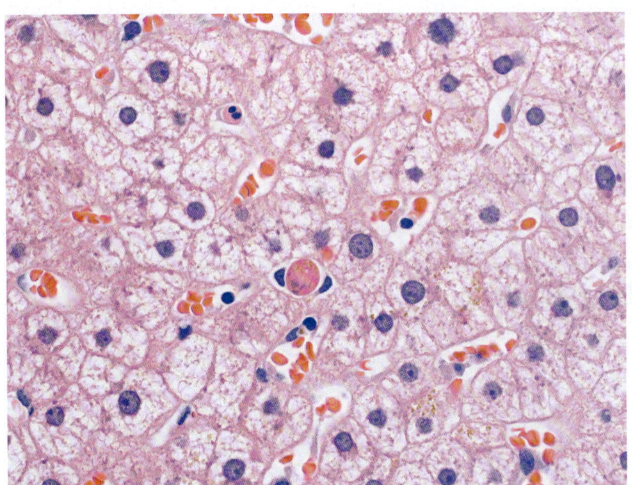

Figure 1.14. **Spotty necrosis.** The lobules showed rare scattered acidophil bodies.

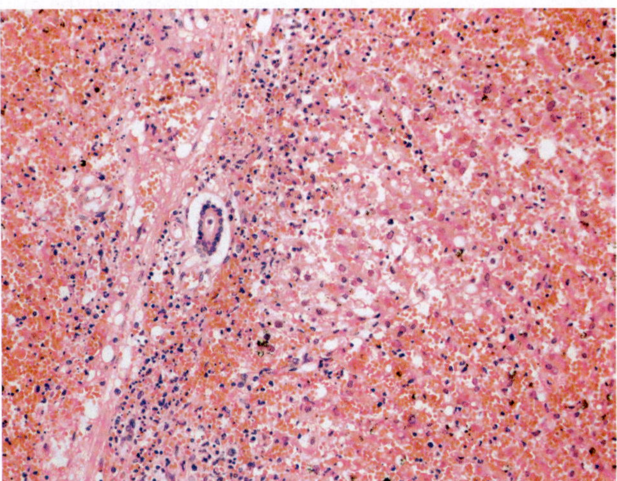

Figure 1.15. **Panacinar necrosis.** In this case of HSV hepatitis, there was extensive necrosis and hemorrhage that extends over many acini, leading to loss of almost all of the parenchyma.

The bland lobular necrosis pattern of injury is distinct from spotty necrosis, which is seen in the hepatitic pattern of injury, where small groups of hepatocytes or individual hepatocytes are necrotic (Fig. 1.14). In contrast, the term bland lobular necrosis indicates larger areas of necrosis. The bland lobular necrosis pattern most often involves zone 3 hepatocytes and multiple hepatic acini in the biopsy specimen. In more severe cases, there will be zone 3 hepatocyte necrosis in most or all of the hepatic acini, and there can be bridging necrosis. While the necrosis typically shows a zone 3 pattern with relative sparing of zones 1 and 2, rarely the necrosis can be focused in zone 1 or zone 2 or, in other cases, show an azonal pattern (no zonation is evident). In more severe cases, larger areas of necrosis can involve all zones and multiple acinar and are described using the term panacinar necrosis or massive necrosis (Fig. 1.15). The pattern of somewhat round, well-circumscribed, but azonal areas of necrosis is called *punched-out necrosis* (Fig. 1.16). This pattern is most commonly viral in origin.

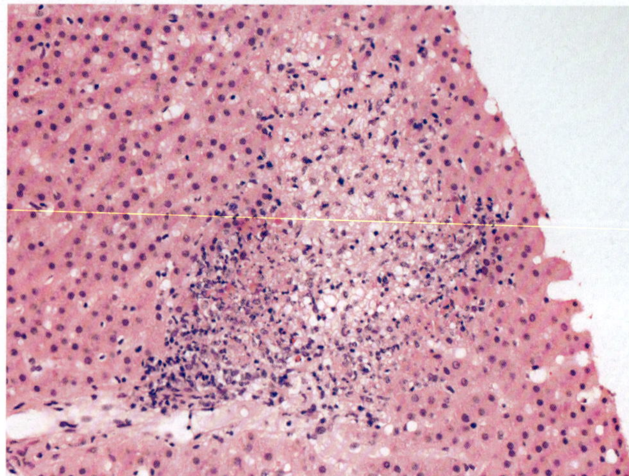

Figure 1.16. **Punched-out necrosis.** In this case of adenovirus hepatitis, the lobules show an azonal, well-circumscribed area of inflammation and necrosis.

In biopsy specimens, it is helpful to provide an estimate of the percent necrosis. An estimate to the nearest 10% will do fine. In some cases, the biopsy will be directed at a discrete lesion, and the bland lobular necrosis pattern will represent a focal change. Almost all of these cases are ischemic related. The differential for random biopsies is much wider, as shown in the checklists.

FATTY LIVER

CHECKLIST: Etiologies of Steatosis/Steatohepatitis

- ☐ Metabolic syndrome
- ☐ Alcohol use
- ☐ Drug effect
- ☐ Many rare genetic conditions such as Wilson disease
- ☐ Cystic fibrosis
- ☐ Elevated cortisol

Fatty liver disease is characterized by fat in the lobules. The fat, or steatosis, can range from minimal to marked. A common approach is to grade the fat as minimal (<5%), mild (5% to 33%), moderate (34% to 66%), and marked (>67%) (Figs. 1.17-1.20). Of course, this system is semiquantitative and nobody expects you to distinguish, for example, between 33% and 34% fat. Instead, your best estimate of the percent of fat is completely satisfactory. Fat estimates are typically made using a 10X or 20X lens. Focus on the macrovesicular steatosis. There always will be some small- and medium-sized droplets of fat too (Fig. 1.21), but focus on the macrovesicular component, which is easier to do if you stick with the 10X or 20X lens. There is no need to separately mention the smaller droplets of fat (Fig. 1.21). Some pathologists cannot resist the temptation and so use terms such as mixed micro- and macrovesicular steatosis, but this is always unnecessary and occasionally troublesome to the clinicians and patients who read these reports and are confused by the terminology, wondering why the pathologist felt it was important to mention the smaller droplets of fat.

Minimal macrovesicular fat is unlikely to be clinically relevant. If there is mild fat or greater, then you will next have to decide if the changes reach the level of steatohepatitis. This decision is made by looking for evidence of active injury, which includes ballooned hepatocytes, more than minimal lobular inflammation, and/or acidophil bodies.

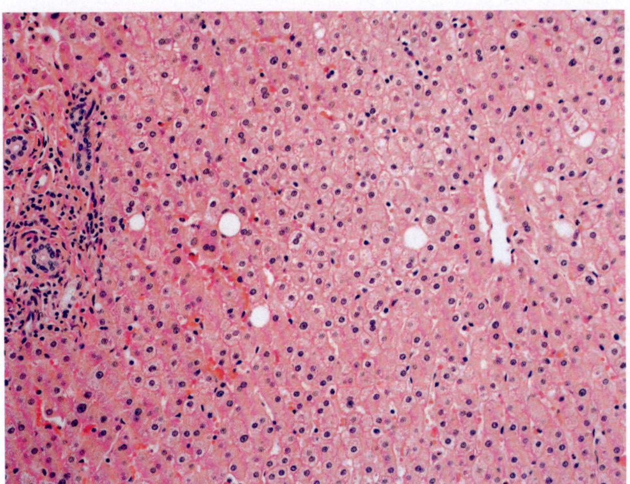

Figure 1.17. Macrovesicular steatosis, minimal. The lobules show less than 5% macrovesicular steatosis.

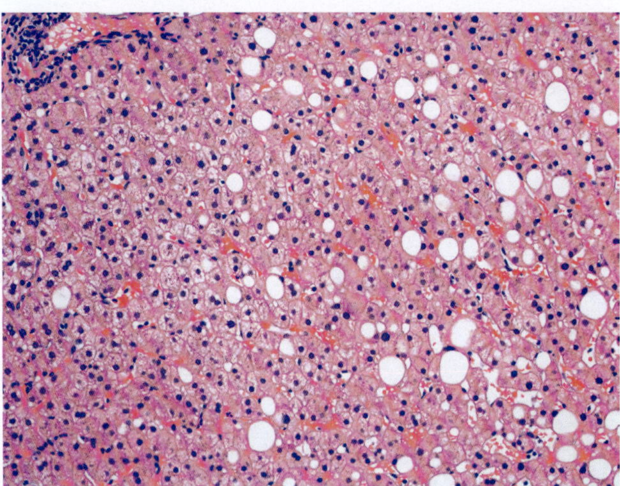

Figure 1.18. Macrovesicular steatosis, mild. The lobules show about 10% macrovesicular steatosis.

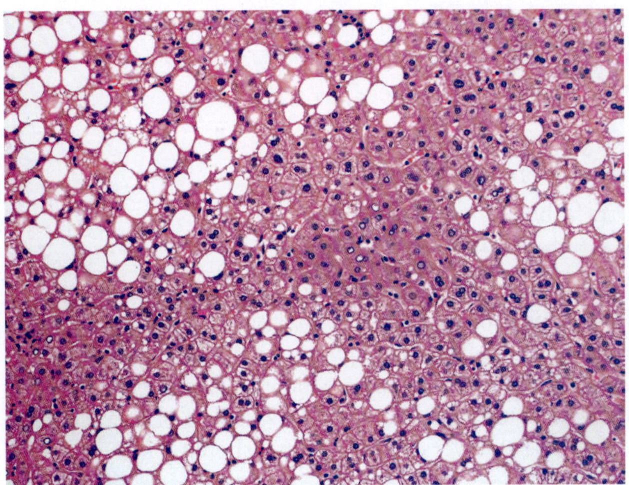

Figure 1.19. Macrovesicular steatosis, moderate. The lobules show about 60% macrovesicular steatosis.

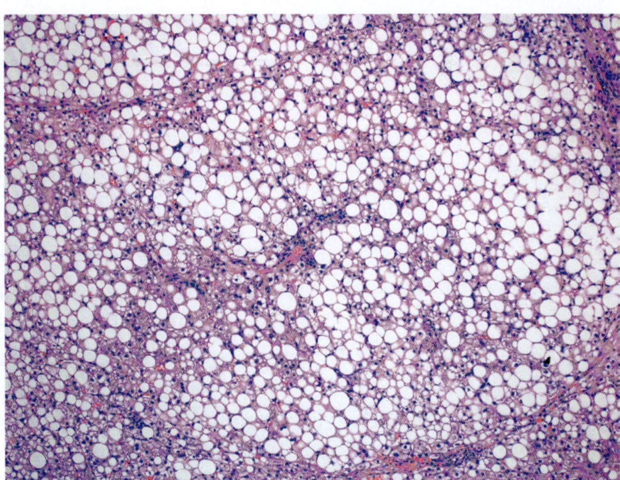

Figure 1.20. Macrovesicular steatosis, marked. The lobules show about 90% macrovesicular steatosis.

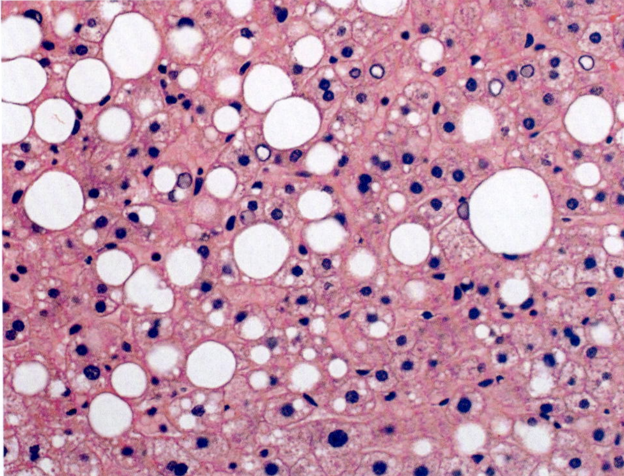

Figure 1.21. Macrovesicular steatosis. In most cases of macrovesicular steatosis, the hepatocytes can also show smaller droplets of fat.

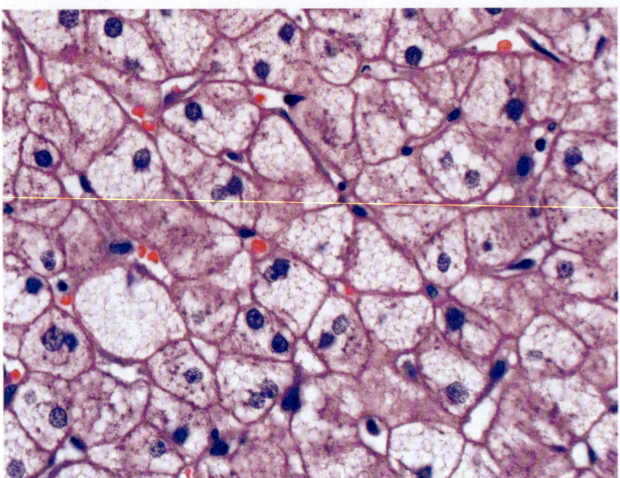

Figure 1.22. **Microvesicular steatosis.** The hepatocytes have a foamy appearance to their cytoplasm that results from numerous droplets of tiny fat that entirely fills the cytoplasm.

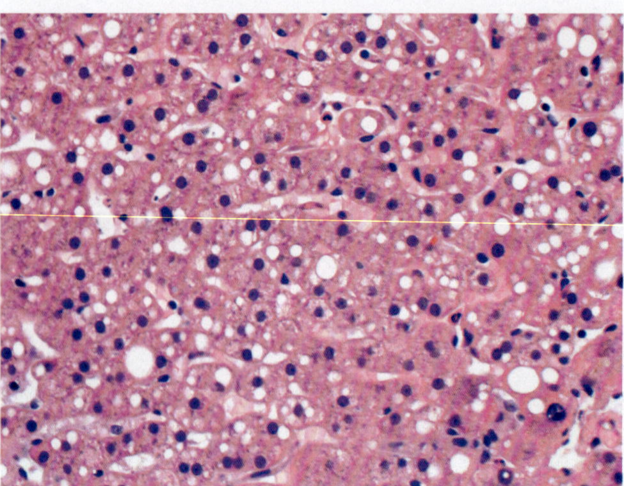

Figure 1.23. **Not microvesicular steatosis.** This pattern is part of macrovesicular steatosis and should not be mistaken for an additional component of microvesicular steatosis.

CHECKLIST: Microvesicular Steatosis

- ☐ Drug effect
- ☐ Acute alcohol foamy degeneration
- ☐ Metabolic defects including fatty liver of pregnancy

A microvesicular pattern of steatosis is very rare, but the hepatocytes are diffusely affected and show numerous tiny droplets of fat in their cytoplasm (Fig. 1.22). This pattern can be subtle on low and medium power, but on high power is generally easy to see. The hepatocyte cytoplasm should be packed with tiny vacuoles. Occasionally, one can encounter cases where a lot of hepatocytes have a few smaller droplets of fat each (Fig. 1.23), usually in the setting of ordinary fatty liver disease, but this should not be mistaken for microvesicular steatosis.

HEPATITIC PATTERN OF INJURY

CHECKLIST: The Hepatitic Pattern

- ☐ Viral hepatitis (hepatotropic viruses A through E)
- ☐ Autoimmune hepatitis
- ☐ Drug reaction

The hepatitic pattern of injury is defined by lymphocytic inflammation in the lobules and/or portal tracts (Fig. 1.24). The degree of inflammation in both the lobules and the portal tracts can range from mild to marked. Moderate or marked lobular inflammation is often accompanied by lobular necrosis (Fig. 1.25). In some diseases, such as autoimmune hepatitis and primary biliary cirrhosis, plasma cells can be prominent in the portal inflammation. Occasional scattered eosinophils are not uncommon and do not have any particular significance when they are sparse (Fig. 1.26). The lobules often show diffuse Kupffer cell hyperplasia (Fig. 1.27). Focal clusters of pigmented histiocytes can also be seen in the lobules and the portal tracts.

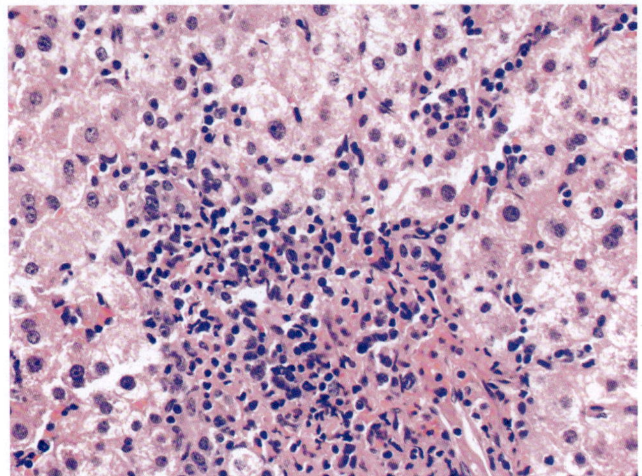

Figure 1.24. **Hepatitic pattern of injury.** The portal tracts and the lobules show mild lymphocytic inflammation.

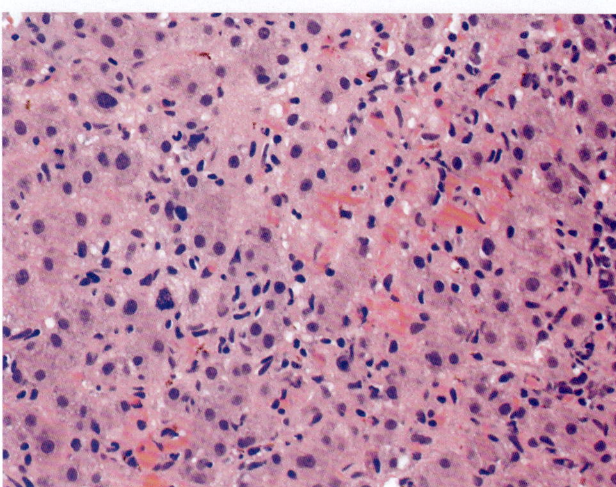

Figure 1.25. **Hepatitic pattern of injury.** There is a moderate lobular hepatitis in this case of a drug reaction.

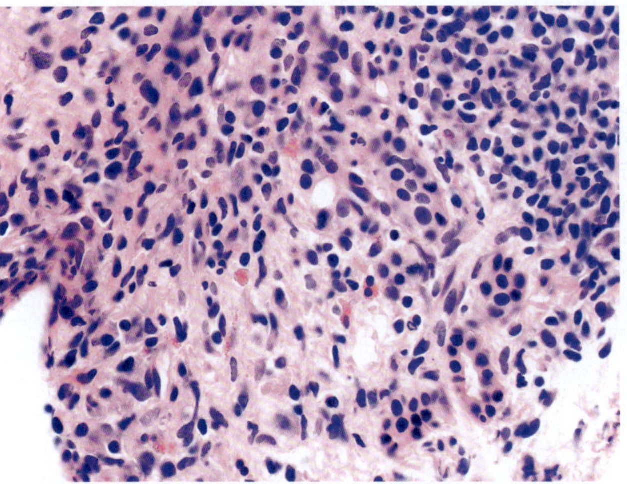

Figure 1.26. **Hepatitic pattern of injury, portal chronic inflammation.** As can be seen in this case of chronic hepatitis C, the portal tract inflammation is predominately lymphocytic but occasional plasma cells or eosinophils are not uncommon and do not have any significance when they are not prominent.

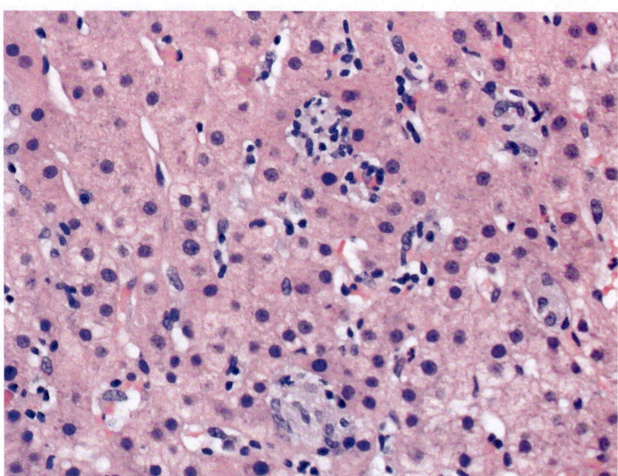

Figure 1.27. **Hepatitic pattern of injury.** Kupffer cell hyperplasia is common with acute liver injury. In this case of resolving hepatitis, the Kupffer cells formed scattered small aggregates. Kupffer cell hyperplasia can be more diffuse when there is more active lobular injury and can be particularly prominent when there is a cholestatic hepatitis.

Of course, other disease patterns frequently have portal and lobular inflammation, but the hepatitic pattern refers to cases where the inflammation is the only pattern or is the predominant pattern. To illustrate these points, a biopsy with mild steatosis, occasional ballooned hepatocytes, and moderate patchy lobular inflammation would be classified as having a pattern typical for moderately active steatohepatitis (Fig. 1.28). On the other hand, a biopsy with mild steatosis but marked lobular inflammation with patchy zone 3 necrosis would be classified as predominately a hepatitic pattern (Fig. 1.29).

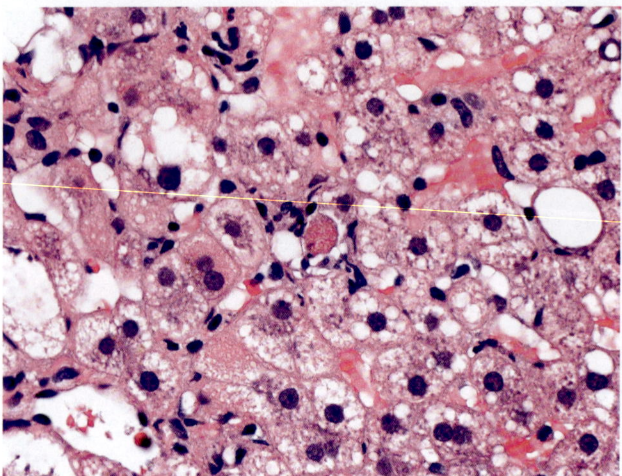

Figure 1.28. **Steatohepatitis.** There is a moderate lobular hepatitis in this case, but the overall pattern was that of moderately active steatohepatitis and not a hepatic pattern.

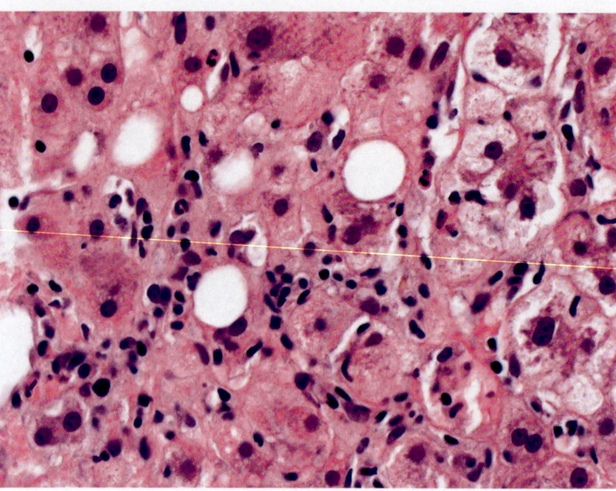

Figure 1.29. **Hepatitic pattern of injury.** This case of acute viral hepatitis B also has some fat, but the predominant pattern of injury is hepatitic and not fatty liver disease.

GIANT CELL HEPATITIS

The giant cell hepatitis pattern shows numerous multinucleated hepatocytes (Fig. 1.30), often with cholestasis and generally mild to moderate hepatitis. The giant cells stain with hepatic markers and typically have 3 to 10 nuclei. A few rare giant cells are not uncommon in many different diseases, but this finding does not qualify for a diagnosis of giant cell hepatitis, which requires the giant cell transformation to be prominent. Giant cell hepatitis is a pattern of injury and can be associated with a variety of injuries, especially in neonates (see Chapter 8). In adults, most cases are idiopathic. Nonspecific elevations in ANA and/or SMA titers are common, but the clinical, serological, and histological findings are rarely if ever that of autoimmune hepatitis.

GRANULOMAS

CHECKLIST: Granulomas

- ☐ Primary biliary cirrhosis
- ☐ Sarcoidosis, CVID, and other systemic granulomatous diseases
- ☐ Drug effect
- ☐ Infection
- ☐ Idiopathic
- ☐ Paraneoplastic

CHECKLIST: Granulomatous Hepatitis Pattern

- ☐ Infection
- ☐ Drug reaction

Granulomas can be found in the portal tracts or the lobules and can be single or numerous. They are most commonly epithelioid and noncaseating, but caseating granulomas are occasionally encountered. Most liver biopsies with granulomas will show a single small granuloma or a few scattered small granulomas, which are epithelioid and noncaseating (Fig. 1.31). In these cases, the granulomas are noted in the report, but the term granulomatous hepatitis is not used. The granulomatous hepatitis pattern of injury shows numerous granulomas and is typically associated with mild or greater lobular inflammation (Fig. 1.32).

The histological findings can provide some clues to the possible etiology of the granulomas, but outside of finding an organism, clinical correlation is always needed. A subset of granulomas will be associated with fibrosis, most commonly in the setting of sarcoidosis (Fig. 1.33). Foreign body granulomas will have visible material in their cytoplasm by light microscopy or by polarization. Granulomas can be associated with other findings typical for a disease. For example, primary biliary cirrhosis can have granulomas. The location of the granulomas (portal tracts vs. lobules) is largely irrelevant.

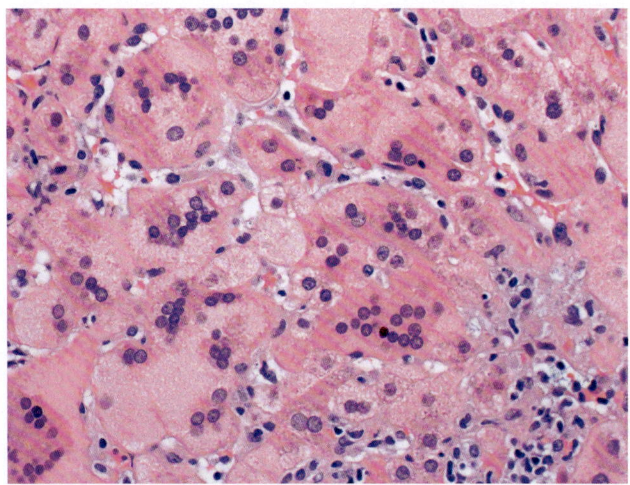

Figure 1.30. **Giant cell hepatitis.** The lobules show prominent giant cell transformation of hepatocytes with mild to focally moderate inflammation.

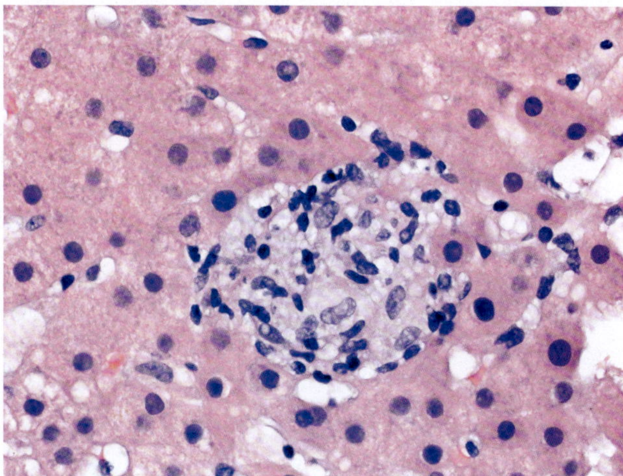

Figure 1.31. **Granulomas.** This liver biopsy showed a few incidental, small, epithelioid granulomas.

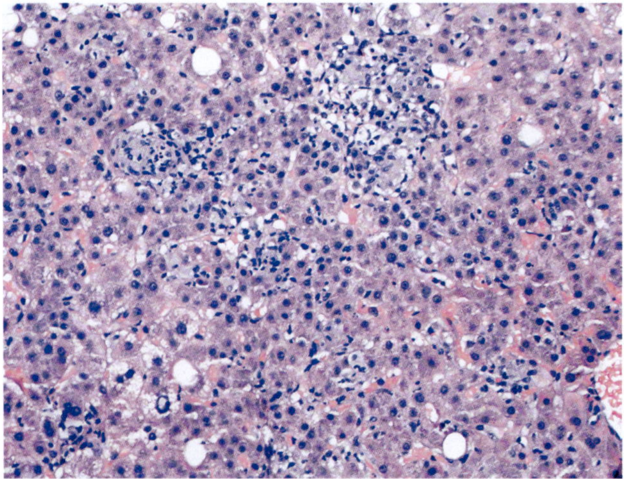

Figure 1.32. **Granulomatous hepatitis.** This biopsy of an acute infectious hepatitis showed numerous lobular granulomas along with moderate lobular hepatitis.

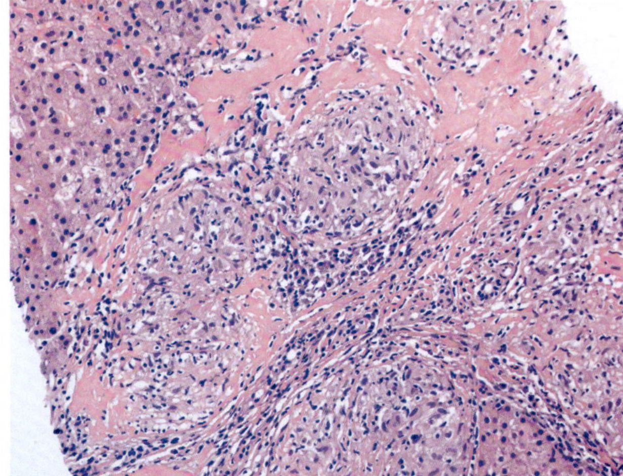

Figure 1.33. **Granulomas, fibrosis.** There was fibrosis associated with granulomas in this case of sarcoidosis. The fibrosis can be seen adjacent to the granulomas and also within the granulomas.

BLAND LOBULAR CHOLESTASIS

CHECKLIST: Bland Lobular Cholestasis Pattern

- ☐ Drug effect
- ☐ Severe systemic illness/sepsis
- ☐ Paraneoplastic syndromes—one example is the Stauffer syndrome, where a subset of patients with carcinomas (usually renal) develop cholestatic liver dysfunction[6-8]

In this pattern, the major finding is lobular cholestasis, without significant inflammation and without changes of biliary obstruction (Fig. 1.34). The bile is typically found in both the hepatocytes and in the bile canaliculi. There is no ductopenia and no evidence for advanced fibrosis.

FAQ: Does the location of the bile have diagnostic value?

Answer: No. The bile can be in hepatocytes or the canaliculi or in proliferating ductules. The location of the bile tends to correlate with the duration and severity of the cholestasis but has no other diagnostic significance. Early and mild cholestasis can be purely hepatocelluar, but most cases have mixed hepatocelluar and canalicular cholestasis. Severe long-standing cholestasis can also have bile located in bile ductules.

Ducular or cholangiolar cholestasis (also called *cholangitis lenta*) is most commonly found in association with severe debilitating illnesses leading to liver dysfunction or with severe long-standing cholestasis. In both situations, individuals are at increased risk for infections and death because of their severe underlying illness, but ductular cholestasis per se does not indicate a person is septic.

FAQ: I thought bile in the proliferating bile ductules (Fig. 1.35) indicated sepsis?

Answer: This is a common misconception that has somehow taken on a life of its own, kind of like fake news. Although the origin of this notion is hard to determine, it seems to have developed in part from a few small case series and the autopsy experience, where prolonged cholestasis and a bit of sepsis is not uncommon in terminally ill patients who die in the hospital.

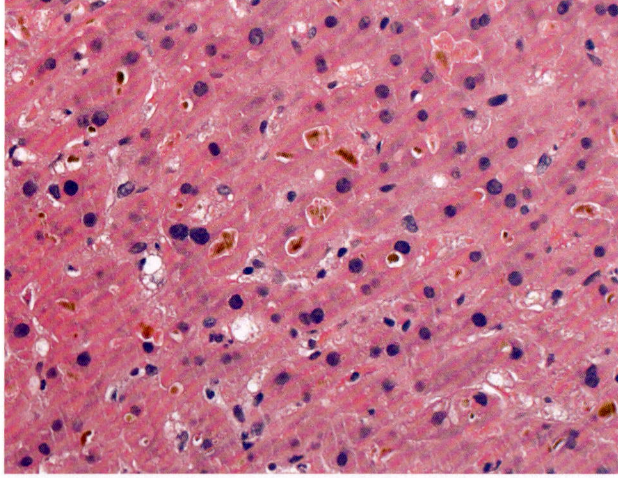

Figure 1.34. **Bland lobular cholestasis.** There is moderate lobular cholestasis in this drug reaction, but there is no significant inflammation and no evidence for biliary obstruction.

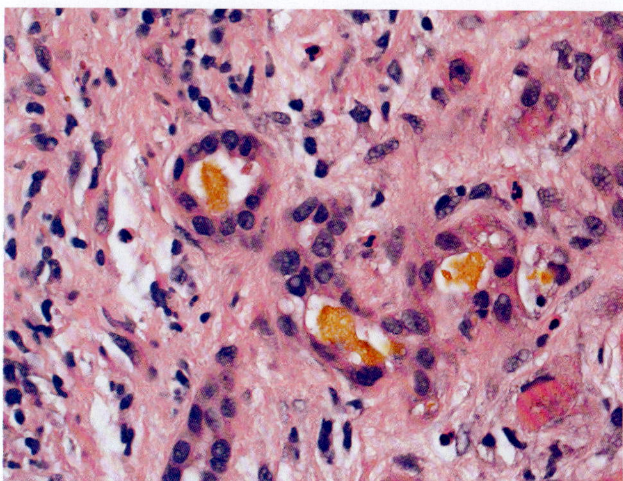

Figure 1.35. **Cholangiolar or bile ductular cholestasis.** This biopsy is from a liver with decompensated cirrhosis from chronic hepatitis C. The liver was deeply cholestatic, but there was no history of sepsis. This pattern is most commonly seen with severe long standing cholestasis from any cause or in chronic cholestasis arising from debilitating illnesses, including many patients who are at increased risk for sepsis. However, this pattern should not be interpreted as indicating the patient is septic.

BILIARY OBSTRUCTION

CHECKLIST: The Biliary Obstruction Pattern

- ☐ Downstream biliary obstruction from strictures, stones, tumors, etc.
- ☐ Ischemic strictures
- ☐ Infectious strictures
- ☐ Mimics of biliary obstruction
    - ○ Vascular outflow disease
    - ○ Severe acute hepatitis
    - ○ MDR3 deficiency

The biliary obstruction pattern is characterized by bile ductular proliferation (Fig. 1.36), mild mixed portal inflammation composed of neutrophils and a few lymphocytes (Fig. 1.37), and occasionally with portal edema (Fig. 1.38). The degree of these changes correlates roughly with the degree and the acuteness of the obstruction, with rapid-onset high-grade acute obstructions showing the most striking changes. The lobules show minimal to mild inflammation. Lobular cholestasis can range from absent to marked, depending on the duration and severity of the obstruction (Fig. 1.39). In cases of long-standing obstruction, bile can also be found in the bile ductules.

Note that a mild patchy bile ductular proliferation is also present to varying degrees in many different disease patterns. In the biliary obstruction pattern, the ductular proliferation and other related changes are the predominant finding, whereas in other disease patterns, the ductular proliferation is a minor component (Fig. 1.40). For example, severe acute viral hepatitis frequently shows mild to moderate bile ductular proliferation, but the major injury is found in the lobules, which show significant inflammation and often areas of confluent necrosis. Vascular outflow disease can also have a mild bile ductular proliferation that mimics biliary tract disease.[9] Inherited bile salt deficiency disease, especially MDR3 deficiency, can also have histological changes that suggest obstruction, especially if there is advanced fibrosis.[10]

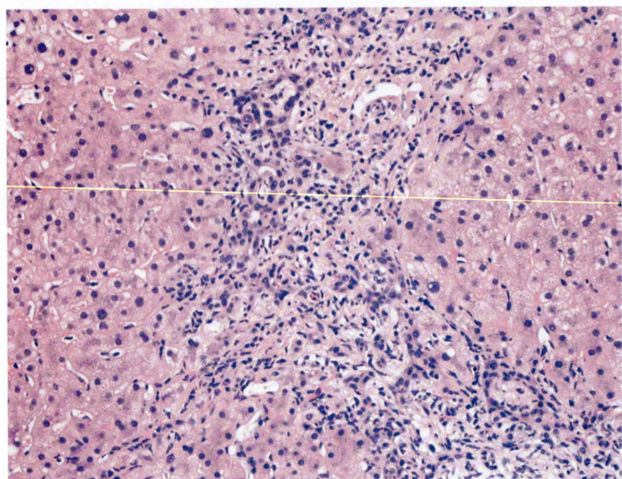

Figure 1.36. **Biliary obstruction pattern.** The portal tract shows a brisk bile ductular proliferation

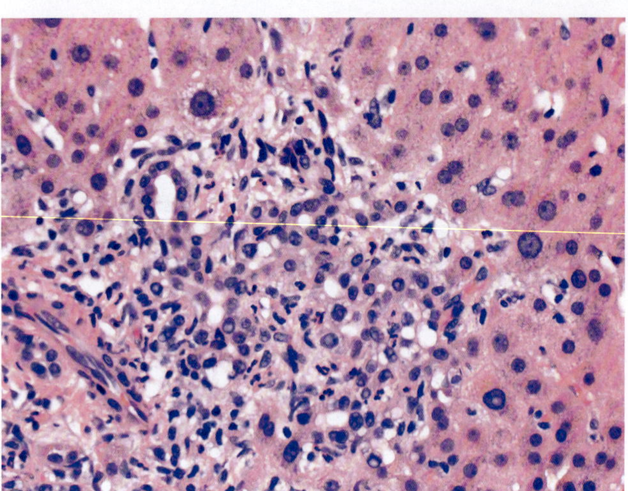

Figure 1.37. **Biliary obstruction pattern.** The ductular proliferation is associated with mixed inflammation including neutrophils, lymphocytes, and occasional eosinophils.

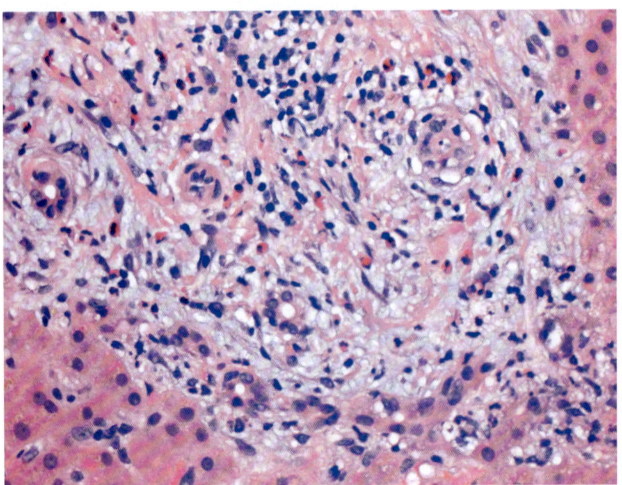

Figure 1.38. **Biliary obstruction pattern.** The portal tract shows mild edema, with light blue gray myxoid material.

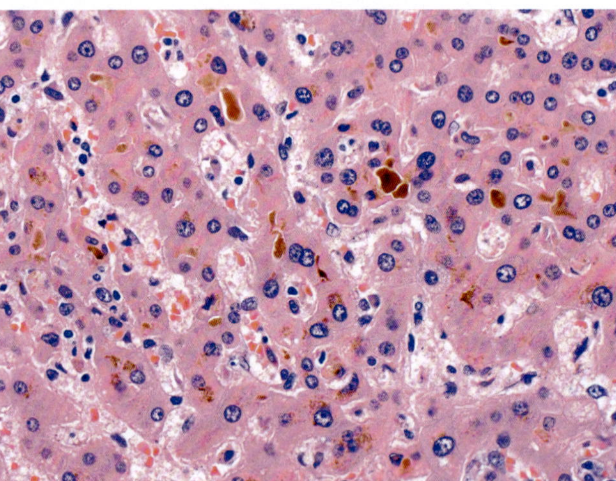

Figure 1.39. **Biliary obstruction pattern.** This liver showed long-standing chronic obstruction due to a cholangiocarcinoma. The lobules show moderate cholestasis.

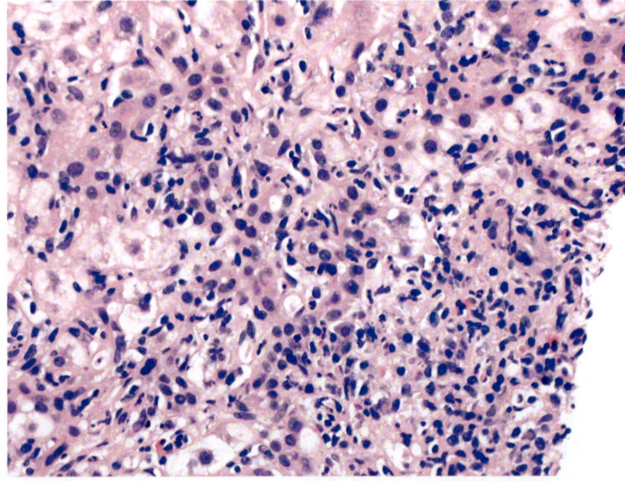

Figure 1.40. **Bile ductular proliferation in a hepatitic pattern.** There is patchy mild bile ductular proliferation in this case of acute hepatitis B, but the predominant pattern is hepatitic.

With chronic biliary obstruction, biopsies can show bile duct duplication (Fig. 1.41) and periductal fibrosis (Fig. 1.42). Periductal fibrosis is very helpful when present but does tend to get over diagnosed, as the normal medium and larger bile ducts of the liver can have a cuff of collagen (Fig. 1.43). Periductal fibrosis can lead in time to complete loss of the bile duct, with replacement of the bile duct by a fibrous scar, a finding called a fibro-obliterative duct lesion (Fig. 1.44). Ductopenia can also develop in time but is not specific for obstruction.

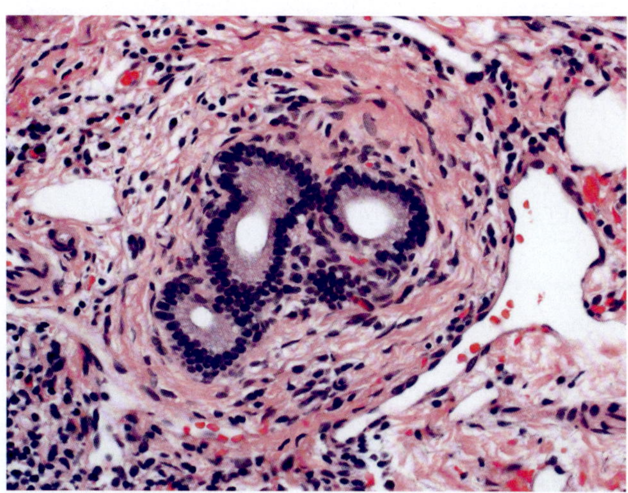

Figure 1.41. **Bile duct duplication.** The portal tracts show a small cluster of bile ducts in this case of primary sclerosing cholangitis.

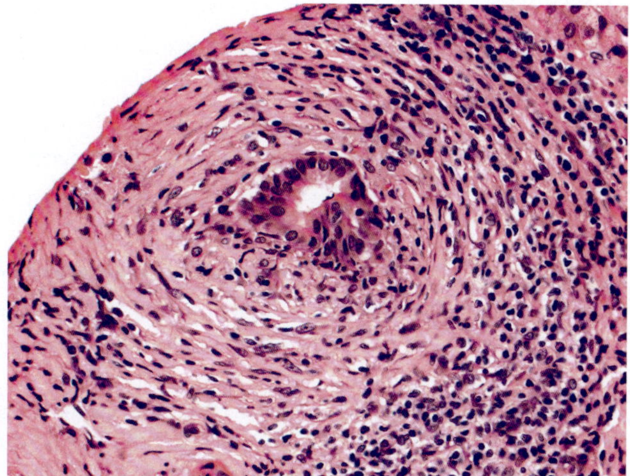

Figure 1.42. **Periductal fibrosis.** This pattern is also called onion skin fibrosis. The bile ducts show a concentric, somewhat laminated cuff of fibrosis.

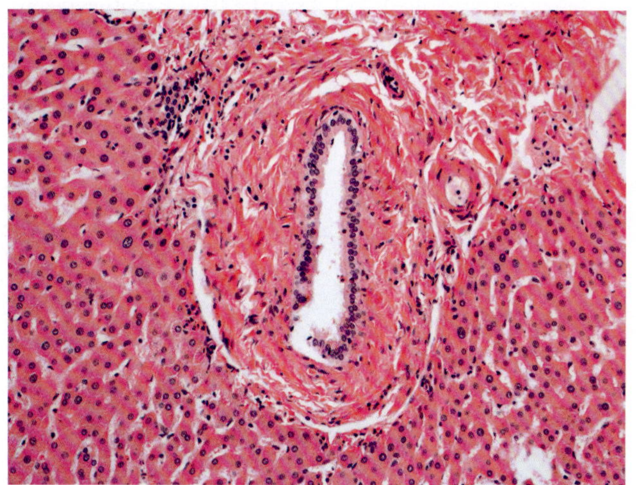

Figure 1.43. **Not periductal fibrosis.** This large portal tract has a normal layer of collagen around the bile duct. Do not mistake this for periductal fibrosis.

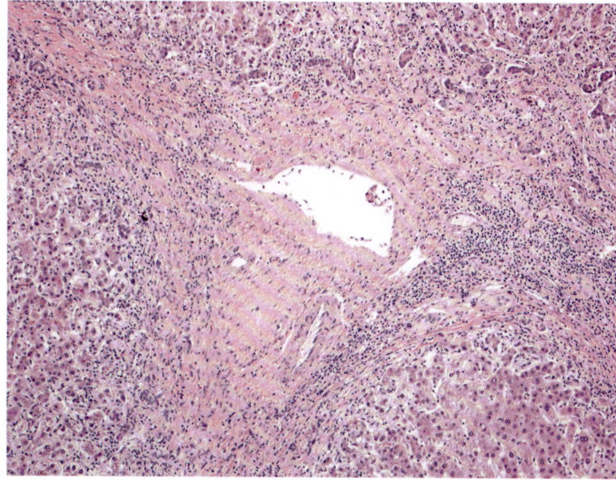

Figure 1.44. **Fibro-obliterative duct lesion.** The bile duct has been replaced by a round scar in this case of end-stage cirrhosis from primary sclerosing cholangitis.

DUCTOPENIA

CHECKLIST: Ductopenia

- ☐ Chronic downstream biliary obstruction from PSC, strictures, stones, tumors, etc.
- ☐ Primary biliary cirrhosis
- ☐ Transplant related, solid organ or bone marrow
    - ○ Chronic liver allograft rejection
    - ○ GVHD
    - ○ Ischemic cholangiopathy
- ☐ Pediatric liver diseases: paucity of intrahepatic bile ducts, inherited bile salt deficiency
- ☐ Drug effect
- ☐ Paraneoplastic syndrome: Hodgkin, peripheral T cell lymphoma
- ☐ AIDS (acquired immunodeficiency syndrome) Most are infection related
- ☐ Idiopathic

Ductopenia is defined by the loss of bile ducts (Fig. 1.45). Sometimes this pattern is called the "vanishing bile duct syndrome" in the literature. In the normal liver, up to 10% of the smallest branches of the portal tracts may not have a bile duct evident on H&E.[11] Thus, the most common definition for ductopenia is that at least 50% of portal tracts should have absent bile ducts, with an adequate biopsy of at least 10 portal tracts. The entire portal tract does not have to be present to be counted toward specimen adequacy, but there should be enough of the portal tract that a bile duct would be evident, if present. As a point of reference, an average needle core biopsy contains 6 complete portal tracts and 3 to 4 nearly complete portal tracts.[11] As the bile ducts and hepatic arteries tend to run close together, you can also look for the arteries to make sure enough of the portal tract is present for scoring.[12] Medium or larger sized portal tracts should always have a bile duct, so if a biopsy happens to sample one of these larger portal tracts, a missing bile duct is always abnormal. A CK7 is an excellent tool to evaluate for ductopenia, and also identifies intermediate hepatocytes (Fig. 1.45). Intermediate hepatocytes are defined by the expression of CK7 and are found in zone 1 hepatocytes in cases of chronic cholestatic liver disease.

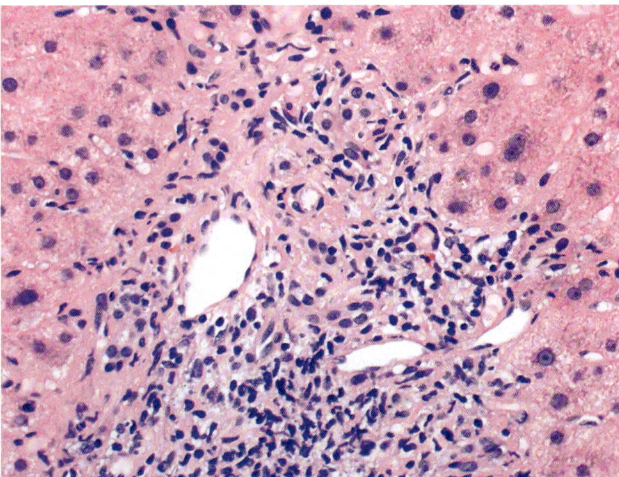

Figure 1.45. Bile duct loss. There is no bile duct in the portal tract (confirmed by CK7 stain). There is mild portal chronic inflammation, but no etiology was identified in this case.

FAQ: What happens if between 50% and 80% of the portal tracts do not have bile ducts?

Answer: In this situation, it is best to report out the findings and indicate that they are suggestive of ductopenia, but are not diagnostic.

PEARLS & PITFALLS

Before making a diagnosis of ductopenia, check the alkaline phosphatase levels. If they are not moderately to markedly elevated, then go back and take another look at the biopsy, as true ductopenia is unlikely. Supplement the H&E findings with CK7 and copper stains. The CK7 will help evaluate ducts and highlight intermediate hepatocytes. Copper deposition is seen in the periportal hepatocytes in most cases of established ductopenia, although it can be quite focal.

CHRONIC BILIARY/CHOLESTATIC INJURY

CHECKLIST: Chronic Biliary/Cholestatic Injury

- □ Chronic downstream biliary obstruction from PSC, other strictures, stones, tumors, etc.
- □ Primary biliary cirrhosis
- □ Drug effect

This pattern has overlap with the biliary obstruction pattern but is a less specific pattern of biliary injury, and the term is used when the overall findings are not sufficient for a confident diagnosis of an obstruction pattern and do not fit for bland lobular cholestasis or ductopenia. Bile ductular proliferation ranges from absent to patchy and mild. The bile ducts proper often look relatively normal, although some cases will show mild bile duct lymphocytosis and injury. There can be mild nonspecific portal inflammation, but lobular inflammation is absent or minimal. Lobular cholestasis is typically absent or sometimes mild. Other findings can include bile duct duplication, periductal fibrosis, and ductopenia.

This pattern of chronic biliary/cholestatic injury is often subtle and the H&E changes can be equivocal so are best supported by CK7 and copper stains. CK7 will help assess for bile duct loss and will identify intermediate hepatocytes (Fig. 1.46). Intermediate hepatocytes are usually in zone 1 but can be more extensive in the lobules in response to severe chronic cholestasis. The periportal hepatocytes can also show cholate stasis, with cell swelling, cytoplasmic clearing, and small fragments of Mallory hyaline (Fig. 1.47). The hepatocytes affected by cholate stasis resemble ballooned hepatocytes, but their location and the overall histological findings are distinct from that of fatty liver disease. Periportal copper deposition also supports a diagnosis of chronic cholestasis (Fig. 1.48), as copper is normally excreted in the bile and chronic elevations in bile salts leads to deposition in zone 1 hepatocytes. Finally, the cirrhotic nodules in biliary cirrhosis can be irregular and vaguely interlocking—sometimes called a jigsaw pattern of cirrhosis—and the cirrhotic nodules can have a rim of edema and cholate stasis at their periphery that really stands out at low power—sometimes called a halo sign (Fig. 1.49).

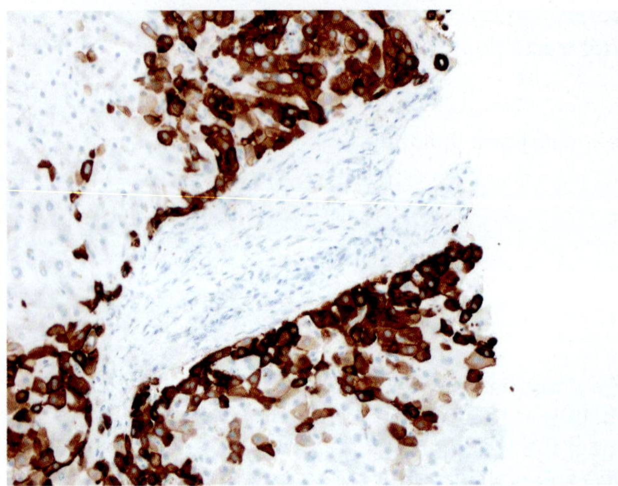

Figure 1.46. **Bile duct loss, CK7 immunostain.** The CK7 shows no bile duct, but does stain zone 1 hepatocytes—called intermediate hepatocytes.

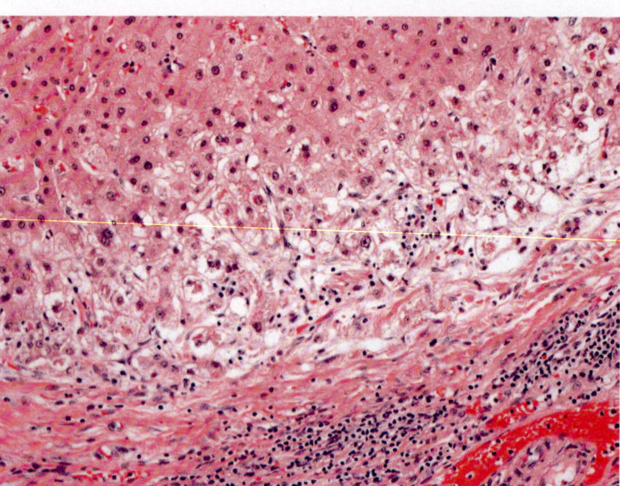

Figure 1.47. **Cholate stasis.** In this case of primary biliary cirrhosis, the zone 1 hepatocytes show mild swelling, cytoplasmic clearing, and Mallory hyaline.

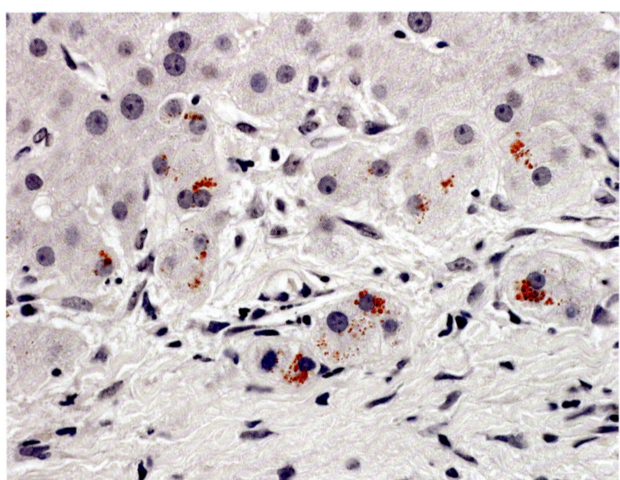

Figure 1.48. **Periportal copper deposition, rhodanine copper stain.** In this case of primary biliary cirrhosis, the zone 1 hepatocytes show mild periportal copper deposition.

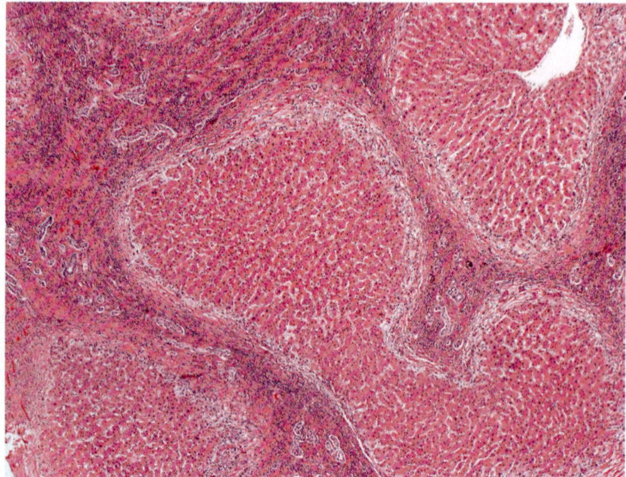

Figure 1.49. **Halo sign.** The cirrhotic nodules are surrounded by cholate stasis, which leads to a "halo" at low power because of cholate stasis.

PEARLS & PITFALLS

With the CK7 stain, a single or rare positive hepatocytes is nonspecific (Fig. 1.50) and does not help support the diagnosis of chronic cholestatic liver injury. A zone 3 pattern of intermediate hepatocytes can be seen with long-standing lobular cholestasis or with vascular outflow disease (Fig. 1.51).

The copper accumulation can be very focal in early cases of chronic cholestatic liver injury, so the stain has to be examined carefully. Copper accumulation in cirrhotic livers can be nonspecific, so the stain is most helpful when there is no or mild fibrosis.

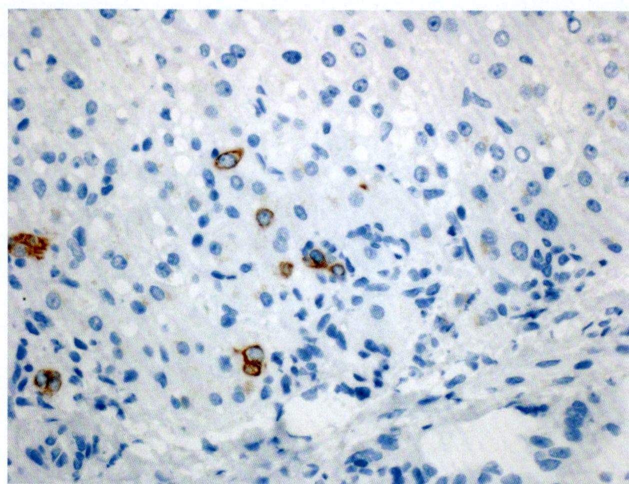

Figure 1.50. CK7, nonspecific rare positive cells. A rare CK7 positive hepatocyte was seen in this wedge biopsy, a nonspecific finding. In the setting of obstruction, there will be larger aggregates or contiguous blocks of positive hepatocytes in zone 1.

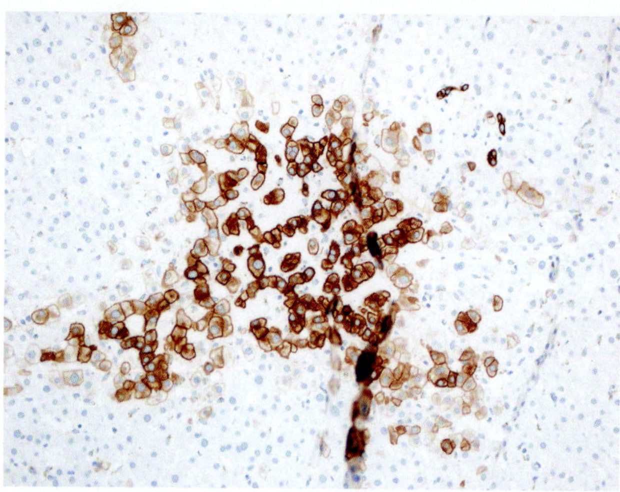

Figure 1.51. CK7, vascular outflow disease. In this case of congestive heart failure, the liver showed only mild zone 3 congestion, but CK7 nicely highlighted zone 3 hepatocytes.

VASCULAR DISEASE

Vascular diseases are classified into hepatic arterial disease, portal vein disease, sinusoidal disease, peliosis hepatis, or hepatic vein disease. The most common pattern is vascular outflow disease, which can result from cardiac disease or thromboses of the hepatic veins or vena cava. Vascular outflow disease also has the most striking findings (Fig. 1.52), with zone 3–predominant sinusoidal dilatation, congestion, and often zone 3 fibrosis. A mild bile ductular proliferation is often seen in the portal tracts (Fig. 1.52).[9] The central veins can also be occluded or scarred in veno-occlusive disease (Fig. 1.53), a pattern now subsumed under the term of sinusoidal obstructive syndrome.

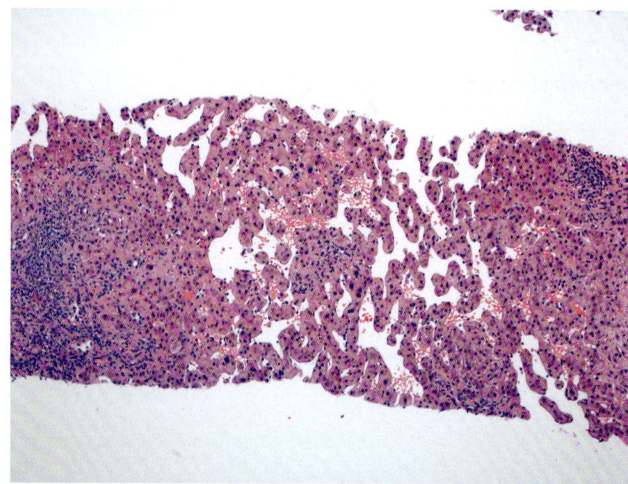

Figure 1.52. Vascular outflow disease. In this case with heart failure, the liver shows marked zone 3 congestion. A trichrome also showed zone 3 fibrosis. The portal tract in the left of the image showed mild bile ductular proliferation.

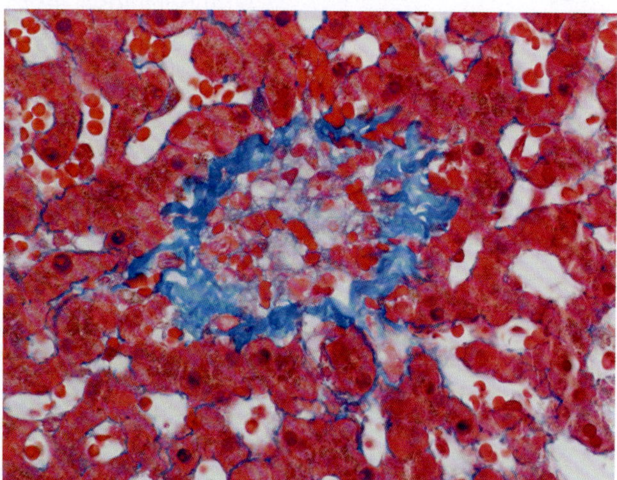

Figure 1.53. Venoocclusive disease, trichrome stain. Sometimes changes in the smallest central veins are easier to see on the trichrome stain. This case is from a drug reaction (herbal remedy).

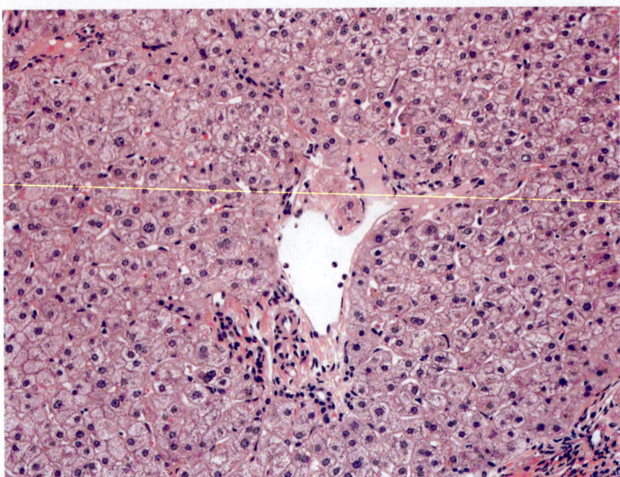

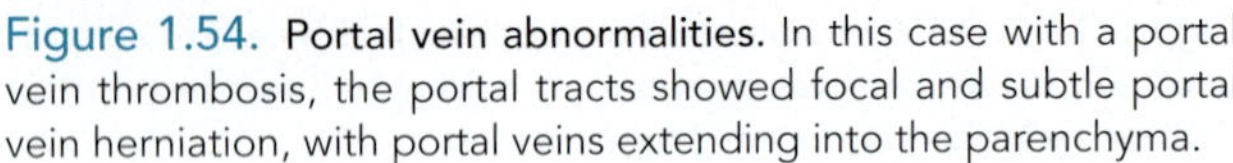

Figure 1.54. **Portal vein abnormalities.** In this case with a portal vein thrombosis, the portal tracts showed focal and subtle portal vein herniation, with portal veins extending into the parenchyma.

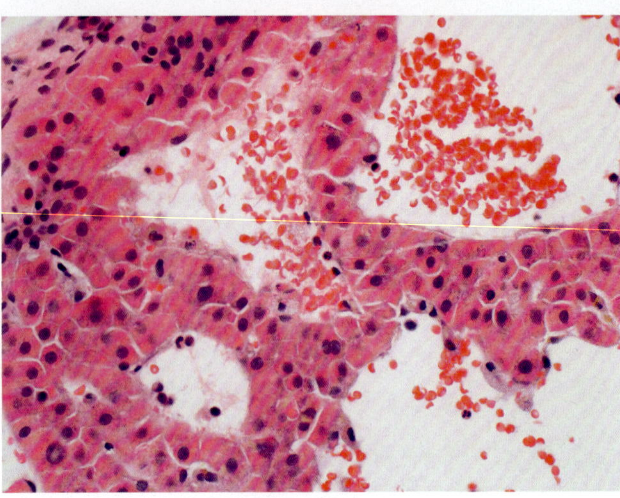

Figure 1.55. **Peliosis hepatis.** The lobules show irregular blood filled cysts in this case of androgen associated peliosis hepatis.

Portal vein disease is considerably more subtle, but the findings revolve around varying degrees of herniation (Fig. 1.54), atrophy, loss, and fibrosis of the portal veins. The lobules will show nodular regenerative hyperplasia in many cases.

Hepatic arterial disease is very uncommon. Low-grade or intermittent arterial obstruction can lead to bland lobular spotty necrosis with little or no inflammation. Acute high-grade obstruction can lead to parenchymal necrosis. Chronic arterial injury can lead to segmental biliary tract disease that closely resembles primary sclerosing cholangitis.

Peliosis hepatis refers to irregular cystlike areas filled with blood (Fig. 1.55). The cystlike spaces do not have an endothelial lining, although there can re-endothelialize in long-standing cases. The cysts are often small, less than 1 mm, but can be up to several cm. The larger cysts can rarely present with hemorrhage, but peliosis hepatis is a histological finding in most cases. Patients can also have portal hypertension. Other organs can also be involved, most commonly the spleen, bone marrow, and lymph nodes.

CHECKLIST: Peliosis Hepatis

- ☐ Debilitating illness
  - Tuberculosis, leprosy
  - AIDS (can be *Bartonella* related)
  - Cancer (most commonly lymphoma/leukemia)
  - Light chain deposition disease
  - Malnutrition
- ☐ Medications
  - Estrogens
  - Androgens
  - Azathioprine

COMBINED PATTERNS

In many liver specimens, elements of more than one pattern of injury are present. In these cases, focus on the major pattern of injury in your assessment. Next, consider the question of whether the second, minor pattern of injury is the one that often co-occurs with the major pattern of injury. For example, marked hepatitis often is accompanied by mild ductular proliferation. In these cases, your report can focus on the major pattern of injury for both the diagnosis and differential. However, if the two patterns do not commonly co-occur together, then both patterns should be given a diagnosis and a differential. As one example, mildly active steatohepatitis does not typically co-occur with significant bile ductular proliferation, so if both patterns are present in a specimen, both should be indicated in the diagnosis and be given differentials in the note/discussion.

CRYPTOGENIC CIRRHOSIS

Cryptogenic cirrhosis is a term used by both clinicians and pathologists. A cirrhotic liver is often biopsied when no definite cause can be determined by serology or clinical findings (clinically cryptogenic). Histological findings can help identify the cause of the cirrhosis in some cases or at least provide a prioritized differential, but many cases remain cryptogenic after full histological and clinical examination. Even when no specific cause is identified, histology can exclude many causes and help narrow the differential.

In this setting, when the histological findings are nonspecific, the final cirrhosis classification is "most likely" or "probable" with a given disease based on the clinical findings. For example, if the patient has the metabolic syndrome and no other risk factors by histology, serology, or clinical findings, then the cirrhosis is classified as probable nonalcoholic fatty liver disease. Likewise, if there is a history of remote but severe alcohol use but no other risk factors, then the cirrhosis is classified as probable alcohol-related cirrhosis, even if there is no active steatohepatitis. Cases with positive autoantibodies but no other risk factors are often classified as probable burned out autoimmune hepatitis.

PEARLS & PITFALLS

Histological examination of the liver is important to rule out recognizable causes of liver disease. Sometimes it can be tempting to push the histology findings too far. These are some examples of findings that are often clues when combined with clinical and serological findings and pitfalls when not:

- Mild macrovesicular steatosis is not a specific finding and does not by itself indicate steatohepatitis was the cause of the cirrhosis but requires clinical correlation with risk factors for the metabolic syndrome or alcohol use.
- Occasional ballooned hepatocytes are not a specific finding and do not in isolation indicate steatohepatitis was the cause of the cirrhosis.
- Pericellular fibrosis in a cirrhotic liver is not a specific finding and does not by itself indicate steatohepatitis was the cause of the cirrhosis.
- Onion-skin fibrosis and/or fibro-obliterative duct lesions do not prove primary sclerosing cholangitis, although they do support a biliary cause for the cirrhosis.
- Alpha-1-antitrypsin globules are most commonly seen in the setting of heterozygosity and do not in isolation prove alpha-1-antitrypsin deficiency as the cause of the cirrhosis (although it could well have been a contributing factor). Homozygosity for alpha-1-antitrypsin deficiency is sufficient alone to cause cirrhosis.
- Moderate iron is common in cirrhotic livers and does not prove hemochromatosis as the cause of the liver disease.
- Mild copper is common in cirrhotic livers and does not prove Wilson disease or biliary cirrhosis as the cause of the liver disease. However, if a specimen has no copper on a properly cut and stained rhodanine stain, then Wilson disease or biliary cirrhosis is less likely.

HEPATOCELLULAR TUMORS

In many cases, the tumor is obvious, while in other cases well-differentiated tumors can blend into the background liver on low power. Clues that can help identify the tumor are the loss of portal tracts (Fig. 1.56), a "clonal appearance" where two distinct populations of cells are present on the biopsy (Fig. 1.57), and arterioles located in the sinusoids (Fig. 1.58). Note that this last finding should not be equated with a definite tumor, as lobular arterialization can be seen in medical liver diseases including fatty liver disease and long-standing portal vein problems.

Once the tumor has been identified, the next steps are to determine if the tumor is benign or malignant and identify the major cell type that comprises the tumor, for example, is the tumor a hepatic proliferation, biliary proliferation, vascular proliferation, etc. Special stains are often used in both of these steps and are detailed in the tumor chapters.

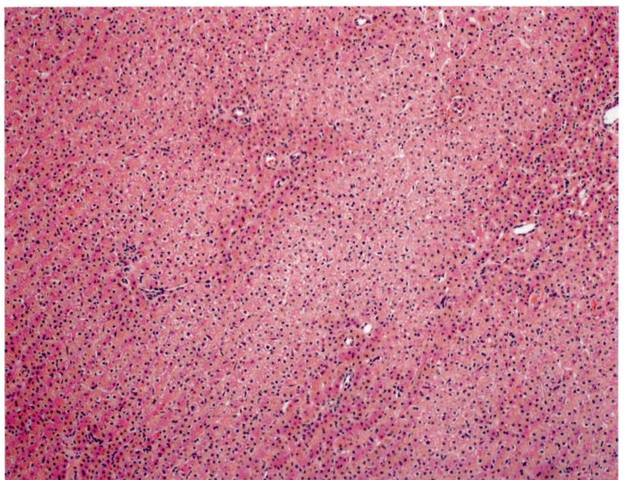

Figure 1.56. **Well-differentiated hepatic tumor.** While the tumor is very well differentiated and the hepatocytes are cytologically normal appearing, the lack of portal tracts identifies this as tumor (from a hepatic adenoma).

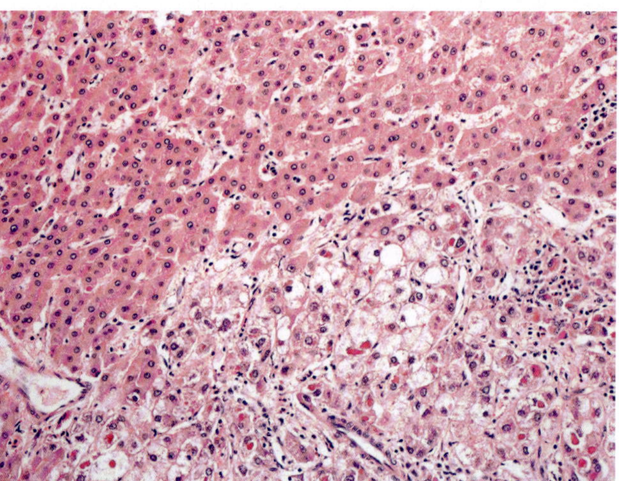

Figure 1.57. **Tumor, clonal appearance.** The hepatocytes in the tumor (lower right) are noticeably different than background liver, with paler cytoplasm and hyaline bodies.

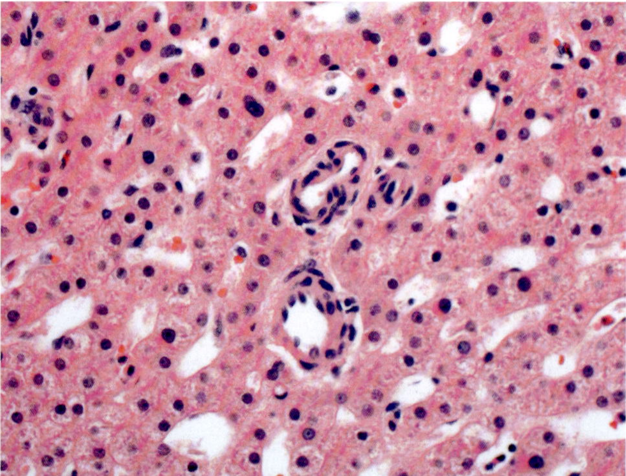

Figure 1.58. **Tumor, aberrant lobular arteries.** The lobules showed scattered naked or aberrant arteries (from a hepatic adenoma).

NEAR MISSES

CASE 1. This liver biopsy was obtained from a 53-year-old woman with "elevated liver enzymes," as per the accompanying clinical information. The biopsy at low power showed mild and rather nonspecific-looking chronic portal inflammation. There was no significant lobular inflammation, no cholestasis, and no fibrosis. It was tempting to sign out the case as nonspecific inflammation with no fibrosis and move on to the many other pending cases. However, on a second look at the biopsy, some but not all of the portal tracts were missing their bile duct (Fig. 1.59). A CK7 was then performed and showed numerous intermediate hepatocytes and confirmed early ductopenia. A phone call to the clinician was made, and the patient had almost normal AST and ALT levels, with an alkaline phosphatase of 330. The biopsy was signed out as mild nonspecific portal chronic inflammation with early bile duct loss and a histological differential that included primary biliary cirrhosis and drug effect. On subsequent testing, the patient's AMA was positive.

Bile duct loss can be very challenging to identify on H&E, especially when it is early and there is mild portal inflammation. In the current case, the diagnosis was strengthened by CK7, which showed intermediate hepatocytes and documented bile duct loss. A copper stain could also have been helpful by showing periportal copper deposition. Correlation with the laboratory testing, which showed a disproportionate elevation in alkaline phosphatase, helped secure the diagnosis.

The differential for ductopenia varies depending on other findings in the liver biopsy. In this case, with mild chronic portal inflammation, the differential is primarily that of primary biliary cirrhosis and drug effect.

CASE 2. A 45-year-old woman with a history of scleroderma was biopsied because of mildly elevated liver enzymes, with AST and ALT in the 60s and an alkaline phosphatase level of 200. Although the enzyme elevations were mild, they were persistent, which led to a liver biopsy. On low power, the biopsy looked essentially normal, with no inflammation, no fatty change, and no fibrosis. Scleroderma can be associated with primary biliary cirrhosis, but there was no significant portal inflammation, no granulomas, and no evidence for bile duct inflammation, injury, or loss. On a careful examination, the portal veins were found to be small and atrophic (Fig. 1.60). There was no nodular regenerative hyperplasia visible on the H&E, but a reticulin stain showed changes consistent with early nodular regenerative hyperplasia.

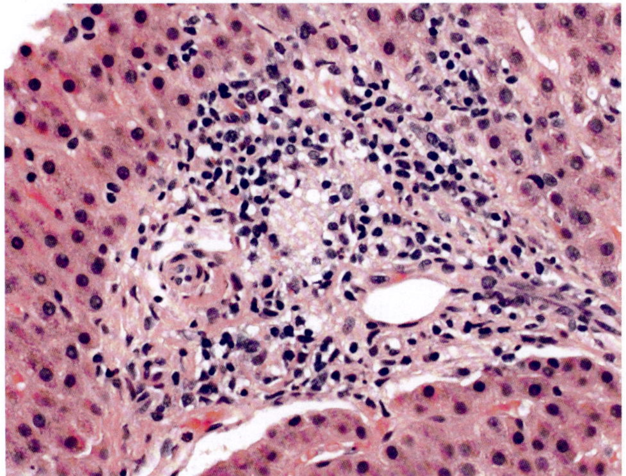

Figure 1.59. **Near miss case 1.** The portal tracts show mild chronic inflammation composed of lymphocytes and histiocytes. The bile duct is missing, an important histological clue that led to the correct diagnosis.

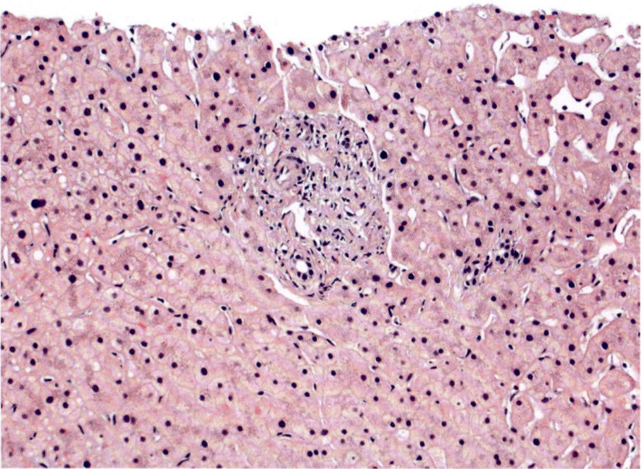

Figure 1.60. **Near miss case 2.** This biopsy looked essentially normal. However, because of the patient's history of scleroderma, it was carefully searched for findings that can be enriched in this patient population. There was no evidence for primary biliary cirrhosis, but the portal veins were noticeable atrophic, and there was mild nodular regenerative hyperplasia.

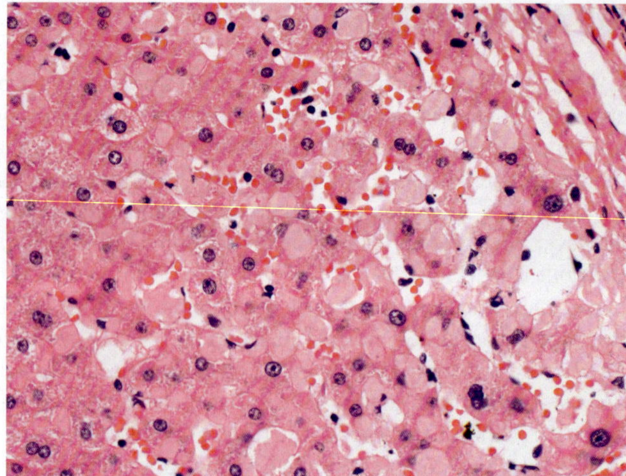

Figure 1.61. Near miss case 3. These distinctive inclusions were found in the background liver of a resection specimen for hepatocellular carcinoma. Work-up showed that these inclusions represent LECT amyloidosis.

Scleroderma and other systemic autoimmune conditions can be associated with portal vein atrophy as well as other changes that fit into the hepatoportal sclerosis pattern of injury. The findings can be very subtle and easily overlooked. In this case, the findings were not evident on low-power examination, but I knew that systemic autoimmune conditions can be associated with a hepatoportal sclerosis pattern of injury, so the portal tracts were carefully examined at medium and high power.

CASE 3. A 61-year-old man had a hepatic resection for a hepatocellular carcinoma. The background liver showed no inflammation, no fatty change, and no fibrosis. However, careful examination of the hepatocytes showed what appeared to be ground glass type inclusions (Fig. 1.61). The inclusions were concentrated in the zone 3 hepatocytes. Hepatitis B ground glass does not have a zonal distribution, and there was no evidence for a chronic hepatitis, making hepatitis B unlikely. Glycogen pseudo–ground glass can have a zone 3 distribution, but the patient was not immunosuppressed and not on medication, other than multivitamins. In addition, the PAS stain was only weakly positive in the inclusions, whereas the inclusions in glycogen pseudo–ground glass are strongly positive. These observations led to the correct diagnosis of Lect2 amyloidosis, which was confirmed on Congo Red and Lect2 immunostaining.

Inclusions in hepatocytes can range from subtle to obvious. Once they are identified, their morphology will suggest the differential, which can then be sorted out by special stains. Lect2 amyloidosis in the liver is often an incidental finding, as seen in this case, but is an important diagnosis to make.

References

1. O'Grady JG, Schalm SW, Williams R. Acute liver failure: redefining the syndromes. *Lancet*. 1993;342:273-275.
2. Singhal A, Vadlamudi S, Stokes K, et al. Liver histology as predictor of outcome in patients with acute liver failure. *Transpl Int*. 2012;25:658-662.
3. Donaldson BW, Gopinath R, Wanless IR, et al. The role of transjugular liver biopsy in fulminant liver failure: relation to other prognostic indicators. *Hepatology*. 1993;18:1370-1376.
4. Miraglia R, Luca A, Gruttadauria S, et al. Contribution of transjugular liver biopsy in patients with the clinical presentation of acute liver failure. *Cardiovasc Intervent Radiol*. 2006;29:1008-1010.
5. Wisell J, Boitnott J, Haas M, et al. Glycogen pseudoground glass change in hepatocytes. *Am J Surg Pathol*. 2006;30:1085-1090.
6. Kranidiotis GP, Voidonikola PT, Dimopoulos MK, Anastasiou-Nana MI. Stauffer's syndrome as a prominent manifestation of renal cancer: a case report. *Cases J*. 2009;2:49.

7. Morla D, Alazemi S, Lichtstein D. Stauffer's syndrome variant with cholestatic jaundice: a case report. *J Gen Intern Med*. 2006;21:C11-C113.

8. Dourakis SP, Sinani C, Deutsch M, Dimitriadou E, Hadziyannis SJ. Cholestatic jaundice as a paraneoplastic manifestation of renal cell carcinoma. *Eur J Gastroenterol Hepatol*. 1997;9:311-314.

9. Kakar S, Batts KP, Poterucha JJ, Burgart LJ. Histologic changes mimicking biliary disease in liver biopsies with venous outflow impairment. *Mod Pathol*. 2004;17:874-878.

10. Alonso EM, Snover DC, Montag A, Freese DK, Whitington PF. Histologic pathology of the liver in progressive familial intrahepatic cholestasis. *J Pediatr Gastroenterol Nutr*. 1994;18:128-133.

11. Crawford AR, Lin XZ, Crawford JM. The normal adult human liver biopsy: a quantitative reference standard. *Hepatology*. 1998;28:323-331.

12. Moreira RK, Chopp W, Washington MK. The concept of hepatic artery-bile duct parallelism in the diagnosis of ductopenia in liver biopsy samples. *Am J Surg Pathol*. 2011;35:392-403.

2 ACUTE AND CHRONIC VIRAL HEPATITIS

CHAPTER OUTLINE

GENERAL CONSIDERATIONS

CHECKLIST: Hepatitis Pattern

- ☐ Viral hepatitis
- ☐ Autoimmune hepatitis
- ☐ Drug effect

Most cases of the acute or chronic hepatitis resulting from the hepatotropic viruses will show a typical hepatitis pattern, with lymphocytic inflammation in the portal tracts and the lobules (Figs. 2.1 and 2.2). In some cases of acute viral hepatitis, plasma cells can also be prominent, closely mimicking autoimmune hepatitis, in particular with acute hepatitis A and B (Fig. 2.3). Thus, in all cases, the final diagnosis of viral hepatitis requires correlation with serological findings, or confirming immunostains, or in situ hybridization.

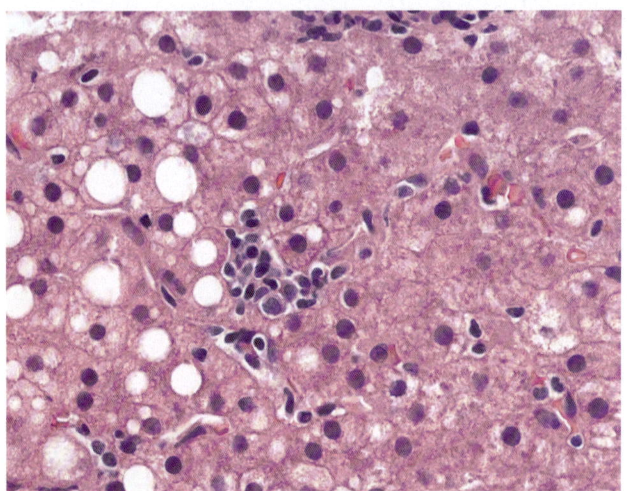

Figure 2.1. **Chronic hepatitis, lobules.** The lobules show mild chronic inflammation in a case of chronic hepatitis C. The inflammation is lymphocytic and shows no zonal pattern.

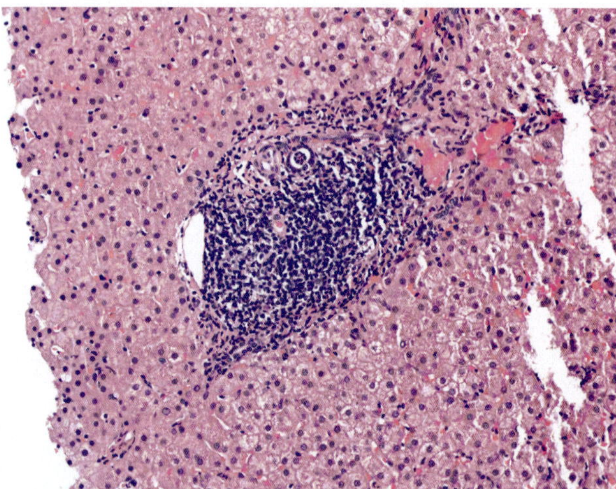

Figure 2.2. **Chronic hepatitis, portal tracts.** This portal tract shows moderate portal chronic inflammation, from a case of chronic hepatitis C.

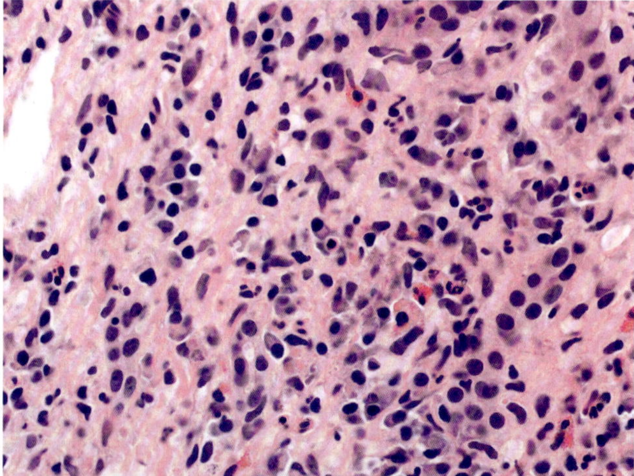

Figure 2.3. **Acute hepatitis B.** The biopsy findings suggested autoimmune hepatitis, but serum HBsAg IgM was positive and the biopsy was positive for HBcAg (strongly) and for HBsAg (weakly) by immunostaining.

In most cases of chronic viral hepatitis, the portal inflammation ranges from mild to moderate and the lobular inflammation ranges from minimal to moderate. The portal inflammation is predominately lymphocytic (Fig. 2.4), but occasional plasma cells and a rare eosinophil or two are common. The lobules will also show scattered, single dead hepatocytes, called spotty necrosis (Fig. 2.5).

Cases of moderate to severe hepatitis commonly show variable cholestasis and Kupffer cell hyperplasia. In addition, severe lobular hepatitis can be associated with confluent necrosis. Confluent necrosis simply means there are larger groups of dead hepatocytes and is used to contrast with spotty necrosis, where single dead cells are scattered in the lobules. In nearly all cases of confluent necrosis, the necrosis starts in zone 3 and, when more severe, leads to bridging necrosis and then to panacinar necrosis, according to the severity of the injury (Fig. 2.6). In very rare cases, a zone 1–predominant pattern of confluent necrosis can be observed, mostly with acute hepatitis A.[1]

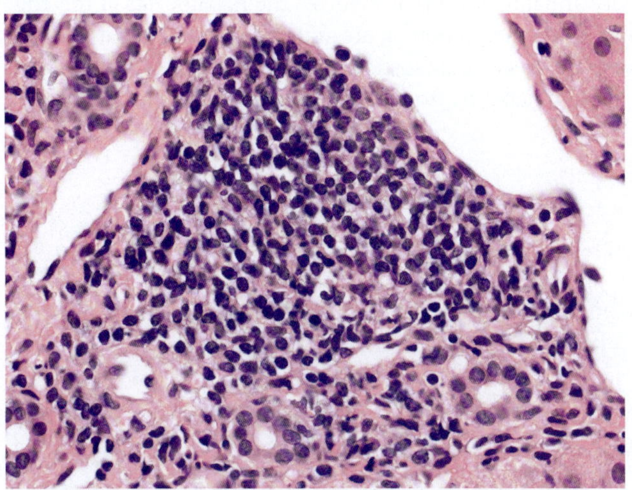

Figure 2.4. **Chronic hepatitis, portal tracts.** The inflammation is mostly lymphocytic.

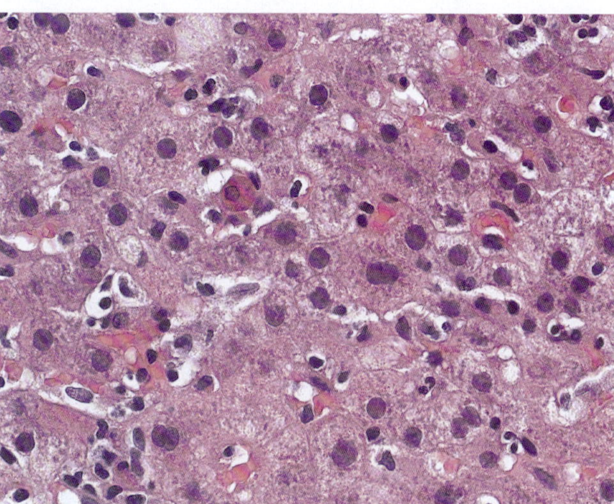

Figure 2.5. **Chronic hepatitis, lobules.** In addition to the inflammation, scattered apoptotic hepatocytes were present in this case of chronic hepatitis C.

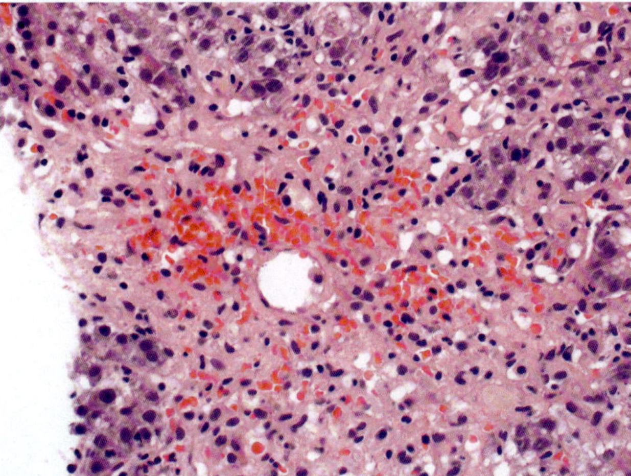

Figure 2.6. **Confluent necrosis.** Confluent zone 3 necrosis is seen in this case of acute autoimmune hepatitis.

DETERMINING ETIOLOGY

In most cases, the histological findings will not reveal the cause of the hepatitis. The final etiology is determined based on serological findings and clinical history, combined with compatible histology. One exception is with hepatitis B, where sensitive and specific immunostains are available (discussed below in the hepatitis B section). In addition, some cases of long-standing chronic hepatitis B can develop ground glass changes in the hepatocytes. Drug effects can show similar pseudo–ground glass changes, so immunostains for HBsAg are needed to confirm the diagnosis of chronic hepatitis B. A few centers also have tissue-based testing for hepatitis C and hepatitis E. Plasma cell-rich inflammation favors autoimmune hepatitis but is not specific (Fig. 2.7) and still requires excluding viral hepatitis and drug effects.

The most common pattern in acute hepatitis, or a flare of chronic hepatitis B, is mild to moderate portal chronic inflammation with moderate lobular activity. The most common pattern in stable chronic viral hepatitis is mild to focally moderate portal chronic inflammation with mild lobular activity. Inflammation that involves the hepatocytes at the edge of the portal tracts is called interface activity in both acute and chronic viral hepatitis (Figs. 2.8 and 2.9). Interface activity has no special diagnostic significance, being found in essentially all cases of moderate or marked hepatitis from any cause and in many cases of mild hepatitis from any cause.

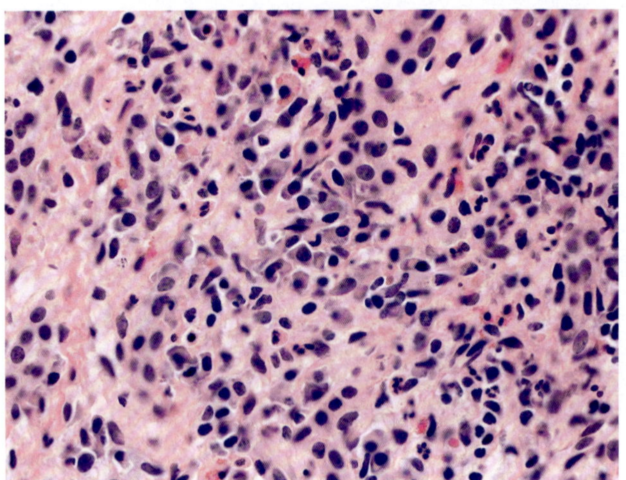

Figure 2.7. **Plasma cell–rich inflammation.** This case of acute hepatitis B showed plasma cell–rich portal inflammation.

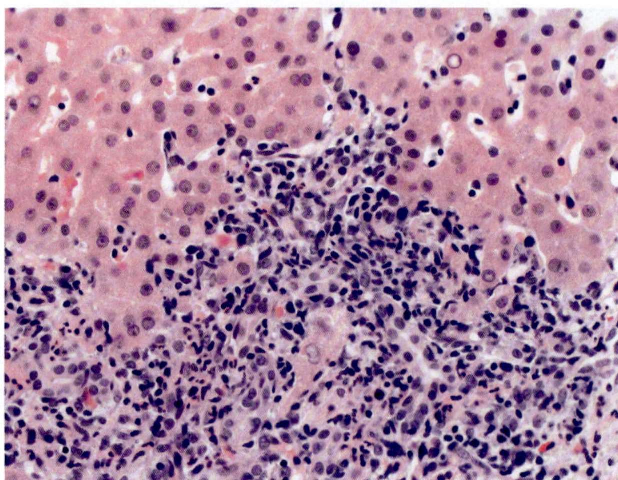

Figure 2.8. **Acute hepatitis, interface activity.** Interface active was patchy but prominent in this case of acute EBV hepatitis.

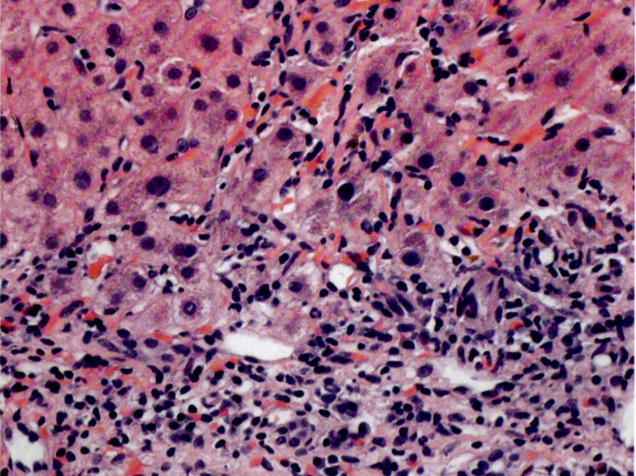

Figure 2.9. **Chronic hepatitis, interface activity.** Brisk interface activity is present in this case of chronic hepatitis C with moderate portal chronic inflammation.

FAQ: Do lymphoid aggregates in the portal tracts suggest chronic hepatitis C as the etiology?

Answer: Nope, they have no value for determining etiology. Also of note, they can be found in both acute and chronic hepatitis and do not indicate chronicity.

FAQ: I was taught that interface hepatitis suggests autoimmune hepatitis as the etiology. Is that true?

Answer: Not true. On the one hand, essentially any cause of inflammatory injury to the liver can have interface activity, including but not limited to autoimmune hepatitis; on the other hand, not all cases of autoimmune hepatitis will have interface activity (i.e., those with mild inflammatory activity) (Fig. 2.10). Nonetheless, you are not to blame for this misunderstanding, as it is one of the more persistent myths in liver pathology, one that is very hard to eradicate. You would think it would die a natural death, as maintaining this belief requires ignoring the literature as well as personal experience (if you are a pathologist), as interface activity is routinely seen in all manner of other diseases. Yet, this belief keeps coming back to life, sort of like a zombie.

ACUTE VERSUS CHRONIC HEPATITIS

The distinction between acute hepatitis and chronic hepatitis in most cases is made using the clinical definition of elevated liver enzymes for 6 months or greater. For most liver biopsy specimens, the question directed to the pathologist is focused more on the etiology, the degree of active injury, and the amount of fibrosis, and less on the exact duration of the hepatitis. However, the presence of definite fibrosis is evidence for a chronic hepatitis. Be aware of the many diagnostic pitfalls in fibrosis evaluation (please also see section below) to avoid overcalling fibrosis.

There is another category of liver injury called *acute-on-chronic hepatitis*, where a case of known chronic hepatitis has either an acute superimposed additional source of injury, or a case of chronic hepatitis has a flare-up. For the latter, the most common causes of chronic hepatitis that can have a flare of more active disease are autoimmune hepatitis and hepatitis B. Examples of acute-on-chronic hepatitis include acute hepatitis D on chronic hepatitis B or superimposed acute hepatitis B on chronic hepatitis C. Another example would be a drug effect superimposed on chronic hepatitis C.

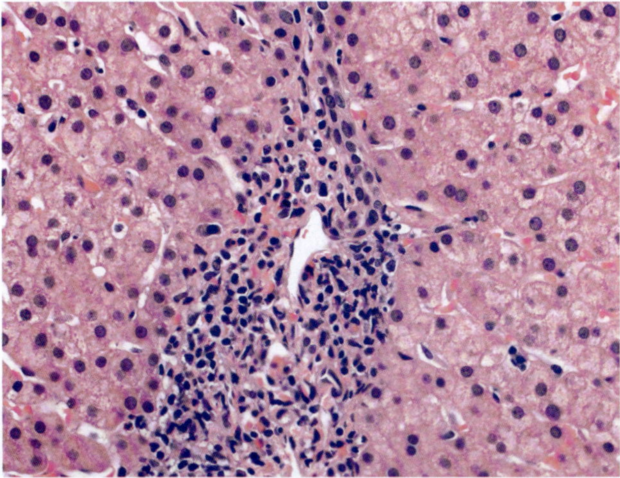

Figure 2.10. **Autoimmune hepatitis, no interface activity.** This case of mildly active autoimmune hepatitis had no interface activity in most of the portal tracts.

FAQ: How do I tell acute hepatitis from chronic hepatitis?

Answer: There can be some histological clues, but in many cases there are none and the distinction is made solely on clinical grounds, with the standard definition being elevated liver enzymes for at least 6 months. Histologically, the presence of definite fibrosis is accepted as evidence for a chronic hepatitis. In addition, a marked lobular hepatitis or diffuse moderate lobular hepatitis indicates either an acute hepatitis or an acute-on-chronic hepatitis, as this degree of lobular inflammation is too injurious to be a chronic process.

Occasionally I have encountered the misunderstanding that the presence of lymphocytic (or lymphoplasmacytic) inflammation in the portal tracts is an indicator of chronic hepatitis. Thus, a case with portal inflammation, or portal predominant inflammation, would be interpreted as having evidence for chronicity. This is simply not true. This misunderstanding seems to arise from a misapplication of the general patterns seen in acute and chronic hepatitis: in acute hepatitis, the inflammation is often lobular predominant, while in chronic hepatitis the inflammation tends to be portal predominant. These general patterns are true enough, but they are very broad and general patterns with many exceptions and do not have sufficient sensitivity or specificity to be clinically useful.

GRADING HEPATITIS

There are many excellent systems designed to grade hepatitis, but you do not need to grade hepatitis using a formal grading schema for clinical care. Grading schemas do not make a pathology report more accurate, as grading introduces its own reproducibility errors. In addition, they are not medically or scientifically more rigorous, as grading schemas largely use numbers as adjectives, for example, "grade 1 of 4" means mild hepatitis, etc. However, if you or your clinical colleagues prefer them, then they are fine to use, as they are mostly compliant with the fundamental medical principle *primum non nocere*, first do no harm.

The Batts–Ludwig grading schema is shown in Table 2.1 as one example of a useful grading system. In this system, the portal inflammation, interface activity, and lobular activity are independently assessed as being minimal, mild, moderate, or marked. Overall, the inflammation in each of these three areas does strongly covary, but when there are discrepancies, the highest grade lesion drives the score. For example, moderate portal chronic inflammation with mild interface activity and mild lobular activity is scored as overall moderate activity, grade 3. When grading, it is easy to slip into the habit of hyphenating inflammatory grades, such as grade 1-2, or 2-3, or 1-4, etc. While this approach is justified occasionally, in most cases you should make your best assessment and assign a single grade.

STAGING HEPATITIS

Specimen adequacy for clinical care depends on both the size of the biopsy and the findings within the specimen. The problem with smaller biopsies is that they tend to under stage fibrosis. In general, a biopsy specimen 10 mm or greater and/or with at least 10 portal tracts is considered adequate. The entire portal tract does not need to be present in adequacy assessments, but there should be enough of the portal tract present to provide useful staging information. While this approach requires some professional judgment, it works quite well in practice. If the H&E or trichrome findings show established cirrhosis, then the biopsy is adequate for staging purposes, even if it is smaller than 10 mm.

Fibrosis staging uses a connective tissue histochemical stain to better visualize fibrosis in the liver. The trichrome stain and the Sirius red stains are the most commonly used stains. The normal liver has collagen present in the portal tracts, but with injury there is new collagen laid down as fibrosis. The normal collagen in the portal tracts is not fibrosis, and by definition all fibrosis in the liver is abnormal. Thus, tautologies such as "no abnormal fibrosis" may be accurate in some sense but come across as a bit awkward and suggest a misunderstanding, perhaps, of the basics.

There are many different formal staging schemas and all work very well (Tables 2.2-2.4). The most common ones are these: Ishak (also known as the modified histology activity index or MHAI), Batts–Ludwig, Scheuer, and METAVIR. For clinical care, none of the systems are better than the others, in large part because they all are more alike than they are different. All chronic viral hepatitis staging systems start with no fibrosis (Fig. 2.11) and then progress to portal fibrosis (Fig. 2.12), next to bridging fibrosis (Fig. 2.13), and end at cirrhosis (Fig. 2.14). The systems vary only in how they subdivide each of these major categories of fibrosis. As one example, some systems will divide portal fibrosis into mild versus moderate, while others do not. Table 2.5 provides a Rosetta stone, allowing a reasonable translation of fibrosis stages in the most common systems. Overall the system with the most unique approach is the Laennec staging system, with its emphasis on the size of the fibrosis bridges and incorporation of the size of cirrhotic nodules (Table 2.6).

TABLE 2.1: Summary of the Batts–Ludwig Grading System

Grade	Definition	Comment
0	No activity	
1	Minimal activity	Portal tracts: up to mild Interface activity: up to focal, minimal Lobular activity: none
2	Mild activity	Portal tracts: up to mild Interface activity: up to mild Lobular activity: up to mild
3	Moderate activity	Portal tracts: up to moderate Interface activity: up to moderate Lobular activity: up to moderate
4	Marked activity	Portal tracts: up to marked Interface activity: up to moderate Lobular activity: up to moderate + confluent necrosis

Batts KP, Ludwig J. Chronic hepatitis. An update on terminology and reporting. *Am J Surg Pathol.* 1995;19:1409-1417.

Note: The highest lesion drives the score. For example, moderate portal chronic inflammation with mild interface activity and mild lobular activity is scored as grade 3.

TABLE 2.2: Batts and Ludwig Staging System

Stage	Definition	Comment
0	No fibrosis	If there is trivial equivocal fibrosis, score as none
1	Portal fibrosis	Can be mild or moderate
2	Periportal fibrosis	• Defined as portal tracts with fine, irregular fibrous extensions that mostly do not extend from portal to portal tract • Rare bridging fibrosis is allowed • No architectural distortion
3	Septal fibrosis	• More than rare bridging fibrosis • Can be portal to portal or portal to central
4	Cirrhosis	Cirrhosis

Batts KP, Ludwig J. Chronic hepatitis. An update on terminology and reporting. *Am J Surg Pathol.* 1995;19:1409-1417.

TABLE 2.3: Summary of the METAVIR Fibrosis Staging System

Stage	Definition	Comment
0	No fibrosis	If there is trivial equivocal fibrosis, score as none
1	Portal fibrosis	Includes all degrees of portal fibrosis
2	Portal tract fibrosis with rare bridging fibrosis	
3	Moderate or marked bridging fibrosis without cirrhosis	
4	Cirrhosis	

Group FMCS. Intraobserver and interobserver variations in liver biopsy interpretation in patients with chronic hepatitis C. The French METAVIR Cooperative Study Group. *Hepatology*. 1994;20:15-20.

TABLE 2.4: Ishak Fibrosis Staging System

Stage	Definition	Comments
0	No fibrosis	• If there is trivial equivocal fibrosis, score as none
1	Portal fibrosis, some portal tracts	• Less than 50% of portal tracts • With or without short fibrous extensions (so-called periportal fibrosis)
2	Portal fibrosis, most portal tracts	• More than 50% of portal tracts with any fibrosis or multiple portal tracts with moderate fibrosis • With or without short fibrous extensions (so-called periportal fibrosis)
3	Mild bridging fibrosis	• Occasional fibrous bridges • Portal to portal bridges
4	Marked bridging fibrosis, numerous fibrous bridges	• Numerous fibrous bridges • Portal to portal bridges or portal to central bridges
5	Fibrous bridges with occasional nodule formation	• Numerous fibrous bridges • Occasional nodule formation • "Early" or "incomplete cirrhosis"
6	Cirrhosis	• Original system allows *probable* or *definite* cirrhosis; in practice, those that are questionable cirrhosis are usually given a 5

Ishak K, Baptista A, Bianchi L, et al. Histological grading and staging of chronic hepatitis. *J Hepatol*. 1995;22:696-699.

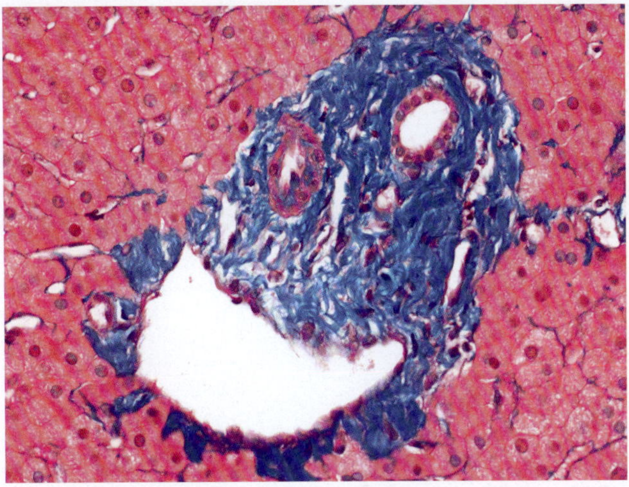

Figure 2.11. No fibrosis, trichrome stain. The normal portal tract has collagen, but there is no fibrosis.

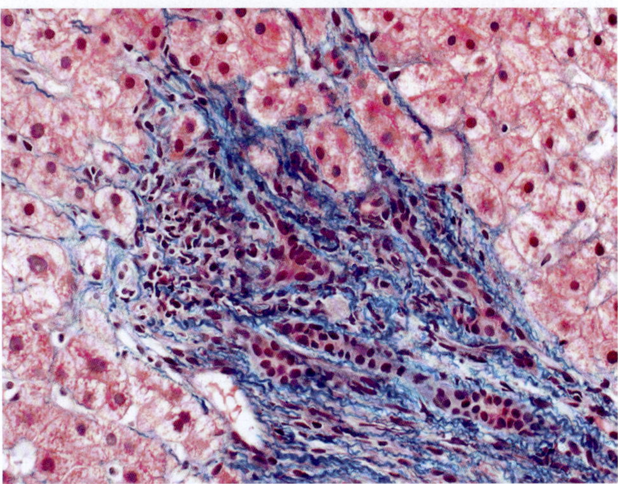

Figure 2.12. Portal fibrosis, trichrome stain. The portal tract shows mild irregular expansion due to fibrosis.

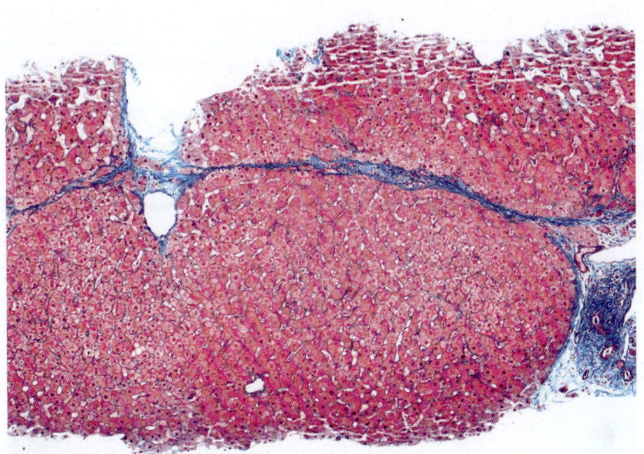

Figure 2.13. Bridging fibrosis, trichrome stain. A thin fibrous bridge extends from a portal tract to a central vein. In most biopsy specimens, the complete bridge is not evident because of the small size of the biopsy, and you will not know if the bridge goes from portal tract to portal tract or from portal tract to central vein. For staging purposes, the distinction is not that relevant.

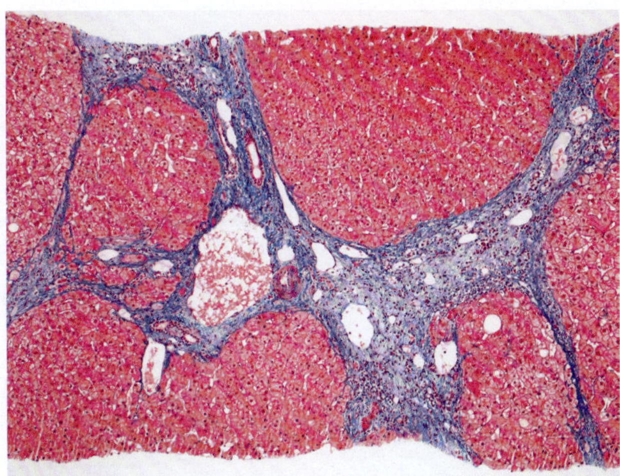

Figure 2.14. Cirrhosis, trichrome. The biopsy shows well-formed nodules of hepatocytes surrounded by bands of fibrosis.

TABLE 2.5: Rosetta Stone for Comparing Fibrosis Staging Systems

Brief Description	Ishak[48] (Modified Histology Activity Index [MHAI])	Knodell[49] (Histology Activity Index [HAI])	METAVIR[47]	Desmet[50]	Scheuer[51]	Batts and Ludwig[46]
None	0	0	0	0	0	0
Mild portal fibrosis	1	1	1	1	1	1
Moderate portal fibrosis	2	1	1	1	1 or 2	1 or 2
Bridging fibrosis	3	3[a]	2	2 or 3[b]	2	2
Extensive bridg-ing with nodularity	4	3	3	2 or 3	3	3
Early cirrhosis	5	3	3	3	3	3
Cirrhosis	6	4	4	4	4	4

[a]Requires two or more portal to portal or portal to central bridges (i.e., one bridge is still considered stage 2, though in common practice this guideline was often not followed).

[b]Stage 3 requires portal to central bridging fibrosis, though in practice stage 3 is commonly used for extensive bridging fibrosis.

TABLE 2.6: Laennec Staging System

Stage	Definition	Description
0	No fibrosis	No fibrosis
1	Minimal fibrosis	Fibrosis can be portal and or sinusoidal. Rare thin fibrous bridges allowed
2	Mild fibrosis	Occasional fibrous bridges
3	Moderate fibrosis	Numerous thin fibrous bridges; can be early nodularity
4A	Mild cirrhosis	Parenchymal nodularity with thin fibrous septa; one broad septum allowed
4B	Moderate cirrhosis	At least two broad septa but no very broad septa; minute nodules in less than half of the biopsy
4C	Severe cirrhosis (at least one very broad septum or more than half of the biopsy composed of minute nodules)	Severe cirrhosis (at least one very broad septum or more than half of the biopsy composed of minute nodules)

Wanless IR, Sweeney G, Dhillon AP, et al. Lack of progressive hepatic fibrosis during long-term therapy with deferiprone in subjects with transfusion-dependent beta-thalassemia. *Blood.* 2002;100:1566-1569 and Kim MY, Cho MY, Baik SK, et al. Histological subclassification of cirrhosis using the Laennec fibrosis scoring system correlates with clinical stage and grade of portal hypertension. *J Hepatol.* 2011;55:1004-1009.

Note: Fibrous septa definitions: thin = not formally defined; broad = less than the average size of the cirrhotic nodules; very broad = thicker than the average size of the cirrhotic nodules.

FAQ: What is the difference between portal fibrosis and periportal fibrosis?

Answer: Mostly, they are synonyms, both referring to fibrosis of the portal tracts that does not reach the level of bridging fibrosis. The terms were used differently a long time ago, when pathologists divided chronic hepatitis cases into *chronic aggressive hepatitis* versus *chronic persistent hepatitis*, but such a distinction is no longer clinically or biologically relevant. However, when these terms were in use, *chronic aggressive hepatitis* was thought to have a worse prognosis and show more interface activity and more irregular portal fibrosis, which was called periportal fibrosis. In contrast, *chronic persistent hepatitis* was thought to have less interface activity and more rounded portal contours, being called portal fibrosis. Once these terms were proposed, they were carefully studied by a large number of papers and generally found to be not useful for clinical care because they did not have reliable power for predicting fibrosis progression or other clinical outcomes. For this reason, this older approach was replaced several decades ago by the current method, where hepatitis is classified by the etiology, the grade of injury, and the degree of fibrosis.

Nonetheless, the term periportal fibrosis lingers on in use, with some pathologists preferring this term when the fibrosis looks "spiky" (Fig. 2.15), but for practical purposes, portal and periportal fibrosis are essentially the same. As one exception, the periportal fibrosis stage in both the Batts–Ludwig staging system and the Scheur staging system includes both portal and early bridging fibrosis.

Overall, fibrosis staging is relatively straightforward in most cases. Discrepancies between pathologists usually arise at the "edges" of the fibrosis stages. For example, one pathologist might feel the trichrome stain is within normal limits, while another might feel there is focal minimal portal fibrosis (Fig. 2.16). Finding entrapped hepatocytes in the portal tracts (Fig. 2.17) would help diagnose mild portal fibrosis, but this finding is not always evident. On the other end of the fibrosis spectrum, the trichrome findings may indicate cirrhosis to one pathologist, while another may think it is not quite cirrhotic. These challenges are probably unavoidable. One reasonable approach is to add into your comment or note some additional description that captures the challenge. For example, you might say this in a note: While the findings are classified as Batts–Ludwig stage 1 of 4 fibrosis, the trichrome stain shows only focal minimal portal fibrosis in a single portal tract.

The other major challenges in fibrosis staging arise when there is marked inflammation (Fig. 2.18), bridging necrosis (Fig. 2.19) or a badly fragmented biopsy specimen (Fig. 2.20). Sometimes a tangential cut of a portal tract can simulate bridging fibrosis (Fig. 2.21), but the smooth regular borders and lack of portal fibrosis elsewhere in the biopsy clarify the diagnosis.

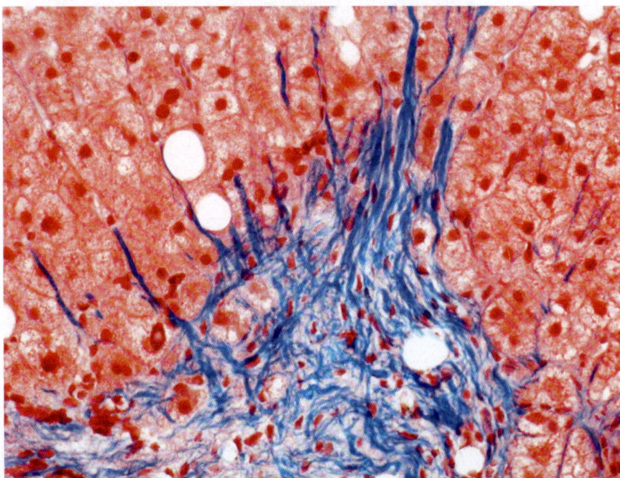

Figure 2.15. **Periportal fibrosis, trichrome stain.** Some staging systems use the term periportal fibrosis. This pattern is essentially the same as portal fibrosis but shows more irregularity to the portal tract.

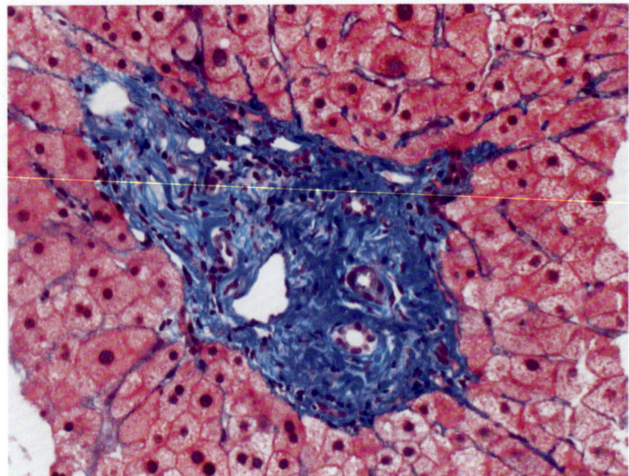

Figure 2.16. **Equivocal portal fibrosis, trichrome stain.** Is there portal tract fibrosis in this single portal tract (the rest of the biopsy was normal)? I thought so but my colleague did not. Instead of arm wrestling to determine who was right, I said in the report that there was focal equivocal portal fibrosis that did not reach the level of stage 1 fibrosis and was best classified as stage 0.

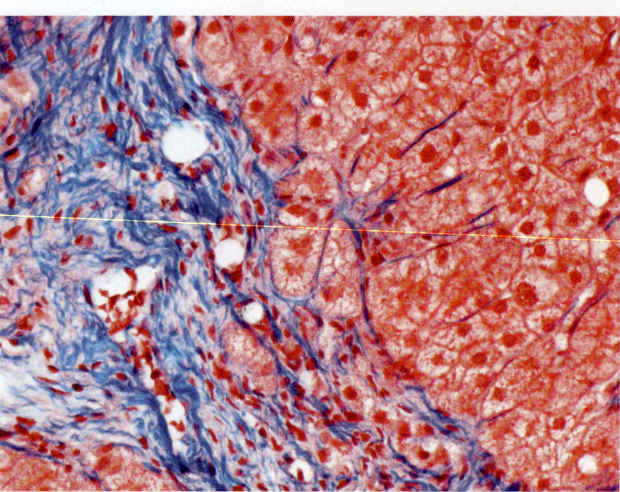

Figure 2.17. **Entrapped hepatocytes, trichrome stain.** This finding supports the diagnosis of mild portal fibrosis. You can also see another example of entrapped hepatocytes in Figure 2.12.

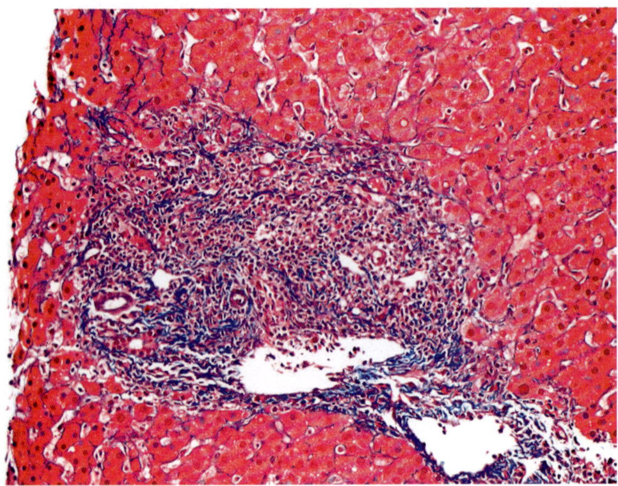

Figure 2.18. **Staging pitfall, marked portal inflammation.** This biopsy showed moderate to marked portal chronic inflammation. The inflammation expands the portal tracts and can sometimes be overcalled as portal fibrosis.

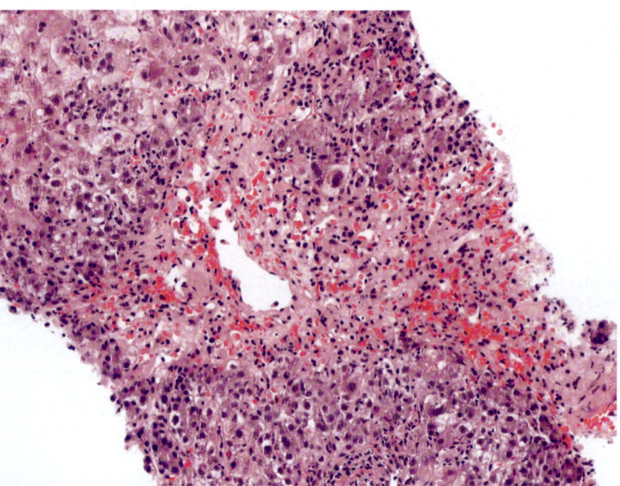

Figure 2.19. **Staging pitfall, bridging necrosis.** In this case of acute hepatitis, there is extensive necrosis in zone 3, causing bridging necrosis in some areas. On trichrome stain, areas of bridging necrosis can mimic bridging fibrosis.

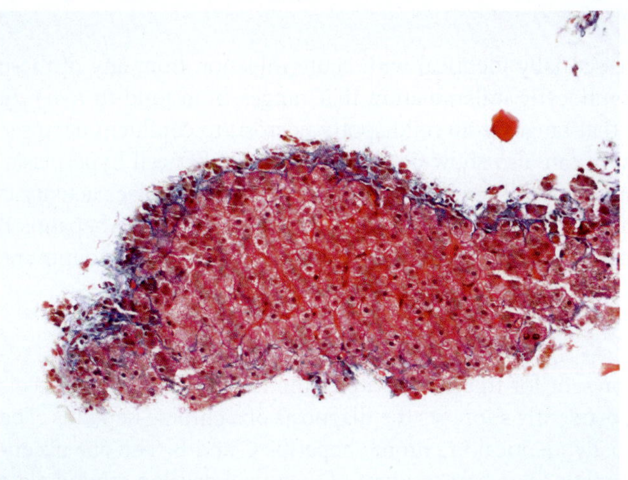

Figure 2.20. Staging pitfall, badly fragmented specimen. This specimen was badly fragmented, and some fragments seemed to have a rim of blue fibrosis, a finding called a *fibrous cap*, tricking the pathologist into staging this biopsy as established cirrhosis.

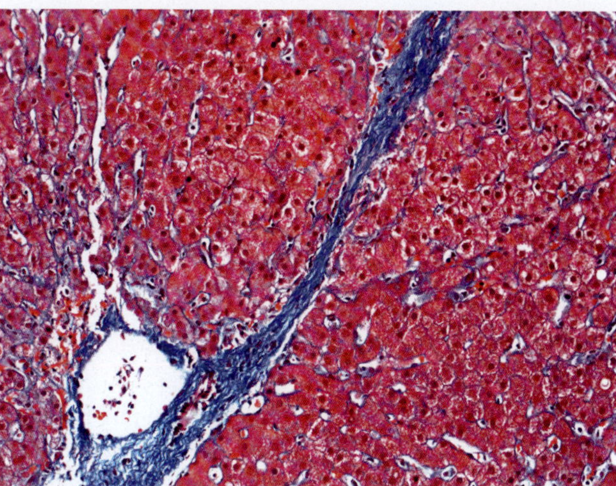

Figure 2.21. Staging pitfall, tangential cut of a normal portal tract. A tangential cut of a normal portal tract can closely mimic a fibrous bridge, but note how thin it is and the lack of inflammation. The rest of the biopsy showed only minimal portal fibrosis, which also helps because significant portal fibrosis precedes the development of bridging fibrosis.

PEARLS & PITFALLS

Fibrosis staging with severe hepatitis has several important pitfalls. Marked portal inflammation can mimic portal fibrosis, and bridging necrosis can mimic bridging fibrosis. Always compare the trichrome staging findings back with the H&E finding to make sure you are not overstaging. If you are not sure of the fibrosis stage, say so and why in the report.

SAMPLE NOTE

Liver needle biopsy: Acute hepatitis B with marked portal and lobular hepatitis with bridging necrosis. There is no evidence for advanced fibrosis. Please see note.

Note. The history of acute hepatitis B is noted (HBV DNA positive by report with recent risk exposure), and the biopsy shows hepatitis with marked portal and lobular inflammation and bridging necrosis. There is expansion of the portal tracts by the marked portal inflammation and mild portal fibrosis cannot be entirely excluded, but there is no evidence for advanced fibrosis or cirrhosis.

SPECIFIC HEPATOTROPIC VIRUSES

GENERAL HISTOLOGY PATTERNS

The known hepatotropic viruses are called hepatitis A through E. These viruses infect primarily or exclusively the liver and all can cause acute hepatitis, while hepatitis B, C, D, and E can lead to chronic hepatitis. Hepatitis D can lead to chronic infection only in patients with hepatitis B infection. Hepatitis E can cause chronic infection in immunosuppressed individuals. While hepatitis A does not cause chronic hepatitis, there are two uncommon disease patterns that can mimic chronic hepatitis: relapsing hepatitis A and hepatitis A with prolonged cholestasis.

Acute Viral Hepatitis

The histological findings are essentially identical with acute infection from any of these viruses. The lobules show lymphocytic inflammation that ranges from mild to marked, and there is hepatocyte injury that ranges from mild spotty necrosis to confluent necrosis. In more severe cases, the lobules can also show cholestasis and Kupffer cell hyperplasia. The inflammation in the portal tracts will range from mild to marked. Interface activity is often present and in general parallels the degree of portal inflammation. Acute hepatitis B and acute hepatitis A can sometimes be plasma cell rich, closely mimicking autoimmune hepatitis.

Chronic Viral Hepatitis

Fibrosis does not have to be present for there to be a chronic hepatitis, but if fibrosis is present, then that finding independently supports the diagnosis of a chronic hepatitis. The histological findings are essentially identical in chronic hepatitis C and B. The one exception is long-standing chronic hepatitis B, where a subset of cases will develop ground glass inclusions within the hepatocytes.

In general, the lobules in chronic hepatitis typically show mild to patchy moderate inflammation, as do the portal tracts (Figs. 2.22 and 2.23). Interface activity is commonly present and tends to parallel the degree of portal inflammation (Fig. 2.24). Other findings can include lymphoid aggregates in the portal tracts, focal mild endothelialitis, and mild bile duct lymphocytosis (Figs. 2.25-2.27). The frequency of the latter two findings depends a great deal on who is sitting at the microscope, but everyone agrees that they can be found occasionally and in general are more common in specimens with moderate or marked portal inflammation. When present, they are a patchy and mild finding and do not have any clinical significance.

The inflammation in the portal tracts is predominately lymphocytic, but there will be occasional eosinophils, histiocytes, and plasma cells. Plasma cells can even be mildly prominent in a subset of cases, typically middle-aged women who have mild elevations in various autoantibody serologies. The chronic viral hepatitis in these patients seems to be triggering hepatitis with some autoimmune hepatitis-like features, but in general most physicians do not consider this pattern to be a viral–autoimmune hepatitis overlap syndrome. Instead, patients are treated for their viral hepatitis and overall seem to have the same clinical course as those with more typical patterns of inflammation.

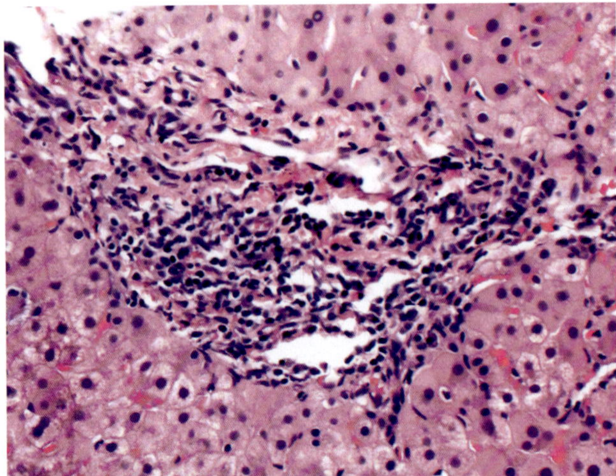

Figure 2.22. Chronic hepatitis B, portal tracts. This case showed mild patchy portal chronic inflammation with minimal lobular activity.

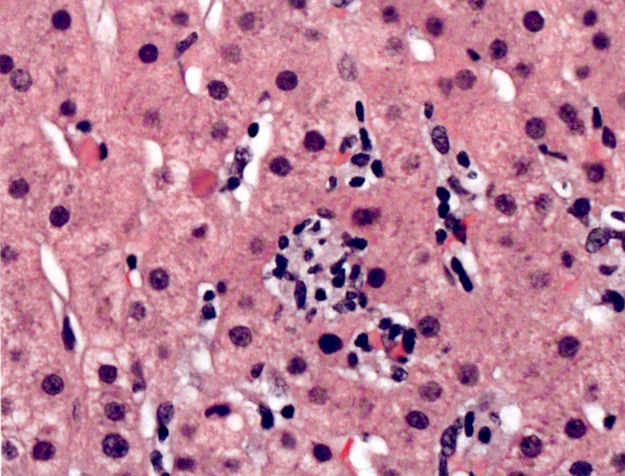

Figure 2.23. Chronic hepatitis, lobular inflammation. This case of chronic hepatitis C shows patchy moderate inflammation.

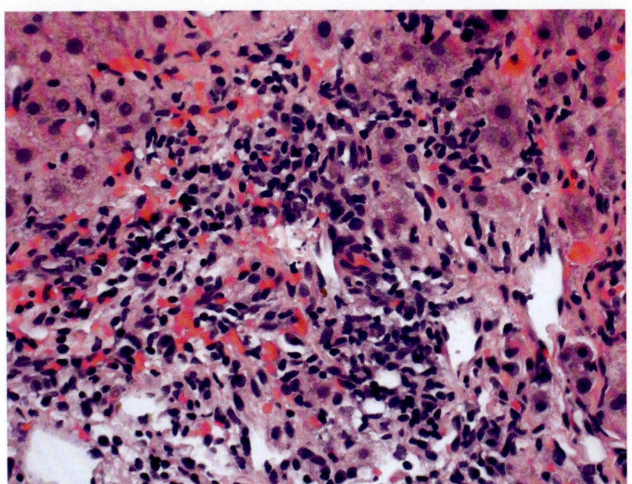

Figure 2.24. **Chronic hepatitis, interface activity.** This case of chronic hepatitis C showed patchy moderate portal chronic inflammation with interface activity.

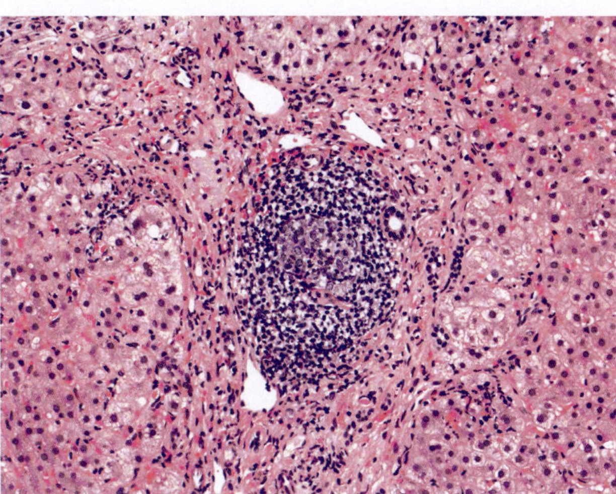

Figure 2.25. **Chronic hepatitis, lymphoid aggregates.** This case of chronic hepatitis showed minimal lobular inflammation and patchy mild portal chronic inflammation with an occasional lymphoid follicle.

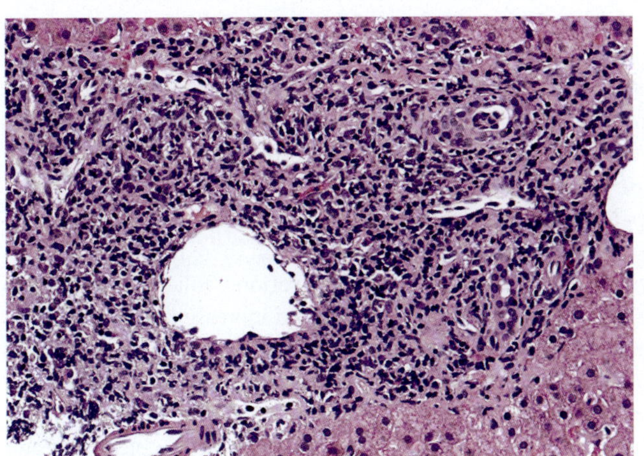

Figure 2.26. **Chronic hepatitis, endothelialitis.** This case of chronic hepatitis C showed patchy endothelialitis of the portal veins in those portal tracts with moderate to marked inflammation.

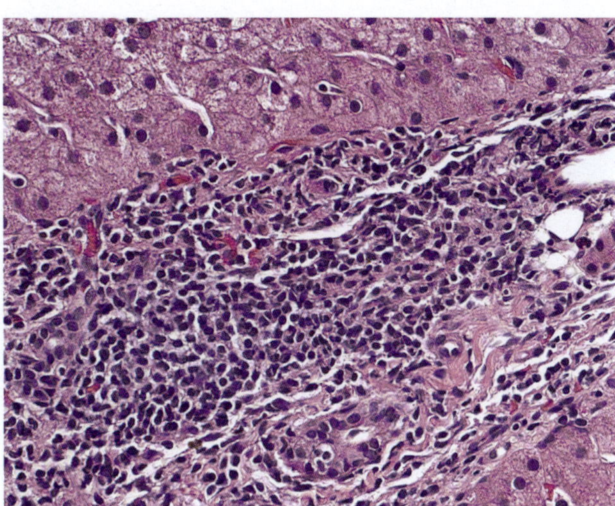

Figure 2.27. **Chronic hepatitis, mild bile duct lymphocytosis without injury.** This case of chronic hepatitis C showed moderate portal inflammation and focal bile duct lymphocytosis.

FAQ: Do lymphoid aggregates suggest chronic hepatitis C as the most likely etiology?

Answer: No. Some studies have found them to be a bit more common in chronic hepatitis C than chronic hepatitis B, but they have no diagnostic value for determining etiology.

FAQ: Do lymphoid follicles in the portal tracts indicate the infection is a chronic hepatitis versus acute hepatitis?

Answer: No. Lymphoid follicles can be present in both acute and chronic hepatitis. They are probably more common in chronic hepatitis but can be present in either and should not be relied to make that distinction, or really any distinction.

HEPATITIS A

KEY POINTS on Biology of Hepatitis A

- RNA virus
- Major routes of transmission: oral fecal most common, also sex and blood born
- Raw sea food consumption is an important risk factor
- Worldwide infection: 1.5 million cases per year
- Incubation: 2-7 weeks
- Chronic infection: no
- Cirrhosis risk: none
- Three patterns of infection: acute (>95%), cholestatic (2%), relapsing (1%)[2]
- Vaccine: yes

An effective vaccine for hepatitis A is available, but the virus remains an important cause of acute hepatitis. With infection, 30% of children have symptoms, compared to 80% of adults. There is no risk for chronic hepatitis A infection, but acute hepatitis A superimposed on chronic hepatitis B or C has a high risk of acute liver failure and death.

Biopsies are only performed when the cause of the acute hepatitis is not clinically evident. The biopsies show a hepatitic pattern with marked portal and lobular inflammation that is often accompanied by necrosis. The necrosis can be mild and have a zone 3 pattern or can be panacinar or massive. Rarely, a zone 1 or 1-2 pattern of necrosis is seen, with sparing of zone 3 (Fig. 2.28). In many cases, the portal inflammation is more prominent than the lobular inflammation.[1,3] The inflammation is predominantly lymphocytic, but plasma cells can be prominent.[3,4] There can be lobular cholestasis and a mild bile ductular proliferation in response to the lobular hepatitis. Fibrosis is not a part of the pathology of hepatitis A infection. If there is fibrosis, then this suggests acute hepatitis A that is superimposed on an additional cause of liver disease.

In addition to the acute hepatitis pattern, hepatitis A infection can have either a relapsing pattern or a cholestatic pattern.[5] The relapsing pattern occurs when there is initial improvement, and sometimes even resolution of the liver enzyme elevations, followed about 3 to 7 weeks later by a second burst of viral replication, with a second increase in liver enzymes. The second phase is clinically and histologically milder than the first phase. The biopsies in the relapsing phase show a hepatitic pattern (Fig. 2.29), with mild to focally moderate lobular inflammation and mild portal inflammation. Necrosis is generally not seen.

The prolonged cholestatic pattern is characterized by a bilirubin that is typically greater than 10 mg/dL at presentation and prolonged cholestasis lasting greater than 12 weeks. Patients also frequently have pruritus, weight loss, diarrhea, and malabsorption.[6] The

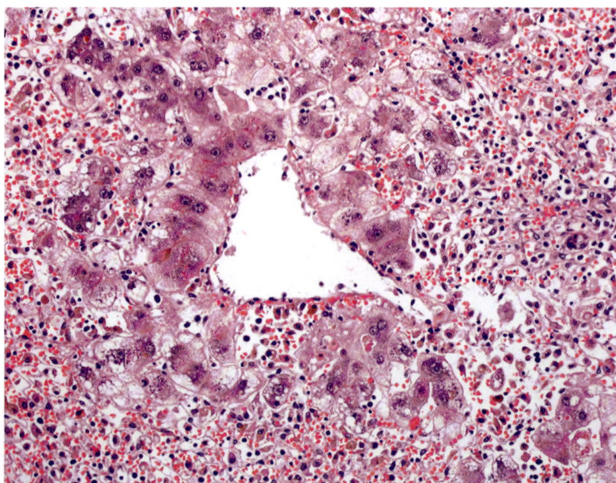

Figure 2.28. Acute hepatitis A, zone 1 pattern of necrosis. In this explanted liver for acute hepatitis A, there was preservation of the zone 3 hepatocytes, with extensive necrosis in zones 1 and 2.

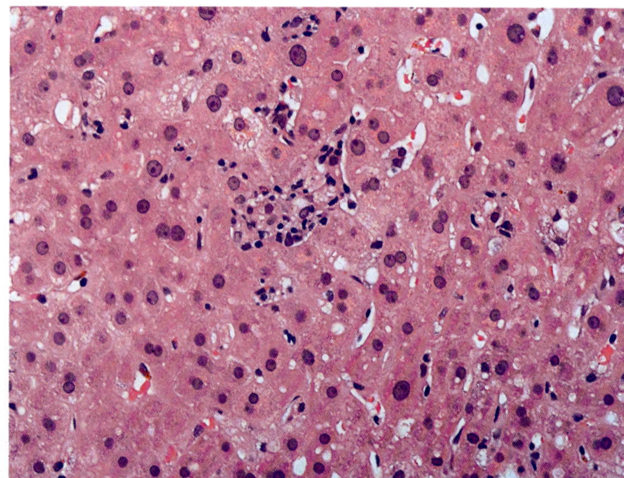

Figure 2.29. Relapsing hepatitis A. The biopsy findings in this case show mild nonspecific lobular hepatitis.

biological explanation is not clear, but from the available information, patients appear to recover without any sequelae. Liver biopsies taken in the prolonged cholestasis phase tend to show a bland lobular cholestatic pattern. The cholestasis is mild and may be accompanied by patchy minimal to mild portal and lobular inflammation. There is no evidence of biliary obstruction.

In all of the different patterns, the histological findings are not specific for hepatitis A. Instead, the diagnosis is made by finding compatible histology along with positive hepatitis A IgM serologies or serum PCR.

HEPATITIS B

KEY POINTS on Biology of Hepatitis B

- DNA virus
- Major routes of transmission: sex, blood born, mother to child
- Worldwide infection: 260 million chronic infections
- Incubation: 2-7 weeks
- Chronic infection: Newborns, 90%; adults 5%
- Cirrhosis risk: 30% in 30 years
- Antiviral therapy: suppresses viral replication but does not cure in most cases
- Vaccine: yes

Biopsies for grading and staging chronic hepatitis B used to be common but now are rare because of the availability of noninvasive testing to determine fibrosis stage. Biopsies are still performed when noninvasive test results are inconsistent with clinical findings or when there is concern for an additional disease process. Acute hepatitis B is only biopsied when the diagnosis is unsuspected or when serological test results are ambiguous, which is not very often.

Acute Hepatitis B

The histology of acute hepatitis B is a hepatic pattern, usually with moderate or marked lobular inflammation (Fig. 2.30), often with zone 3 necrosis and sometimes with more severe bridging or panacinar necrosis. The inflammation is predominately lymphocytic but can be plasma cell rich, mimicking autoimmune hepatitis. The lobules show scattered acidophil bodies and Kupffer cell hyperplasia. With moderate or severe hepatitis, the lobules can show cholestasis. Ground glass hepatocytes will be absent, being found only with chronic hepatitis B infection. Immunostains for HBcAg tend to show lots of positive nuclei (Fig. 2.31), while immunostains for HBsAg will be negative or show weak and patchy staining that is often membranous (Fig. 2.32).[7]

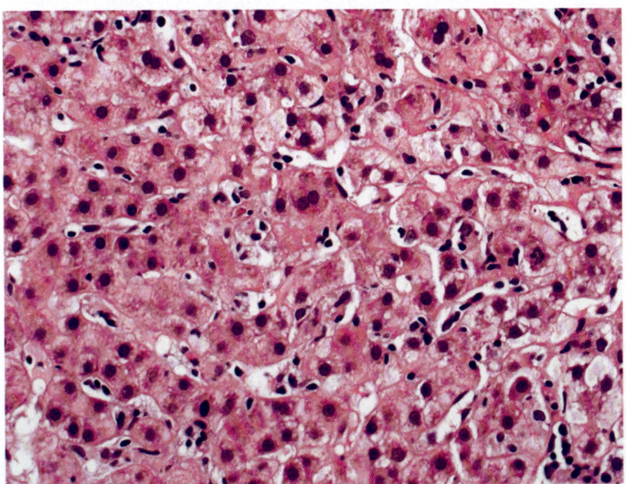

Figure 2.30. **Acute hepatitis B.** Moderate lobular hepatitis is seen.

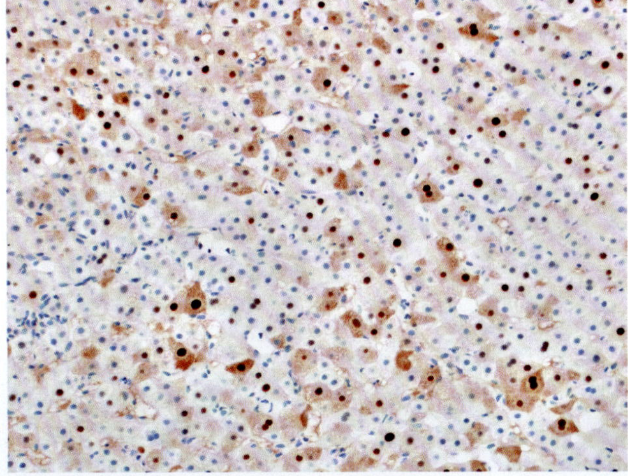

Figure 2.31. **Acute hepatitis B, HBcAg.** The hepatocytes show nuclear and cytoplasmic staining.

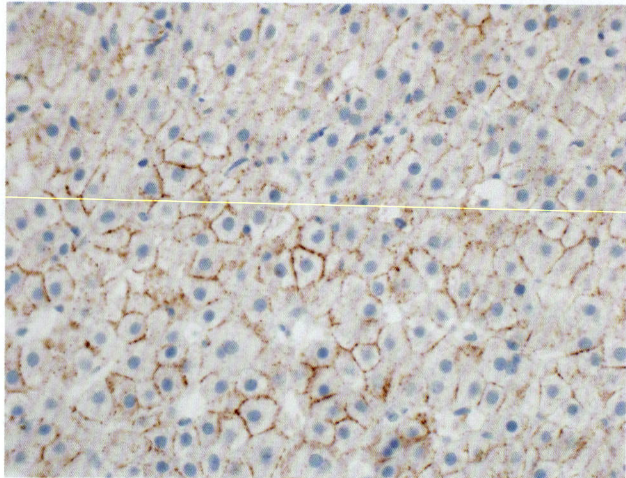

Figure 2.32. **Acute hepatitis B, HBsAg.** Instead of the usual cytoplasmic staining, the hepatocytes in this case show membranous staining.

Chronic Hepatitis B

For clinical purposes, chronic hepatitis B infection is divided into several broad phases or categories[8]: immunotolerant hepatitis B, chronic hepatitis B, inactive HBsAg carrier state, and resolved hepatitis B (Table 2.7). These categories have only a few broad pathology correlates, and their main value is in guiding clinical treatment decisions. Nonetheless, it can be useful to be familiar with them when discussing patients with your clinical colleagues. Not included in this table is the possibility of an HBV flare. Chronic hepatitis B infections can have sporadic flares of increased viral replication. These flares are identified clinically when there is a spike in viral replication associated with increased ALT levels, commonly defined as ALT elevations that spiked at least 2X more than the baseline value, often reaching more than 10X the upper limit of normal. The differential for an HBV flare includes hepatitis D virus (HDV) superinfection or other superimposed liver injuries. On histology, an HBV flare shows moderate to marked lobular hepatitis, often with patchy zone 3 necrosis.

In general, the biopsy findings in chronic hepatitis B show a hepatitic pattern that can range from minimal to marked inflammation depending on the degree of viral replication and the extent of the immune response. The chronic hepatitis shows no distinguishing features that can be used to separate hepatitis B infection from other causes of hepatitis. In most cases, both the portal chronic inflammation and the lobular inflammation are either mild or moderate. Severe lobular hepatitis is unusual in chronic hepatitis B and suggests an HBV flare, HDV superinfection, or other superimposed hepatic injury. Interface activity is common, and its frequency and extent tend to correlate with the degree of portal inflammation. Discrete lymphoid aggregates are present in the portal tracts in 10% to 20% of cases.[9] In addition, in approximately 10% of cases the bile ducts show mild lymphocytic inflammation and reactive epithelial changes (Poulsen lesion) but are without significant bile duct injury.[9] Studies that compared large groups of biopsies from patients with chronic hepatitis B to chronic hepatitis C found that lymphoid aggregates and bile duct lymphocytosis are somewhat more common in hepatitis C compared to hepatitis B, but these observations are not diagnostically useful because there is too much overlap, and serological testing, not histology, is the foundation for diagnosing viral hepatitis. Incidental, small epithelioid granulomas are found in about 1% to 2% of biopsies for chronic hepatitis B.[10,11]

A chronic hepatitis that also has ground glass change in the hepatocytes strongly suggests chronic hepatitis B, though drug effects can show similar changes, a finding called pseudo–ground glass inclusions, so immunostaining or serological confirmation of hepatitis B is still required. The ground glass inclusions in chronic hepatitis B are found only in a subset of patients with long-standing chronic infection (Fig. 2.33). They are not found with acute hepatitis B. The ground glass inclusions result from the accumulation of badly mutated viruses that produce proteins that are not readily secreted and perhaps also prevent other normal proteins from being secreted.[12,13] Ground glass hepatocytes can also be identified on

Shikata orcein stain and Victoria blue stain, but immunostains for HBsAg are more sensitive and specific. HBsAg will be positive in many hepatocytes that do not show ground glass change. The staining is cytoplasmic in most cases, but in cases with higher viral replication, the staining can be membranous, though membranous staining is not specific for high viral replication per se and also appears to depend to some degree on the antibody used.

An additional H&E finding called sanded glass nuclei is rarely seen and can be challenging to confidently identify (Fig. 2.34) but is seen in cases with high viral replication.[14–17] The hepatocyte nuclei accumulate HBcAg, which gives the nucleus a smudgy glassy look. Immunostains are positive for HBcAg. Sometimes HDV superinfection can also give similar changes,[18] so immunostains for HBcAg and correlation with other serological findings are important.

TABLE 2.7: Clinically Defined Phases of Chronic Hepatitis B Infection

Phase	Simplified Summary	Typical Biopsy Findings[a]
Immunotolerant phase • Serology: HBsAg positive, HBeAg positive • Serum DNA levels : 5 to 12 log • AST/ALT levels: normal or near normal	***Active infection with little active liver damage***	**Inflammation**: minimal to mild **Fibrosis**: absent, occasionally mild portal fibrosis **Immunostains**: HBsAg positive; HBcAg positive
Immunoactive phase, also called immune clearance phase • Serology: HBsAg positive, HBeAg positive or negative • Serum DNA levels: >5 log when HBeAg positive, but lower when HBeAg negative • AST/ALT levels: elevated; may be persistent or intermittent	***Active infection with active liver damage because the body is trying to clear the infection***	**Inflammation**: mild to moderately active hepatitis. Hepatitis can be severe during a flare of viral replication **Fibrosis**: range from none to cirrhosis **Immunostains**: HBsAg positive; HBcAg positive
Inactive carrier state, also called nonreplicative phase or immune control phase • Serology: HBsAg positive, HBeAg negative, HBeAb positive • Serum DNA levels < 4 log • AST/ALT levels: normal or near normal	***Ongoing infection, but active liver damage is reduced to low levels***	**Inflammation**: minimal to mild **Fibrosis**: range from none to cirrhosis **Immunostains**: HBsAg rare positive cells; HBcAg negative to rare cells
Resolved hepatitis B, also called cleared hepatitis B • History: known prior acute or chronic HBV infection or serological evidence with HBcAb positivity + HBsAb positivity • Serology: HBsAg negative, HBeAg negative • Serum DNA levels: negative • AST/ALT levels: normal	***Infection has been cleared and there is little or no ongoing inflammation/damage to the liver***	**Inflammation**: none to minimal **Fibrosis**: range from none to cirrhosis **Immunostains**: HBsAg negative; HBcAg negative

(Continued)

TABLE 2.7: Clinically Defined Phases of Chronic Hepatitis B Infection (Continued)

Phase	Simplified Summary	Typical Biopsy Findings[a]
Occult hepatitis B (subset of resolved hepatitis B cases) • History: known prior acute or chronic HBV infection or serological evidence with HBcAb positivity + HBsAb positivity • Serology: HBsAg negative, HBeAg negative • Serum DNA levels: negative on routine testing; specialized ultrasensitive testing can be positive • HBV DNA in liver tissue: positive • AST/ALT levels: normal or minimal elevated (may still have enzyme flares)	***Infection is latent in the liver; replication flares are rare but can be triggered by immunosuppression or other factors***	**Inflammation**: none to minimal **Fibrosis**: range from none to cirrhosis **Immunostains**: HBsAg may show rare positive cells; HBcAg negative

[a]Note: Biopsy findings for any category can vary widely, but "typical" findings are listed in this section.
Cases of acute hepatitis B (individuals with less than 6 months of HBsAg) are not part of this classification system.

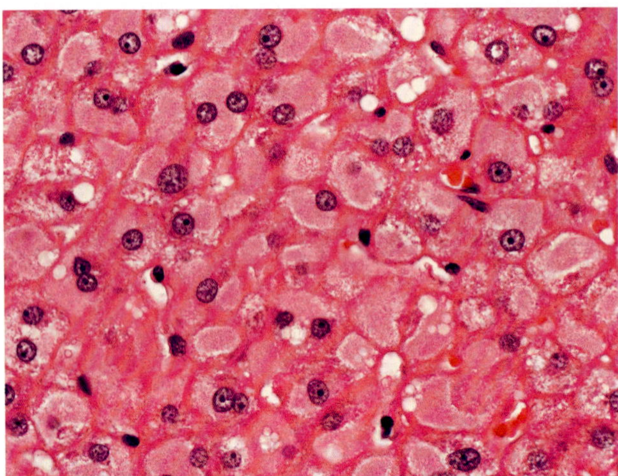

Figure 2.33. **Chronic hepatitis B, ground glass hepatocytes.** Numerous ground glass hepatocytes are seen. The ground glass change fills the entire cytoplasm leading to a light gray inclusion–like change.

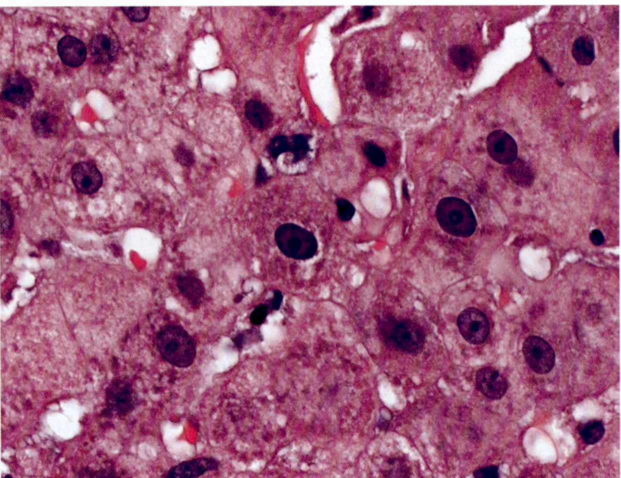

Figure 2.34. **Chronic hepatitis B, sanded glass nuclei.** The hepatocyte in the center of the image has a glassy almost homogenous appearance to its nucleus.

Immunostains for Hepatitis B

Immunostains for HBsAg or HBcAg work very well but are not needed when the diagnosis of hepatitis B has been made on clinical grounds. Their staining characteristics are discussed above and in Table 2.7, but in brief, HBsAg is typically a cytoplasmic and/or membranous stain (Figs. 2.35 and 2.36), with the membranous staining correlating broadly with higher levels of viral replication. HBsAg staining can be found in both benign hepatocytes and in hepatocellular carcinoma. In any given hepatocyte, the cytoplasmic staining can be diffuse and homogenous, show a tram-track-like pattern, or have a distinct granular staining pattern. Acute hepatitis B can be negative for HBsAg in the early course of infection. In chronic hepatitis B, HBsAg positive cells can be scattered or organized into distinct nodule-like areas (Fig. 2.37). The number of positive cells varies from just a few to more than 50%.

Ignoring the distinct clusters of positive cells, which are more commonly seen in cases of long-standing viral infection with advanced fibrosis, the extent of cytoplasmic staining correlates roughly with the overall degree of viral replication.

HBcAg stains benign hepatocytes and sometimes hepatocellular carcinomas. HBcAg staining is nuclear and/or cytoplasmic (Fig. 2.38). Cytoplasmic staining for HBcAg is more likely when viral replication levels are high.[15-17] HBcAg stains are typically positive in acute hepatitis B infection, and in chronic hepatitis B the number of positive nuclei correlates roughly with the degree of viral replication. In chronic viral hepatitis with low levels of viral replication, HBcAg can be negative on liver biopsies or show only rare positive cells. Finally, bile ducts can occasionally show rare cells positive for HBcAg.

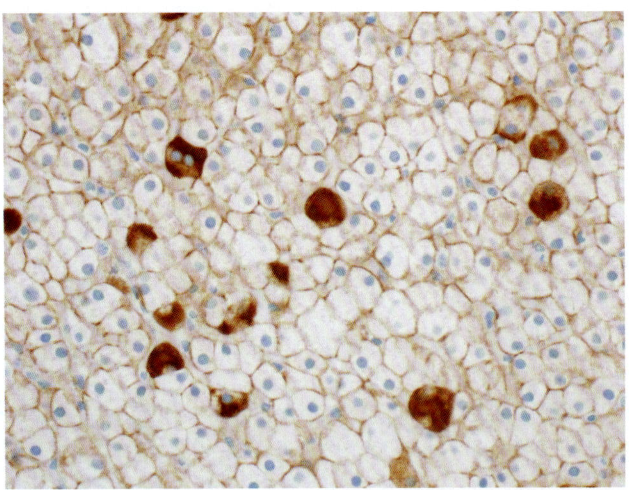

Figure 2.35. **Chronic hepatitis B, HBsAg.** Scattered single positive cells are seen throughout the lobules. The hepatocytes also show a more generalized membranous staining pattern. This membranous pattern can be associated with higher levels of viral replication, but the correlation is not perfect and other technical factors may play a role such as antibody and antibody titer.

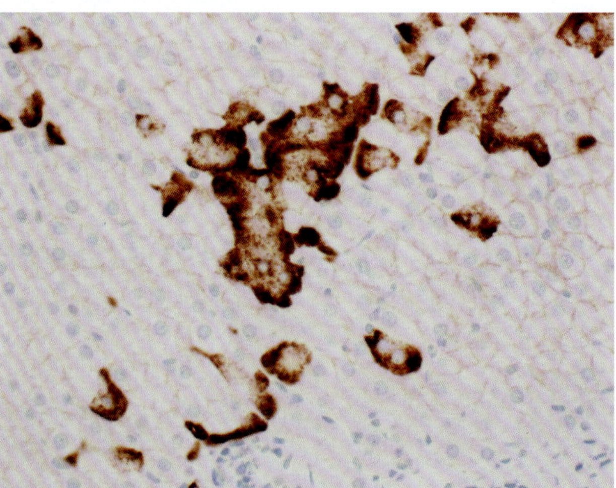

Figure 2.36. **Chronic hepatitis B, HBsAg.** Strong cytoplasmic and weak membranous staining is seen in this case of long-standing chronic hepatitis B with cirrhosis.

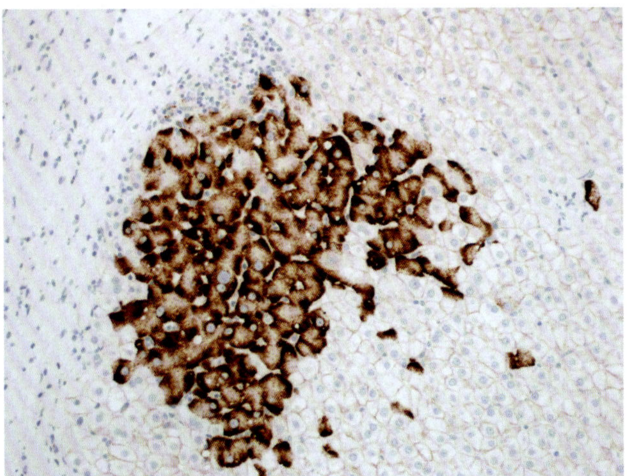

Figure 2.37. **Chronic hepatitis B, HBsAg.** In cirrhotic livers, aggregates of positive staining hepatocytes are common, sometimes called a *clonal pattern*.

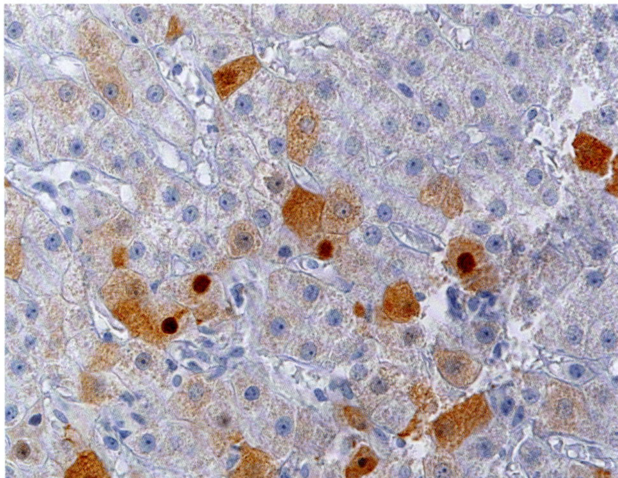

Figure 2.38. **Chronic hepatitis B, HBcAg.** There is both nuclear staining and cytoplasmic staining in this case. Cytoplasmic staining is more common in cases with higher levels of viral replication.

Large Cell Change

Large cell change can be found in any cirrhotic liver and less commonly in noncirrhotic livers (Fig. 2.39). In noncirrhotic livers, large cell change is more common with chronic HBV infection, but this finding is not specific and can be seen with many conditions.

With large cell change, the biopsy shows small patches or aggregates of hepatocytes with nuclear changes that stand out at low power, including mild hyperchromasia, pleomorphism, and sometimes multinucleation. Despite these nuclear changes, the hepatocytes retain a normal or near normal N:C ratio. The precise mechanism for large cell change is not clear, but large cell change is associated with DNA damage.[19-22] Molecular biology studies also indicate that large cell change is genetically heterogeneous. In most cases, the changes appear to be degenerative or senescent, while in a subset of cases the changes may be directly premalignant.

Hepatocellular Carcinoma

Chronic hepatitis B infection is an important risk factor for hepatocellular carcinoma. Hepatocellular carcinomas can arise in both cirrhotic and noncirrhotic livers. The hepatocellular carcinomas do not have any specific morphological findings but can stain positive for HBsAg.

HEPATITIS D INFECTION

KEY FEATURES on Biology of Hepatitis D

- RNA virus
- Major routes of transmission: sex, bloodborne
- Worldwide infection: 20 million, but there is wide regional variation; overall about 5% of all chronic HBV infected individuals also have chronic HDV
- Incubation: 4 to 8 weeks
- Two basic patterns of infection: HDV superinfection of the liver with chronic HBV; HDV and HBV coinfection (acute infections occur at the same time)
- Chronic infection: 90% with superinfection; 2% with coinfection
- Cirrhosis risk: with superinfection, 70% in 10 years; with coinfection, 20% in 10 years
- Antiviral therapy: suppresses viral replication but does not cure in most cases
- Vaccine: no, but HBV vaccine also prevents HDV infection

HDV infections require hepatitis B infection because HDV relies on HBsAg to package its own nucleic acids. Thus, HDV can either infect the liver at the same time as HBV (coinfection) or infect a liver that already has chronic hepatitis B infection (superinfection). Superinfection has a higher risk of acute liver failure, chronic HDV infection, and accelerated fibrosis progression.

HDV/HBV coinfection shows a typical pattern of acute hepatitis without any distinguishing features. Likewise, HDV superinfection shows an acute-on-chronic hepatitis pattern without any distinguishing features. The clinical and histological differential will include a flare of the underlying hepatitis B infection, but with an HBV flare, the HBV DNA levels are significantly elevated above their baseline; while with HDV superinfection, the HBV DNA levels are not increased and are often decreased. The diagnosis in most centers is made by serological testing for HDV. Immunostains are also useful when available. Chronic HDV/HBV coinfection can lead to more rapid fibrosis progression, but the inflammation patterns are similar to that of HBV infection alone (Fig. 2.40).

HEPATITIS C

KEY FEATURES on Biology of Hepatitis C

- RNA virus
- Major routes of transmission: bloodborne, sex
- Worldwide infection: 71 million
- Incubation: 2 weeks to 6 months

- Chronic infection: ~80%
- Cirrhosis risk: 30% in 30 years
- Antiviral therapy: cure in 90+% of cases with new direct-acting antiviral agents
- Historically when interferon was the main treatment, genotyping was important as IL28 b genotype predicts response rate for interferon-based therapy: CC better than CT better than TT
- Vaccine: no

Hepatitis C can cause acute and chronic hepatitis. Acute hepatitis is usually subclinical but can be symptomatic, especially in the elderly. In this setting, the biopsies show a typical acute hepatitis pattern and can be cholestatic (Fig. 2.41).[23] There is moderate to marked lobular hepatitis and mild to moderate portal inflammation. The portal tracts can also show a reactive bile ductular proliferation that resembles biliary obstruction (Fig. 2.42).[23]

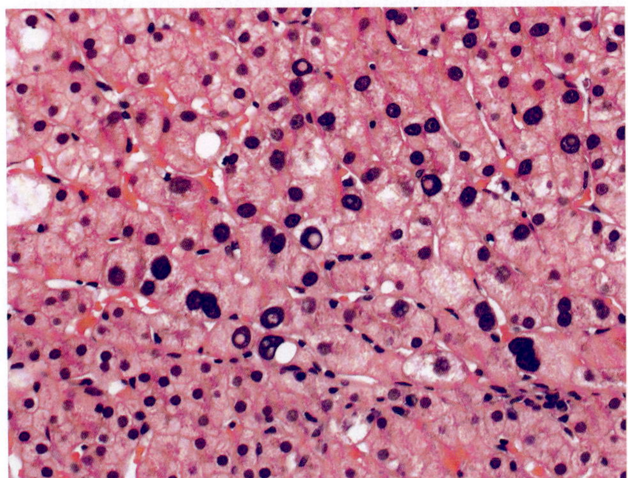

Figure 2.39. **Chronic hepatitis B, large cell change.** In large cell change, hepatocytes stand out at low power. They have enlarged hyperchromatic nuclei, but a largely preserved N:C ratio. This finding is not specific for hepatitis B, but does seem to be more common than in chronic hepatitis C.

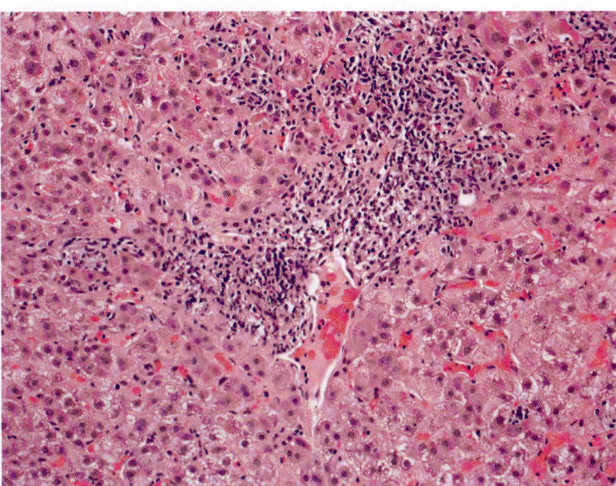

Figure 2.40. **Chronic hepatitis B/ hepatitis D infection.** The biopsy showed patchy moderate portal chronic inflammation and mild lobular activity, with no features that would distinguish this case from ordinary hepatitis B. HDV testing was performed for clinical reasons (patient was from an area of the world with a high prevalence of HDV).

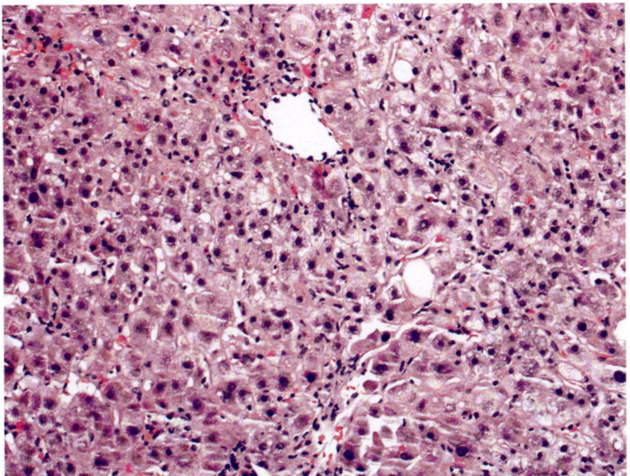

Figure 2.41. **Acute hepatitis C.** The lobules showed moderate hepatitis with mild cholestasis.

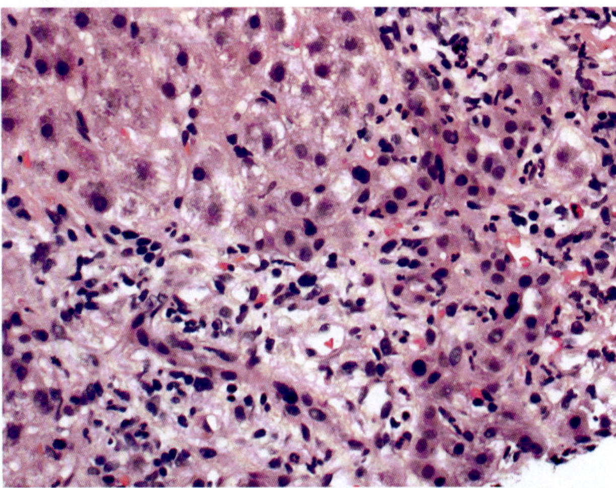

Figure 2.42. **Acute hepatitis C.** The portal tracts showed a bile ductular proliferation that mimicked biliary obstruction.

Grading and staging chronic hepatitis C used to be a common indication for liver biopsy, as antiviral therapy was expensive and the response rate was about 50%, so therapy was commonly initiated only when the biopsy showed advanced fibrosis (bridging fibrosis or cirrhosis). With the development of modern antiviral therapies and the introduction of noninvasive measures of fibrosis, biopsies for grading and staging chronic hepatitis C are now rare. Biopsies are still performed if there is a significant discordance between clinical findings and noninvasive markers of fibrosis or if there is concern for an additional disease superimposed onto the chronic hepatitis C.

Untreated chronic hepatitis C typically shows mild (~30% of cases) to moderate portal chronic inflammation (~65% of cases) with minimal to mild lobular hepatitis (65%) (Figs. 2.43 and 2.44).[24] Heavier lobular inflammation is less common, with about 30% of cases showing patchy moderate lobular hepatitis and 5% showing patchy marked lobular hepatitis.[24] Diffuse marked portal inflammation, marked lobular hepatitis, or zone 3 necrosis suggest an additional superimposed liver injury (Fig. 2.45). Correlation with liver enzymes pattern is also very helpful, as a recent spike in liver enzymes supports the likelihood of a superimposed liver injury. Likewise, lobular cholestasis suggests an additional injury unless there is decompensated cirrhosis.

Other nonspecific findings of no strong clinical significance include mild bile duct lymphocytosis, mild focal endothelialitis of either the portal or central veins, and focal giant cell transformation of hepatocytes.[23,25,26] The giant cell transformation can be persistent on subsequent biopsies[25] but is not associated with more aggressive disease. What causes the giant cell change is unknown. Lymphoid aggregates can be found in the portal tracts, with or without germinal centers, but also have no diagnostic significance. Interface activity tends to correlate with the degree of portal inflammation (Fig. 2.46). Interface activity has no special diagnostic or prognostic information over that of inflammation in the portal tracts or lobules but is commonly included in formal systems for grading the amount of inflammation in hepatitis C–infected livers.

Fatty liver disease is a common finding in chronic hepatitis C (Fig. 2.47) and can reflect the metabolic syndrome, alcohol use, drug effect, or viral genotype. HCV genotype 3 is associated with macrovesicular steatosis, in particular if the patient also has risk factors for the metabolic syndrome. The fatty liver disease should be evaluated separately from the chronic hepatitis C, including the amount of fat, steatosis versus steatohepatitis, and presence or absence of pericellular fibrosis.

Approximately 5% of biopsies will also show small incidental granulomas.[27,28] The granulomas are epithelioid, noncaseating, and found in either the portal tracts (most commonly) or the lobules. Stains for organisms such as AFB and GMS stains are negative, and their etiology is typically unclear even after full clinical and histological evaluation. In subsequent biopsies, the granulomas are commonly still present, but they do not have any strong clinical significance.

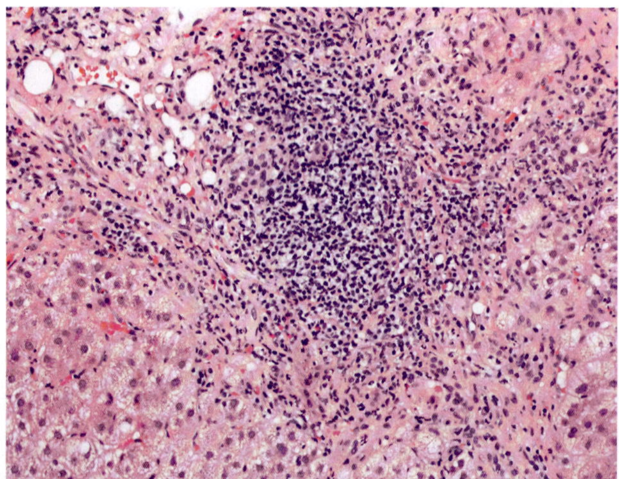

Figure 2.43. Chronic hepatitis C, portal inflammation. This biopsy showed patchy moderate portal chronic inflammation and mild lobular activity.

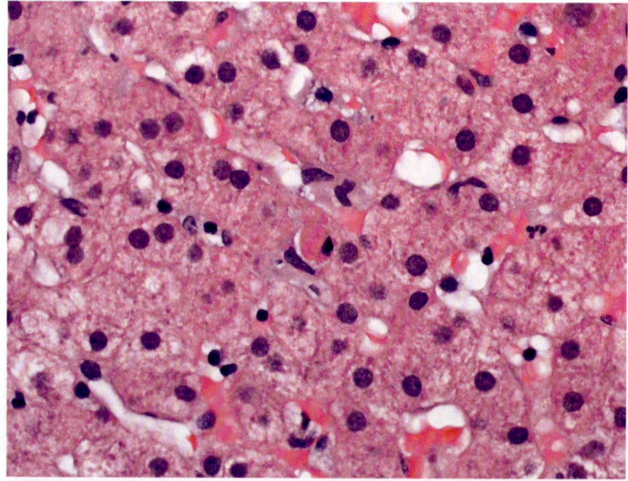

Figure 2.44. Chronic hepatitis C, lobular inflammation. This case showed very mild patchy lobular hepatitis. An acidophil body can be seen in the center of the image.

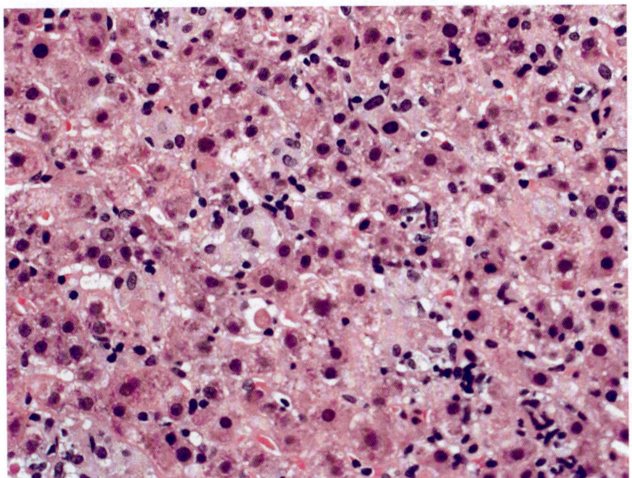

Figure 2.45. **Chronic hepatitis C, too much lobular inflammation.** In this case of chronic hepatitis C, the lobules showed diffuse moderate lobular hepatitis—too much for typical chronic hepatitis C. The liver enzymes have also showed a recent flare above background. The cause was suspected to be a drug reaction based on clinical findings.

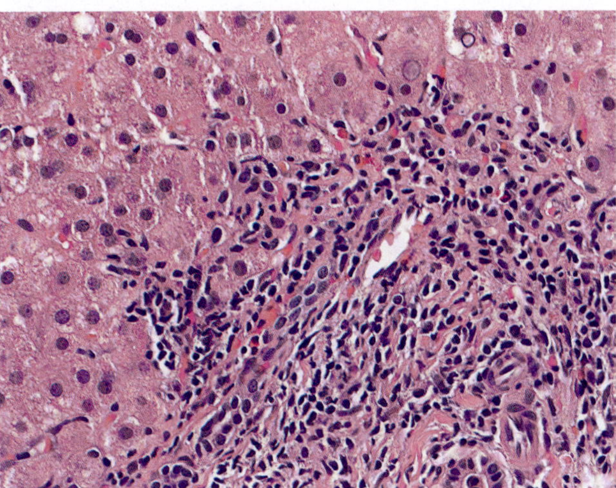

Figure 2.46. **Chronic hepatitis C, interface activity.** This case showed moderate interface activity. The interface activity is seen as inflammation and injury to the hepatocytes that are adjacent to the portal tract. The portal tract in this case also shows moderate portal chronic inflammation.

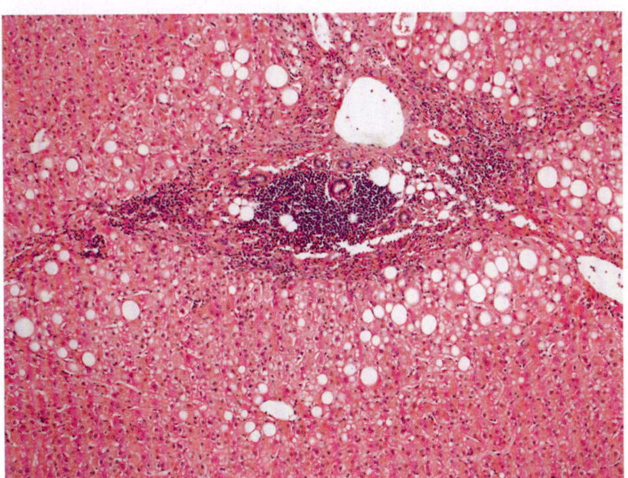

Figure 2.47. **Chronic hepatitis C, macrovesicular steatosis.** This patient had both chronic hepatitis C genotype 3 and mild obesity.

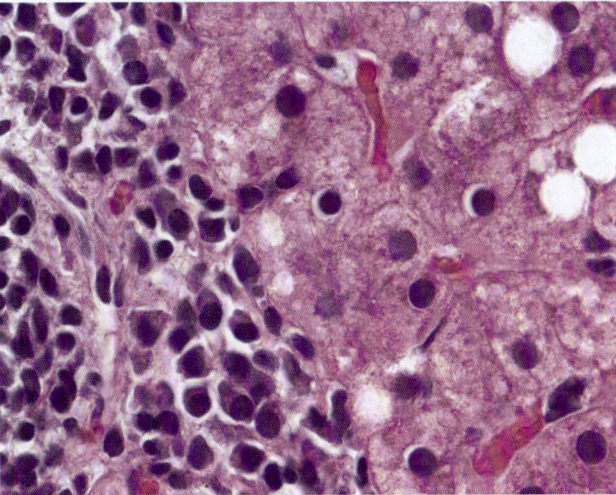

Figure 2.48. **Chronic hepatitis C, plasma cell rich portal inflammation.** A few of the portal tracts in this case have plasma cell–rich inflammation, but the patient had no other serological or histological evidence for autoimmune hepatitis.

The inflammation in the portal tracts is predominately lymphocytic, but rare plasma cells are commonly present (Fig. 2.48). In about 5% of cases, plasma cells can show a mild, patchy prominence, with more plasma cells than is usual in chronic hepatitis C, but less than is typical in autoimmune hepatitis. This finding has also been linked to low titer serum autoantibodies,[29] but does not appear to represent a true autoimmune hepatitis. These cases respond to antiviral therapy in the expected manner and do not leave behind an underlying autoimmune hepatitis. Thus, this pattern of injury should not be classified as an overlap of chronic hepatitis C and autoimmune hepatitis. In some publications, the term "hepatitis C with autoimmune features" is used to describe these cases, but this term is confusing to almost everyone and should be avoided. A true autoimmune hepatitis can occur but is very uncommon in individuals with chronic hepatitis C. When present, it will show the typical clinical, serological, and histological findings of autoimmune hepatitis that are seen outside the setting of chronic hepatitis C, with elevated serum IgG levels, high titer autoantibodies such as ANA and/or ASMA, plasma cell–rich inflammation in the portal tracts, and moderate to marked lobular hepatitis. Of note, isolated elevations in serum autoantibodies, without compelling histological findings, should not be used to suggest a coexisting autoimmune hepatitis, as 15% of individuals with ordinary chronic hepatitis C are positive for ANA antibodies, 34% for smooth muscle antibodies, and 0.5% for anti-LKM antibodies.[30]

Hepatitis C is a recognized risk factor for both hepatocellular carcinoma and cholangiocarcinoma. Hepatitis C can cause hepatocellular carcinoma even if the liver is noncirrhotic,[31] though the risk increases substantially once the liver is cirrhotic. Explanted livers should be carefully searched for tumor nodules. In addition, about 2% of liver explants show bile duct dysplasia.[32] The dysplasia is usually low grade and most commonly affects the medium and larger sized bile ducts in the liver hilum or the larger segmental branches of the biliary tree.

FIBROSING CHOLESTATIC HEPATITIS B AND C

CHECKLIST: Fibrosing Cholestatic Hepatitis B and C

- ☐ Immunosuppressed individuals
- ☐ High levels of viral replication
- ☐ Biopsies with bile ductular proliferation and lobular cholestasis can mimic biliary obstruction
- ☐ Inflammation tends to be relatively sparse

Immunosuppressed individuals with chronic hepatitis C or chronic hepatitis B can show a distinctive pattern of injury that results from very high levels of viral replication. This injury pattern is thought to result from direct viral injury rather than the immune system. Viral levels are often greater than 30 million copies per mL for HCV. Patients can be immunosuppressed from bone marrow or solid organ transplantation, human immunodeficiency virus (HIV), or other causes. The biopsies show a cholestatic pattern of injury that can closely resemble biliary obstruction, with a brisk bile ductular proliferation and moderate to marked lobular cholestasis (Fig. 2.49). In fact, imaging of the biliary tree is indicated before a diagnosis of fibrosing cholestatic hepatitis is finalized. The inflammation can be relatively mild in both the portal tracts and the lobules. The zone 1 hepatocytes in particular show swelling with a cholate stasis pattern of injury. A trichrome stain shows portal fibrosis and pericellular fibrosis of the zone 1 hepatocytes. When left untreated, there can be rapid fibrosis progression to cirrhosis.

The diagnosis is usually evident when (1) there is a history of immunosuppression, (2) the viral nucleic acid levels in the serum are very high, and (3) the full injury pattern is present on biopsy (lobular cholestasis, hepatocyte swelling, ductular proliferation, portal and pericellular fibrosis). However, there are many cases that do not have all of the histological

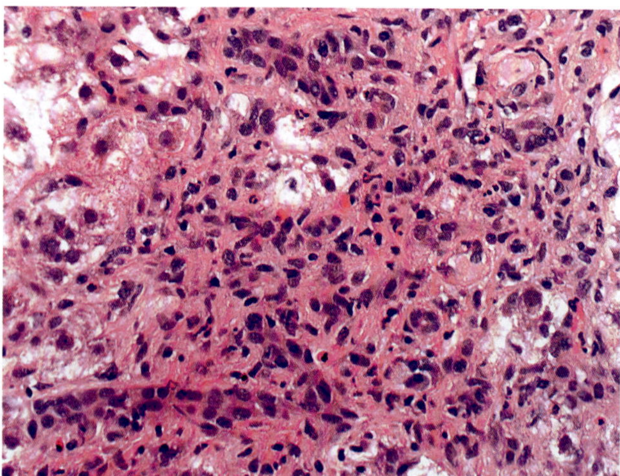

Figure 2.49. **Fibrosing cholestatic hepatitis C.** The portal tracts show bile ductular proliferation and fibrosis with relatively little inflammation.

changes, with the histology falling somewhere in between that of ordinary chronic viral hepatitis and that of fibrosing cholestatic viral injury. This middle group of cases does not have a good name, but most cases improve with reduced immunosuppression, consistent with the changes being part of the early spectrum of fibrosing cholestatic hepatitis. The histological differential typically includes ordinary viral hepatitis with a superimposed cholestatic injury such as a drug effect or biliary obstruction, and these possibilities should also be excluded before a final diagnosis of early cholestatic fibrosing viral hepatitis.

HEPATITIS E VIRAL INFECTION

KEY FEATURES on Biology of Hepatitis E

- RNA virus
- Major routes of transmission: oral–fecal, undercooked meat
- Worldwide infection: 20 million per year
- Incubation: 2 to 10 weeks
- Chronic infection: yes, but only in immunosuppressed individuals
- Vaccine: no (available only in some parts of Asia)

Hepatitis E virus (HEV) is transmitted by the oral–fecal route or by eating undercooked meat. In places in the world that do not have adequate safe drinking water, most infections are transmitted when there is fecal contamination of the water source and can lead to large epidemics of infection. These illnesses are caused by HEV genotypes 1 and 2. Pregnant women are at high risk of liver failure, with a fatality rate of 5%. In contrast, endemic HEV is caused by HEV genotype 3, and the most common infection route is eating undercooked pork,[33] especially pork liver, or eating undercooked wild game.[34] However, in many cases a specific infection source is not identified. Endemic infections are mostly likely to cause acute hepatitis in older males,[33] where infection can be mistaken for a drug reaction.[35] Infections in younger healthy individuals are usually asymptomatic. Infections do not lead to chronic HEV infection in immunocompetent individuals, but there can be prolonged infections in the elderly. However, individuals with immunosuppression from solid organ transplantation, especially liver transplants, can develop chronic hepatitis.

The histology of acute HEV infection is similar to the histology of acute hepatitis A, B, and C, with a lymphocytic hepatitis pattern that is often cholestatic.[36-38] The sinusoids can also show a mild prominence in neutrophils.[36,38] In most cases, the hepatitis is mild (Fig. 2.50), but it can be more severe. Overall, the hepatitis is not very specific, so your best chance of making this diagnosis is to remember that HEV is in the histological differential for acute cholestatic hepatitis, especially in older aged individuals. The diagnosis can be secured by serum IgM positivity, serum PCR testing for HEV, or by staining tissue for viral nucleic acids with in situ hybridization (Fig. 2.51) or viral proteins with immunohistochemistry.[39] In terms of antibody testing, IgM antibodies to HEV are detectable for 1 to 3 months after acute infection. In contrast, IgG antibodies are detectable for many years after exposure and in some individuals for life.

Chronic hepatitis E occurs only in the setting of immunosuppression, in particular with organ transplants, where it presents as an unexplained chronic hepatitis.[40-42] While uncommon, cases of chronic HEV have also has been reported with HIV infection, with cancer chemotherapy,[33] and in the elderly without other causes of immunsuppresion.[43]

The histological findings in all of these cases are not very specific, and many other diagnoses are typically considered before chronic HEV is diagnosed, such as drug reaction or other viral infections. Chronic HEV infection typically shows mild nonspecific lobular hepatitis with minimal or absent cholestasis and mild portal chronic.

NONHEPATOTROPIC VIRUSES

A number of systemic viral infections can also involve the liver, with liver injury sometimes taking prominence at presentation. These infections are all rare, but the most common in nontropical areas of the world are Epstein–Barr virus (EBV), cytomegalovirus (CMV),

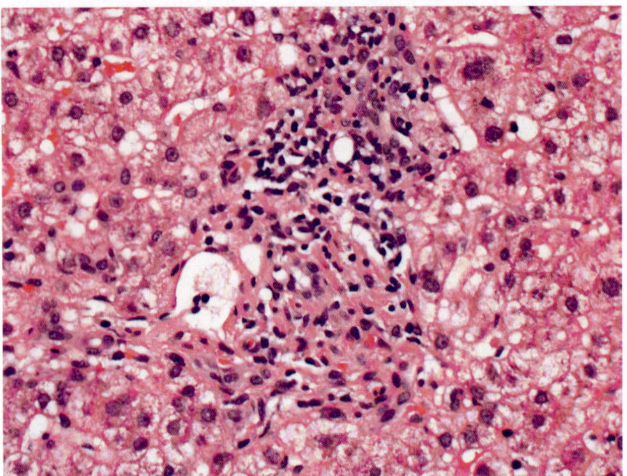

Figure 2.50. **Chronic hepatitis E.** After liver transplantation, this person developed a long-standing, unexplained chronic hepatitis. The liver was biopsied several times but never showed much more than very mild nonspecific chronic hepatitis.

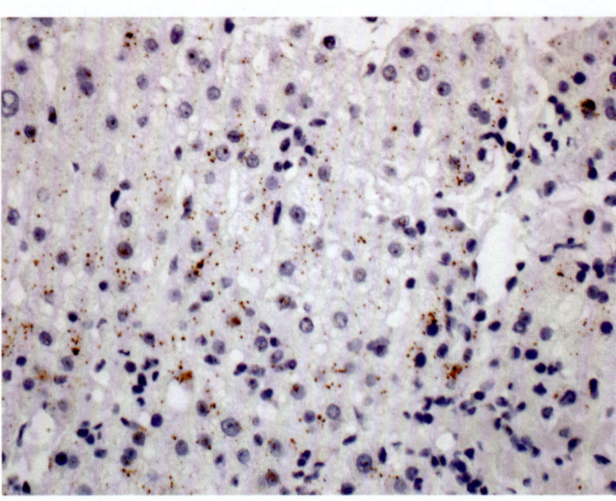

Figure 2.51. **Chronic hepatitis E in situ hybridization.** The hepatitis show patchy staining by HEV in situ hybridization.

herpes simplex virus (HSV), and adenovirus. Immunosuppression from any cause is an important risk factor for all of these viral infections. The most common nonhepatotropic viral infections in immunocompetent individuals are EBV and HSV.

EPSTEIN–BARR VIRUS (EBV)

EBV infection of the liver tends to look like an ordinary and rather nondescript hepatitis, with mild to moderate portal and lobular inflammation (Figs. 2.52-2.54). The virus does not infect hepatocytes, but rather B lymphocytes and rarely T lymphocytes, so there is relatively little hepatocyte injury even when there is striking lobular inflammation. The lobular inflammation can be predominately sinusoidal, sometimes leading to a "beading" appearance of the lymphocytes. However, this beaded appearance is not very sensitive or specific, so EBV infection should be considered whenever there is an unexplained hepatitis in younger individuals (teens, young adults) or in immunosuppressed individuals. EBV in situ hybridization is an important tool to confirm the diagnosis (Fig. 2.55).

CYTOMEGALOVIRUS (CMV)

CMV infection occurs almost exclusively in immunosuppressed patients, with only rare case reports of infection in the immunocompetent. In both cases, the patient can present with fulminant hepatitis. Most immunosuppressed patients present with an acute flair in liver enzymes. The histological findings can be subtle (Fig. 2.56), so it is best to do an immunostain whenever there is clinical or histological concern for CMV infection. In more severe cases, the infection can be histologically obvious (Fig. 2.57), with viral inclusions in endothelial cells and less commonly in hepatocytes or bile duct epithelial cells. The infection can be accompanied by various degrees of inflammation and hepatocyte necrosis. Small sinusoidal clusters of neutrophils can sometimes be numerous with CMV infection, a finding called a neutrophilic microabscess. However, single or a few small neutrophilic microabscesses are also common in other inflammatory conditions of the liver and so are not specific for CMV infection.

ADENOVIRUS, HERPES SIMPLEX VIRUS (HSV), AND VARICELLA ZOSTER VIRUS (VZV)

These viral infections are very rare and tend to present with fulminant liver failure. All of these infections are most commonly identified in immunosuppressed patients, though fulminant HSV can also present in otherwise immunocompetent individuals.[44,45] When HSV presents as fulminant hepatitis, mucocutaneous lesions are often absent.

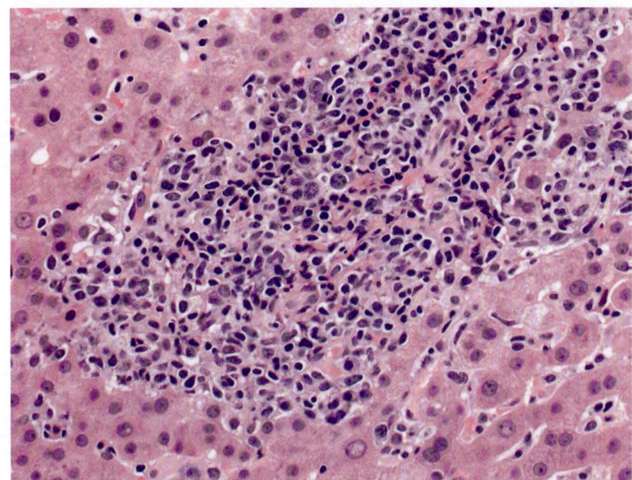

Figure 2.52. **EBV hepatitis.** The portal tracts show diffusely moderate chronic inflammation. The inflammation is mostly lymphocytes, but there also are plasma cells, histiocytes, and rare eosinophils.

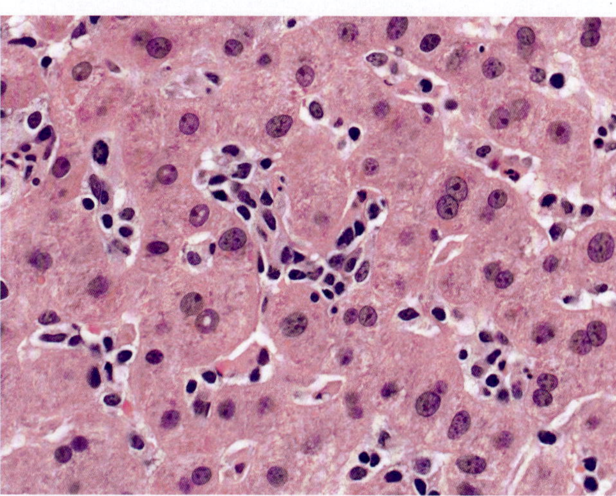

Figure 2.53. **EBV hepatitis.** The lobules show patchy dense sinusoidal infiltrates of lymphocytes with relatively little hepatocyte injury.

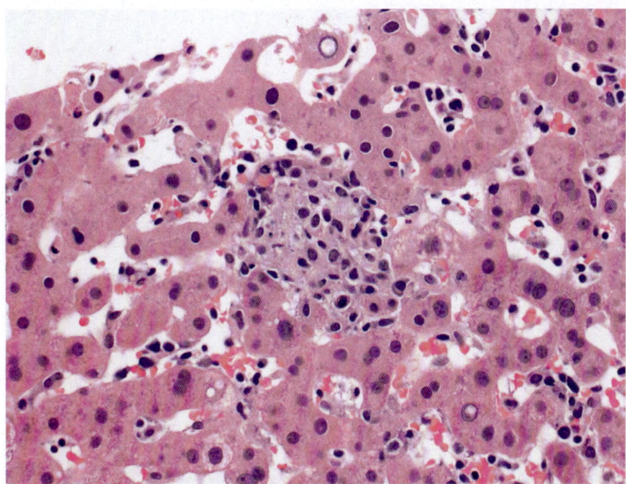

Figure 2.54. **EBV hepatitis.** Rare granulomas are also present in the lobules.

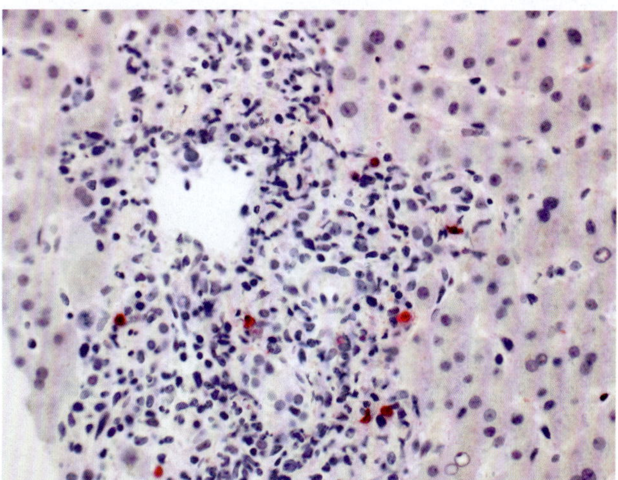

Figure 2.55. **EBV hepatitis in situ hybridization.** Scattered positive cells are seen. In most cases of EBV, the number of infected cells is relatively small compared to the density of the inflammation.

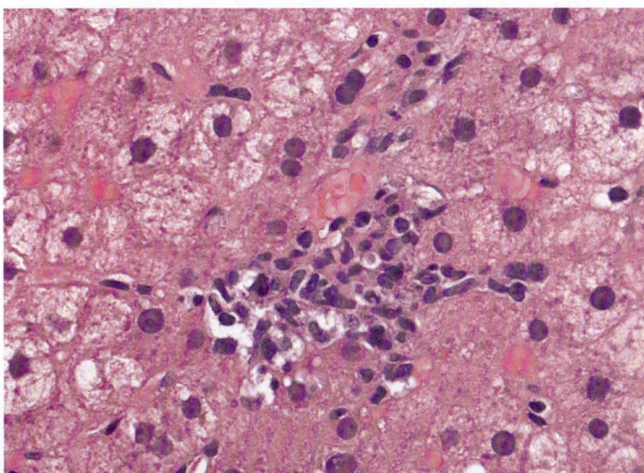

Figure 2.56. **CMV hepatitis.** This case of CMV hepatitis had patchy lobular inflammation and the diagnosis was made by positive CMV staining. Even in retrospect, viral inclusions were not evident on H&E.

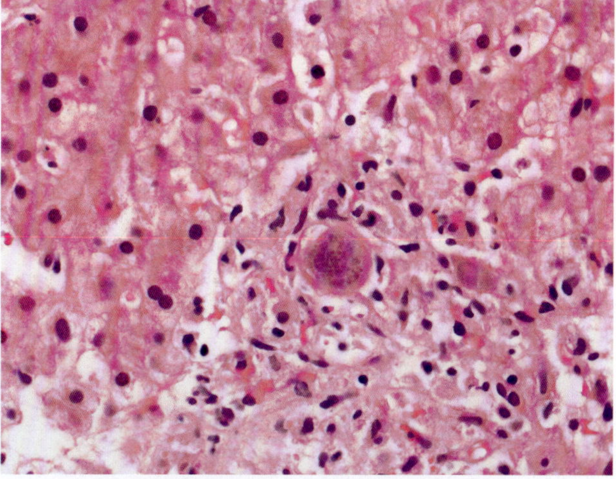

Figure 2.57. **CMV hepatitis.** In contrast to the case in Figure 2.56, numerous easily identified viral inclusions are seen in this case.

The histological findings in all of these infections tend to be similar, with large irregular areas of inflammatory necrosis that do not have zonal patterns. The necrotic areas tend to have sharp borders with the inflamed nonnecrotic areas, a finding that is described as "punched-out" necrosis (Figs. 2.58 and 2.59). The inflammation accompanying the necrosis can be variable, depending on the immunosuppression levels and on the interval from infection to histological examination. Viral inclusions are best identified at the edges of the necrotic lesions, in the hepatocytes that still look largely viable (Figs. 2.60 and 2.61). The inclusions can be subtle, so immunostains are important tools to rule out infection whenever large irregular areas of necrosis are encountered (Fig. 2.62).

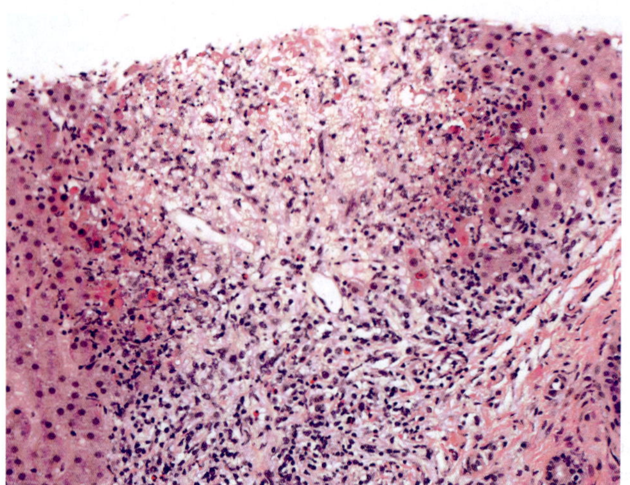

Figure 2.58. **Adenovirus hepatitis.** A well-circumscribed area of inflammatory necrosis is seen, a pattern called *punched out* necrosis.

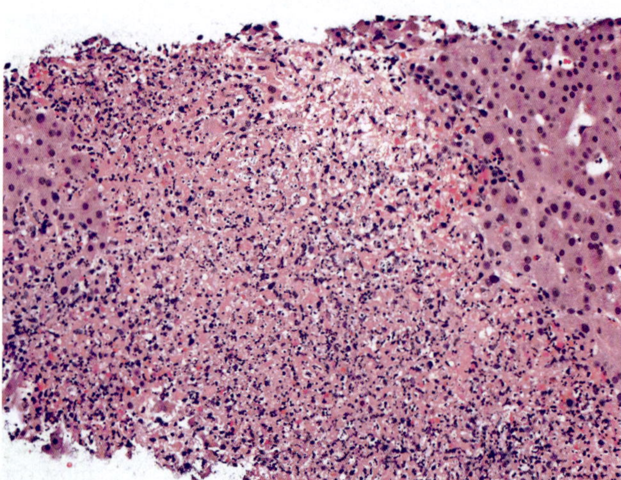

Figure 2.59. **HSV hepatitis.** A pattern of punched out necrosis is seen in this case of HSV infection.

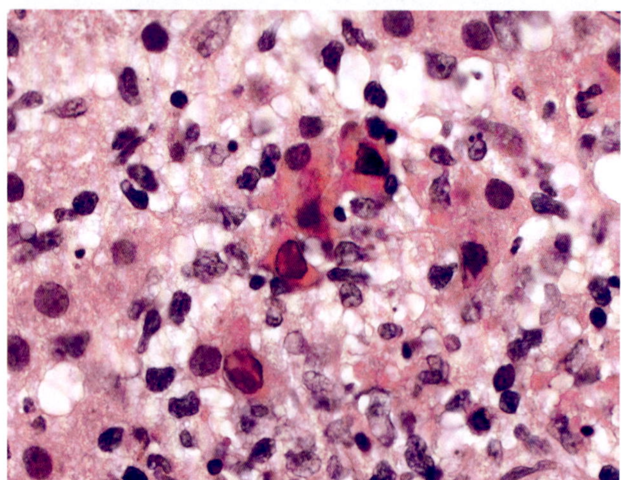

Figure 2.60. **Adenovirus hepatitis, inclusions.** The infected hepatocytes show glassy nuclear chromatin with a condensation of nuclear chromatin at the periphery.

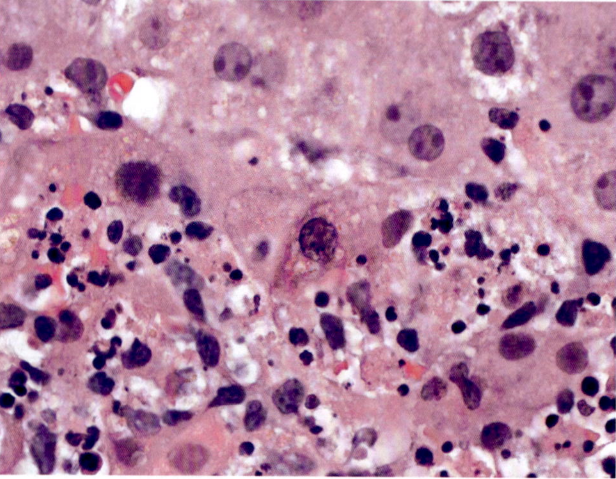

Figure 2.61. **HSV hepatitis, viral inclusions.** The infected hepatocytes show mottled purple glassy nuclei with a rim of chromatin at the edges. The inclusions can be challenging to confidently identify on H&E. They can also look like other viral infections, such as adenovirus (see Fig. 2.60).

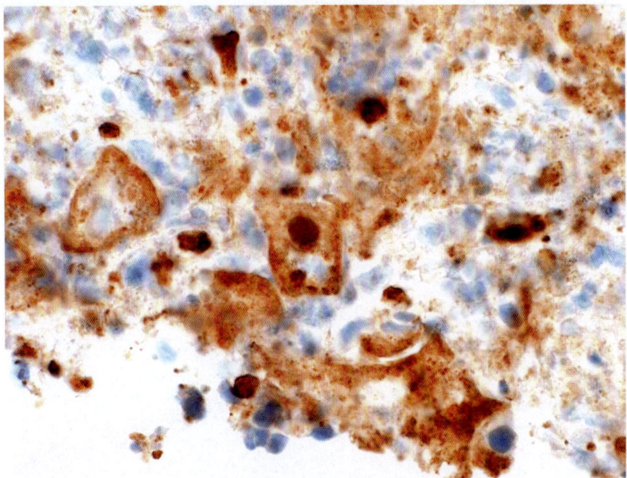

Figure 2.62. **HSV hepatitis, HSV immunostain.** An immunostain shows nuclear and cytoplasm positivity.

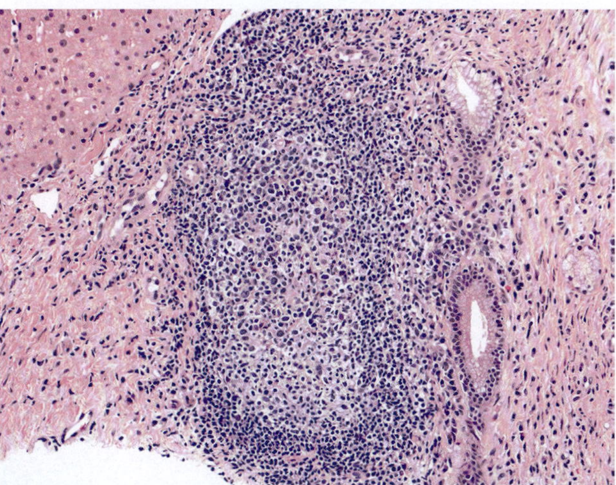

Figure 2.63. **Near miss case 1.** Lymphoid aggregates mimicking chronic hepatitis. This biopsy showed a mild patchy hepatitis that resulted from a drug reaction. A lymphoid aggregate is prominent in this portal tract.

NEAR MISSES

CASE 1. A 42-year-old man presented with elevated liver enzymes, with AST and ALT levels in the low 100s and a minimally elevated alkaline phosphatase. The biopsy showed patchy moderate portal chronic inflammation with mild lobular activity and no fibrosis. The case had been signed out as chronic hepatitis, most consistent with viral hepatitis C because of scattered lymphoid aggregates. Subsequent viral testing was negative, so the case was sent out in consultation.

On review, the overall pattern had been recognized correctly—the biopsy did show patchy moderate portal chronic inflammation with mild lobular activity. There were two portal tracts with lymphoid aggregates, one of which is shown here (Fig. 2.63). There was no fibrosis and no other distinguishing features. Additional medical records were obtained, and there was a strong temporal association with starting a new medication. This association had been recognized clinically, so the drug had been stopped and the enzymes normalized by the time the biopsy arrived for review, which made the diagnosis of "most consistent with a drug effect" relatively straightforward.

From a pathology perspective, this case illustrates several important points. First, the pattern of "more inflammation in the portal tracts than the lobules" does not indicate a person has chronic hepatitis. Secondly, lymphoid aggregates in the portal tracts do not indicate a diagnosis of chronic hepatitis C. Thirdly, the final disease diagnosis almost always requires correlating the clinical, laboratory, and histological findings. Fourth, the process of revisiting a histological diagnosis because of new clinical or laboratory findings is an important part of patient care. It can be a bit uncomfortable sometimes when a diagnosis has to be modified or clarified in some fashion, but this same process of refining a diagnosis based on additional testing is the same model used in all diagnostically focused medical specialties.

CASE 2. A woman in her 30s presented with a skin rash, muscle pain, jaundice, and markedly elevated liver enzymes. She was mildly obese but otherwise in good health and not taking any medications. She had returned from a vacation to Singapore several days before becoming ill. Testing for HAV, HBV, and HCV was negative. An ANA was mildly positive, while ASMA was negative.

The biopsy showed well-defined punched-out areas of necrosis in a background of fatty liver disease (Fig. 2.64). The punched areas were somewhat azonal, with only an equivocal predilection for zone 3 regions. There was no fibrosis. The punched-out areas of necrosis suggested viral infection such as HSV or adenovirus. However, immunostains and serologies were negative, so the biopsy was signed out descriptively with a differential that included primarily viral infection versus toxin exposure. The biopsy ruled out autoimmune

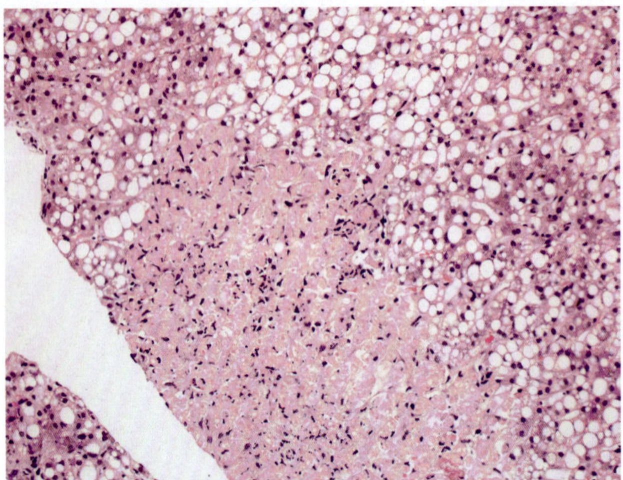

Figure 2.64. **Near miss case 2, dengue fever.** The biopsy shows an irregular area of confluent necrosis.

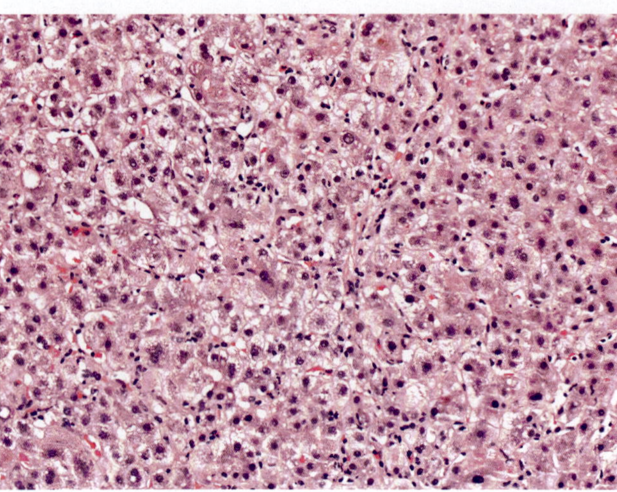

Figure 2.65. **Near miss case 3, acute hepatitis C.** The biopsy shows a mild cholestatic hepatitis.

hepatitis and showed no findings to suggest any alternative to viral infection versus toxin exposure. Subsequent serologies for dengue fever (IgM) were positive.

Dengue fever is transmitted by mosquitoes and is endemic in some tropical areas of the world. The incubation period ranges from several days up to two weeks, which fits well with the recent travel history in this case. This case illustrates the importance of considering travel history when evaluating a biopsy. The world is much smaller now because travel is so common, leading to potential disease exposures that may not be evident when you are sitting at the microscope. This case also illustrates the fundamental role of pathology: identify patterns of injury, accurately report the degree of injury (grade) and the amount of fibrosis (stage), and provide a prioritized differential.

CASE 3. A 64-year-old man previously in normal health presented with a month-long history of progressive jaundice, malaise, and fatigue. At first presentation, AST was 1100 and ALT 1400, but enzymes decreased spontaneously by week two, to 563 and 830, respectively. The alkaline phosphatase was mildly elevated at 190. Antinuclear antibody and anti–smooth muscle antibodies were negative. Hepatitis C and hepatitis B antibodies were negative.

The biopsy showed a cholestatic hepatitis, with mild lobular chronic inflammation (Fig. 2.65), patchy moderate portal chronic inflammation, and no fibrosis. There was no evidence for biliary obstruction. There was no plasma cell enrichment in the hepatitis. The case was signed out with a differential of primarily acute viral infection versus drug effect. Subsequent serum testing was positive for hepatitis C RNA, and hepatitis C antibodies developed.

This case reminds us that viral hepatitis B and C can present with acute hepatitis. These viruses are usually encountered as chronic infections, but acute infections can be clinically symptomatic, especially in the older aged individuals. During a brief window period following acute infection, serologies can be negative. Liver biopsies can provide important information to direct subsequent clinical and laboratory testing.

References

1. Abe H, Beninger PR, Ikejiri N, Setoyama H, Sata M, Tanikawa K. Light microscopic findings of liver biopsy specimens from patients with hepatitis type A and comparison with type B. *Gastroenterology*. 1982;82:938-947.
2. Kwon SY, Park SH, Yeon JE, et al. Clinical characteristics and outcomes of acute hepatitis a in Korea: a nationwide multicenter study. *J Korean Med Sci*. 2014;29:248-253.
3. Okuno T, Sano A, Deguchi T, et al. Pathology of acute hepatitis A in humans. Comparison with acute hepatitis B. *Am J Clin Pathol*. 1984;81:162-169.
4. Teixeira MR, Weller IV, Murray A, et al. The pathology of hepatitis A in man. *Liver*. 1982;2:53-60.
5. Cuthbert JA. Hepatitis A: old and new. *Clin Microbiol Rev*. 2001;14:38-58.

6. Gordon SC, Reddy KR, Schiff L, Schiff ER. Prolonged intrahepatic cholestasis secondary to acute hepatitis A. *Ann Intern Med*. 1984;101:635-637.

7. Su IJ, Kuo TT, Liaw YF. Hepatocyte hepatitis B surface antigen. Diagnostic evaluation of patients with clinically acute hepatitis B surface antigen-positive hepatitis. *Arch Pathol Lab Med*. 1985;109:400-402.

8. Lok AS, McMahon BJ. Chronic hepatitis B: update 2009. *Hepatology*. 2009;50:661-662.

9. Rozario R, Ramakrishna B. Histopathological study of chronic hepatitis B and C: a comparison of two scoring systems. *J Hepatol*. 2003;38:223-229.

10. Tahan V, Ozaras R, Lacevic N, et al. Prevalence of hepatic granulomas in chronic hepatitis B. *Dig Dis Sci*. 2004;49:1575-1577.

11. Goldin RD, Levine TS, Foster GR, Thomas HC. Granulomas and hepatitis C. *Histopathology*. 1996;28:265-267.

12. Wang HC, Wu HC, Chen CF, Fausto N, Lei HY, Su IJ. Different types of ground glass hepatocytes in chronic hepatitis B virus infection contain specific pre-S mutants that may induce endoplasmic reticulum stress. *Am J Pathol*. 2003;163:2441-2449.

13. Schirmacher P, Schauss D, Dienes HP. Intracellular accumulation of incompletely processed transforming growth factor-alpha polypeptides in ground glass hepatocytes of chronic hepatitis B virus infection. *J Hepatol*. 1996;24:547-554.

14. Serinoz E, Varli M, Erden E, et al. Nuclear localization of hepatitis B core antigen and its relations to liver injury, hepatocyte proliferation, and viral load. *J Clin Gastroenterol*. 2003;36:269-272.

15. Son MS, Yoo JH, Kwon CI, et al. Associations of expressions of HBcAg and HBsAg with the histologic activity of liver disease and viral replication. *Gut Liver*. 2008;2:166-173.

16. Milani S, Ambu S, Patussi V, et al. Serum HBV DNA and intrahepatic hepatitis B core antigen (HBcAg) in chronic hepatitis B virus infection: correlation with infectivity and liver histology. *Hepatogastroenterology*. 1988;35:306-308.

17. Ramakrishna B, Mukhopadhya A, Kurian G. Correlation of hepatocyte expression of hepatitis B viral antigens with histological activity and viral titer in chronic hepatitis B virus infection: an immunohistochemical study. *J Gastroenterol Hepatol*. 2008;23:1734-1738.

18. Moreno A, Ramon y Cajal S, Marazuela M, et al. Sanded nuclei in delta patients. *Liver*. 1989;9:367-371.

19. Lee RG, Tsamandas AC, Demetris AJ. Large cell change (liver cell dysplasia) and hepatocellular carcinoma in cirrhosis: matched case-control study, pathological analysis, and pathogenetic hypothesis. *Hepatology*. 1997;26:1415-1422.

20. Marchio A, Terris B, Meddeb M, et al. Chromosomal abnormalities in liver cell dysplasia detected by comparative genomic hybridisation. *Mol Pathol*. 2001;54:270-274.

21. Park YN. Update on precursor and early lesions of hepatocellular carcinomas. *Arch Pathol Lab Med*. 2011;135:704-715.

22. Niu ZS, Niu XJ, Wang WH, Zhao J. Latest developments in precancerous lesions of hepatocellular carcinoma. *World J Gastroenterol*. 2016;22:3305-3314.

23. Johnson K, Kotiesh A, Boitnott JK, Torbenson M. Histology of symptomatic acute hepatitis C infection in immunocompetent adults. *Am J Surg Pathol*. 2007;31:1754-1758.

24. Bedossa P, Poynard T. An algorithm for the grading of activity in chronic hepatitis C. The METAVIR Cooperative Study Group. *Hepatology*. 1996;24:289-293.

25. Micchelli ST, Thomas D, Boitnott JK, Torbenson M. Hepatic giant cells in hepatitis C virus (HCV) mono-infection and HCV/HIV co-infection. *J Clin Pathol*. 2008;61:1058-1061.

26. Moreno A, Perez-Elias MJ, Quereda C, et al. Syncytial giant cell hepatitis in human immunodeficiency virus-infected patients with chronic hepatitis C: 2 cases and review of the literature. *Hum Pathol*. 2006;37:1344-1349.

27. Snyder N, Martinez JG, Xiao SY. Chronic hepatitis C is a common associated with hepatic granulomas. *World J Gastroenterol*. 2008;14:6366-6369.

28. Ozaras R, Tahan V, Mert A, et al. The prevalence of hepatic granulomas in chronic hepatitis C. *J Clin Gastroenterol*. 2004;38:449-452.

29. Yee LJ, Kelleher P, Goldin RD, et al. Antinuclear antibodies (ANA) in chronic hepatitis C virus infection: correlates of positivity and clinical relevance. *J Viral Hepat*. 2004;11:459-464.

30. Clifford BD, Donahue D, Smith L, et al. High prevalence of serological markers of autoimmunity in patients with chronic hepatitis C. *Hepatology*. 1995;21:613-619.

31. Yeh MM, Daniel HD, Torbenson M. Hepatitis C-associated hepatocellular carcinomas in non-cirrhotic livers. *Mod Pathol*. 2010;23:276-283.

32. Torbenson M, Yeh MM, Abraham SC. Bile duct dysplasia in the setting of chronic hepatitis C and alcohol cirrhosis. *Am J Surg Pathol*. 2007;31:1410-1413.

33. Hoofnagle JH, Nelson KE, Purcell RH. Hepatitis E. *N Engl J Med*. 2012;367:1237-1244.

34. Legrand-Abravanel F, Kamar N, Sandres-Saune K, et al. Characteristics of autochthonous hepatitis E virus infection in solid-organ transplant recipients in France. *J Infect Dis*. 2010;202:835-844.

35. Davern TJ, Chalasani N, Fontana RJ, et al. Acute hepatitis E infection accounts for some cases of suspected drug-induced liver injury. *Gastroenterology*. 2011;141:1665-1672 e1-9.

36. Malcolm P, Dalton H, Hussaini HS, Mathew J. The histology of acute autochthonous hepatitis E virus infection. *Histopathology*. 2007;51:190-194.

37. Moucari R, Bernuau J, Nicand E, et al. Acute hepatitis E with severe jaundice: report of three cases. *Eur J Gastroenterol Hepatol*. 2007;19:1012-1015.

38. Peron JM, Danjoux M, Kamar N, et al. Liver histology in patients with sporadic acute hepatitis E: a study of 11 patients from South-West France. *Virchows Arch*. 2007;450:405-410.

39. Gupta P, Jagya N, Pabhu SB, Durgapal H, Acharya SK, Panda SK. Immunohistochemistry for the diagnosis of hepatitis E virus infection. *J Viral Hepat*. 2012;19:e177-e183.

40. Kamar N, Selves J, Mansuy JM, et al. Hepatitis E virus and chronic hepatitis in organ-transplant recipients. *N Engl J Med*. 2008;358:811-817.

41. Pischke S, Suneetha PV, Baechlein C, et al. Hepatitis E virus infection as a cause of graft hepatitis in liver transplant recipients. *Liver Transpl*. 2010;16:74-82.

42. Haagsma EB, van den Berg AP, Porte RJ, et al. Chronic hepatitis E virus infection in liver transplant recipients. *Liver Transpl*. 2008;14:547-553.

43. Liu L, Liu Y. Analysis of acute to chronic hepatitis E: 6-10 year follow-up. *Hepatogastroenterology*. 2011;58:324-325.

44. Ono A, Hayes CN, Akamatsu S, Imamura M, Aikata H, Chayama K. Retrospective identification of Herpes Simplex 2 virus-associated acute liver failure in an immunocompetent patient detected using whole transcriptome shotgun sequencing. *Case Reports Hepatol*. 2017;2017:4630621.

45. Abbo L, Alcaide ML, Pano JR, Robinson PG, Campo RE. Fulminant hepatitis from herpes simplex virus type 2 in an immunocompetent adult. *Transpl Infect Dis*. 2007;9:323-326.

46. Batts KP, Ludwig J. Chronic hepatitis. An update on terminology and reporting. *Am J Surg Pathol*. 1995;19:1409-1417.

47. Group FMCS. Intraobserver and interobserver variations in liver biopsy interpretation in patients with chronic hepatitis C. The French METAVIR Cooperative Study Group. *Hepatology*. 1994;20:15-20.

48. Ishak K, Baptista A, Bianchi L, et al. Histological grading and staging of chronic hepatitis. *J Hepatol*. 1995;22:696-699.

49. Knodell RG, Ishak KG, Black WC, et al. Formulation and application of a numerical scoring system for assessing histological activity in asymptomatic chronic active hepatitis. *Hepatology*. 1981;1:431-435.

50. Desmet VJ, Gerber M, Hoofnagle JH, Manns M, Scheuer PJ. Classification of chronic hepatitis: diagnosis, grading and staging. *Hepatology*. 1994;19:1513-1520.

51. Scheuer PJ. Classification of chronic viral hepatitis: a need for reassessment. *J Hepatol*. 1991;13:372-374.

52. Wanless IR, Sweeney G, Dhillon AP, et al. Lack of progressive hepatic fibrosis during long-term therapy with deferiprone in subjects with transfusion-dependent beta-thalassemia. *Blood*. 2002;100:1566-1569.

53. Kim MY, Cho MY, Baik SK, et al. Histological subclassification of cirrhosis using the Laennec fibrosis scoring system correlates with clinical stage and grade of portal hypertension. *J Hepatol*. 2011;55:1004-1009.

NONVIRAL INFECTIONS OF THE LIVER 3

CHAPTER OUTLINE

INTRODUCTION

CHECKLIST: Nonviral Infections of the Liver

- ☐ Parasitic
  - ○ Strong regional variations in types of organisms and frequency of infection
- ☐ Fungal
  - ○ Strong regional variations in immunocompetent individuals (for example histoplasmosis and the Ohio river valley)
  - ○ Immunosuppression is an important risk factor
- ☐ Bacterial
  - ○ Wide number of organisms
  - ○ Main patterns: large abscess, small microabscess, or numerous small clusters of sinusoidal histiocytes

The infections in this chapter are often very hard to diagnosis. Special stains are an important tool (Table 3.1), but organisms are often sparse or absent, and you may have to give a prioritized differential for a pattern of injury that suggests infection, with the diagnosis eventually determined by serologic or microbiology testing. Viral infections and granulomatous infections are considered separately in their own chapters.

TABLE 3.1: Special Stains Used to Identify Organisms

Organism	Stains	Comment
Fungi	Gomori methenamine silver (GMS) PAS Alcian Blue/ mucicarmine	GMS also stains some bacteria such as *Actinomyces* and *Nocardia*. Alcian blue/mucicarmine can be used to stain the mucoid capsule of *Cryptococcus neoformans*.
General bacteria	Gram-Weigert Brown-Hopps Giemsa	Gram-positive organisms are blue. Gram-negative organisms are either negative (Gram-Weigert) or red (Brown-Hopps). Brown-Hopps also stains *Rickettsia*. Geimsa is best for *Leishmania* and *Plasmodium*. *Plasmodium* can be seen in peripheral blood smears but not in most liver biopsy specimens.
Acid-fast bacteria	Kinyoun/Ziehl-Neelsen Fite	Mycobacteria will be red/purple while non–acid-fast bacteria will be blue. Fite is best for identifying *Nocardia* and *Mycobacterium leprae*.
Spirochetes	Warthin–Starry Dieterle Steiner stains	Many different types of bacteria are positive on silver stain, so morphology of the organism is important to identify a spirochete.
Specific immunostains	*T. pallidum* *T. whippelii*	*T. pallidum* also stains other spirochetes and perhaps other nonspirochete bacteria, so correlation with serum findings is important.

PARASITIC INFECTIONS

ECHINOCOCCOSIS

This parasitic infection shows two basic patterns in the liver. The first is the most common and the one we memorized in medical school: cystic echinococcosis, which is caused by *Echinococcosis granulosus* and forms large abscesses in the liver that are filled with grungy material. The liver cysts tend to grow very slowly and over time can become very large. The cysts are lined by an outer pericyst that consists of a hyalinized layer of fibrosis with relatively little inflammation. The cyst wall, when well preserved, also shows a thin acellular middle layer and an inner germinal layer (Fig. 3.1). In most cases, the outer layer is the easiest to see. The cyst fluid has a granular brown appearance on H&E stain (Fig. 3.2) and can contain remnants of dead parasites, especially the hooklets (Fig. 3.2). Infections are most common in individuals involved in raising sheep, especially if they also have working dogs, as sheep serve as intermediate hosts and dogs as the most common definitive host, becoming infected when they eat infected sheep viscera. The infected dogs shed parasite eggs in their stool, which can then contaminate food and water consumed by people. The diagnosis is usually made by imaging studies and by serology, but not by biopsy, as a ruptured cyst can lead to anaphalytic shock.

The second pattern of infection is called alveolar echinococcosis and is caused by *Echinococcosis multilocularis*. The disease is often transmitted by contact with wild animals, in particular fox and coyotes. This pattern shows a range of findings from small cysts[1] to necrotizing granulomatous inflammation without the well-formed cyst walls (Fig. 3.3). Trichrome stains, PAS, or Gomori methenamine silver (GMS) stains are very useful in highlighting degenerating parasite forms (Fig. 3.4).[1]

SCHISTOSOMIASIS

Schistosomiasis infections result from several species of trematodes. The infection results from drinking or swimming in contaminated water. The organism is able to penetrate the skin or intestinal mucosa and then migrates to the portal veins. In the portal veins, they mate and secrete thousands of eggs, many of which get entrapped in the portal veins, eliciting an inflammatory response. In general, most diagnoses are made using stool or urine samples or serology. Serology does not indicate active infection, only exposure. Organisms are shed only intermittently, so multiple stool and urine samples are usually tested.

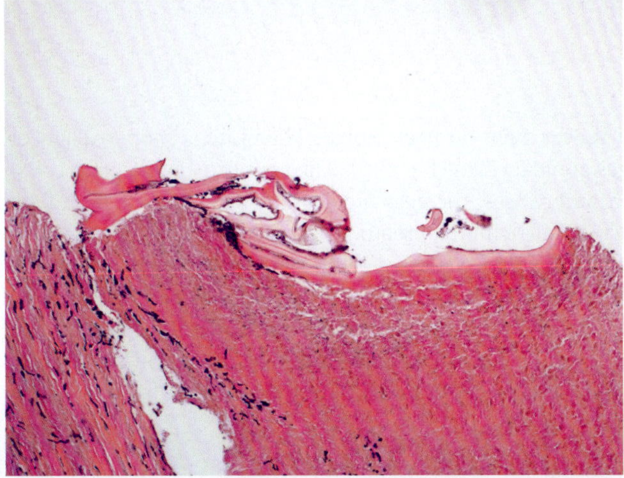

Figure 3.1. *Echinococcus granulosus.* All three layers of the cyst are evident in this image. There is an outer layer of hyalinized fibrosis, a thin acellular middle layer, and an inner germinal layer.

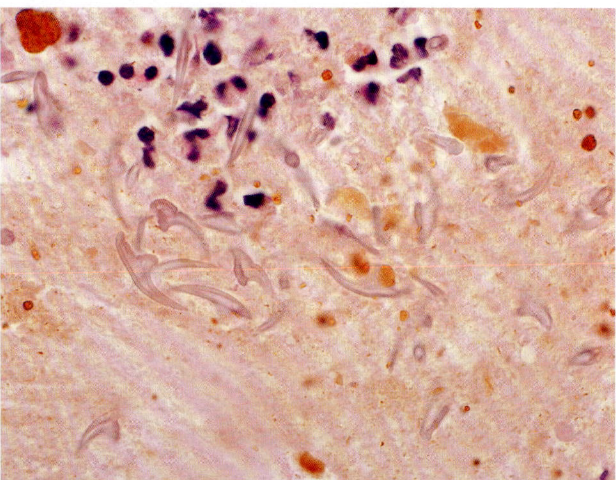

Figure 3.2. *Echinococcus granulosus.* A large cyst was resected, and the center showed a grungy brown granular material. In some fields, numerous hooklets were present.

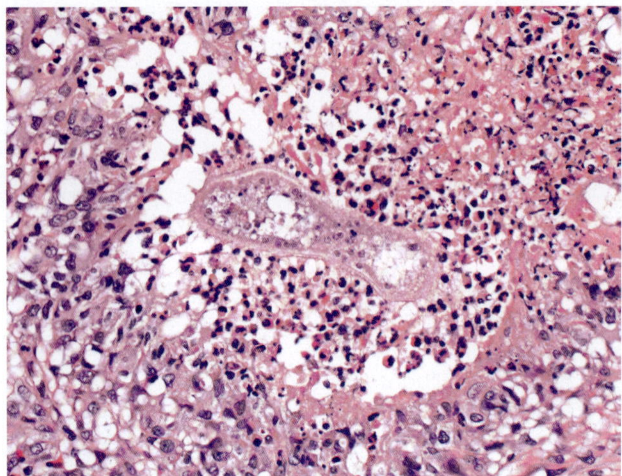

Figure 3.3. ***Echinococcus multilocularis.*** This case showed necrotizing granulomatous inflammation, without well-formed cyst walls. A degenerated parasite is present in the middle of the image, but this was a rare finding in a much larger mass of necrotizing inflammation.

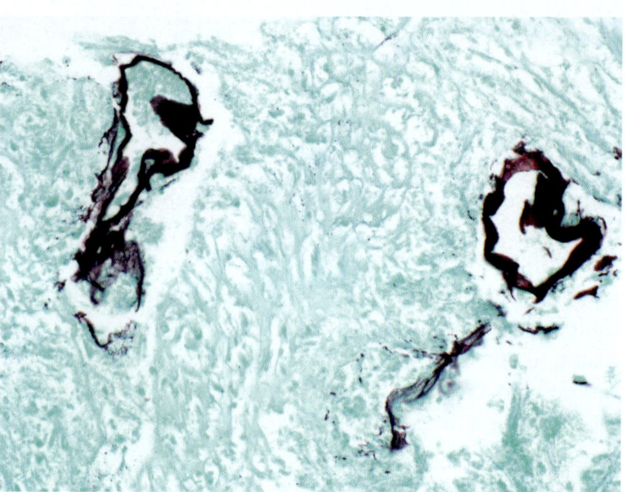

Figure 3.4. ***Echinococcus multilocularis.*** The trichrome stain was very helpful in highlighting the occasional degenerating parasites.

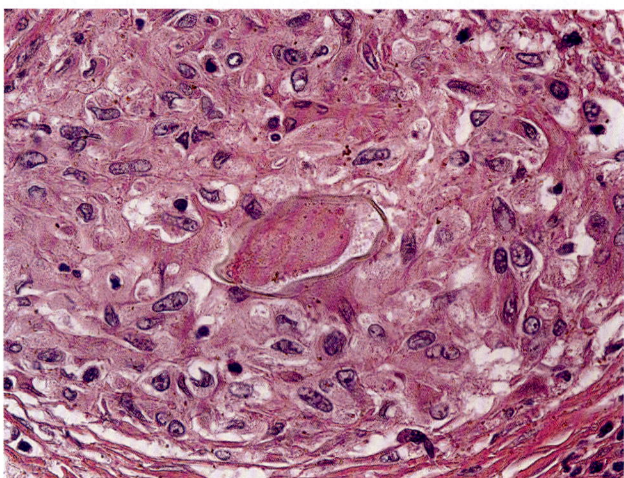

Figure 3.5. **Schistosomiasis.** A schistosomiasis egg has a granulomatous reaction.

The adult worms are rarely, if ever, seen on liver biopsy. Therefore, a biopsy diagnosis is made in most cases when eggs are identified (Fig. 3.5). The eggs can elicit a giant cell or granulomatous reaction, but in other cases, the eggs are present with little or no inflammatory response. Rarely, an eosinophil-rich inflammatory response has been observed.[2] In most cases, the eggs are degenerated, so speciation is challenging. Histologically, the eggs have distinctive, thin, retractile edges that stand out as foreign-type material. The portal tracts can show phlebitis and sometimes a distinctive scarring of the portal veins and portal tracts, called *Symmers pipestem fibrosis*, where fibrosis leads to chunky round portal tracts and sclerotic portal veins.[3] In many cases, individuals will have additional liver pathology, such as chronic viral hepatitis.[4]

TICK-BORNE DISEASES

CHECKLIST: Tick-Borne Diseases

- ☐ Bacterial
  - ○ Ehrlichiosis, caused by *Ehrlichia* and *Anaplasma*
  - ○ Lyme disease, caused by the spirochete, *Borrelia burgdorferi*
  - ○ Rocky Mountain spotted fever, caused by *Rickettsia rickettsia*, a gram-negative intracellular bacteria
  - ○ Relapsing fever, caused by *Borrelia spirochetes*
  - ○ Tularemia, caused by *Francisella tularensis*
- ☐ Viral
  - ○ Colorado tick fever, caused by Colorado tick fever virus
- ☐ Protozoal
  - ○ Babesiosis, caused by *Babesia*

Tick-borne infections result from a variety of different organisms. In some cases, there is a solid history of a tick bite and characteristic clinical findings, but in many cases, the diagnosis is very challenging to make. The clinical signs and symptoms are variable and often vague and nonspecific. However, gastrointestinal (GI) findings are often present, including nausea, vomiting, abdominal pain, and diarrhea. Liver disease is generally not a primary clinical manifestation of any of the tick-borne infections, but mild hepatomegaly is common, and the liver is typically involved microscopically, in particular with the bacterial infections. Essentially all known tick-borne diseases can lead to liver enzyme elevations.[5]

At the histological level, the changes in tick-borne diseases have not been well defined, so the findings in an average case, as well as the range of findings for different infectious organisms, are poorly understood. Overall, most of the reported findings are mild and nonspecific. They primarily include mild portal and lobular lymphocytic inflammation,[5,6] Kupffer cell hyperplasia, and occasionally granulomas.[7-9] Clusters of lobular macrophages and small lobular abscesses have also been reported. In cases of *ehrlichiosis*, reports have described discrete well-circumscribed foci of lymphocytes and macrophages (often 50 to 100 cells in size) that are associated with foci of hepatocyte dropout.[10,11] Cholestasis can be seen in cases with severe illness.

In Rocky Mountain spotted fever, the organisms infect endothelial cells and the liver can show vasculitis. Although the histological findings can be mild and nonspecific, some cases show moderate portal inflammation with prominent neutrophilic inflammation,[12,13] along with portal vein vasculitis and fibrin thrombi.

In tularemia, the liver often shows small abscesses measuring 1 to 2 mm in size. The abscesses have a central focus of necrosis and a thin rim of mixed neutrophils, lymphocytes, and macrophages.[14-17]

In essentially all cases, the infection is finally identified by serology or PCR studies. Liver biopsies can be helpful in raising the possibility of an infectious cause and in ruling out other disease patterns, but organisms are only rarely identified. In Lyme disease, some studies report that spirochetes can be found on Dieterle silver stains and/or immunostains.[6,9,18] In *ehrlichiosis*, the organisms infect monocytes or granulocytes, and they are best identified on peripheral blood smears.[19]

BACTERIAL INFECTIONS

CHECKLIST: Injury Patterns With Bacterial Infections of the Liver

There are four major patterns

- ☐ Generalized Kupffer cell hyperplasia plus numerous Kupffer cell aggregates ("microgranulomas") in the lobules
  - ○ Leptospirosis
  - ○ Listeriosis
  - ○ Salmonellosis
  - ○ Tularemia
- ☐ Small microabscesses with central necrosis/neutrophils and rim of macrophages
  - ○ Tularemia
  - ○ Listeriosis
- ☐ Abscess
  - ○ Can evolve in time to a pseudotumor pattern
  - ○ Irregularly shaped abscess with palisading histiocytes suggests bartonella henselae
- ☐ Inflammatory pseudotumor pattern
  - ○ *T. pallidum*

A number of bacterial infections of the liver all lead to a similar constellation of findings, with mild nonspecific portal and lobular inflammation with a disproportionate Kupffer cell hyperplasia, often forming small Kupffer cell aggregates or nodules in the lobules. There can be subtle differences in the histology of these infections (see checklist), but there tends to be a lot more overlap than distinct findings between the various patterns of bacterial infections. Nonetheless, the most important aspect is to recognize this pattern and suggest further evaluation for these bacterial organisms, such as culture or other microbiological testing on blood specimens.

SYPHILIS

CHECKLIST: Injury Patterns With *Treponema pallidum*

- ☐ Diffuse sinusoidal fibrosis (neonates with congenital syphilis)
- ☐ Giant cell hepatitis pattern (neonates with congenital syphilis)
- ☐ Mild nonspecific inflammation with Kupffer cell hyperplasia
- ☐ Inflammatory pseudotumor pattern
- ☐ Gumma pattern

Syphilis is caused by *Treponema pallidum*, and the liver can be involved in any of the stages of syphilis. The diagnosis of syphilis is made by serological studies in most cases, but occasionally the diagnosis is first made on liver biopsy. Congenital infection or infection in immunosuppressed individuals is more likely to involve the liver than acquired syphilis. The findings in congenital syphilis were described many years ago, but there are relatively little recent data on histological changes in this setting. However, the classic pattern is mild sinusoidal lymphocytosis and diffuse sinusoidal fibrosis. Organisms are easily found on immunostain or Warthin Starry, although immunostains are generally much easier to read. Other cases can show a neonatal giant cell hepatitis pattern[20] or paucity of intrahepatic bile ducts.[21]

In acquired syphilis, the findings are generally mild, and in some cases, the biopsy can look essentially normal.[22,23] In most cases, the biopsy will show mild nonspecific portal and lobular chronic inflammation with Kupffer cell hyperplasia.[23,24] Epithelioid granulomas are occasionally present and are noncaseating. Rarely, the findings can mimic autoimmune

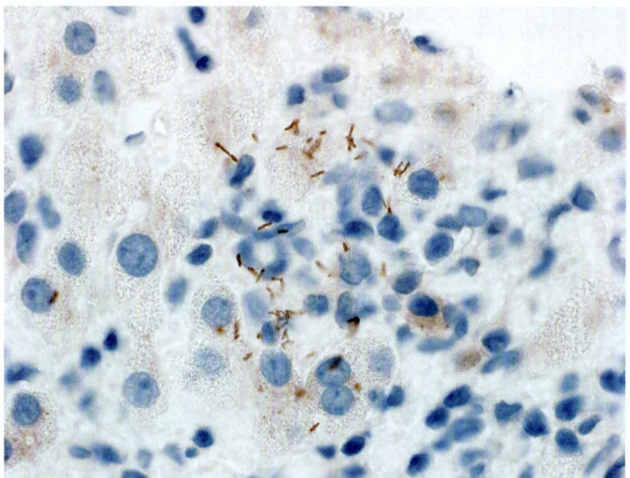

Figure 3.6. *Treponema pallidum* **immunostain.** The organisms are nicely highlighted. The Immunostain is not entirely specific, as it can cross-react with other spirochetes, so serological testing is necessary for confirmation.

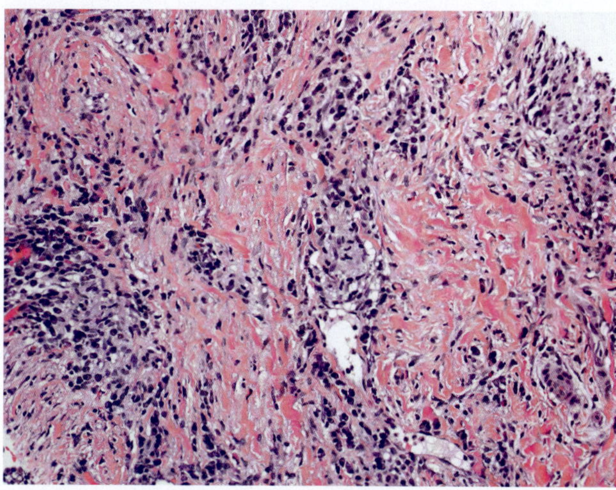

Figure 3.7. ***Treponema pallidum*, inflammatory psuedotumor.** This case presented as a mass lesion composed of inflamed fibrous tissue. The inflammation was a bit plasma cell rich but overall looked like an ordinary inflammatory pseudotumor. An immunostain for *Treponema pallidum* was positive (see preceding image).

hepatitis with moderate portal chronic inflammation containing prominent plasma cells.[25] Because the findings are nonspecific, special stains for organisms are needed to make the diagnosis. The number of organisms is typically small, but with an adequate biopsy, spirochetes can often be found, even when the histological changes are very mild. *T. pallidum* immunostains are much more sensitive than silver stains but are not entirely specific, as *T. pallidum* immunostains can also be positive with other spirochetes (Fig. 3.6). Thus, serological testing is needed to confirm the diagnosis.

Finally, late syphilis can present with mass lesions formed by gummas or inflammatory pseudotumors. The gumma is very rarely encountered but looks similar to an abscess. There is a central zone of necrosis and a surrounding rim of inflamed fibrous tissue. The central necrosis tends to be more fibrotic than a bacterial abscess and, most helpful as a diagnostic clue, can contain small islands of necrotic hepatocytes. Inflammatory pseudotumors can also present in late syphilis and are presumed to represent more fibrotic gummas. The histological findings are similar to any other inflammatory pseudotumor, with fibrosis admixed with lymphocytes, plasma cells, and often small numbers of eosinophils and neutrophils (Fig. 3.7).[26]

WHIPPLE DISEASE

Whipple disease results from infection with *Tropheryma whipplei*, a gram-positive organism. Liver involvement is part of systemic disease. Whipple disease is extremely rare, and there are a lot more clinical requests to rule out Whipple disease in the liver than there are actual cases. However, this makes sense as the infection tends to be slowly progressive, and the diagnosis is very difficult to make, as patients tend to have nonspecific findings of arthralgia, weight loss, diarrhea, and abdominal pain.[27]

The histological findings are broadly similar to those seen in the GI tract, with clusters of PAS-positive foamy macrophages involving the lobules and/or the portal tracts. Epithelioid granulomas can also be seen.[28,29] The background liver tends to show mild nonspecific portal chronic inflammation. The lobules also can show mild nonspecific inflammation, along with a mild more generalized Kupffer cell hyperplasia.[30,31] In cases with significant malnutrition from small bowel disease, the liver can also show fatty liver disease.[32] Many larger medical centers have either immunostains (Fig. 3.8) or PCR testing to establish a tissue-based diagnosis.

ACTINOMYCOSIS

Actinomyces is part of the normal flora of the GI tract and the female genital tract but can cause abscesses in the liver, usually in immunocompetent individuals. Overall the organism is of low pathogenicity, so infections tend to present with mild and nonspecific

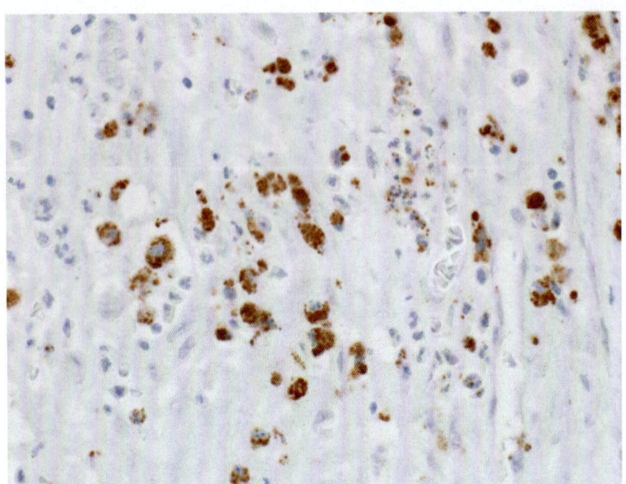

Figure 3.8. **Whipple immunostain.** This case of Whipple disease is from the small bowel, but the organisms are nicely highlighted by the immunostain. At Mayo clinic, a tissue diagnosis is confirmed using PCR, which works very well but is not as photogenic.

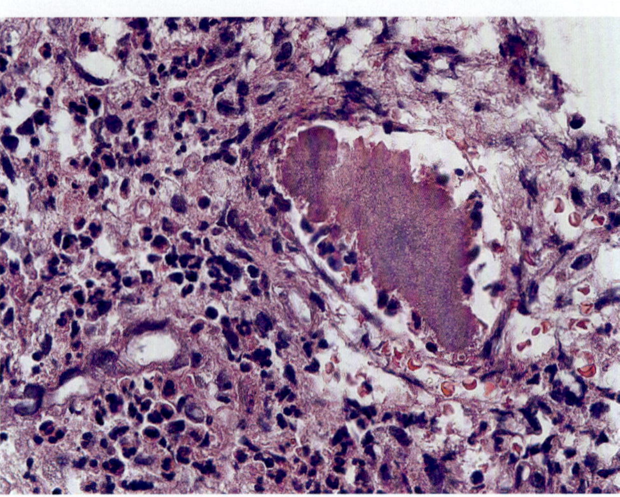

Figure 3.9. ***Actinomyces* abscess.** The *Actinomyces* organisms are clustered into a sulfur granule, a small purple nodule in the upper right of the image.

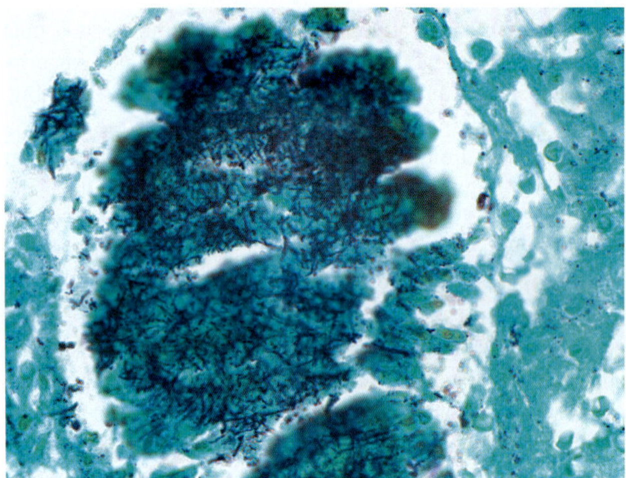

Figure 3.10. ***Actinomyces* abscess, Gomori methenamine silver (GMS) stain.** The *Actinomyces* organisms are GMS positive.

clinical findings. Liver disease is most commonly part of multiorgan infections, but there can be infections localized to the liver. Localized infections commonly form mass lesions that can be single (2/3 of cases) or multiple (1/3 of cases) and often closely mimic hepatic tumors.[33,34] They can be very large, up to 11 cm.

The histological findings in mass-forming lesions range from changes typical for a hepatic abscess to findings typical of an inflammatory pseudotumor. The organism is a filamentous bacteria, so it can mimic fungal infections, but the bacteria is thinner than fungal hyphae and tends to grow in large clumpy colonies. The best place to find them is in the necrotic center of the abscess. The large colonies of *Actinomyces* often surround sulfur granules, and these stand out as purple in color on H&E stain (Fig. 3.9). Sulfur granules are present in about 2/3 of biopsy specimens.[33] *Actinomyces* are GMS positive (Fig. 3.10), usually gram positive, and Fite negative. In contrast, *Nocardia*, which have a similar filamentous morphology, are also GMS positive but are Fite negative. *Nocardia* does not grow in the distinct clumps found in most *Actinomyces* infections. About a third of *Actinomyces* abscesses are polymicrobial,[33] so other organisms can be seen on bacterial stains.

LIVER ABSCESSES

Hepatic abscesses present as mass lesions. As the abscesses become more fibrotic, the imaging findings are not always typical and biopsies are often performed. The most common clinical associations include chronic biliary tract disease or immunosuppression.[35] Colon cancer has an increased risk for hepatic abscesses, even without metastatic disease.[36] The infection is usually bacterial (pyogenic) in origin, but mixed bacterial and fungal abscesses are common. In adults, the most common organisms are streptococcal or *Pseudomonas* species, while in children, the most common organism is *Staphylococcus aureus*.[37]

A biopsy core (Fig. 3.11) that goes from the liver parenchyma into the abscess center shows first the benign reactive liver parenchyma with nonspecific inflammation and bile ductular proliferation; next a layer or rind of inflamed, fibrotic tissue; and finally small bits of necrotic debris, usually at the edge of the biopsy cores (Fig. 3.12). The inflammation in the abscess rind is primarily lymphocytic, but histiocytes, plasma cells, and sometimes neutrophils can all be present. The inflamed fibrotic edge commonly has admixed reactive bile ductules and small islands of residual hepatocytes. Fibroblasts and myofibroblasts can be prominent. In many cases with central necrotic debris, bacteria can be identified on special stains (Fig. 3.13), but the best way to identify organisms is to submit tissue for culture, as special stains are often negative and do not allow bacterial speciation. GMS stains for fungal organisms are also important because mixed infections are common.

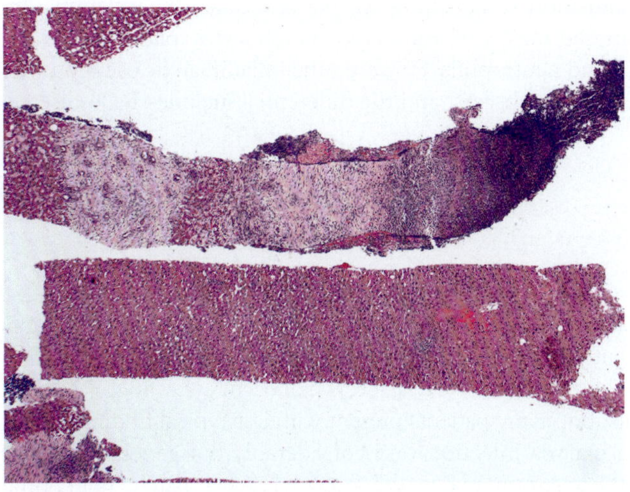

Figure 3.11. **Liver abscess.** The biopsy shows almost-normal background liver, a fibrotic rind, and an inner core of necrotic debris.

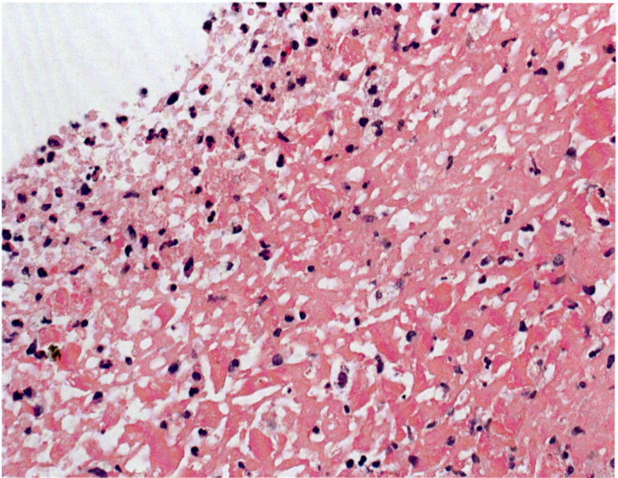

Figure 3.12. **Liver abscess.** The necrotic center of an abscess shows mixed inflammation, fibrin, and hemorrhage. Cultures showed this abscess was caused by *Klebsiella pneumoniae.*

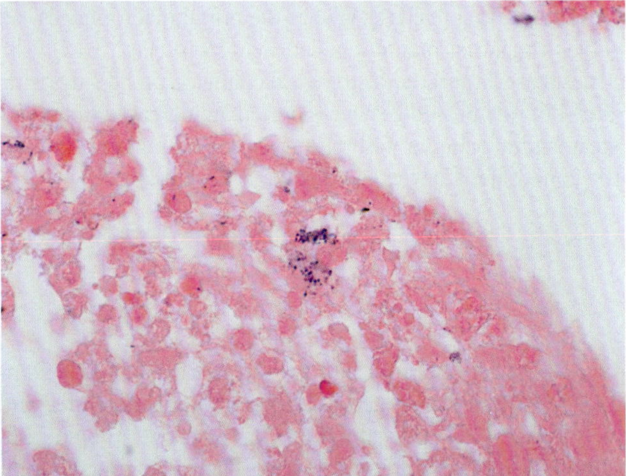

Figure 3.13. **Liver abscess, Gram-Weigert stain.** Occasional small clusters of gram-positive cocci were seen in the necrotic center this hepatic abscess.

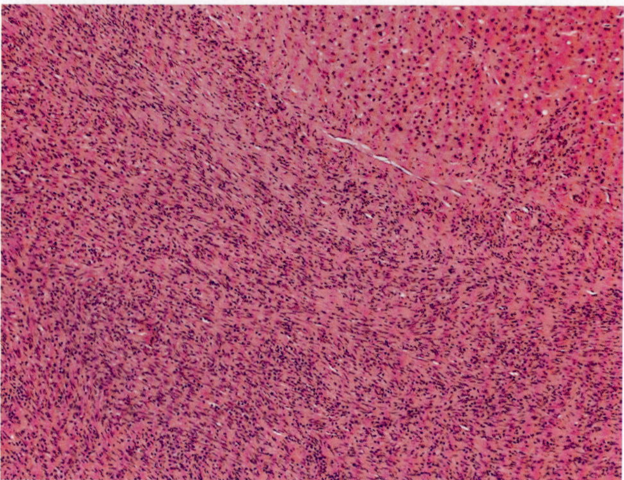

Figure 3.14. **Inflammatory psuedotumor.** This inflammatory pseudotumor is composed mostly of fibroblasts and admixed lymphocytes and plasma cells. The adjacent liver is present in the upper right of the image. Tissue culture of this inflammatory pseudotumor was positive for *Bacteroides fragilis*.

In time, the abscess can transition to an end-stage pattern called an inflammatory pseudotumor (Fig. 3.14), composed mostly of fibroblasts, lymphocytes, plasma cells, and occasional admixed eosinophils and neutrophils. However, the inflammatory pseudotumor pattern is not specific for an end-stage abscess, and the differential includes IgG4 disease, syphilis, and Hodgkin disease.

MALARIA

Malaria results from infection of red blood cells by the protozoan *Plasmodium*, which is transmitted by the anopheline mosquito. There are four malarial species: *falciparum*, *vivax*, *malariae*, and *ovale*. The classic clinical presentation is cyclic fevers that occur every 48 to 72 hours, often preceded by shaking chills, but many patients present with less typical findings.

The histological changes in malaria infection vary considerably but generally show a similar pattern to infections of the liver from many other nonviral causes: patchy mild portal chronic (rarely moderate or severe) with inflammation composed mostly of lymphocytes. The lobules generally show mild Kupffer cell hyperplasia, but in some cases, the Kupffer cells are more prominent and demonstrate hemophagocytosis. The lobules can show cholestasis if the patient is very sick. In malaria, the Kupffer cells as well as the portal macrophages can accumulate a distinctive brown–black malarial pigment called hemozoin (Fig. 3.15). The actual organisms are not seen in most cases[38] and the histological changes can be surprising mild, even with fatal cases.[38,39] Some but not all studies have reported an increased frequency and degree of macrovesicular steatosis in patients with clinically severe malaria. In fatal cases, hemorrhagic necrosis of the zone 3 hepatocytes has also been described.[38]

NEAR MISSES

CASE 1. A 59-year-old man vacationed in the tropics of South America and did extensive fresh water fishing. Soon after returning home, he developed high fevers, chills, and rigors. After about a week, he felt better without treatment other than over-the-counter medications but became sick again with similar symptoms 3 weeks later. This time he went to his physician, where mild jaundice and elevated liver enzymes were noted, leading to a liver biopsy. The biopsy showed mild nonspecific portal inflammation along with lobular cholestasis, generalized Kupffer cell hyperplasia, and scattered large clusters of Kupffer

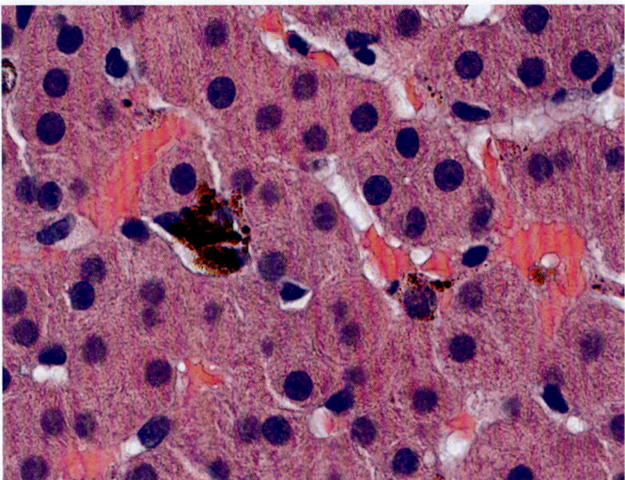

Figure 3.15. Malaria. The Kupffer cells have a distinctive brown–black malarial pigment called hemozoin.

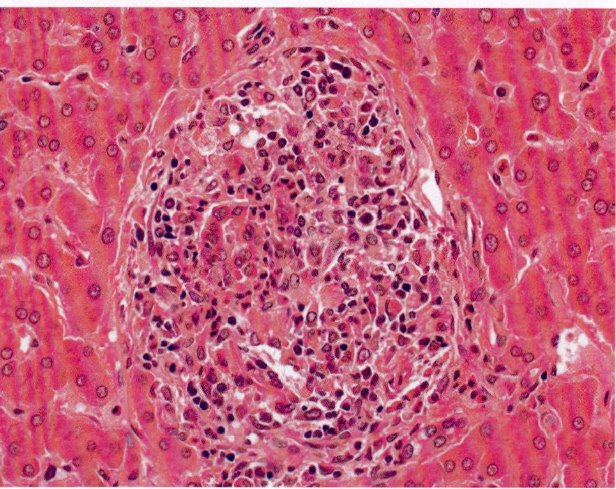

Figure 3.16. Near miss case 1, leptospirosis. This case of leptospirosis shows discohesive granulomas.

cells/histiocytes that suggested cholestatic and discohesive granulomas (Fig. 3.16). Gram, AFB, and GMS stains were negative. The case was signed out descriptively noting that the pattern of cholestasis, Kupffer cell hyperplasia, and granuloma-like foci of histiocytes suggested a bacterial or fungal infection, especially in light of the clinical presentation. The report also indicated that there was no evidence for a significant hepatitis to suggest viral infection or autoimmune hepatitis and no evidence for biliary obstruction.

The diagnosis was made several days later after an infectious disease consult led to testing for leptospirosis. Leptospirosis is caused by spirochete bacteria called *Leptospira*. Leptospirosis is endemic in the tropics, where fresh water sports such as swimming or fishing are major risk factors.[40] Most infections are asymptomatic, but infections are more likely to be symptomatic in the elderly. The infection is often biphasic, as seen in this case, and severe infections can lead to jaundice, renal failure, and hemorrhagic complications.[41,42] Cases with jaundice are also referred to as Weil disease.

In retrospect, the clinical history and the histological findings were very typical for leptospirosis, but the rarity of this disease outside of tropical areas led to diagnostic challenges. The basic histological pattern seen in this case was mild cholestasis, Kupffer cell hyperplasia, and larger aggregates of Kupffer cells. This constellation of findings can be seen in many bacterial infections and is not specific for leptospirosis.

CASE 2. A 24-year-old man presented with an incidentally discovered liver mass, and a biopsy was performed. There was no other clinical information available at the time of signout. The biopsy showed what looked to be an abscess, with a small focus of inflammatory exudate adjacent to a rim of inflamed fibrous tissue. The inflammation in some areas showed a striking enrichment for eosinophils (Fig. 3.17). The striking eosinophilia was, however, quite patchy. There was only a small amount of background liver, which looked essentially normal.

Examination of the inflammatory exudate showed no hooklets or other parasite forms, and bacterial and fungal stains were negative. The case was signed out as showing no evidence for malignancy and overall being most consistent with an abscess, with a note that the prominent eosinophils were of uncertain significance but raised the possibility of a parasite. Serological studies were subsequently positive for *Fasciola* (*Fasciola hepatica* or common liver fluke).

Most infections result from contaminated water, especially eating raw water plants such as watercress or water lettuce. The source of infection in this case was never clearly identified. *Fasciola* is a trematode that infects the liver and can lead to clinical presentations characterized by biliary obstruction, pancreatitis, or masslike lesions of the liver.[43,44] The diagnosis is made in most cases by serology or by fecal analysis for ova and parasites. However, presentation with masslike lesions in the liver can lead to liver biopsy.

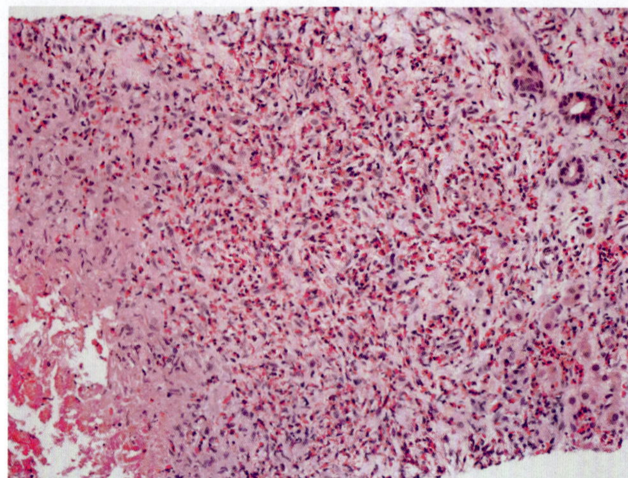

Figure 3.17. Near miss case 2, *Fasciola hepatica*. The biopsy shows an eosinophil-rich abscess.

References

1. Atanasov G, Benckert C, Thelen A, et al. Alveolar echinococcosis-spreading disease challenging clinicians: a case report and literature review. *World J Gastroenterol*. 2013;19:4257-4261.
2. Guangjin S, Mingdao J, Qiyang L, Hui X, Jiangming H, Xiaomei Y. Study on histopathology, ultrasonography and some special serum enzymes and collagens for 38 advanced patients of schistosomiasis japonica. *Acta Trop*. 2002;82:235-246.
3. Voieta I, de Queiroz LC, Andrade LM, et al. Imaging techniques and histology in the evaluation of liver fibrosis in hepatosplenic schistosomiasis mansoni in Brazil: a comparative study. *Mem Inst Oswaldo Cruz*. 2010;105:414-421.
4. Li Y, Chen D, Ross AG, et al. Severe hepatosplenic schistosomiasis: clinicopathologic study of 102 cases undergoing splenectomy. *Hum Pathol*. 2011;42:111-119.
5. Zaidi SA, Singer C. Gastrointestinal and hepatic manifestations of tickborne diseases in the United States. *Clin Infect Dis*. 2002;34:1206-1212.
6. Goellner MH, Agger WA, Burgess JH, Duray PH. Hepatitis due to recurrent lyme disease. *Ann Intern Med*. 1988;108:707-708.
7. Chavanet P, Pillon D, Lancon JP, Waldner-Combernoux A, Maringe E, Portier H. Granulomatous hepatitis associated with lyme disease. *Lancet*. 1987;2:623-624.
8. Zanchi AC, Gingold AR, Theise ND, Min AD. Necrotizing granulomatous hepatitis as an unusual manifestation of lyme disease. *Dig Dis Sci*. 2007;52:2629-2632.
9. Middelveen M, McClain S, Bandoski C, et al. Granulomatous hepatitis associated with chronic borrelia burgdorferi infection: a case report. In: *Biology and Environmental Science Faculty Publications Vol. Paper.* 33. 2014.
10. Sehdev AE, Dumler JS. Hepatic pathology in human monocytic ehrlichiosis. Ehrlichia chaffeensis infection. *Am J Clin Pathol*. 2003;119:859-865.
11. Sosa-Gutierrez CG, Solorzano-Santos F, Walker DH, Torres J, Serrano CA, Gordillo-Perez G. Fatal monocytic ehrlichiosis in woman, Mexico, 2013. *Emerg Infect Dis*. 2016;22:871-874.
12. Adams JS, Walker DH. The liver in Rocky Mountain spotted fever. *Am J Clin Pathol*. 1981;75:156-161.
13. Jackson MD, Kirkman C, Bradford WD, Walker DH. Rocky mountain spotted fever: hepatic lesions in childhood cases. *Pediatr Pathol*. 1986;5:379-388.
14. Case records of the Massachusetts General Hospital. Weekly clinicopathological exercises. Case 22-2001. A 25-year-old woman with fever and abnormal liver function. *N Engl J Med*. 2001;345:201-205.
15. Gourdeau M, Lamothe F, Ishak M, et al. Hepatic abscess complicating ulceroglandular tularemia. *Can Med Assoc J*. 1983;129:1286-1288.
16. Ortego TJ, Hutchins LF, Rice J, Davis GR. Tularemic hepatitis presenting as obstructive jaundice. *Gastroenterology*. 1986;91:461-463.

17. Lamps LW, Havens JM, Sjostedt A, Page DL, Scott MA. Histologic and molecular diagnosis of tularemia: a potential bioterrorism agent endemic to North America. *Mod Pathol*. 2004;17:489-495.

18. Duray PH, Steere AC. Clinical pathologic correlations of lyme disease by stage. *Ann N Y Acad Sci*. 1988;539:65-79.

19. Hamilton KS, Standaert SM, Kinney MC. Characteristic peripheral blood findings in human ehrlichiosis. *Mod Pathol*. 2004;17:512-517.

20. Shet TM, Kandalkar BM, Vora IM. Neonatal hepatitis–an autopsy study of 14 cases. *Indian J Pathol Microbiol*. 1998;41:77-84.

21. Sugiura H, Hayashi M, Koshida R, Watanabe R, Nakanuma Y, Ohta G. Nonsyndromatic paucity of intrahepatic bile ducts in congenital syphilis. A case report. *Acta Pathol Jpn*. 1988;38:1061-1068.

22. Wright DJ, Berry CL. Letter: liver involvement in congenital syphilis. *Br J Vener Dis*. 1974;50:241.

23. Terry SI, Hanchard B, Brooks SE, McDonald H, Siva S. Prevalence of liver abnormality in early syphilis. *Br J Vener Dis*. 1984;60:83-86.

24. Pareek SS. Liver involvement in secondary syphilis. *Dig Dis Sci*. 1979;24:41-43.

25. Khambaty M, Singal AG, Gopal P. Spirochetes as an almost forgotten cause of hepatitis. *Clin Gastroenterol Hepatol*. 2015;13:A21-A22.

26. Hagen CE, Kamionek M, McKinsey DS, Misdraji J. Syphilis presenting as inflammatory tumors of the liver in HIV-positive homosexual men. *Am J Surg Pathol*. 2014;38:1636-1643.

27. Arnold CA, Moreira RK, Lam-Himlin D, De Petris G, Montgomery E. Whipple disease a century after the initial description: increased recognition of unusual presentations, autoimmune *comorbidities,* and therapy effects. *Am J Surg Pathol*. 2012;36:1066-1073.

28. Torzillo PJ, Bignold L, Khan GA. Absence of PAS-positive macrophages in hepatic and lymph node granulomata in Whipple's disease. *Aust N Z J Med*. 1982;12:73-75.

29. Saint-Marc Girardin MF, Zafrani ES, Chaumette MT, Delchier JC, Metreau JM, Dhumeaux D. Hepatic granulomas in Whipple's disease. *Gastroenterology*. 1984;86:753-756.

30. Cho C, Linscheer WG, Hirschkorn MA, Ashutosh K. Sarcoidlike granulomas as an early manifestation of Whipple's disease. *Gastroenterology*. 1984;87:941-947.

31. Viteri AL, Stinson JC, Barnes MC, Dyck WP. Rod-shaped organism in the liver of a patient with Whipple's disease. *Dig Dis Sci*. 1979;24:560-564.

32. Schultz M, Hartmann A, Dietmaier W, Woenckhaus M, Lock G. Massive steatosis hepatis: an unusual manifestation of Whipple's disease. *Am J Gastroenterol*. 2002;97:771-772.

33. Yang XX, Lin JM, Xu KJ, et al. Hepatic actinomycosis: report of one case and analysis of 32 previously reported cases. *World J Gastroenterol*. 2014;20:16372-16376.

34. Kanellopoulou T, Alexopoulou A, Tanouli MI, et al. Primary hepatic actinomycosis. *Am J Med Sci*. 2010;339:362-365.

35. Huang CJ, Pitt HA, Lipsett PA, et al. Pyogenic hepatic abscess. Changing trends over 42 years. *Ann Surg*. 1996;223:600-607; discussion 7-9.

36. Qu K, Liu C, Wang ZX, et al. Pyogenic liver abscesses associated with nonmetastatic colorectal cancers: an increasing problem in eastern Asia. *World J Gastroenterol*. 2012;18:2948-2955.

37. Mishra K, Basu S, Roychoudhury S, Kumar P. Liver abscess in children: an overview. *World J Pediatr*. 2010;6:210-216.

38. Rupani AB, Amarapurkar AD. Hepatic changes in fatal malaria: an emerging problem. *Ann Trop Med Parasitol*. 2009;103:119-127.

39. Whitten R, Milner DA, Yeh MM, Kamiza S, Molyneux ME, Taylor TE. Liver pathology in Malawian children with fatal encephalopathy. *Hum Pathol*. 2011;42:1230-1239.

40. van de Werve C, Perignon A, Jaureguiberry S, Bricaire F, Bourhy P, Caumes E. Travel-related leptospirosis: a series of 15 imported cases. *J Trav Med*. 2013;20:228-231.

41. Talwani R, Gilliam BL, Howell C. Infectious diseases and the liver. *Clin Liver Dis*. 2011;15:111-130.

42. Haake DA, Levett PN. Leptospirosis in humans. *Curr Top Microbiol Immunol*. 2015;387:65-97.

43. Yilmaz B, Koklu S, Gedikoglu G. Hepatic mass caused by Fasciola hepatica: a tricky differential diagnosis. *Am J Trop Med Hyg*. 2013;89:1212-1213.

44. Kaya M, Bestas R, Cetin S. Clinical presentation and management of Fasciola hepatica infection: single-center experience. *World J Gastroenterol*. 2011;17:4899-4904.

GRANULOMAS AND GRANULOMATOUS DISEASE 4

CHAPTER OUTLINE

OVERVIEW

Granulomas are aggregates of activated macrophages (Fig. 4.1). There are a number of terms to master as you read the literature on granulomas (Table 4.1). These terms are not always used consistently in the literature, but Table 4.1 provides a useful approach, one that is followed by most authors. One key point is that granulomas should not be confused or conflated with microgranulomas, which are small clusters of 2 to 3 macrophages that frequently accompany lobular hepatitis from any cause (Figs. 4.2 and 4.3). Moreover, it is best not to mix up the terms *granuloma* and *granulomatous hepatitis*. Granulomatous hepatitis has numerous granulomas, which are often less well formed, plus an additional component of lymphocytic hepatitis. These definitions work well only when used with common sense. For example, a case of typical autoimmune hepatitis that also has one or two small granulomas should not be called granulomatous hepatitis, even though it has both granulomas and hepatitis. Instead, it should be called autoimmune hepatitis with one or two small granulomas. Finally, you can use the terms *granulomas* and *granulomata* interchangeably for cases with more than one granuloma, depending on how sophisticated you are feeling.

The most common causes for granulomas in Europe, United States, and Canada are shown in Table 4.2.[1-5] Studies from other parts of the world often show a higher frequency of infectious granulomas and a lower frequency of primary biliary cirrhosis and sarcoidosis,[6] underscoring the importance of knowing the major risk factors for granulomas for the area of the world in which the patient lives or previously lived. Granulomas remain idiopathic in 35% of cases, despite full clinical and histological work-up.

FAQ: Does the location of the granulomas (portal tracts vs. lobules) matter?

Answer: No. All diseases with granulomas, perhaps with the exception of those focused on the hepatic arteries, can have granulomas in either or both the portal tracts and the lobules.

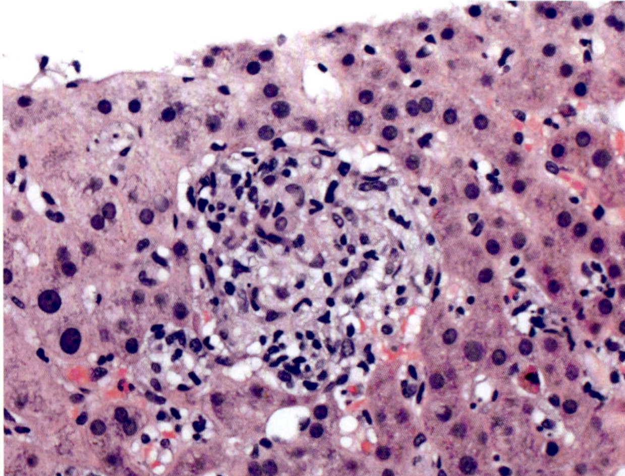

Figure 4.1. **Granuloma.** This is a typical granuloma. It is composed of an epithelioid cluster of histiocytes with admixed lymphocytes. There is no necrosis.

TABLE 4.1: Granuloma Terminology

Term	Comment
Microgranulomas	• Small cluster of lobular macrophages cleaning up a site of prior injury. • PASD positive • Not the same as a granuloma • Often helpful to not use the term microgranuloma in your report because they can be confused with granulomas
Granuloma	• Meant to convey that the biopsy shows typical granulomas • Discrete cluster of epithelioid histiocytes • PASD negative, mostly

Poorly formed granuloma	• Meant to convey that the histological findings strongly suggest granulomas (and the relevant differential), but typical epithelioid granulomas are not present
	• The poorly formed granuloma is composed of a vague cluster of histiocytes, but it typically does not stand out from the background inflammation in the same distinct way of a granuloma
	  • The aggregate of histiocytes is not as well demarcated
	  • The histiocytes are often less epithelioid and commonly more foamy

Granulomatous inflammation	• Meant to convey the finding of loose aggregates of histiocytes, without well-formed granulomas • Can be part of a florid duct lesion • Can be seen with brisk lobular hepatitis, typically as part of a drug reaction • The term can be confused with granulomatous hepatitis, so I generally prefer to not use this term in clinical reports
Granulomatous hepatitis	• Meant to convey the idea of a significantly active hepatitis that also has lots of granulomas • Granulomas will range from epithelioid and well formed to loose and poorly formed • Often a lobular cholestatic component

Granulomatous disease	• Meant to convey the idea of any disease pattern that is characterized by granulomas
	  • Infectious causes: tuberculosis, fungal, parasites
	  • Systemic diseases: Primary biliary cirrhosis, sarcoidosis, common variable immunodeficiency, Crohn disease
	  • This term is very broad and its usually better to use a more specific term when possible

APPROACH TO DIAGNOSIS

Many different diseases lead to granulomas in the liver, so a systematic approach can be helpful. First start with the clinical information, looking for relevant history such as an occupational or hobby risk, a new medication, a clinical diagnosis of sarcoidosis or other systemic granulomatous diseases, or living in areas known to be endemic for infections that cause granulomas—such as living in the Ohio river valley where histoplasmosis is endemic.

Next, examine the granulomas. Central necrosis strongly suggests infection (Fig. 4.4). However, remember that larger granulomas can have central hyalinization, which often mimics necrosis (Fig. 4.5). Fibrotic granulomas suggest sarcoidosis (Fig. 4.6). Granulomas should be polarized for foreign material (Figs. 4.7 and 4.8). The yield is very low, but the test is fast and cheap. The granulomas should also be examined by

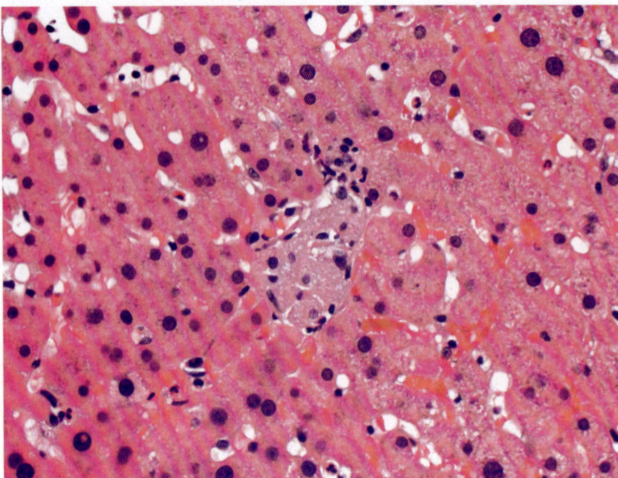

Figure 4.2. **Microgranuloma.** This small cluster of lobular histiocytes represents a small foci of prior lobular injury and is not the same as a granuloma.

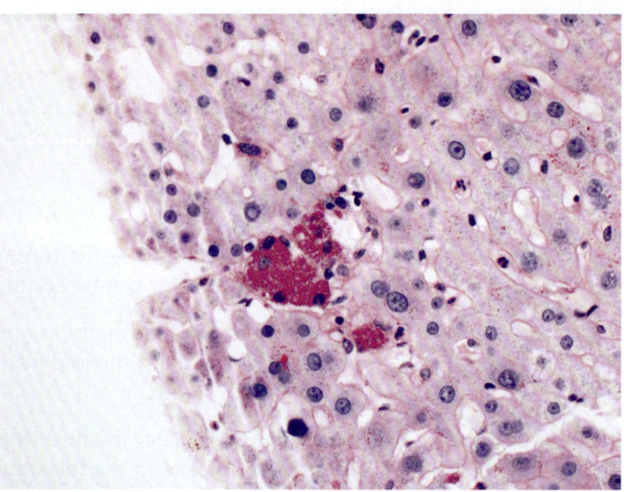

Figure 4.3. **Microgranuloma, PASD stain.** Microgranulomas are typically positive on PASD stains. Most true granulomas are not.

TABLE 4.2: Most Common Causes of Granulomas

Disease	Frequency (%)
Primary biliary cirrhosis	45
Idiopathic	35
Sarcoidosis	10
Infection	5
Drugs	3
Other	2

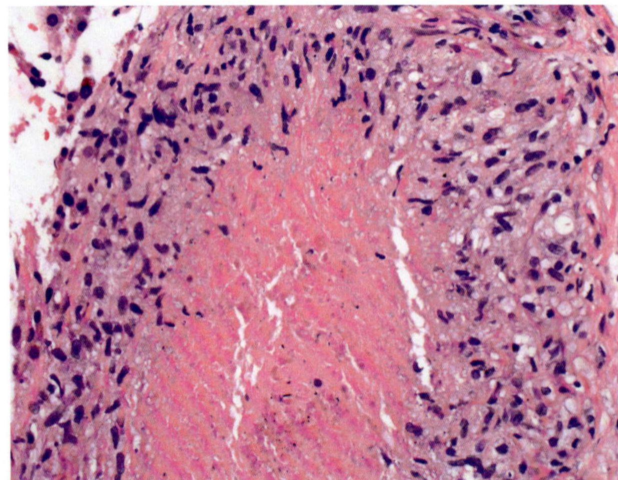

Figure 4.4. **Granuloma with central necrosis.** This pattern is also cased *caseating* and almost always results from infections.

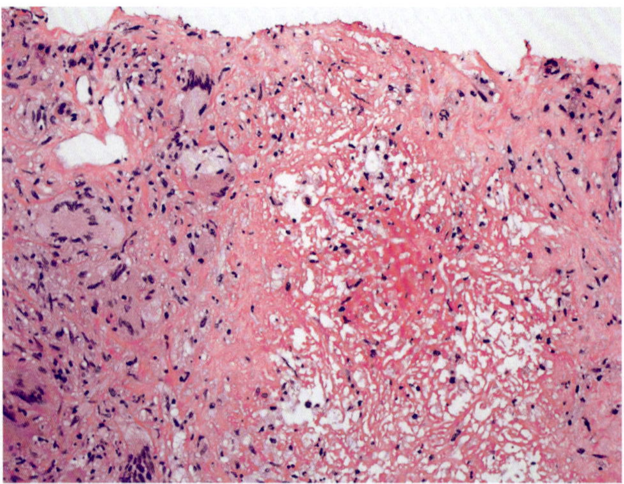

Figure 4.5. **Granuloma with central hyalinization.** This pattern is often mistaken for necrosis but instead represents nonspecific central hyalinization, a finding common in many larger granulomas. The hyalinized area lacks the nuclear/cellular debris of true necrosis and tends to be more eosinophilic and glassy in appearance.

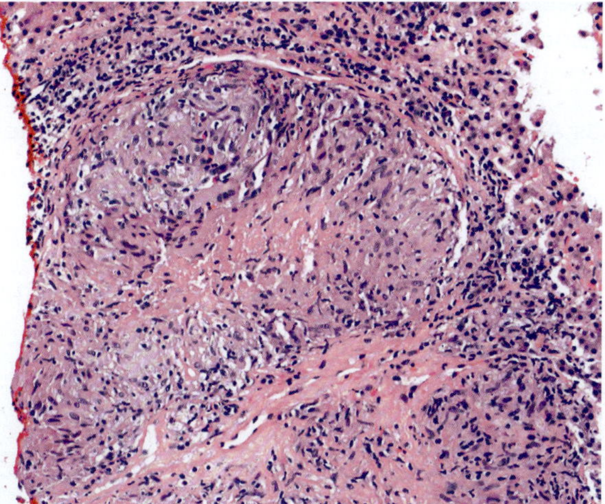

Figure 4.6. **Granuloma with fibrosis.** The granuloma in this case of sarcoidosis is associated with intragranuloma and perigranuloma fibrosis. This pattern is not entirely specific for sarcoidosis, so clinical correlation is still required. This pattern is also not sensitive, as many granulomas in sarcoid will lack the fibrosis. Whether this is completely true is unclear, but the fibrotic granulomas are thought to represent older granulomas and the ones without fibrosis younger granulomas.

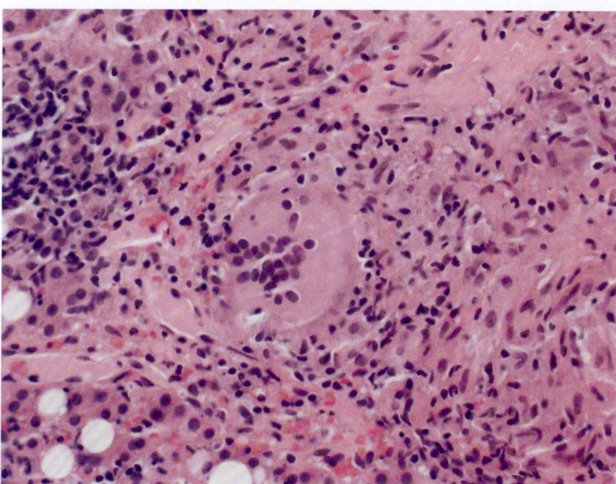

Figure 4.7. **Granuloma with foreign body material.** This granuloma was found in person with a history of chronic hepatitis C and injection drug use.

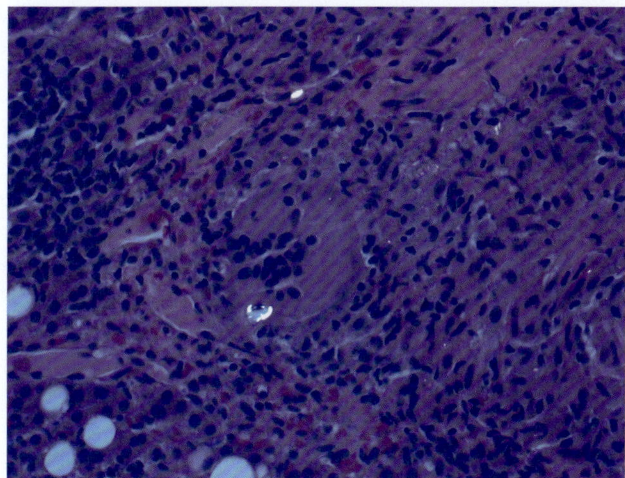

Figure 4.8. **Granuloma with foreign body material, polarized light.** The foreign material polarizes (same case as above).

stains for acid fast bacilli and fungi. Once again, the yield is very low in most centers, but they have a high impact on patient care when positive. In patients who have follow-up biopsies for known diseases with granulomas, such as primary biliary cirrhosis, AFB and fungal stains are not necessary when stains were performed on prior biopsies, except for when the granulomas in the follow-up biopsy specimen are caseating or show other unusual features.

Next, determine if the granulomas are associated with active injury to a structure in the liver, such as arteries or bile ducts. Finally, examine the biopsy for other findings, such as hepatitis, cholestasis, or ductopenia, which can provide important clues to the etiology.

CHECKLIST: Granulomas Associated With Anatomic Structures

Granulomas and arteritis

- ☐ Vasculitis diseases such as ANCA-associated vasculitis,[7] polyarteritis nodosa, and giant cell arteritis[8,9]

Granulomas associated with phlebitis

- ☐ Sarcoidosis
- ☐ Drug reaction
- ☐ Shisotsomaisis—granulomatous response to the eggs

Granulomas associated with bile duct injury

- ☐ Primary biliary cirrhosis
- ☐ Drug reaction
- ☐ Hodgkin lymphoma (can also be associated with ductopenia)

TYPES OF GRANULOMAS

FIBRIN RING GRANULOMA

CHECKLIST: Fibrin Ring Granulomas

Infections

- ☐ Coxiella burneti (Q-fever)[10,11]
- ☐ Epstein–Barr Virus[12]
- ☐ Hepatitis A[13,14]
- ☐ Toxoplasmosis[15]
- ☐ Cytomegalovirus (CMV)[1]
- ☐ Leishmaniasis[16,17]

Drugs

- ☐ Allopurinol[17–19]
- ☐ Checkpoint inhibitors (cancer therapy)[20]

Fibrin ring granulomas have a central droplet of fat that is surrounded by a thin and sometimes attenuated ring of pink fibrin and then by an outer layer of epithelioid histiocytes (Figs. 4.9 and 4.10). In an individual biopsy, not all of the granulomas will be fibrin ring granulomas, with many granulomas showing an ordinary epithelioid morphology. While first coming to prominence with Q-fever, fibrin ring granulomas are found in many different conditions. Regardless of the cause, the liver essentially always shows a background of macrovesicular steatosis. For this reason, it seems likely that an acute hepatitis from any cause that is superimposed on a background of fatty liver disease is a better explanation for fibrin ring granulomas, rather than a specific agent.

FIBROTIC GRANULOMA

These are epithelioid granulomas that have fibrosis within the granuloma or have an aggregate of granulomas in a fibrotic matrix. This pattern is most commonly associated with sarcoidosis. To my knowledge, the sensitivity and specificity of this pattern for sarcoidosis has not been formally studied, but it appears to be strong, although not perfect, with greater specificity than sensitivity.

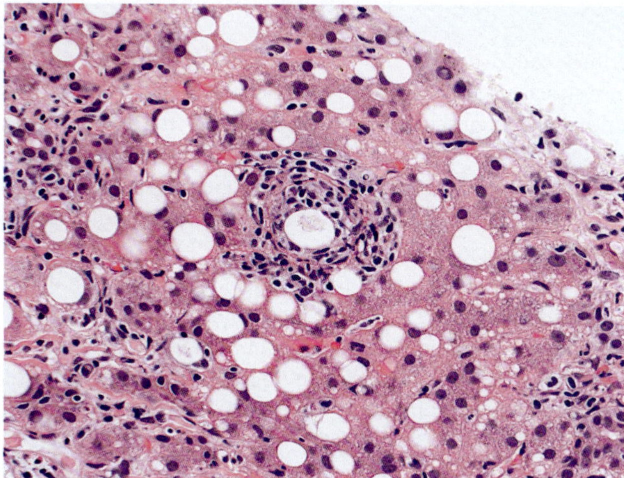

Figure 4.9. **Fibrin ring granuloma.** A Fibrin ring granuloma shows a central droplet of fat. Fibrin ring granulomas are usually small in size and are never caseating. In essentially all cases the background liver also shows fatty liver disease, regardless of the etiology of the granulomas.

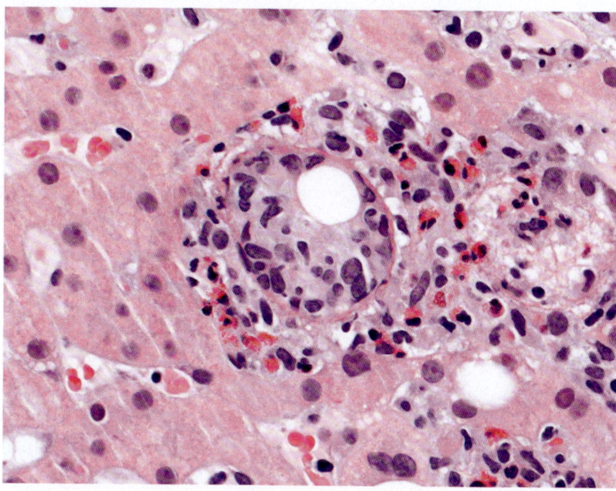

Figure 4.10. **Fibrin ring granuloma.** Fibrin ring granulomas at higher power show a central droplet of fat and histiocytes surrounded by a thin rim of fibrin and an outer layer of ordinary epithelioid histiocytes and lymphocytic/eosinophilic inflammation.

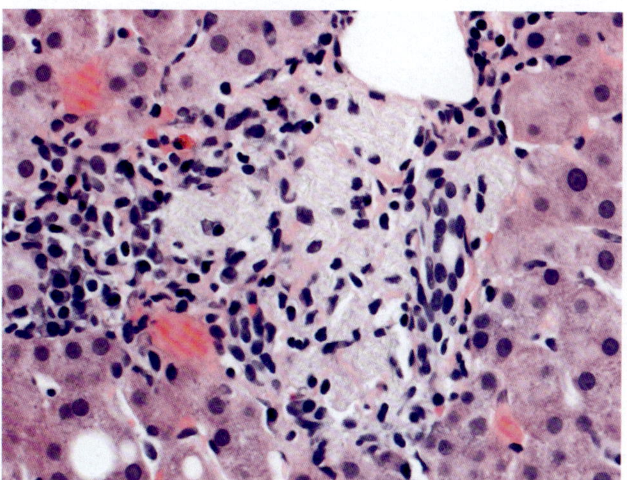

Figure 4.11. **Talc granuloma.** A cluster of histiocytes show talc in the portal tracts in a patient with a history of injection drug use. Well-formed granulomas were not present and usually are not with talc deposition.

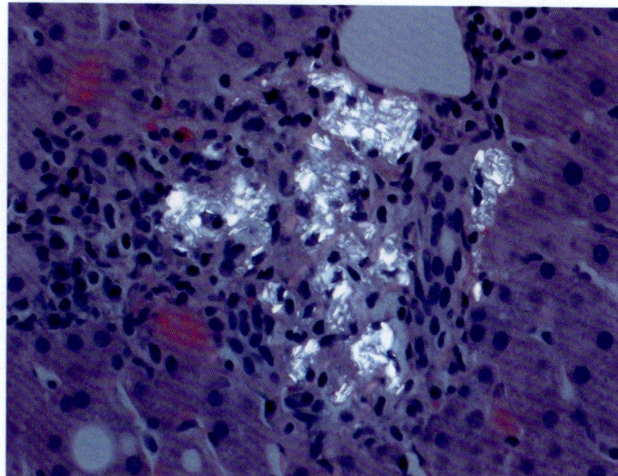

Figure 4.12. **Talc granuloma, polarized light.** Same image field as above. The talc shows strong polarization.

FOREIGN BODY GRANULOMA

These granulomas have visible foreign material by light microscopy. Sometimes the foreign material is evident on H&E but does not polarize; sometimes foreign material is both seen on H&E and polarizes; and sometimes foreign material is seen only with polarization. Foreign body granulomas most commonly result from prior medical procedures—such as surgical foam, prior peritonitis from hollow viscous rupture, such as a rupture appendix or prior injection drug use—most commonly leading to Talc powder deposits (Figs. 4.11 and 4.12). With any of these causes there can be multiple granulomas, and not every granuloma will have foreign material, but if most do, then that is acceptable as foreign body granulomas. Pigmented macrophages can also be seen in a subset of individuals with joint replacements and are thought to represent titanium (Fig. 4.13). These pigmented macrophages do not form granulomas and are an incidental finding. Sometimes this material can mimic malarial pigment.

LIPOGRANULOMA

Lipogranulomas are also sometimes called lipid granulomas and are made up of a loose cluster of foamy histiocytes, often associated with focal fibrosis (Fig. 4.14). Lipogranulomas are usually found with fatty liver disease[21,22] or with chronic hepatitis C.[21] In these diseases, they have a frequency of about 10% to 20%.[21,23] In fatty liver disease, they tend to be more common in steatosis than steatohepatitis[23] and more common in alcohol versus nonalcohol fatty liver disease,[24] but overall they have no diagnostic relevance. Most lipogranulomas are located next to central veins or in portal tracts.

While lipogranulomas are commonly associated with focal fibrosis, they are not a driver of fibrosis per se. They are technically granulomas, but have a completely different clinical significance (none) compared with other granulomas, so the term lipogranuloma is of little value in your surgical pathology report and, in some cases, can do a disservice by confusing clinicians and patients. Interestingly, they have a frequency of about 45% in canine livers, but there too have no clinical significance.[25]

MINERAL OIL GRANULOMA

Mineral oil granulomas look exactly like lipogranulomas, but instead of being associated with fatty liver disease, they are derived from mineral oil used as a food additive.[26,27] Like lipogranulomas, they can be associated with focal mild fibrosis, but have no clinical significance. Most of the time, mineral oil granulomas are classified together with lipogranulomas during research studies because they cannot be separated based on H&E findings alone lipogranulomas are more common.

NECROTIZING GRANULOMA

These granulomas are defined by central necrosis (Fig. 4.15). They are almost always infectious, usually bacterial or fungal. The central areas of necrosis typically have a granular, grungy appearance—in contrast to smooth or fibrillary hyalinization that can be seen in larger granulomas with central hyalinization. Granulomas with central hyalinization tend to be larger and are not enriched for infectious causes compared with ordinary epithelioid granulomas.

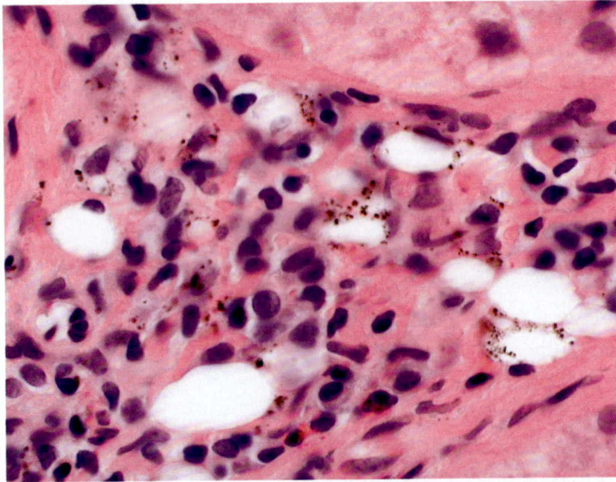

Figure 4.13. **Portal macrophages with titanium pigment.** Dark brown–black pigment is seen. The patient had a history of a knee replacement. Titanium will be negative on iron stain.

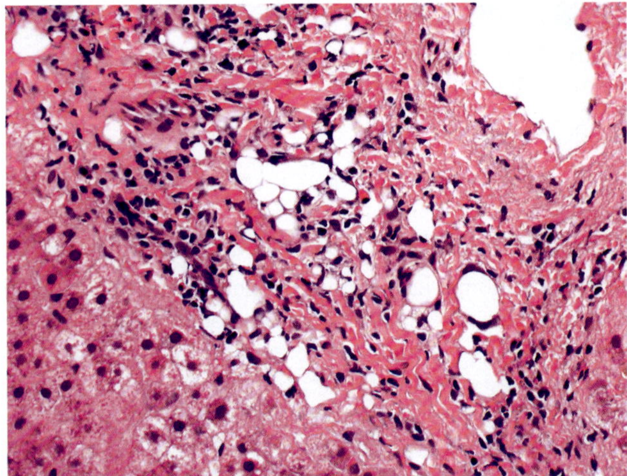

Figure 4.14. **Lipogranuloma.** The portal tract in this case of nonalcoholic fatty liver disease shows a cluster of lipid laden macrophages, mild chronic inflammation, and focal fibrosis.

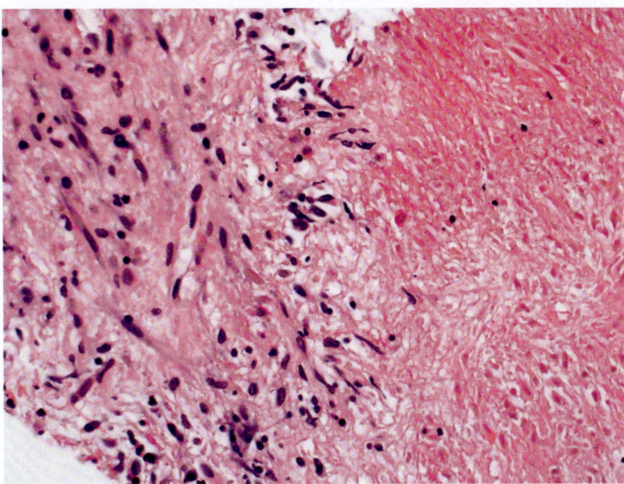

Figure 4.15. **Granuloma with central necrosis.** This biopsy is from a person with Crohn disease, but this granuloma is inconsistent with Crohn disease. AFB and GMS stains were negative, but the granuloma is almost certainly infectious in origin.

SPECIFIC GRANULOMATOUS DISEASES

MYCOBACTERIUM TUBERCULOSIS

CHECKLIST: *Mycobacterium tuberculosis* Clinical Tests

- ☐ Mantoux test (PPD): A positive test does not distinguish between active and latent infections. It is controversial whether testing is useful in individuals who have been vaccinated with BCG (bacillus Calmette–Guerin) because of high false-positive rates.
- ☐ QuantiFERON-TB Gold blood test: Measures interferon gamma after blood samples are exposed to *M. tuberculosis* proteins. A positive test does not distinguish between active and latent infections.

Most mycobacterial infections encountered in surgical pathology are from *Mycobacterium tuberculosis*. While the incidence is slowly decreasing, infection continues to be one of the leading causes of death worldwide. Serological findings are used to identity exposure but do not indicate active infection.

The histological findings vary widely but tend to cluster into several distinct patterns. Granulomatous disease is characterized by varying sized epithelioid granulomas (Figs. 4.16 and 4.17), some with central caseating necrosis. The frequency of necrosis in granulomas is about 60%.[28] The granulomas are usually accompanied by mild nonspecific portal and lobular inflammation. Other patterns that have been reported include peliosis hepatis,[29] nonspecific hepatitis, and fatty change.[28] Miliary tuberculosis refers to cases that have numerous small caseating and/or noncaseating granulomas, where the granulomas are typically less than 5 mm but still visible by imaging or gross examination. This term is most commonly use to describe lung disease but also occurs in the liver.[30] Rarely, cases can have a biliary obstruction pattern, due either to biliary strictures or to compression of the bile duct by enlarged hilar lymph nodes.[31]

BACILLUS CALMETTE–GUERIN AND OTHER *MYCOBACTERIUM* INFECTIONS

BCG therapy (live bovine tuberculosis bacillus) is used to tread bladder cancer and sometimes leads to granulomas in the liver (Fig. 4.18).[28] The granulomas are noncaseating and can range from a few granulomas identified as incidental findings to numerous granulomas causing clinical symptoms such as fevers or jaundice.[28,32]

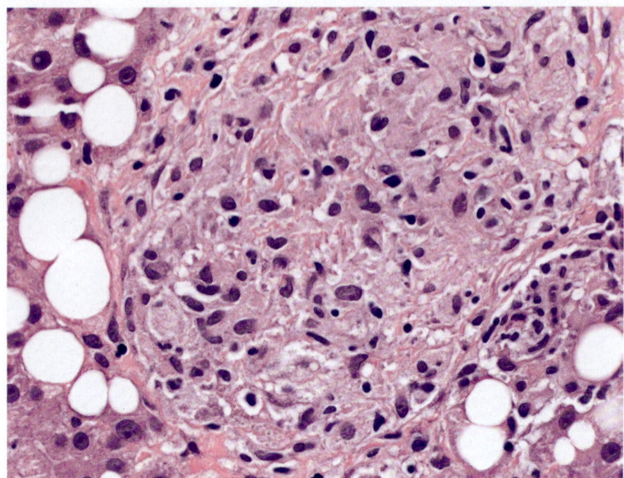

Figure 4.16. **Granuloma, *Mycobacteria tuberculosis*.** Many of the granulomas in cases of *M. tuberculosis* are not caseating.

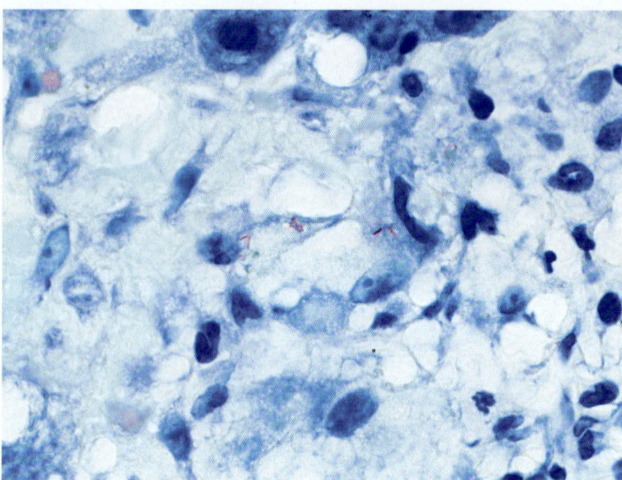

Figure 4.17. **Granuloma, *Mycobacteria tuberculosis*, acid fast stains.** Rare, beaded, rod shaped organisms are seen.

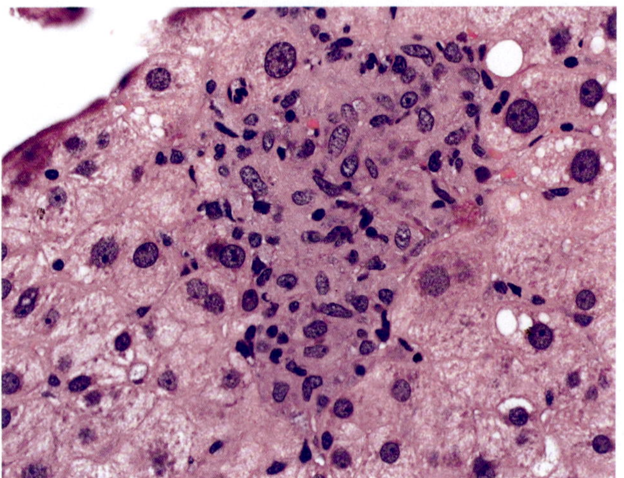

Figure 4.18. **Bacillus Calmette–Guerin (BCG).** In this case, the patient developed fever and elevated liver enzymes following BCG therapy to tread bladder cancer. A liver biopsy shows numerous granulomas and mild portal and lobular lymphocytic inflammation.

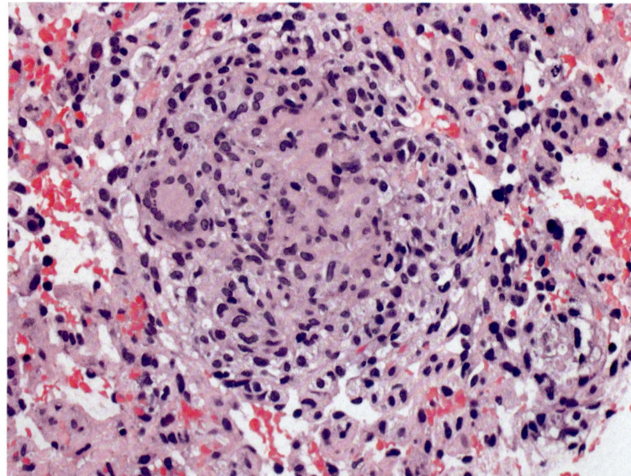

Figure 4.19. ***Mycobacterium chimaera.*** The liver biopsy showed numerous noncaseating granulomas.

Other *Mycobacterium* infections include *Mycobacterium intracellulare, Mycobacterium avium*, and *Mycobacterium chimaera* (Fig. 4.19). These infections can cause granulomatous disease in immunosuppressed individuals. *Mycobacterium avium-intracellulare* occurs primarily in end-stage HIV (human immunodeficiency virus) infection or with other severe forms of immunosuppression. The infection tends to show clusters of foamy macrophages in the sinusoids and the portal tracts, without well-formed epithelioid granulomas. The histiocytes are strongly PAS positive and AFB stains shows large numbers of organisms. However, organisms can be sparse in cases with less severe immunosuppression.

MYCOBACTERIUM LEPRAE

Leprosy is caused by *Mycobacterium leprae* and leads primarily to skin disease and injury to the peripheral nerves. The incubation period after initial exposure can be as long as several decades, so the sources of infection and routes of transmission are often hard to determine. Known reservoirs for *Mycobacterium leprae* include primates and some armadillo species.

The liver disease can manifest as distinct epithelioid granulomas, a pattern called tuberuculoid leprosy, or show aggregates of foamy histiocytes in the lobules and portal tracts, a disease pattern called lepromatous leprosy (Fig. 4.20). The Fite stain is the best stain to identify organisms, which tend to be rare in the tubercuolid pattern and numerous in lepromatous pattern (Fig. 4.21). The relative frequency of tuberuculoid versus lepromatous patterns of leprosy varies with geography, presumably representing differences in the environment, host genetics, or different species of *Mycobacterium*.[33] The tuberuculoid pattern of leprosy is more common in India and Africa, while the lepromatous pattern is more common in Mexico.

FUNGAL INFECTIONS

Patterns of liver injury in fungal infections can range from large necrotizing granulomas to old fibrotic granulomas. In addition to the granulomas, the background liver commonly shows mild nonspecific portal and lobular inflammation but sometimes can show moderate portal and lobular inflammation, resembling a chronic hepatitis (Fig. 4.22). Fungal organisms are best identified with special stains such as GMS (Fig. 4.23) or PAS. In the United States, the most common fungal infection of the liver in immunocompetent individuals is histoplasmosis, although immunosuppressed individuals can have other infections such as *Candida* or *Aspergillus*. *Histoplasmosis* is caused by the fungus *Histoplasma capsulatum*. Infections result from inhaling organisms that are found in the soil, in particular soil that is contaminated by bird or bat droppings. Most infections occur in the Ohio River valley or the lower Mississippi river valley. Infections are largely asymptomatic but can lead to flulike symptoms or nonspecific upper respiratory tract disease. Most symptomatic disease involves

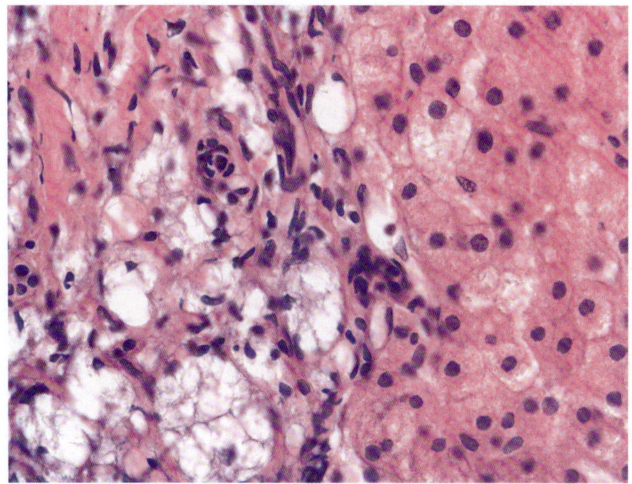

Figure 4.20. **Lepromatous leprosy.** Numerous foamy macrophages are present in the portal tracts. Similar changes were seen in the lobules.

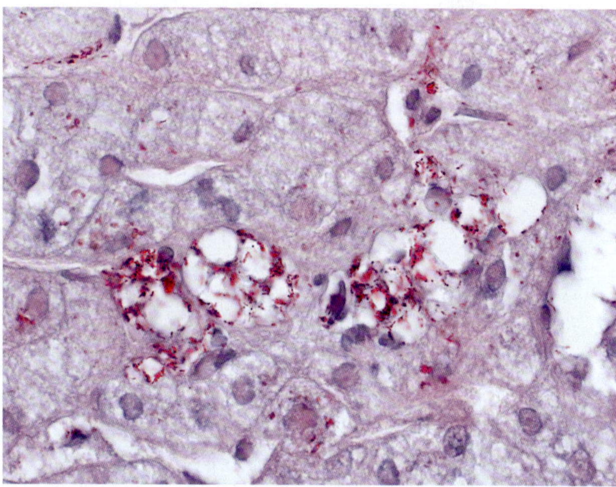

Figure 4.21. **Lepromatous leprosy, Fite stain.** Numerous organisms are seen in clusters of foamy lobular macrophages.

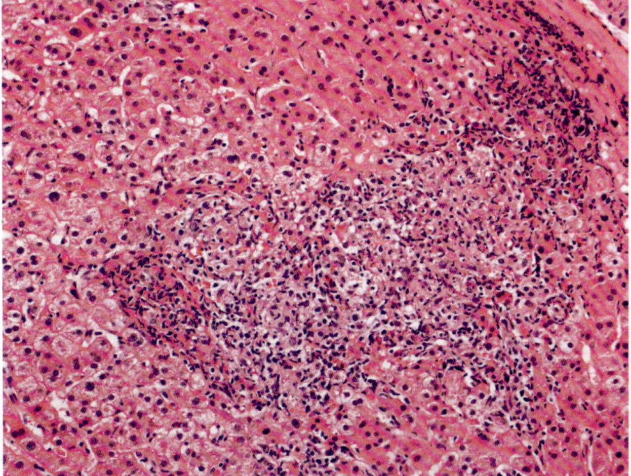

Figure 4.22. **Granulomatous hepatitis from histoplasmosis.** The liver showed moderate lobular hepatitis and numerous granulomas.

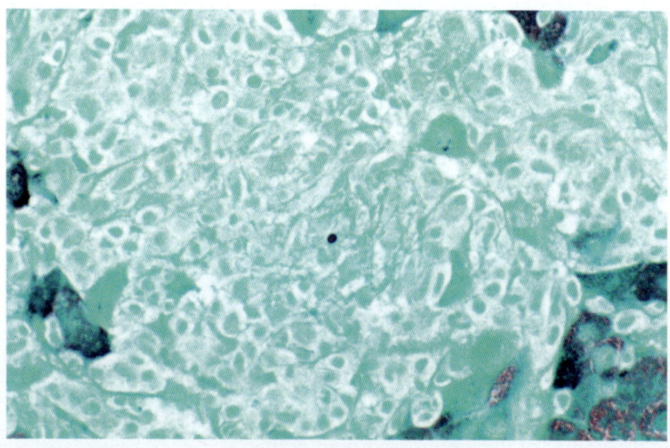

Figure 4.23. **Histoplasmosis, GMS stain.** Despite the numerous granulomas, organisms are sparse.

the lungs and can lead to chronic cavitary lung disease. Infections can also spread outside the lungs, leading to fibrosing mediastinitis, gastrointestinal tract disease, and liver disease.

Liver involvement in immunocompetent individuals leads to lymphohistiocytic inflammation in the portal tracts and Kupffer cell hyperplasia in the sinusoids.[34] Well-formed granulomas are rare to absent, with most cases showing poorly formed lymphohistiocytic nodules. Organisms are more commonly identified by special stains when individuals have active clinical symptoms. In contrast, organisms are sparse to absent when granulomas are an incidental finding in liver biopsies performed for other clinical reasons. Over time, granulomas heal and become fibrotic and often become calcified.

PARASITES

Granulomas can develop in response to parasites, in particular parasite eggs. Schistosomiasis is the most common granulomatous parasite in the liver (Fig. 4.24). Schistosomiasis can also lead to granulomatous phlebitis and a dense heavy portal fibrosis called Symmers fibrosis.

SARCOIDOSIS

Sarcoidosis is a systemic granulomatous disease of unknown etiology that tends to affect younger individuals (age less than 40 years) and is more common in individuals of Scandinavian descent, particularly Sweden and Iceland. However, all ethnic groups can be affected. Overall, the disease tends to be more aggressive in those of African descent.

A final diagnosis of sarcoidosis always requires clinical correlation; the biopsy findings are never sufficient in isolation. Hepatic granulomas are present in about 75% of individuals. In most cases, the liver disease is clinically silent, but mild liver disease can be evident in about 20% of individuals. Severe liver disease is uncommon.

Histologically, the most common pattern is clusters of granulomas in the portal tracts associated with fibrosis (Fig. 4.25). The lobules also have occasional granulomas, although they tend to be single and not associated with fibrosis (Fig. 4.26). The portal tracts and the lobules also commonly show mild nonspecific inflammation. Asteroid and Schaumann bodies are rare in sarcoidal granulomas of the liver and are not specific anyway. The larger granulomas can show central hyalinization but not true caseating necrosis.

In addition to granulomas, sarcoidosis can show several additional rare findings. First, some cases will also show a biliary obstruction pattern when enlarged hilar lymph nodes compress the hilar bile ducts. In other cases, the ducts can be actively injured by granulomatous inflammation.[35] Over time, some of these cases with a biliary pattern can become ductopenic.[36,37] A second uncommon pattern shows granulomatous phlebitis. Portal vein phlebitis can lead to portal vein atrophy, fibrosis, and loss, with subsequent changes of

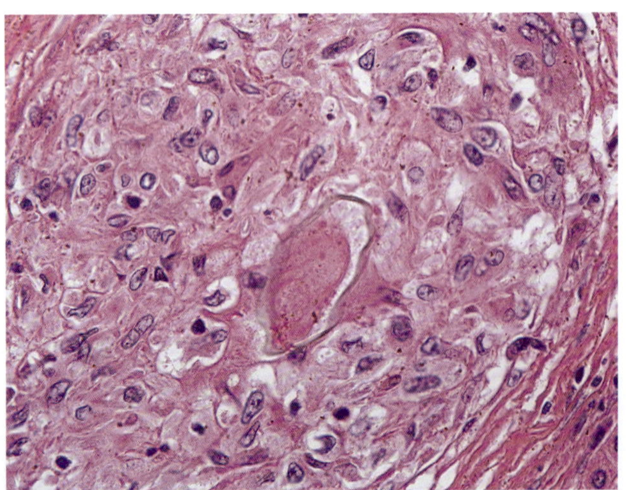

Figure 4.24. Schistosomiasis. A schistosomiasis organism is seen in the center of this epithelioid granuloma.

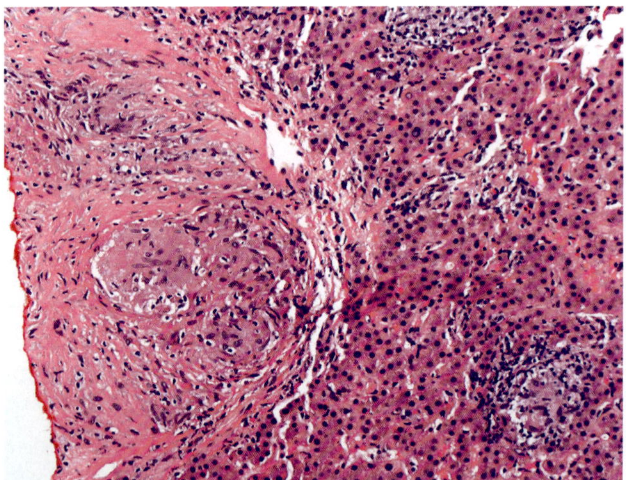

Figure 4.25. Sarcoidosis. Fibrotic granulomas can be seen in the portal tract at the left of the image. Several smaller lobular granulomas are present in the right half of the image. As seen in this case, lobular granulomas often do not show fibrosis.

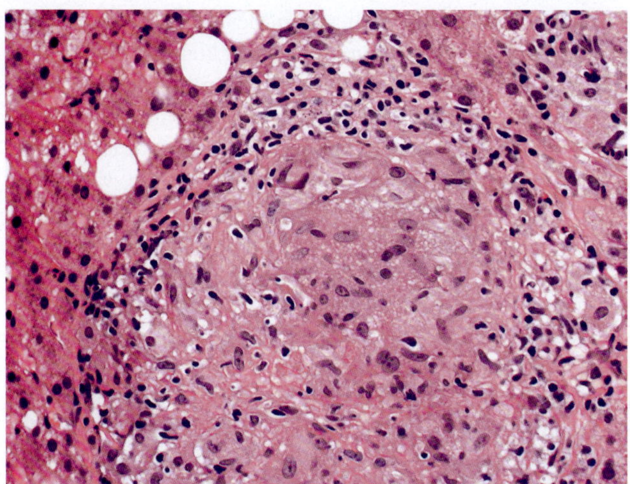

Figure 4.26. **Sarcoidosis.** In this case, the portal tracts contained multiple epithelioid granulomas. Fibrosis can be seen at the edges of the granulomas.

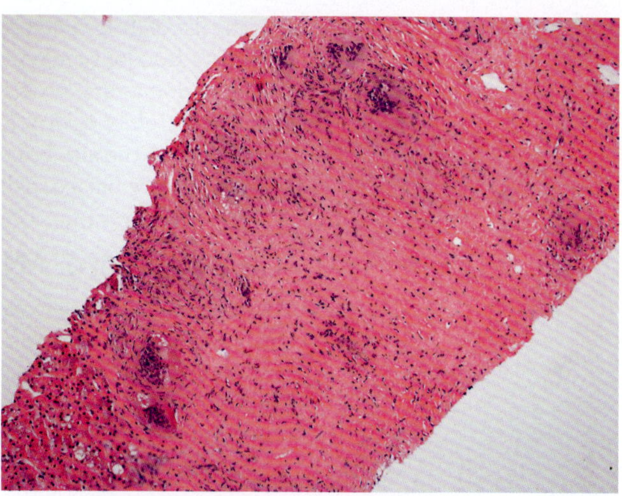

Figure 4.27. **Sarcoidoma.** An area of confluent granulomas and fibrosis formed a mass lesion.

nodular regenerative hyperplasia. The phlebitis pattern can also show more typical sarcoidal epithelioid granulomas in the portal tracts and lobules, but overall these two patterns are quite distinct—enough so that it suggests distinct pathogenesis. Finally, rare cases can present with a mass lesion that results from a large consolidated aggregate of fibrotic granulomas (Fig. 4.27), a finding sometimes called a *sarcoidoma*.[38] Advanced fibrosis including cirrhosis is rare but has been described.[39-41]

COMMON VARIABLE IMMUNODEFICIENCY (CVID)

About 20% of Common variable immunodeficiency (CVID) patients have mildly elevated liver enzymes.[42] The liver is typically not biopsied unless the diagnosis of CVID is unknown or the liver enzyme elevations are higher than usual. The biopsies show mild to focally moderate nonspecific portal and lobular inflammation, often mild fatty change and scattered small epithelioid granulomas.[43] The granulomas can be found in the portal tracts and the lobules. Organism stains are negative in most cases but should still be performed. Nodular regenerative hyperplasia is also a common finding.[43]

CROHN DISEASE

Crohn disease is discussed here but the most common liver injury pattern associated with Crohn disease in surgical pathology specimens is primary sclerosing cholangitis. Clinical survey studies show liver enzymes are elevated in 10% to 20% of Crohn disease patients,[44,45] usually with a mild and nonspecific pattern, except when there is coexisting primary sclerosing cholangitis. The frequency of liver enzyme elevations is similar in both Crohn disease and ulcerative colitis.[44] Excluding cases with primary sclerosing cholangitis, the overall patterns of liver injury has not been well studied but generally shows mild nonspecific portal and lobular inflammation, sometimes with mild fatty change.[46] Granulomas are rare but can be seen.

DRUG REACTIONS

CHECKLIST: Drugs and Granulomas Not an Exhaustive List of Course, but Examples of Drugs That Commonly Cause Granulomas When They Cause a Drug Reaction.

- ☐ Allopurinol
- ☐ penicillins
- ☐ phenothiazines
- ☐ phenlybutazine

The list of drugs that can cause granulomas is not endless, but nearly so. Nonetheless, a few drug reactions are typically associated with granulomas (see checklist). In most cases, the granulomas are associated with significant portal and lobular hepatitis, and the granulomas are often poorly formed. Well-formed epithelioid granulomas without minimal inflammation can also be encountered but are less common. Rare drug reactions can closely mimic primary biliary cirrhosis.

GRANULOMAS AND NEOPLASMS

Granulomas can be associated with a variety of tumors including convenitonal hepatocellular carcinoma,[3,4] fibrolamellar carcinoma, cholangiocarcinoma,[3] metastatic tumors,[2] and lymphoma.[3,5] In rare cases, the granulomas appear to be a response to the tumor itself, but in most cases, they are likely an incidental finding. In general, no specific tumor or general type of tumor has a strong tendency to elicit granulomas.

Overall, the lymphoma most strongly linked to granulomas is Hodgkin's disease, with cases reported of hepatic granulomas preceding Hodgkin disease by months to years. The granulomas can be small, epithelioid, and otherwise nondescript, usually in a background of mild portal and lobular hepatitis, or can show a more inflamed granulomatous hepatitis pattern.[47,48] Other organs, such as the bone marrow, can also have granulomas preceding a diagnosis of Hodgkin lymphoma.

OTHER CAUSES

There is a very long list of additional rare associations between granulomas and other diseases. In none of these diseases are the granulomas characteristic and in most cases the granulomas could just as well be an incidental finding. These included chronic viral hepatitis B, chronic viral hepatitis C, autoimmune hepatitis,[4-6] polymyalgia rheumatic,[5] juvenile chronic arthritis,[5] gout,[2] vasculitis,[4] graft versus host disease,[5] and jejuno–ileal bypass surgery.[5]

Rheumatoid nodules are not technically granulomas but can involve the liver[49] and be misinterpreted as a granuloma. They have a central zone that is eosinophilic and composed of fibrin and sometimes necrosis, with a rim of palisading histiocytes and an outer layer of lymphoplasmacytic inflammation (Figs. 4.28 and 4.29). Older lesions can become more sclerotic.

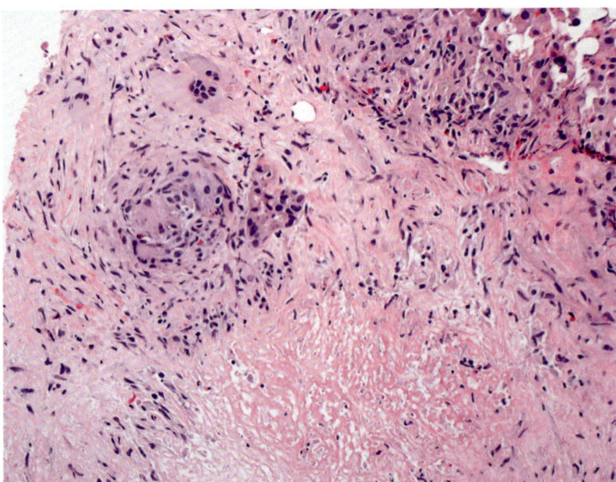

Figure 4.28. Rheumatoid nodules. This rheumatoid nodule shows an eosinophilic center composed of fibrin and fibrosis, with a rim of palisading histiocytes.

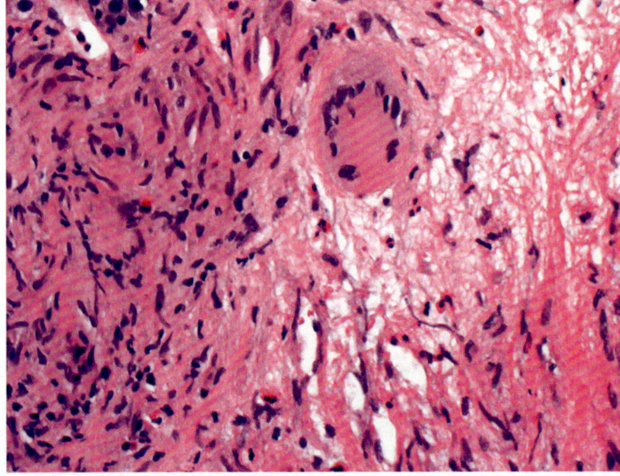

Figure 4.29. Rheumatoid nodules. Scattered multinucleated giant cells are located at the periphery of the nodule.

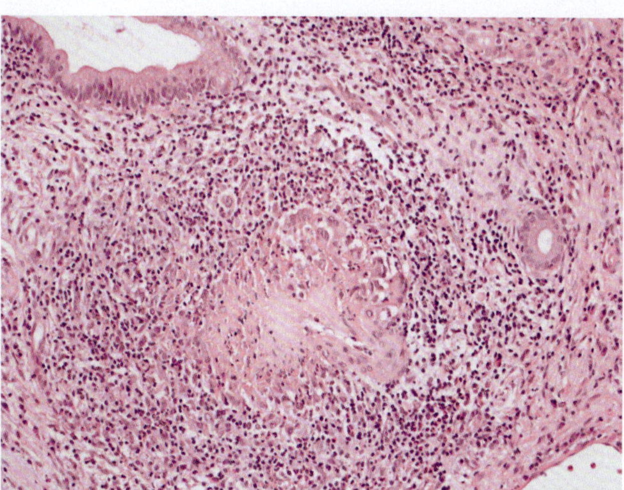

Figure 4.30. **Near miss, case 1, necrotizing arteritis.** The necrotizing arteritis in this case at first suggested necrotizing granulomas.

NEAR MISSES

CASE 1. A liver biopsy in a 39-year-old man with new onset fevers and rash showed moderate mixed portal inflammation as well as mild patchy lobular inflammation. In several portal tracts, there appeared to be necrotic granulomas (Fig. 4.30). AFB and GMS stains were negative. On rereview, the lesions that looked like necrotic granulomas were not actually granulomas, but were instead necrotizing arteritis. Several clues led to the correct diagnosis. One clue was that only a single granuloma was present in each affected portal tracts, and they were always adjacent to the bile ducts. In addition, the hepatic arteries were missing in these portal tracts. Subsequent work-up established a diagnosis of polyarteritis nodosa.

Polyarteritis nodosa can occur at any age, but most patients are men in their 40s and 50s. Most cases are idiopathic. Historically, about one-third of polyarteritis nodosa cases were associated with hepatitis B or other infections, but in current classification systems, such cases are separated into their own category of infection related vasculitis.[50] Patients commonly have fevers, weight loss, skin rashes, peripheral neuropathy, and muscle and joints pain. Renal disease is common, but lung disease is not.

The most characteristic lesion when polyarteritis nodosa involves the liver is necrotizing arteritis. Other common findings include nodular regenerative hyperplasia.[51,52] Polyarteritis nodosa can also lead to ischemic biliary strictures of the extrahepatic and largery intrahepatic bile ducts, which can in turn lead to a variety of changes on peripheral needle biopsy, including bile ductular proliferation and onion-skinning fibrosis.[52]

References

1. Drebber U, Kasper HU, Ratering J, et al. Hepatic granulomas: histological and molecular pathological approach to differential diagnosis–a study of 442 cases. *Liver Int*. 2008;28:828-834.
2. McCluggage WG, Sloan JM. Hepatic granulomas in Northern Ireland: a thirteen year review. *Histopathology*. 1994;25:219-228.
3. Turhan N, Kurt M, Ozderin YO, Kurt OK. Hepatic granulomas: a clinicopathologic analysis of 86 cases. *Pathol Res Pract*. 2011;207:359-365.
4. Dourakis SP, Saramadou R, Alexopoulou A, et al. Hepatic granulomas: a 6-year experience in a single center in Greece. *Eur J Gastroenterol Hepatol*. 2007;19:101-104.
5. Gaya DR, Thorburn D, Oien KA, Morris AJ, Stanley AJ. Hepatic granulomas: a 10 year single centre experience. *J Clin Pathol*. 2003;56:850-853.
6. Geramizadeh B, Jahangiri R, Moradi E. Causes of hepatic granuloma: a 12-year single center experience from Southern Iran. *Arch Iran Med*. 2011;14:288-289.
7. Kurata A, Nishimura Y, Yamato T, et al. Systemic granulomatous necrotizing vasculitis in a MPO-ANCA-positive patient. *Pathol Int*. 2004;54:636-640.

8. Heneghan MA, Feeley KM, DeFaoite N, Little MP, O'Gorman TA. Granulomatous liver disease and giant-cell arteritis. *Dig Dis Sci*. 1998;43:2164-2167.
9. Litwack KD, Bohan A, Silverman L. Granulomatous liver disease and giant cell arteritis. Case report and literature review. *J Rheumatol*. 1977;4:307-312.
10. Pellegrin M, Delsol G, Auvergnat JC, et al. Granulomatous hepatitis in Q fever. *Hum Pathol*. 1980;11:51-57.
11. Jang YR, Shin Y, Jin CE, et al. Molecular detection of coxiella burnetii from the formalin-fixed tissues of Q fever patients with acute hepatitis. *PLoS One*. 2017;12:e0180237.
12. Nenert M, Mavier P, Dubuc N, Deforges L, Zafrani ES. Epstein-Barr virus infection and hepatic fibrin-ring granulomas. *Hum Pathol*. 1988;19:608-610.
13. Yamamoto T, Ishii M, Nagura H, et al. Transient hepatic fibrin-ring granulomas in a patient with acute hepatitis A. *Liver*. 1995;15:276-279.
14. Ruel M, Sevestre H, Henry-Biabaud E, Courouce AM, Capron JP, Erlinger S. Fibrin ring granulomas in hepatitis A. *Dig Dis Sci*. 1992;37:1915-1917.
15. Marazuela M, Moreno A, Yebra M, Cerezo E, Gomez-Gesto C, Vargas JA. Hepatic fibrin-ring granulomas: a clinicopathologic study of 23 patients. *Hum Pathol*. 1991;22:607-613.
16. Moreno A, Marazuela M, Yebra M, et al. Hepatic fibrin-ring granulomas in visceral leishmaniasis. *Gastroenterology*. 1988;95:1123-1126.
17. Khanlari B, Bodmer M, Terracciano L, Heim MH, Fluckiger U, Weisser M. Hepatitis with fibrin-ring granulomas. *Infection*. 2008;36:381-383.
18. Vanderstigel M, Zafrani ES, Lejonc JL, Schaeffer A, Portos JL. Allopurinol hypersensitivity syndrome as a cause of hepatic fibrin-ring granulomas. *Gastroenterology*. 1986;90:188-190.
19. Stricker BH, Blok AP, Babany G, Benhamou JP. Fibrin ring granulomas and allopurinol. *Gastroenterology*. 1989;96:1199-1203.
20. Everett J, Srivastava A, Misdraji J. Fibrin ring granulomas in checkpoint inhibitor-induced hepatitis. *Am J Surg Pathol*. 2017;41:134-137.
21. Zhu H, Bodenheimer HC, Clain DJ, Min AD, Theise ND. Hepatic lipogranulomas in patients with chronic liver disease: association with hepatitis C and fatty liver disease. *World J Gastroenterol*. 2010;16:5065-5069.
22. Delladetsima JK, Horn T, Poulsen H. Portal tract lipogranulomas in liver biopsies. *Liver*. 1987;7:9-17.
23. Kleiner DE, Brunt EM, Van Natta M, et al. Design and validation of a histological scoring system for nonalcoholic fatty liver disease. *Hepatology*. 2005;41:1313-1321.
24. Morita Y, Ueno T, Sasaki N, et al. Comparison of liver histology between patients with non-alcoholic steatohepatitis and patients with alcoholic steatohepatitis in Japan. *Alcohol Clin Exp Res*. 2005;29:277S-281S.
25. Isobe K, Nakayama H, Uetsuka K. Relation between lipogranuloma formation and fibrosis, and the origin of brown pigments in lipogranuloma of the canine liver. *Comp Hepatol*. 2008;7:5.
26. Boitnott JK, Margolis S. Saturated hydrocarbons in human tissues. 3. Oil droplets in the liver and spleen. *Johns Hopkins Med J*. 1970;127:65-78.
27. Carlton WW, Boitnott JK, Dungworth DL, et al. Assessment of the morphology and significance of the lymph nodal and hepatic lesions produced in rats by the feeding of certain mineral oils and waxes. Proceedings of a pathology workshop held at the Fraunhofer Institute of Toxicology and Aerosol Research Hannover, Germany, May 7-9, 2001. *Exp Toxicol Pathol*. 2001;53:247-255.
28. Amarapurkar A, Agrawal V. Liver involvement in tuberculosis–an autopsy study. *Trop Gastroenterol*. 2006;27:69-74.
29. Sanz-Canalejas L, Gomez-Mampaso E, Canton-Moreno R, Varona-Crespo C, Fortun J, Dronda F. Peliosis hepatis due to disseminated tuberculosis in a patient with AIDS. *Infection*. 2014;42:185-189.
30. Tajiri T, Tate G, Makino M, et al. Autopsy cases of miliary tuberculosis: clinicopathologic features including background factors. *J Nippon Med Sch*. 2011;78:305-311.
31. Amarapurkar DN, Patel ND, Amarapurkar AD. Hepatobiliary tuberculosis in Western India. *Indian J Pathol Microbiol*. 2008;51:175-181.
32. Leebeek FW, Ouwendijk RJ, Kolk AH, et al. Granulomatous hepatitis caused by Bacillus Calmette-Guerin (BCG) infection after BCG bladder instillation. *Gut*. 1996;38:616-618.

33. Han XY, Seo YH, Sizer KC, et al. A new *Mycobacterium* species causing diffuse lepromatous leprosy. *Am J Clin Pathol*. 2008;130:856-864.

34. Lamps LW, Molina CP, West AB, Haggitt RC, Scott MA. The pathologic spectrum of gastrointestinal and hepatic histoplasmosis. *Am J Clin Pathol*. 2000;113:64-72.

35. Ishak KG. Sarcoidosis of the liver and bile ducts. *Mayo Clin Proc*. 1998;73:467-472.

36. Farouj NE, Cadranel JF, Mofredj A, et al. Ductopenia related liver sarcoidosis. *World J Hepatol*. 2011;3:170-174.

37. Nakanuma Y, Kouda W, Harada K, Hiramatsu K. Hepatic sarcoidosis with vanishing bile duct syndrome, cirrhosis, and portal phlebosclerosis. Report of an autopsy case. *J Clin Gastroenterol*. 2001;32:181-184.

38. Devaney K, Goodman ZD, Epstein MS, Zimmerman HJ, Ishak KG. Hepatic sarcoidosis. Clinicopathologic features in 100 patients. *Am J Surg Pathol*. 1993;17:1272-1280.

39. Ennaifer R, Ayadi S, Romdhane H, et al. Hepatic sarcoidosis: a case series. *Pan Afr Med J*. 2016;24:209.

40. Fetzer DT, Rees MA, Dasyam AK, Tublin ME. Hepatic sarcoidosis in patients presenting with liver dysfunction: imaging appearance, pathological correlation and disease evolution. *Eur Radiol*. 2016;26:3129-3137.

41. Ungprasert P, Crowson CS, Simonetto DA, Matteson EL. Clinical characteristics and outcome of hepatic sarcoidosis: a population-based study 1976-2013. *Am J Gastroenterol*. 2017;112:1556-1563.

42. Hermaszewski RA, Webster AD. Primary hypogammaglobulinaemia: a survey of clinical manifestations and complications. *Q J Med*. 1993;86:31-42.

43. Fuss IJ, Friend J, Yang Z, et al. Nodular regenerative hyperplasia in common variable immunodeficiency. *J Clin Immunol*. 2013;33:748-758.

44. Cappello M, Randazzo C, Bravata I, et al. Liver function test abnormalities in patients with inflammatory bowel diseases: a hospital-based survey. *Clin Med Insights Gastroenterol*. 2014;7:25-31.

45. Broome U, Glaumann H, Hellers G, Nilsson B, Sorstad J, Hultcrantz R. Liver disease in ulcerative colitis: an epidemiological and follow up study in the county of Stockholm. *Gut*. 1994;35:84-89.

46. Eade MN, Cooke WT, Williams JA. Liver disease in Crohn's disease. A study of 100 consecutive patients. *Scand J Gastroenterol*. 1971;6:199-204.

47. Kanbay M, Altundag K, Gur G, Boyacioglu S. Non-Hodgkin's lymphoma presenting with granulomatous hepatitis and hemophagocytosis. *Leuk Lymphoma*. 2006;47:767-769.

48. Aderka D, Kraus M, Avidor I, Sidi Y, Weinberger A, Pinkhas J. Hodgkin's and non-Hodgkin's lymphomas masquerading as "idiopathic" liver granulomas. *Am J Gastroenterol*. 1984;79:642-644.

49. Smits JG, Kooijman CD. Rheumatoid nodules in liver. *Histopathology*. 1986;10:1211-1213.

50. Ozen S. The changing face of polyarteritis nodosa and necrotizing vasculitis. *Nat Rev Rheumatol*. 2017;13:381-386.

51. Nakanuma Y, Ohta G, Sasaki K. Nodular regenerative hyperplasia of the liver associated with polyarteritis nodosa. *Arch Pathol Lab Med*. 1984;108:133-135.

52. Goritsas CP, Repanti M, Papadaki E, Lazarou N, Andonopoulos AP. Intrahepatic bile duct injury and nodular regenerative hyperplasia of the liver in a patient with polyarteritis nodosa. *J Hepatol*. 1997;26:727-730.

DRUG-INDUCED LIVER INJURY 5

CHAPTER OUTLINE

OVERVIEW

Drug-induced liver injury (DILI) is a common form of liver injury. The most common causes of DILI in adults are acetaminophen, antibiotics, central nervous system agents, antihypertensive agents, dietary supplements, and antidiabetic agents.[1] In children the most common causes are antibiotics and central nervous system agents.[2] In most cases, the temporal correlation between beginning a new drug and the development of liver enzyme elevations, or other clinical findings of hepatitis, quickly points to a drug reaction, and such cases are rarely biopsied. In surgical pathology, DILI tends to be enriched for (1) newly released drugs because of limited clinical experience with their toxicity profile; (2) herbal remedies because the patients may not report their use to the clinical team; or (3) complicated clinical scenarios because multiple agents in the patient's clinical history could have led to liver injury.

DILI can lead to different patterns of liver injury, and these patterns tend to broadly reflect the main mechanism of injury. DILI can be classified as direct toxin injuries, allergic (hypersensitivity) drug reactions, or idiosyncratic drug reactions. Of these, idiosyncratic drug reactions are by far the most common type seen in surgical pathology specimens. In contrast, both allergic reactions and toxin-related injuries are usually diagnosed without a liver biopsy because of their distinct clinical findings.

There are several excellent resources when evaluating a liver biopsy for a possible DILI. Of course, books are an excellent starting point, but they cannot include all possible causes or patterns of DILI, so also consider searching PubMed, commercial databases, or the Livertox website, http://livertox.nih.gov/.

GENERAL APPROACH

It is fairly well known by pathologists that drug reactions can show almost any pattern of liver injury and this sometimes leads to a nihilistic approach, where a pathologist includes a drug reaction in the differential of most of their medical liver biopsy reports. At the other end of the spectrum, pathologists can become too dogmatic that a biopsy with a potential drug reaction needs to show exactly the same changes found in text book images or internet images. It is true that the histological findings in DILI for any given drug tend to have a typical pattern of injury, but most patterns of injury are neither very sensitive nor specific. For this reason, in most cases there is limited value in being too dogmatic that a specific drug must show a specific pattern of injury. A more balanced approach is generally better, having a high index of suspicion for a drug reaction when (1) there is clinical evidence that would support a drug reaction, (2) the biopsy findings have no better explanation, and (3) the biopsy findings are broadly in line with the changes expected for that drug.

Some examples might help illustrate these points. Example 1: A patient starts a cancer drug that is new to the market and 10 days later develops liver enzyme elevations. Viral serologies are negative. A biopsy shows a hepatitic pattern of injury (Fig. 5.1). This case would fit well for a likely drug reaction. Example 2: A biopsy is performed to evaluate for possible acetaminophen toxicity and shows a hepatitic pattern of injury (Fig. 5.2), instead of a bland lobular necrosis pattern of injury. In this case there is likely a better diagnosis than acetaminophen toxicity. Example 3: A patient starts a new antibiotic and 7 days later has new-onset enzyme elevations 5X the upper limit of normal. Viral and autoimmune serologies are negative. A liver biopsy shows mostly lobular hepatitis with only mild portal inflammation (Fig. 5.3). The pictures in your text book suggest the injury pattern should be less hepatitic and more portal inflammation with duct-focused injury. Putting everything together, this still would be consistent with a drug reaction.

Temporal associations are very helpful in assessing for possible DILI. The most straightforward temporal associations are with direct toxins, such as acetaminophen, because liver toxicity is both time and dose dependent. However, most drug reactions

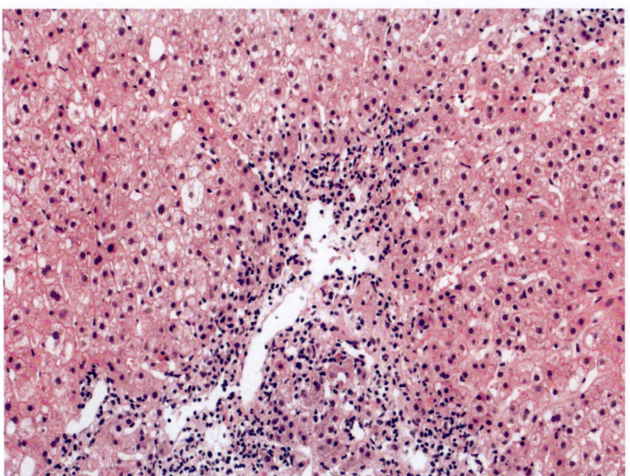

Figure 5.1. Drug reaction, hepatitic pattern. The biopsy shows lobular inflammation and injury. This pattern would fit well for an idiosyncratic drug reaction, even if drug-induced liver injury (DILI) is not well described in a newly marked drug.

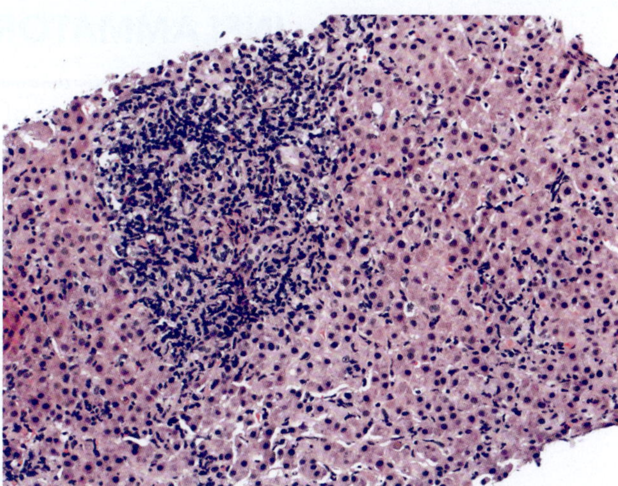

Figure 5.2. Drug reaction, hepatitic pattern. The biopsy shows portal and lobular inflammation and injury (from a case of minocycline drug-induced liver injury [DILI]). This pattern would fit well for an idiosyncratic drug reaction but not a toxin, such as acetaminophen toxicity.

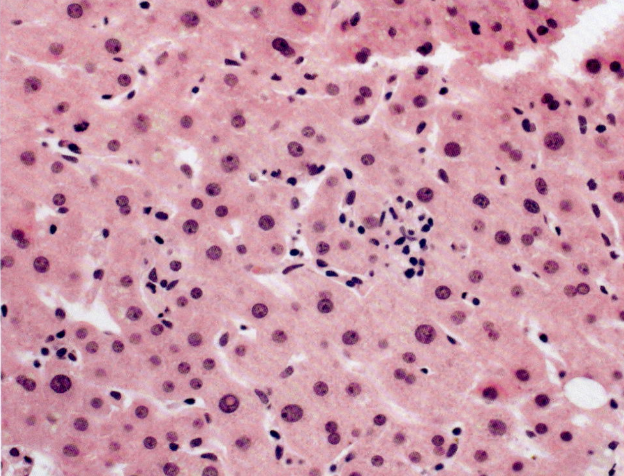

Figure 5.3. Drug reaction, hepatitic pattern. This drug reaction resulted from amoxicillin. Amoxicillin classically shows more of a cholangitic pattern of injury, but in this case, all other causes were excluded and the liver enzymes normalized after stopping the medication.

are idiosyncratic and thus are not dose related. For idiosyncratic drug reactions, the clinicians or the patient may have discontinued the medication days to weeks before the biopsy, so both current and recently discontinued medicines should be evaluated as possible causes of the DILI. Most idiosyncratic drug reactions occur within the first several weeks after starting the medication, but rare cases can develop months or longer after starting a new medication.

In the end, a diagnosis of DILI is made when there is a compatible exposure, compatible histological findings, and other potential causes are excluded. Despite best practices, some cases diagnosed as DILI turn out to have another cause that only becomes evident with additional clinical or laboratory findings. This is particularly true with idiosyncratic DILI, where the histological findings are best considered to be "most consistent with DILI" and not to be "biopsy-proven DILI." To illustrate this point, acute viral hepatitis can closely mimic drug reactions and are sometimes only retrospectively identified in cases previously classified as DILI.[1,3]

INFLAMMATORY PATTERNS OF INJURY

CHECKLIST: Patterns of Injury

- ☐ Idiosyncratic reactions
  - ○ Hepatitic pattern, including resolving hepatitis pattern
  - ○ Cholangitic pattern
  - ○ Bland lobular cholestasis pattern
  - ○ Granuloma pattern
- ☐ Toxic injury
  - ○ Bland necrosis, most commonly zone 3 pattern of necrosis
- ☐ Allergic
  - ○ Hepatitic pattern with numerous eosinophils
- ☐ Other patterns
  - ○ Isolated hyperammonemia
  - ○ Hypervitaminosis A
  - ○ Glycogen pseudo–ground glass inclusions
  - ○ Glycogenic hepatopathy
  - ○ Microvesicular steatosis
  - ○ Macrovesicular steatosis
  - ○ Ductopenia

IDIOSYNCRATIC DRUG REACTIONS

Most drug reactions encountered in surgical pathology are idiosyncratic. A diagnosis of DILI requires (1) a history of exposure to the drug; (2) a clinically compatible correlation with the onset of the liver injury; and (3) exclusion of other causes as thoroughly as possible.

Serological findings are important to rule out other causes of liver injury, but there are no positive tests that are helpful in confirming a diagnosis of DILI. Likewise, positive serology for ANA or SMA does not exclude DILI, as rare cases of DILI can be associated with elevated serum autoantibodies (Table 5.1). Clinically, most cases of idiosyncratic DILI present within 4 to 6 weeks of starting the medication, but rare cases have been reported that developed months to years after using a medication.

Overall, the most common DILI histological patterns are that of a nonspecific hepatitis or bland lobular cholestasis (Fig. 5.4). In the hepatitic pattern, the inflammation can range from mild to marked. The lobular hepatitis can show a zone 3 accentuation in some cases (Fig. 5.5), but this pattern is not specific for etiology, also being found in some cases of autoimmune hepatitis and viral hepatitis. The lobular hepatitis can be accompanied by lobular cholestasis (Fig. 5.6). In cases of more severe DILI, there can be zone 3 or panacinar

TABLE 5.1: Common Causes of DILI That Resemble Autoimmune Hepatitis on Histology and Can Have Positive Autoantibody Serology

Drug	Comments
Minocycline[49]	Antibiotic used to treat acne
Methyldopa[50]	Antihypertensive
Clometacin[51]	NSAID
Nitrofurantoin[49]	Antibiotic used to treat urinary tract infections

DILI, drug-induced liver injury; NSAID, nonsteroidal anti-inflammatory drug.

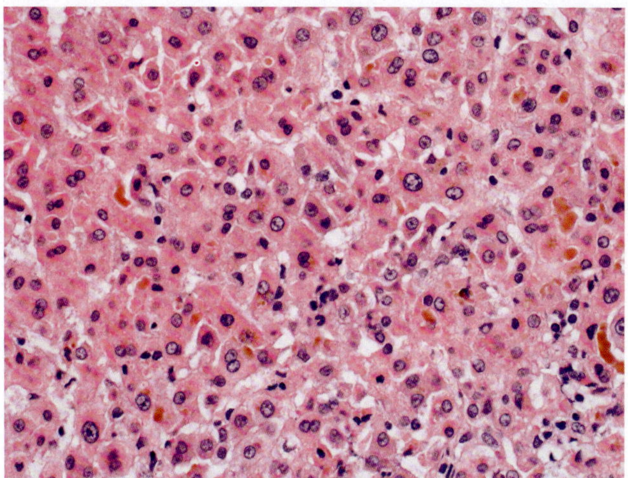

Figure 5.4. **Drug reaction, bland lobular cholestasis pattern.** This drug reaction (from the use of body building supplements with androgens) led to moderate lobular cholestasis with minimal inflammatory changes.

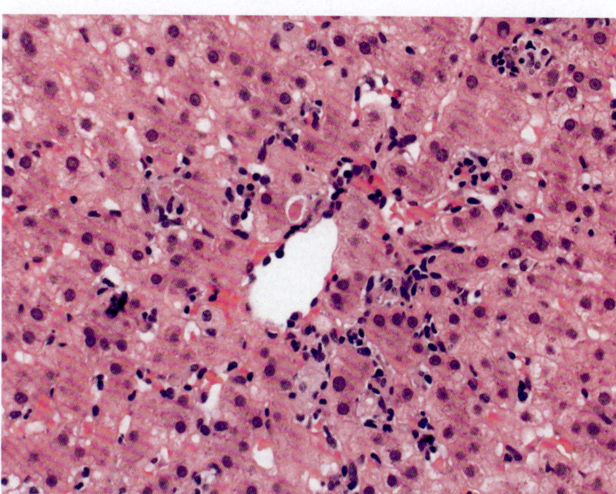

Figure 5.5. **Drug reaction, hepatitic pattern with zone 3 accentuation.** This pattern of lobular hepatitis with a zone 3 prominence is not specific for etiology and can be seen in a subset of cases of drug-induced liver injury (DILI), autoimmune hepatitis, and viral hepatitis. This case resulted from the use of a herbal remedy.

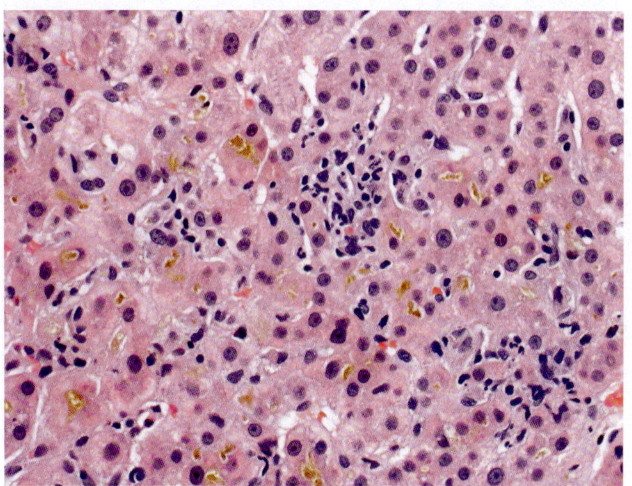

Figure 5.6. **Drug reaction, hepatitic pattern with lobular cholestasis.** This case of drug-induced liver injury (DILI) resulted from nitrofurantoin and showed a moderate lobular hepatitis with marked lobular cholestasis.

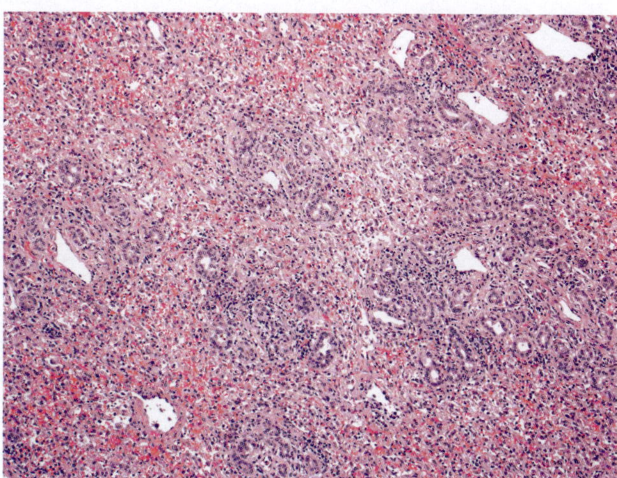

Figure 5.7. **Drug reaction, hepatitic pattern.** This case of severe drug-induced liver injury (DILI) resulted from isoniazid therapy and showed extensive, panacinar lobular necrosis.

necrosis (Fig. 5.7). Interface activity is common and tends to correlate with the degree of portal inflammation. The inflammation is predominately lymphocytic but plasma cells are common and can be prominent (Fig. 5.8) (Table 5.1). Likewise, occasional scattered eosinophils are common (Fig. 5.9) but eosinophilic rich inflammation is rare outside of an allergic drug reaction. If an allergic drug reaction has been excluded, then other diseases with eosinophil-rich inflammation should also be excluded, including Hodgkin lymphoma, mast cell disease, Langerhans histiocytosis, and Rosia Dorfman disease.

The recent increase in the use of monoclonal antibody therapies to treat cancer has also led to a number of idiosyncratic hepatitic patterns of DILI. One example is ipilimumab, a monoclonal antibody that activates the immune system by blocking the action of the receptor CTLA-4. This allows the immune system to be more active against the tumor but can also lead to a hepatitic pattern of DILI (Fig. 5.10). The biopsies can show a panlobular hepatitis pattern or a zone 3–predominant hepatitis pattern.[4,5] Another example is infliximab, a monoclonal antibody against TNF alpha, that can lead to an autoimmune-like hepatitis pattern of DILI, one that can also be associated with positive serum ANA and ASMA autoantibodies.[6]

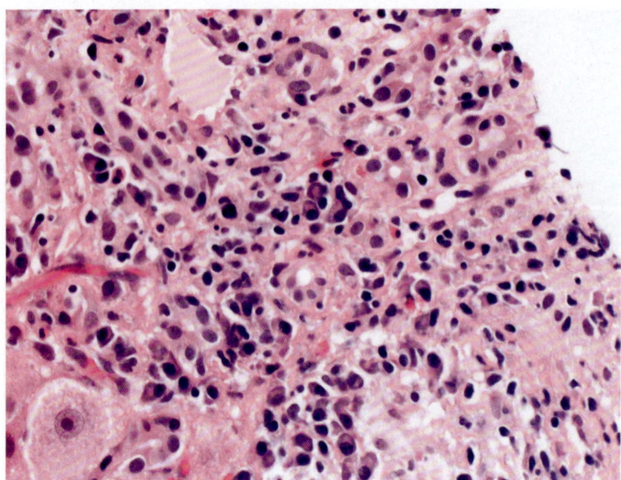

Figure 5.8. **Drug reaction, hepatitic pattern with prominent plasma cells.** The histological findings in this case suggested the possibility of autoimmune hepatitis.

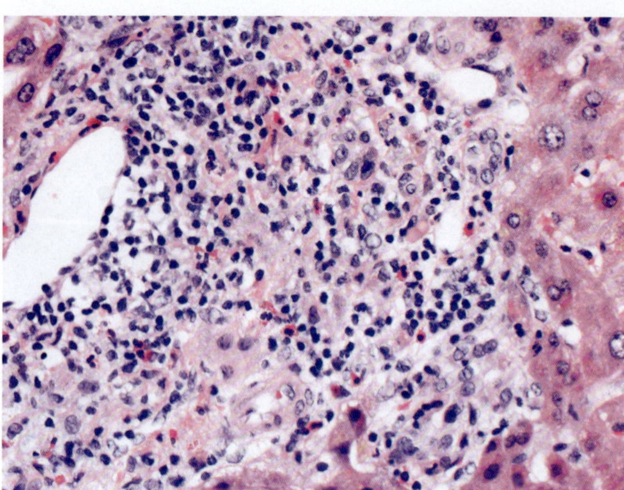

Figure 5.9. **Drug reaction, hepatitic pattern with occasional eosinophils.** This hepatitic pattern of drug-induced liver injury (DILI) showed focal and mildly prominent eosinophils, but overall this degree of eosinophilia is nonspecific for etiology.

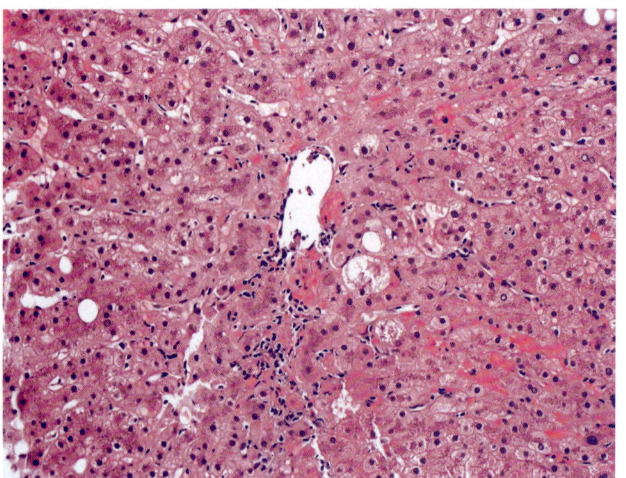

Figure 5.10. **Drug reaction, hepatitic pattern.** This case of ipilimumab-induced drug-induced liver injury (DILI) showed mild lobular hepatitis with a zone 3 accentuation.

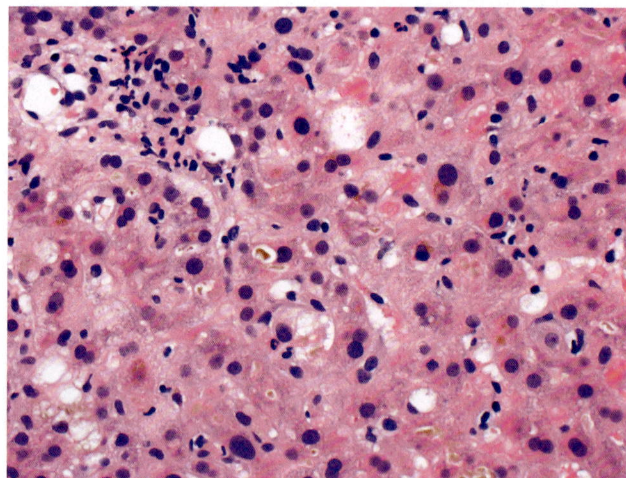

Figure 5.11. **Drug reaction, bland lobular cholestasis pattern.** A case of trenbolone-associated DILI shows moderate lobular cholestasis with minimal inflammatory changes. Trenbolone is a powerful androgen.

The bland lobular cholestasis pattern (Fig. 5.11) usually shows mild to moderate lobular cholestasis with little or no portal or lobular inflammation. Ductular proliferation is also minimal to absent. The liver biopsy should also be carefully examined to rule out drug-induced ductopenia. A CK7 or other keratin stain can be very helpful in excluding ductopenia.

The cholangitic pattern shows portal inflammation with active bile duct injury (Fig. 5.12). The portal inflammation is predominately lymphocytic but occasional eosinophils and neutrophils are common. The bile ducts show active inflammation and injury, usually mild. Focal and mild bile ductular proliferation can also be seen. Antibiotics are the most common cause of this DILI pattern.

In the granuloma pattern of injury, granulomas tend to be either sparse, well-formed, and epithelioid (Fig. 5.13) or more numerous, poorly formed, and associated with brisk lobular inflammation (Fig. 5.14). The granulomas in either case are nonnecrotizing (which would suggest infection) and are not associated with fibrosis (which would suggest sarcoidosis). The location of the granulomas—portal versus lobular—is not helpful in determining etiology. In all cases, infection should be excluded as best as possible with special stains and by serologies. The granulomas should also be polarized for foreign material.

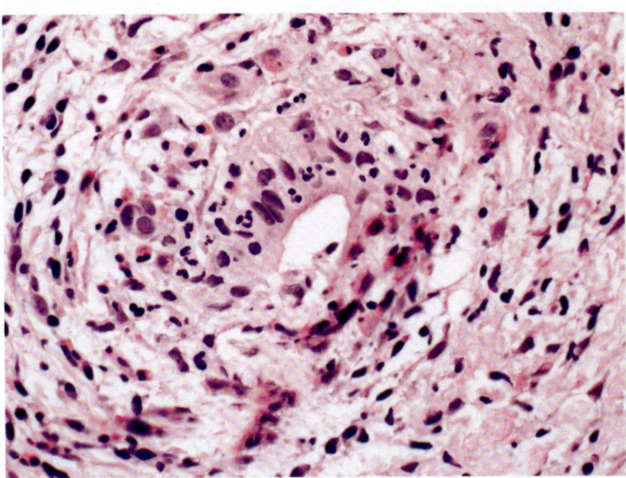

Figure 5.12. **Drug reaction, cholangitic pattern.** A case of amoxicillin-associated drug-induced liver injury (DILI) shows neutrophil rich inflammation and destruction of a bile duct.

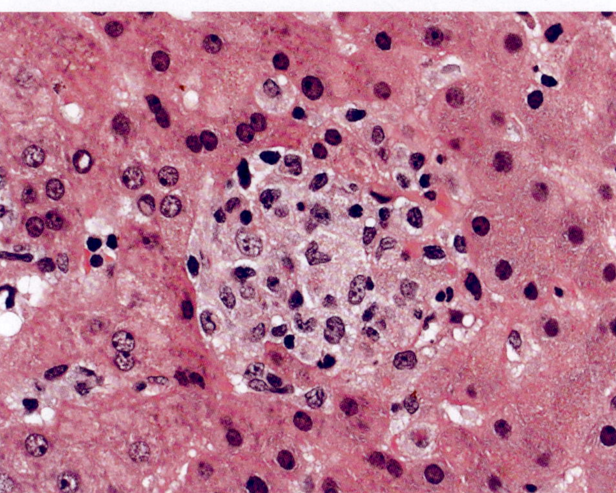

Figure 5.13. **Drug reaction, granulomas.** This case of drug-induced liver injury (DILI) showed occasional well-formed lobular granulomas.

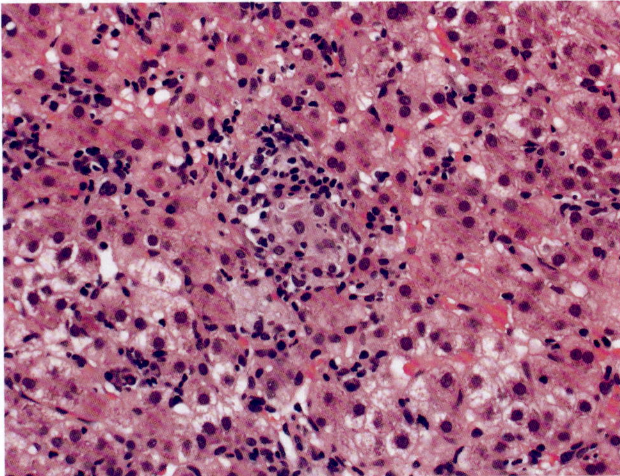

Figure 5.14. **Drug reaction, granulomas.** This case of drug-induced liver injury (DILI) resulted from a herbal remedy and showed marked lobular hepatitis with scattered poorly formed granulomas.

Liver fibrosis is largely inconsistent with an idiosyncratic drug reaction, regardless of the pattern of injury, and suggests an underlying liver disease that may have a superimposed drug reaction or a different process entirely.

RESOLVING PATTERN OF HEPATITIS

The resolving hepatitis pattern of injury is not very specific, but many biopsies that show this pattern end up being idiosyncratic drug reactions. The lobules show occasional scattered pigmented macrophages and minimal to absent inflammation in both the portal tracts and lobules (Fig. 5.15). Occasionally, the portal tracts will continue to show mild nonspecific lymphocytic inflammation. In most cases with the resolving hepatitis pattern, the patient's medication list was modified to eliminate the most likely causes of DILI before the biopsy was obtained and the biopsy shows changes representing clean-up and repair from the prior injury. The changes can be subtle and are often easiest to see on the PASD stain, which will highlight the pigmented macrophages. Immunostains for Ki-67 also tend to show a mild but definite increase in hepatocyte proliferation as part of the reparative process. In cases that initially had a cholestatic pattern of injury or a mixed hepatitic/cholestatic pattern, lobular cholestasis can also be seen, usually mild and patchy.

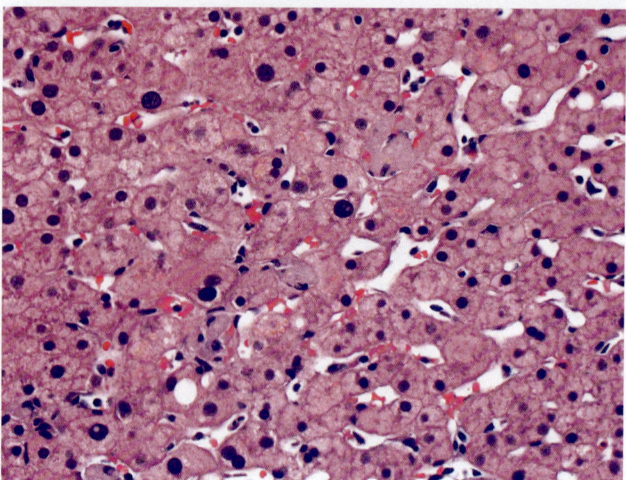

Figure 5.15. **Drug reaction, resolving hepatitis pattern.** In this case, the drug was stopped 6 days before the liver biopsy, and the liver showed no inflammation, only scattered pigmented macrophages.

DIRECT TOXINS

CHECKLIST: Toxins With Zone 1 Pattern of Necrosis

- ☐ Halothane toxicity (zone 3 necrosis more typical)
- ☐ Ferrous iron toxicity
- ☐ White phosphorous toxicity
- ☐ Industrial chemicals such as allyl alcohol
- ☐ Cocaine

CHECKLIST: Toxins With Zone 2 Pattern of Necrosis

- ☐ Laboratory solvents such as dioxane
- ☐ Heavy metals such as berrylium

CHECKLIST: Toxins With Zone 3 Pattern of Necrosis

- ☐ Acetaminophen
- ☐ Alpha-methyl dopa
- ☐ Chloroform
- ☐ Halothane
- ☐ Mushrooms
- ☐ Industrial chemicals such as urethane
- ☐ Cocaine

By definition, direct toxins lead to liver injury in a reproducible and dose-dependent manner. This, however, does not mean that every person gets the exact same degree of injury, only that the degree of injury correlates strongly with dose and duration. By far, acetaminophen is the most common example of a direct toxin injury, but other causes include mushroom poisoning and miscellaneous household and industrial chemicals. An exposure of more than 7.5 g of acetaminophen is usually needed to cause toxicity, with severe injury seen at levels of 15 to 25 g. However, injury can be seen at lower doses when there also

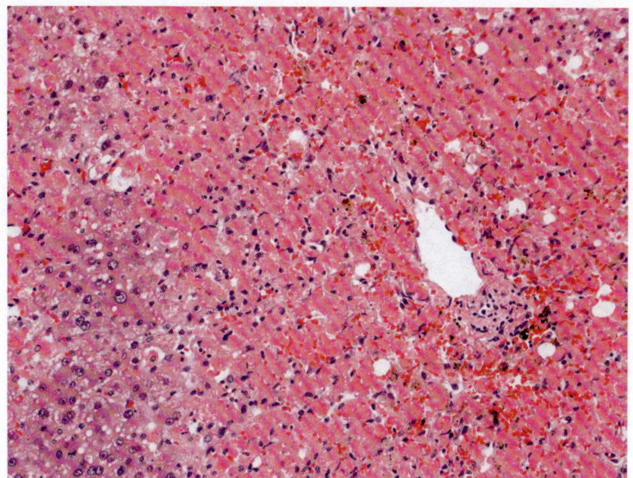

Figure 5.16. **Drug reaction, toxic injury with a zone 3 pattern of necrosis.** This case of acetaminophen drug-induced liver injury (DILI) shows zone 3 necrosis. The central vein in the right middle of the image is surrounded by thick rim of dead hepatocytes. Viable hepatocytes are seen on the left of the image.

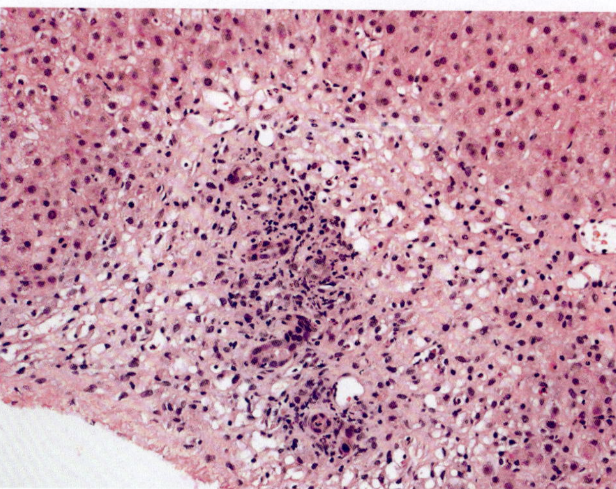

Figure 5.17. **Drug reaction (probable), toxic injury with a zone 1 pattern of necrosis.** The biopsy in this case showed a zone 1 pattern of necrosis. The portal tracts show mild mixed inflammation and mild bile ductular proliferation and were surrounded by a rim of necrosis. The cause was never definitely identified but was thought to be toxin exposure.

is chronic alcohol consumption,[7] fatty liver disease,[8] sleep apnea (commonly present with obesity),[9] or use of drugs that stimulate the P-450 enzyme system, such as isoniazid or phenytoin.[7] Acetaminophen toxicity can be effectively treated with N-Acetylcysteine in the first 24 hours of presentation.

Histologically, the toxic pattern of injury shows bland hepatocyte necrosis with little inflammation. The necrosis in most cases has a zone 3 pattern (Fig. 5.16), but rare and exotic poisons can preferentially lead to zone 1 (Fig. 5.17) or zone 2 necrosis (see checklists).[10,11] In many cases, the cause is not clinically evident at the time of biopsy and requires a careful history that includes work-related and medication-related exposures. Regardless of the toxin, severe injury can lead to panacinar necrosis, where no residual zonation is evident.

ALLERGIC TYPE DRUG REACTIONS

Allergic drug reactions are almost never biopsied because the clinical findings tend to include hives, wheezing, and peripheral eosinophilia that begins within a few hours to days following the start of the new medication. However, if biopsied, the liver shows eosinophil-rich inflammation in the portal tracts and lobules (Fig. 5.18). The eosinophil-rich inflammation will be fairly diffuse.

CHECKLIST: DRESS Syndrome Symptoms

- ☐ Fever of greater than 38°C
- ☐ Rash
- ☐ Lymphadenopathy in at least two locations
- ☐ Peripheral eosinophilia
- ☐ Peripheral thrombocytopenia
- ☐ Peripheral lymphocytosis or lymphopenia
    - ○ Lymphocytes often show cytological atypia

The DRESS syndrome is a rare severe systemic drug reaction with a mortality of up to 10%.[12] The acronym stands for drug reaction with eosinophilia and systemic symptoms. In contrast to most allergic type drug reactions, the DRESS syndrome typically develops later, often three weeks or more following use of the triggering medication. Furthermore,

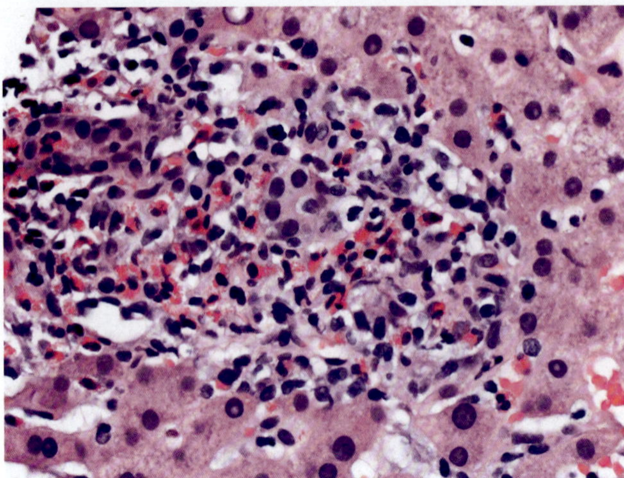

Figure 5.18. **Drug reaction, hepatitic pattern with prominent eosinophils.** Eosinophils were focally prominent in most of the portal tracts of this drug reaction

symptoms can continue for several weeks after the triggering medication is stopped. The liver is commonly involved and biopsies (only rarely performed) show moderate to marked portal eosinophilia along with lobular inflammation that is rich in eosinophils. There can be zone 3 or panacinar liver necrosis in severe cases. One case with zone 1 necrosis has also been reported.[13] Other findings include epithelioid granulomas and lymphocytic cholangitis.[13] There is a very long list of drugs associated with the DRESS syndrome, but common drugs include carbamazepine (27% of cases), allopurinol (11%), lamotrigine (6%), phenobarbital (6%), nevirapine (5%) phenytoin (4%), and abacavir (3%).[14]

PEARLS & PITFALLS

Eosinophils in a liver biopsy specimen can lead to a misdiagnosis of a drug reaction. Of note, eosinophils are routinely present with the hepatitic pattern of injury, regardless of the cause. The eosinophils may even be focally prominent in a portal tract or two. However, these changes are part of the ordinary hepatic pattern of injury and should not be overcalled as indicating a drug reaction. When there truly is an allergic type drug reaction, you will not miss it because the eosinophils will be very prominent.

Another pitfall occurs when patients have a peripheral eosinophilia due to other causes, and a liver biopsy shows increased numbers of eosinophils in the sinusoids. This pattern also does not necessarily suggest an allergic type drug reaction, as there are many causes of peripheral eosinophilia.

OTHER PATTERNS OF INJURY

ISOLATED HYPERAMMONEMIA

Rarely, patients can present with isolated levels of serum ammonia, prompting a biopsy to rule out advanced cirrhosis. The most common causes of this pattern of DILI are valproic acid[15] or infusion of high-dose 5-fluorouracil for chemotherapy.[16] On histology the biopsy is essentially normal, although there can be minimal nonspecific inflammatory changes and sometimes minimal fatty changes (Fig. 5.19). Other diseases that also cause isolated hyperammonemia includes urea cycle defects,[17] portosystemic shunt,[18] or infection—often urinary tract—with urease producing bacteria.[19,20]

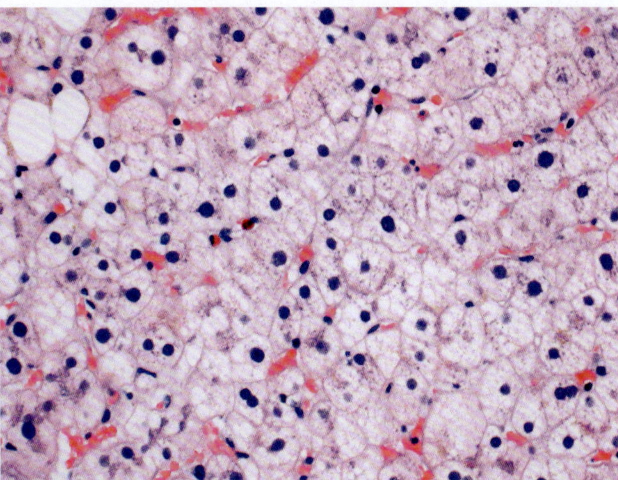

Figure 5.19. **Drug reaction, isolated hyperammonemia.** This drug-induced liver injury (DILI) resulted from valproic acid. The patient presented with isolated hyperammonemia, and the biopsy showed only minimal fatty change with no significant inflammation and no fibrosis.

HYPERVITAMINOSIS A

Too much vitamin A can lead to liver injury with either an acute or chronic presentation. Acute toxicity is rare but results from very high doses of vitamin A, usually >100 times the RDA.[21] Clinical findings with acute toxicity include severe headache, nausea, vertigo, blurred vision, muscle pain, and skin desquamation with alopecia. Liver biopsies are not usually necessary for the diagnosis. On the other hand, chronic toxicity usually requires at least 6 months of exposure with doses >10 times the RDA. Essentially all of these cases result from taking too much preformed vitamin A from vitamins, dietary supplements, or rarely eating too much liver of certain animals such as moose or polar bear. Topical Retin-A has also been associated with stellate cell hyperplasia, the main histological manifestation of hypervitaminosis A.[22] The good news is that eating lots of vegetables is not a risk factor, even those vegetables rich in beta carotenes, as the body tightly controls the conversion of beta carotenes to vitamin A.

With chronic hypervitaminosis A, patients typically present with mild but persistent AST and ALT elevations. In many cases, the patient is unaware that they are taking excessive doses of vitamin A, as it is a component of a general vitamin or nutritional supplement.

The liver biopsy findings are very subtle and are easily missed because the biopsy appears essentially normal in most cases. However, careful examination will show scattered hyperplastic stellate cells, engorged by tiny lipid vacuoles in their cytoplasm (Figs. 5.20 and 5.21). The rest of the biopsy is usually essentially normal, although nodular regenerative hyperplasia has been reported.[23] In most cases there is no fibrosis, as fibrosis requires years to decades of chronic exposure.[23] However, if present, a pericellular-predominant pattern of fibrosis can be seen.

PEARLS & PITFALLS

Most cases submitted for consultation as possible stellate cell hyperplasia are not stellate cell hyperplasia, and even a lot of data in published papers on stellate cell hyperplasia are probably incorrect. In both of these settings, pathologists were tricked, falling into one of two major diagnostic pits.

First, and most importantly, Kupffer cell hyperplasia tricks many pathologists by mimicking stellate cell hyperplasia. Kupffer cell hyperplasia is common in cholestatic liver disease and in most cases of moderate to marked hepatitis. Kupffer cells are considerably bigger than stellate cells in general, but depending on the cut, they can mimic stellate cells. They often have bubbly appearing cytoplasm, further adding to the confusion. Even experienced pathologists can be tricked. For example, studies that list all kinds of associations with stellate cell hyperplasia, from drug reactions, to chronic viral hepatitis, to autoimmune hepatitis, to biliary tract disease, illustrate this point nicely. Thankfully, the overall histological patterns of injury will guide you away from this diagnostic pit in most cases. In addition, Kupffer cell hyperplasia is more diffuse and striking than stellate cell hyperplasia. If in doubt, use a CD68 immunostain to identify the Kupffer cells.

Secondly, if you wait until midafternoon and look for a long time at almost any slide and squinch up your eyes just right, you can often convince yourself that there just may be a stellate cell or two visible on H&E. However, these kinds of observations almost never hold true when you look at the slide again the next morning. As a good rule of thumb, if you cannot see a reasonable number of stellate cells on H&E, typically >10 even in a modestly sized biopsy, typically with at least one per high power field, then be careful as you might be close to the edge of the pit.

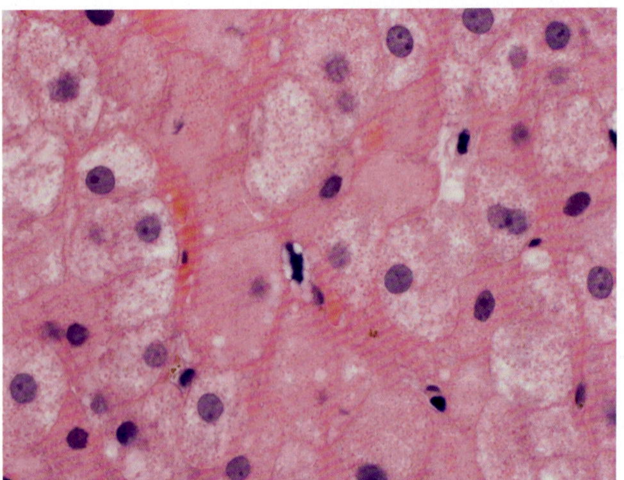

Figure 5.20. **Drug reaction, hypervitaminosis A.** The findings are subtle, but several stellate cells are evident. The stellate cells have hyperchromatic nuclei with numerous tiny cytoplasmic bubbles that often lead to indentations in their nuclei.

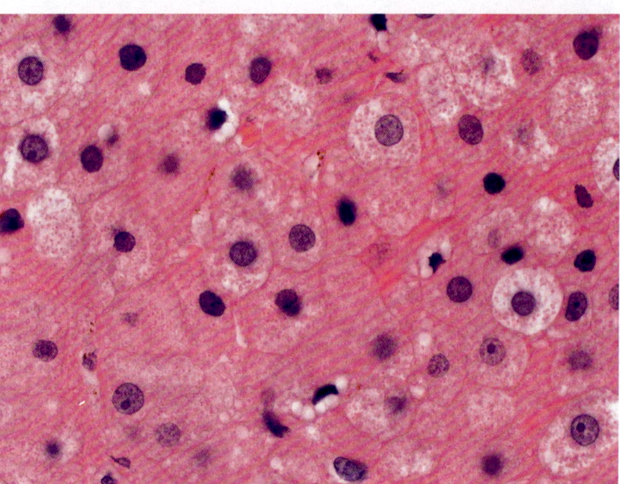

Figure 5.21. **Drug reaction, hypervitaminosis A.** Another example of stellate cell hyperplasia.

Unfortunately, there are no reliable immunostains to identify stellate cells, and the diagnosis is based on subtle H&E findings. Immunostains for smooth muscle actin often highlight sinusoidal cells when there is stellate cell hyperplasia (Fig. 5.22), but the use of this stain has not been well studied as a diagnostic tool. Overall, it seems to be more sensitive than specific. In any case, the diagnosis requires the typical H&E findings and should not be based solely on smooth muscle actin staining.

The clinical team should retake the clinical history, looking for exogenous sources of vitamin A. Of note, blood testing for vitamin A (retinol) is clinically useful primarily to detect vitamin A deficiency and not vitamin A excess. While elevated retinol levels can be seen in the setting of excess vitamin A intake, serum levels can also be normal because a large proportion of vitamin A is bound to plasma proteins and is not detected in routinely used serum tests.[24]

GLYCOGEN PSEUDO–GROUND GLASS CHANGES

Glycogen pseudo–ground glass change is associated with mildly elevated liver enzymes, but it does not lead to progressive liver injury. The ground glass–like changes are commonly persistent on subsequent biopsies, but there is no evidence that these changes lead to fibrosis. Most cases are seen in immunosuppressed individuals who are taking multiple medications. However, no single drug or class of drugs seems to be directly responsible, and at this time, the precise cause of the change remains unclear. The etiology is probably even more complicated, as glycogen pseudo–ground glass change can rarely be seen in individuals on single medications and in those who are not clearly immunosuppressed.

Glycogen pseudo–ground glass change leads to distinctive round hepatocyte inclusions (Fig. 5.23) that resemble the ground glass changes that are seen in some cases of

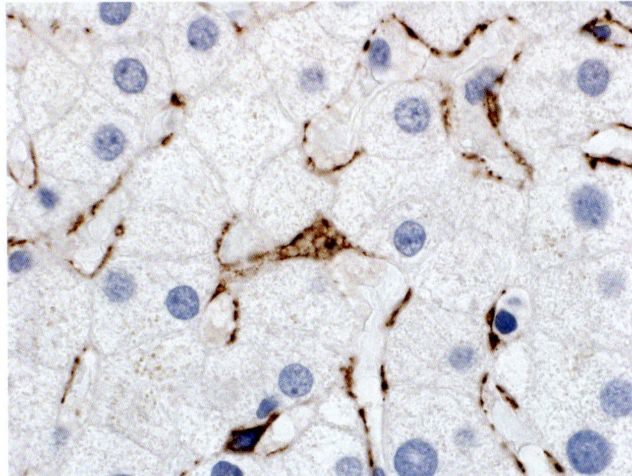

Figure 5.22. **Drug reaction, hypervitaminosis A, immunostain for smooth muscle actin.** An immunostain for smooth muscle actin shows diffuse sinusoidal staining. The specificity and sensitivity of this stain has not been well established, but it can be helpful. It should not be the only diagnostic finding, as H&E changes are the foundation for the diagnosis of stellate cell hyperplasia.

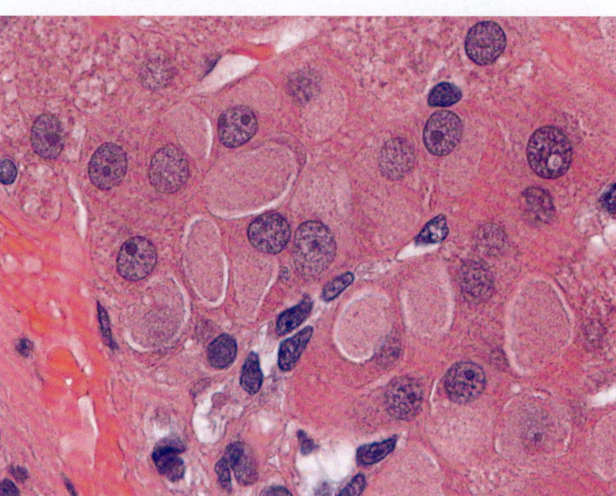

Figure 5.23. **Drug reaction, glycogen pseudo–ground glass change.** The hepatocytes contain single large amphophilic inclusions that fill the cytoplasm.

long-standing chronic hepatitis B infection.[25] Each affected hepatocyte has a single large amphophilic inclusion. The inclusions are glycogen rich, so are PAS positive and diastase sensitive. By electron microscopy, the inclusions are associated with smooth endoplasmic reticulum proliferation containing glycogen with an abnormal folding pattern.[25-27]

The histological differential for glycogen pseudo–ground glass change is primarily chronic hepatitis B–associated ground glass. The histological findings are essentially identical, so immunostains for hepatitis B surface antigen should be performed. Negative hepatitis B serology makes hepatitis B infection unlikely, but serological findings alone do not completely exclude HBV,[28] so immunostains are still important. The histological differential in theory also includes other drug effects such as cyanamide (used as an alcohol deterrent in some countries), genetic disorders such as LaFora bodies, fibrinogen storage disease, glycogen storage disease type IV, and reactive changes associated with uremia. However, at a practical level, the clinical situations are so distinct that there is rarely, if ever, any real question as to the classification of the inclusions (Table 5.2).

OTHER DRUG-INDUCED SMOOTH ENDOPLASMIC RETICULUM PROLIFERATIONS

In addition to glycogen pseudo–ground glass, two other drug-induced changes are associated with striking smooth endoplasmic reticulum proliferations that are evident on H&E. Neither is very common. Both can be associated with mild liver enzyme elevations, but overall they do not appear to cause much injury and have not been associated with fibrosis. Thus, these changes may be more of an adaptive change than an injury pattern. The first pattern is called *induced hepatocytes*, where the cytoplasm shows a diffuse gray homogenous change, but there are no well-developed inclusions (Fig. 5.24). The extent of the cytoplasmic changes are variable, ranging from milder cases that can show a zone 3 accentuation of affected hepatocytes to more severe case where essentially all hepatocyte are involved. Overall, the induced hepatocyte pattern of injury is most commonly seen with the use of phenobarbital and barbiturates.[29]

A second pattern is similar in many ways to induced hepatocytes, but leads to a distinctive "two-tone" appearance to the hepatocytes (Figs. 5.25 and 5.26), with about half of the cytoplasm showing the normal cytoplasmic color, while the other half shows smooth endoplasmic reticulum proliferation. The prominent endoplasmic reticulum proliferation can affect either side of the hepatocyte, sometimes the side next to the bile canaliculi and in other cases the side near the sinusoids. Too few cases have been reported to know if there are any strong clinical or medication associations.

TABLE 5.2: Differential for Pseudo–Ground Glass Inclusions in Hepatocytes

Type of Inclusion	PAS	PASD	HBsAg	Other Stains
Glycogen pseudo–ground glass	Positive	Sensitive	Negative	
Hepatitis B ground glass	Positive	Sensitive	**Positive**	
Cyanamide	Positive	Sensitive	Negative	
Fibrinogen	**Negative**	Not applicable	Negative	Fibrinogen positive
Type IV glycogen storage disease	Positive	Partially sensitive	Negative	Colloidal iron negative
LaFora	Positive	**Diastase resistant**	Negative	Colloidal iron positive
Uremia	Positive	Sensitive	Negative	

The diastase reaction can vary between laboratories, so the results are not always consistent. PAS stains are also useful when they are negative, suggesting fibrinogen storage disease.

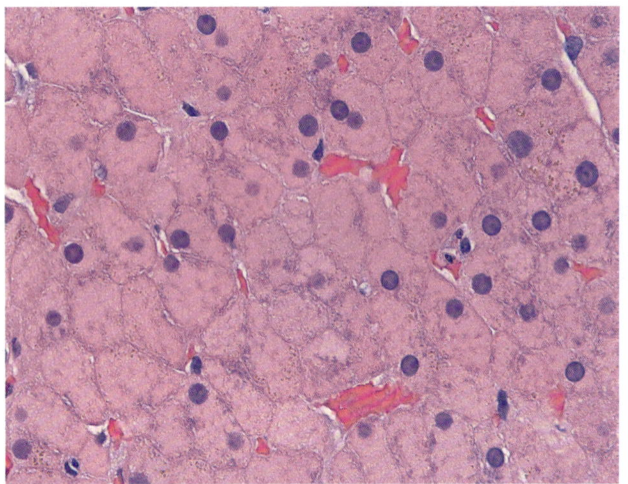

Figure 5.24. **Drug reaction, induced hepatocytes.** The hepatocytes in this case of phenobarbital drug-induced liver injury (DILI) show a diffuse glassy cytoplasmic change without well-defined inclusions.

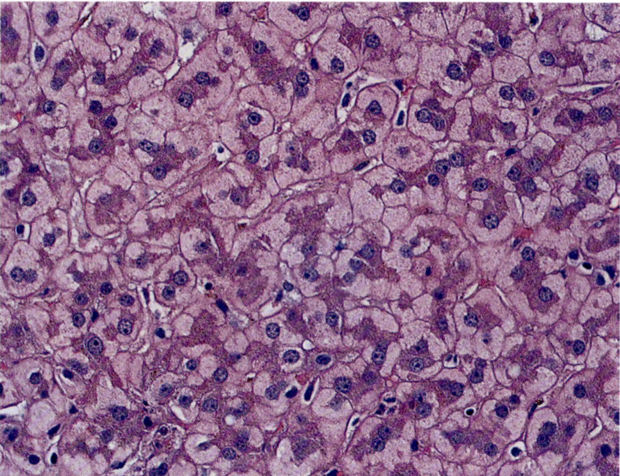

Figure 5.25. **Drug reaction, "two-tone" hepatocytes.** The hepatocytes have a distinctive appearance with each cell having two colors: (1) pale cytoplasm with (2) a purple accentuation around the bile canaliculi.

GLYCOGENIC HEPATOPATHY

In this pattern of injury, the hepatocytes show abundant pale cytoplasm as a result of glycogen accumulation (Fig. 5.27). In most cases of DILI with a glycogenic hepatopathy pattern of injury, the changes are seen after a bolus of ccorticosteroids for treatment of either autoimmune hepatitis or allograft liver rejection. The overall findings are histologically very similar to the pattern of injury seen in glycogenic hepatopathy that results from poorly controlled diabetes mellitus. With drug-induced glycogenic hepatopathy, the liver glycogenosis is usually more subtle than diabetes mellitus–associated glycogenic hepatopathy and often shows a zone 3 accentuation. With drug-induced glycogenic hepatopathy, hepatic enzymes and the histological findings quickly return to baseline in a few days.

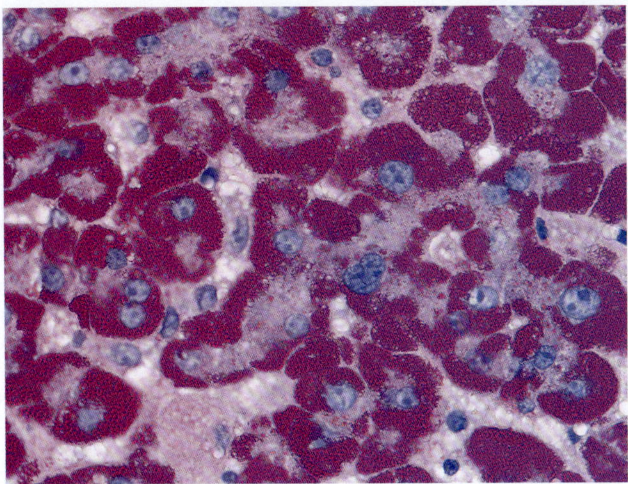

Figure 5.26. **Drug reaction, "two-tone" hepatocytes, PAS stain.** The PAS stain highlights the parts of the cytoplasm that were pale gray on H&E, same case as Figure 5.25.

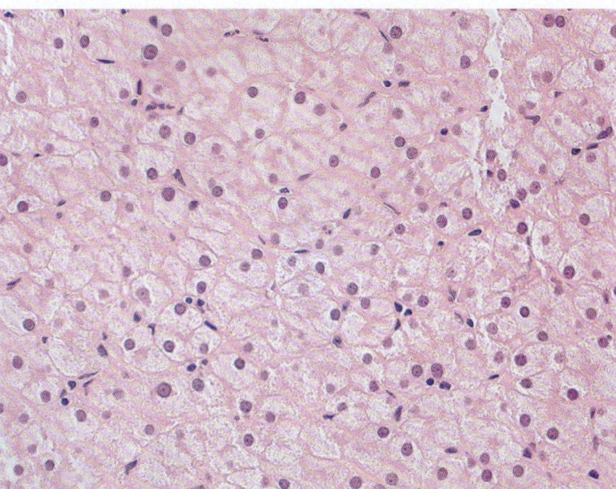

Figure 5.27. **Drug reaction, glycogenic hepatopathy.** The hepatocytes show diffuse clear cell change that resulted from glycogen accumulation after the use of high-dose corticosteroids.

MACROVESICULAR STEATOSIS

Many different drugs have been associated with macrovesicular steatosis and/or steatohepatitis, but in most cases, the patients have other risk factors for fatty liver disease and it is challenging to precisely ascribe the correct percentage of blame on the drug. In many cases, there appears to be a synergistic effect between the drug and other risk factors for fatty liver disease. Examples of drugs that have primarily a synergist effect include estrogens, tamoxifen, and nifedipine. One study estimated that 2% of all cases of nonalcoholic fatty liver disease resulted from DILI.[30] In general, most drugs cause steatosis rather than steatohepatitis, but there are exceptions. For example, amiodarone and irinotecan can cause steatohepatitis with fat, ballooned hepatocytes, and Mallory hyaline.

Fatty liver disease develops in up to 4% of individuals on chronic amiodarone therapy.[31,32] Amiodarone is one of the rare drugs that has a very long half-life and becomes concentrated in the liver over time. The risk for fatty liver disease is driven by the duration of therapy and total accumulated dose and not so much by the current dosage. In most cases, fatty liver disease does not develop until there has been at least a year of use.[30] Histologically, the balloon cells and Mallory hyaline tend to be much more striking than the macrovesicular steatosis (Figs. 5.28 and 5.29) and can suggest alcoholic liver disease.[33] In fact, some cases have mostly hepatocyte ballooning with only minimal fatty change. Overall, the portal and lobular inflammation is patchy, mild, and mostly lymphocytic.

Chemotherapy can also lead to fatty liver disease, a pattern sometimes called CASH, which stands for chemotherapy-associated steatohepatitis. Most cases of CASH arise in individuals who also have risk factors for the metabolic syndrome,[34] indicating a synergistic effect between the metabolic syndrome and chemotherapy. The most common chemotherapy association is with irinotecan and oxaliplatin.[35-37] Most cases of CASH are found in the background livers of resected colorectal metastases. The fatty liver disease is histologically identical to that arising in other settings; other than that additional changes of sinusoidal dilation may also be present if there also is chemotherapy-associated sinusoidal obstruction syndrome. The lobules can show anywhere from mild to marked steatosis, and some cases will show additional changes of steatohepatitis. Steatohepatitis, especially if there is a significant lobular inflammation component, is associated with increased morbidity and mortality after partial hepatectomy of the liver for metastases.[37]

MICROVESICULAR STEATOSIS

Microvesicular steatosis results from mitochondrial injuries that impair normal lipid metabolism, leading to numerous tiny vacuoles that fill the hepatocyte cytoplasm. The injury can be diffuse within the lobules, but milder cases often show a zone 3 accentuation. Focal macrovesicular steatosis is also common, but the microvesicular component

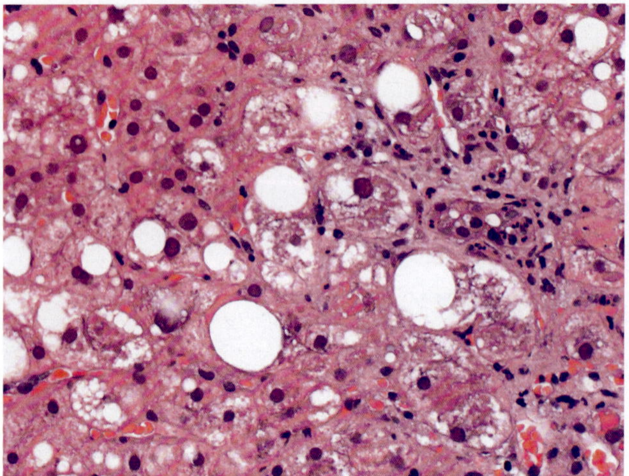

Figure 5.28. **Drug reaction, amiodarone.** The hepatocytes show mild macrovesicular steatosis with numerous ballooned hepatocytes and abundant Mallory hyaline.

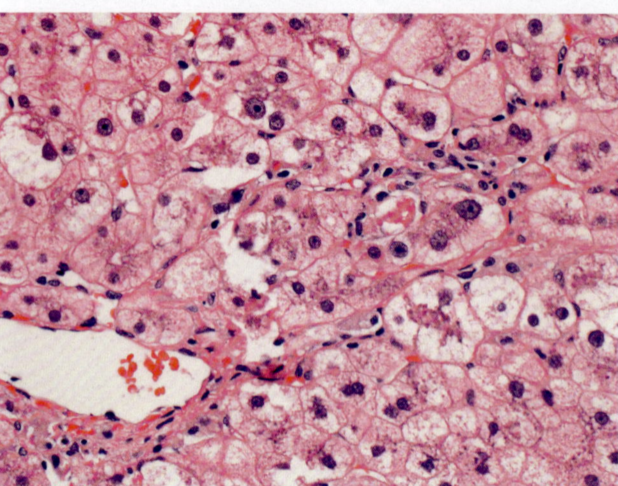

Figure 5.29. **Drug reaction, amiodarone.** Another case shows almost no steatosis but numerous ballooned hepatocytes and abundant Mallory hyaline.

should be striking for this diagnosis. The most common drugs causing this pattern of injury are valproic acid, tetracycline, and zivodine. The histological differential also includes acute fatty liver of pregnancy and acute foamy alcoholic degeneration, but the clinical settings are distinct, and this theoretical differential is rarely a practical concern.

PHOSPHOLIPIDIOSIS

Some of the drugs that cause fatty liver disease also cause a pattern of injury called phospholipidosis. This pattern of injury can also be an isolated finding, without a background of steatosis. In either case, the Kupffer cells are hyperplastic and have a foamy appearance to their cytoplasm (Figs. 5.30 and 5.31). The degree of phospholipidosis in any given biopsy will vary from subtle to striking. Cases with striking findings are the most likely to lead to diagnostic challenges, as they can sometimes mimic a storage disorder. However, the clinical context and the background liver findings will point to the correct diagnosis. Phospholipidosis results from the accumulation of lamellar inclusions in lysosomes, and some authors feel it is more likely to be an adaptive change rather than a true injury pattern. In any case, when it is prominent I still include the finding in the pathology report. The list of drugs associated with phospholipidosis is very long,[38] but examples include amiodarone, perhexiline maleate, and diethylaminoethoxyhexestrol.

DUCTOPENIC PATTERN

This pattern of DILI is defined by reduced numbers of bile ducts. They do not have to be all gone, but in general at least 50% of the portal tracts should be missing their bile ducts. The disease begins with loss of the smallest branches of the biliary tree and then progress to include many of the medium-sized branches. The largest bile ducts are typically still present in livers with ductopenia, although they are hardly ever sampled on a peripheral needle biopsy. The liver biopsy often shows other mild and nonspecific changes including patchy portal chronic inflammation and sometimes mild fatty changes. Cholate stasis is not uncommon, but cholestasis is not present in most cases until there has been long-standing and severe bile duct loss.

Immunostains are strongly recommended to support the diagnosis. A CK7 will help identify bile ducts (reduced in ductopenia) and intermediate hepatocytes (present in ductopenia), as well as a copper stain, which will show periportal copper deposition in most cases. Also, the serum alkaline phosphatase levels are invariably elevated when there is established ductopenia.

The biopsy should also be searched for findings that would suggest an alternative diagnosis to DILI-related ductopenia. These changes include more than focal and minimal bile

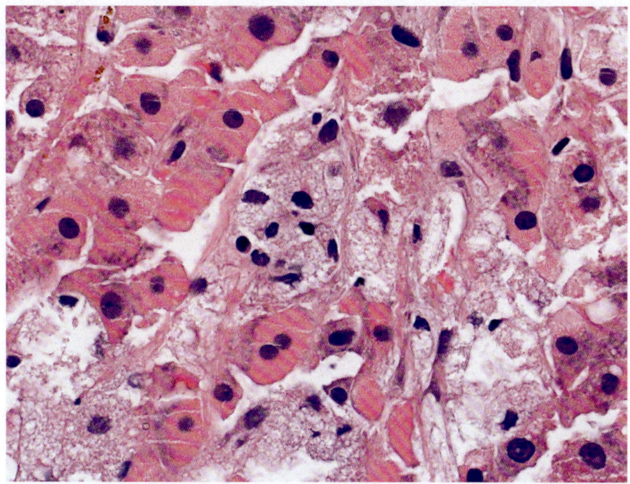

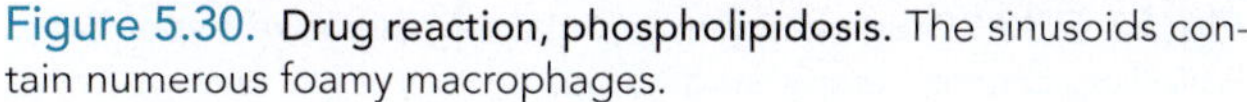

Figure 5.30. **Drug reaction, phospholipidosis.** The sinusoids contain numerous foamy macrophages.

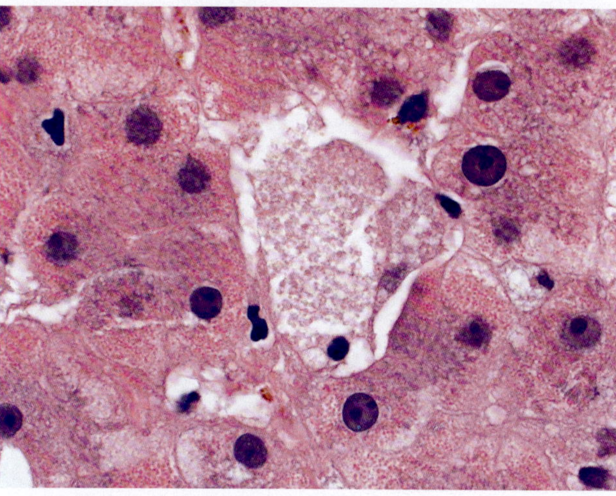

Figure 5.31. **Drug reaction, phospholipidosis.** A higher power view of the foamy macrophages in the sinusoids.

ductular proliferation, florid bile duct lesions, bile duct duplication, onion skinning fibrosis, or fibro-obliterative duct lesions. Also, fibrosis is not part of the typical DILI pattern of ductopenia, so any degree of significant fibrosis suggests an additional or alternative source of liver injury.

VASCULAR CHANGES ASSOCIATED WITH DILI

There are a number of different vascular patterns of injury that have been associated with DILI. These injury patterns tend to fall into one of four major categories: (1) veno-occlusive/sinusoidal obstructive injury; (2) nodular regenerative hyperplasia; (3) sinusoidal congestion; (4) and peliosis hepatis.

The veno-occlusive/sinusoidal obstructive injury pattern is most commonly associated with chemotherapy or with herbal remedies. Oxaliplatin is one of the more common chemotherapy agents that has been associated with a sinusoidal obstructive injury pattern, and the changes often can be identified in the background livers of resection specimens for metastatic colon adenocarcinoma. The liver parenchyma shows variable zone 3 sinusoidal dilatation and congestion (Fig. 5.32). The zone 3 hepatocytes can also show mild atrophy and changes of nodular regenerative hyperplasia may be present.[34,35,39] The central veins are often within normal limits, but occasional occlusions by loose collagen might be found.

The nodular regenerative hyperplasia pattern of injury is also most commonly found with chemotherapy or other drugs that cause vascular injury with little inflammation (Fig. 5.33). Sinusoidal dilation is not a specific pattern of injury, of course, but can be a result of DILI, especially estrogens (Fig. 5.34). The peliosis hepatis pattern (Fig. 5.35) has been associated primarily with estrogen, androgens, azathioprine, and corticosteroids.

MEDICATIONS ASSOCIATED WITH FIBROSIS

Most cases of DILI do not lead to fibrosis. There are many case reports, small case series, and event registry–based studies that have linked all kinds of DILI to fibrosis, but in most cases, the evidence is not compelling, as affected individuals also have comorbidities that are known to be fibrogenic, such as the metabolic syndrome or autoimmune hepatitis. Nonetheless there are a few medications that have been strongly linked to a risk for fibrosis, in particular methotrexate (discussed in chapter 6, Fatty Liver Disease) and amiodarone (discussed above).

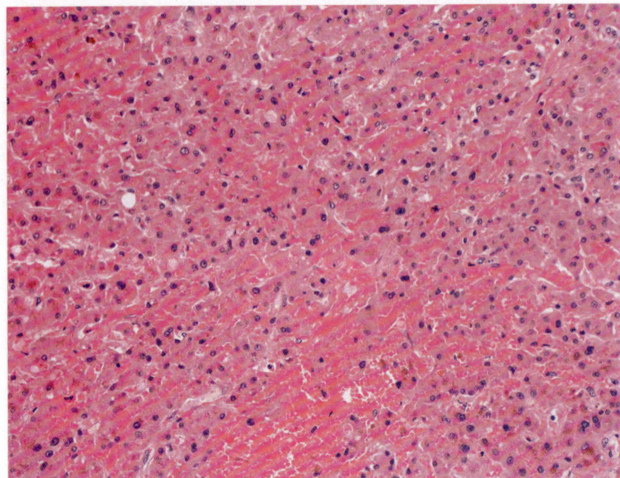

Figure 5.32. Drug reaction, VOD. The liver parenchyma shows mild zone 3 sinusoidal dilatation and congestion in this case of Oxaliplatin-associated veno-occlusive disease.

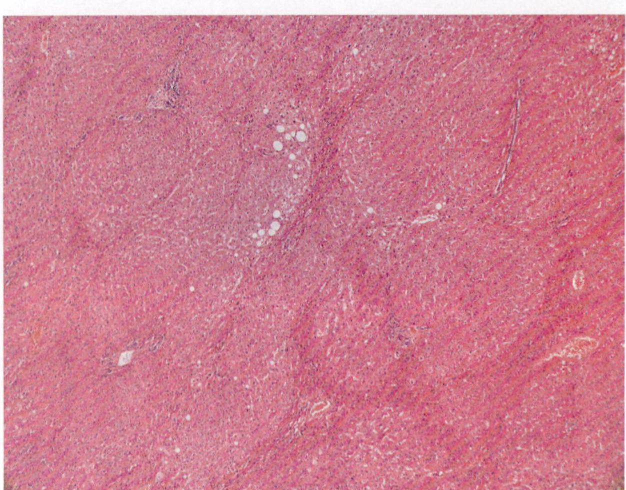

Figure 5.33. Drug reaction, nodular regenerative hyperplasia. Following chemotherapy, surgery was performed to remove a metastatic deposit of colon carcinoma. The background liver showed nodular regenerative hyperplasia.

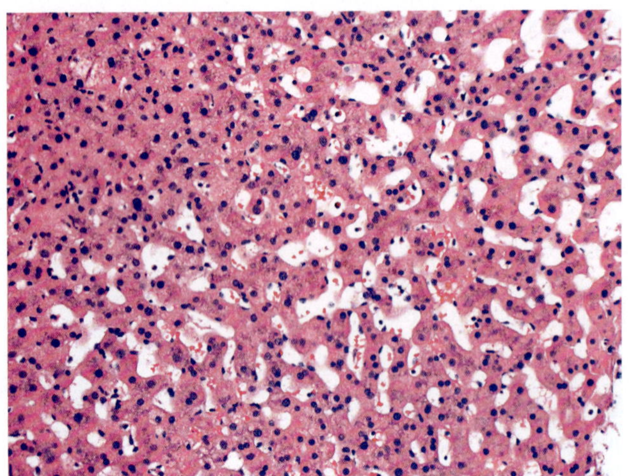

Figure 5.34. Drug reaction, sinusoidal dilatation. Following the start of oral contraception, a patient presented with hepatomegaly and mildly elevated liver enzymes. The biopsy showed patchy moderate sinusoidal dilation.

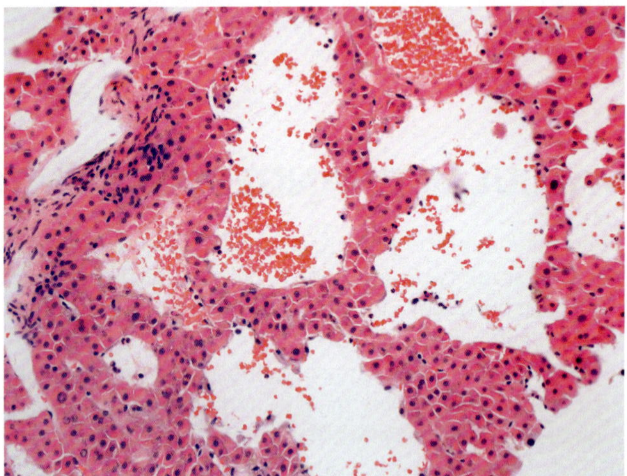

Figure 5.35. Drug reaction, peliosis hepatis. The lobules show dilated, blood-filled spaces unlined by endothelial cells. This case resulted from androgen use.

NEAR MISSES

CASE 1. A 57-year-old woman had mild but persistent elevations in AST and ALT, approximately 2X ULN, with minimally elevated total bilirubin levels and nearly normal alkaline phosphate levels. Viral and autoimmune serologies were negative. She was taking no medications. She was otherwise healthy and was in fact very health conscious in terms of diet and exercise.

The biopsy showed mild lobular inflammation along with pigmented lobular macrophages (Fig. 5.36), consistent with ongoing mildly active hepatitis. There was mild patchy portal chronic inflammation. The inflammation in the lobules and portal tracts was lymphocytic, with no plasma cell enrichment. There were no findings to suggest any other pattern of injury, so the case was signed out as a mild nonspecific hepatitis. Since viral infection and autoimmune hepatitis studies were all negative, and since the patient was not taking any medications, the differential was felt to include the possibility of inflammation of the small bowel, such as can be seen with Crohn disease or celiac disease. However, follow-up studies were negative for inflammation of the gastrointestinal (GI) tract. The clinicians requested rereview of the biopsy, which identified nothing additional. At the next

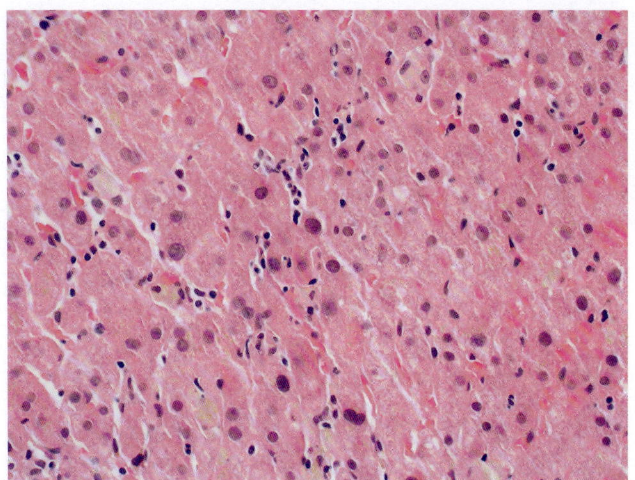

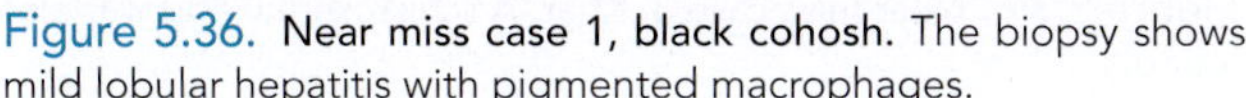

Figure 5.36. **Near miss case 1, black cohosh.** The biopsy shows mild lobular hepatitis with pigmented macrophages.

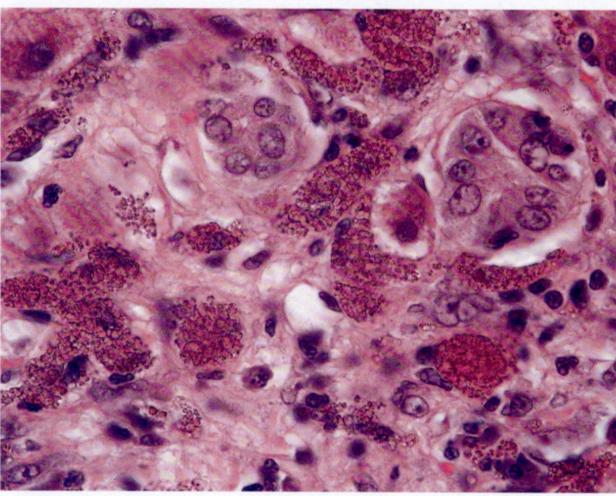

Figure 5.37. **Near miss case 2, Thorotrast.** The granular foreign material is Thorotrast.

clinical visit, a careful history taking revealed that the patient was using black cohosh tea and black cohosh pills as a remedy for menopausal symptoms. Liver enzymes normalized after stopping the herbal remedy.

Black cohosh can lead to liver injury, where it usually shows a hepatitic pattern of injury. The hepatitis can be severe, leading to liver failure.[40] Sometimes, the clinical presentation and histological findings can mimic autoimmune hepatitis.[41] This case illustrates the importance of considering herbal remedies as a cause of liver injury, even when the patient reports the use of no medications.

CASE 2. An 80-year-old man presented with a liver mass. A biopsy showed a cholangiocarcinoma, which subsequently underwent resection. In the background of the cholangiocarcinoma were focal clusters of macrophages with foreign material (Fig. 5.37). Iron and copper stains were negative. The specimen was signed out as cholangiocarcinoma, with a comment in the microscopic description about clusters of macrophages with foreign material. The case was subsequently presented at tumor board. There it emerged that the patient had a remote history of intestinal vascular anomalies, which were diagnosed as a child. A review of the histology recognized the material as Thorotrast.

Thorotrast is a thorium-based radioactive contrast agent that was used in imaging studies, particularly for angiography, from the 1930s up through the 1950s. Unfortunately, thorium dioxide particles are retained in reticulendothelial system of the body, in many cases for life, and can continue to emit radioactive particles, leading to malignancies, in particular angiosarcomas and cholangiocarcinoma.[42,43]

CASE 3. A 49-year-old man presented with reflux symptoms, and endoscopy showed reflux disease as well as esophageal varices. Subsequent workup showed a low platelet count and splenomegaly. Viral serologies and autoimmune studies were negative. There was an equivocal history of alcohol use. A liver biopsy was obtained. The biopsy showed cirrhosis. The portal tracts showed patchy moderate portal chronic inflammation (Fig. 5.38), along with mild patchy lobular inflammation. Plasma cells were mildly prominent in a few of the portal tracts. There was no evidence for fatty liver disease. An incidental degenerating parasitic egg, consistent with schistosomiasis, was also found (Fig. 5.39). There were no other significant histological findings, and the case was signed out descriptively.

After the pathology report had been signed out, more information became available. The patient was an immigrant from Ethiopia who regularly chewed Khat leaves. Khat is a mild stimulant and chronic use shows a strong and dose-dependent association with the development of chronic liver disease.[44] Patients can present with either acute[45,46] or chronic hepatitis with advanced fibrosis.[47,48] The histological findings of Khat use have not been well described but mostly show a nonspecific hepatitis pattern of injury that can range from mild to severe. In some cases, plasma cells can be focally prominent. Fibrosis can range from none to cirrhosis.

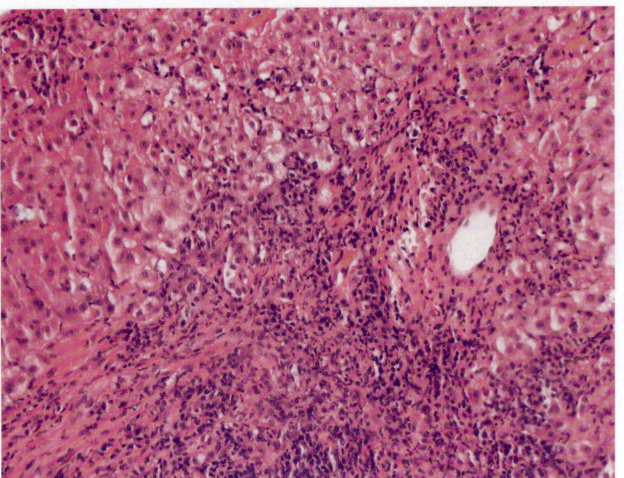

Figure 5.38. **Near miss case 3, Khat.** There is patchy moderate portal and mild lobular chronic inflammation.

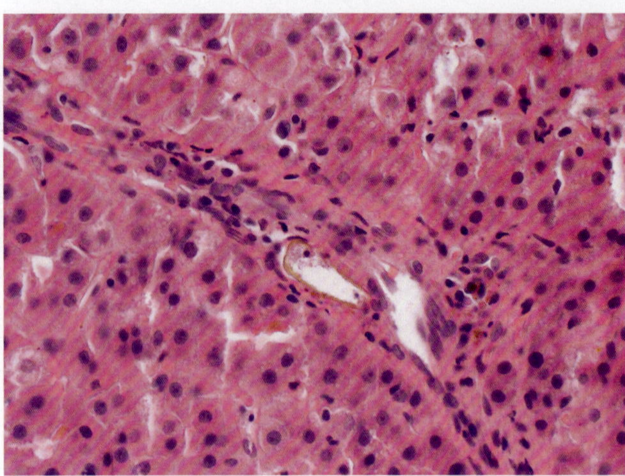

Figure 5.39. **Near miss case 3, Khat.** A schistosomal egg was also found.

References

1. Chalasani N, Fontana RJ, Bonkovsky HL, et al. Causes, clinical features, and outcomes from a prospective study of drug-induced liver injury in the United States. *Gastroenterology*. 2008;135:1924-1934, 34 e1-4.
2. Molleston JP, Fontana RJ, Lopez MJ, Kleiner DE, Gu J, Chalasani N. Characteristics of idiosyncratic drug-induced liver injury in children: results from the DILIN prospective study. *J Pediatr Gastroenterol Nutr*. 2011;53:182-189.
3. Davern TJ, Chalasani N, Fontana RJ, et al. Acute hepatitis E infection accounts for some cases of suspected drug-induced liver injury. *Gastroenterology*. 2011;141:1665-1672 e1-9.
4. Johncilla M, Misdraji J, Pratt DS, et al. Ipilimumab-associated hepatitis: clinicopathologic characterization in a series of 11 cases. *Am J Surg Pathol*. 2015;39:1075-1084.
5. Kleiner DE, Berman D. Pathologic changes in ipilimumab-related hepatitis in patients with metastatic melanoma. *Dig Dis Sci*. 2012;57:2233-2240.
6. Germano V, Picchianti Diamanti A, Baccano G, et al. Autoimmune hepatitis associated with infliximab in a patient with psoriatic arthritis. *Ann Rheum Dis*. 2005;64:1519-1520.
7. Yoon E, Babar A, Choudhary M, Kutner M, Pyrsopoulos N. Acetaminophen-induced hepatotoxicity: a comprehensive update. *J Clin Transl Hepatol*. 2016;4:131-142.
8. Michaut A, Moreau C, Robin MA, Fromenty B. Acetaminophen-induced liver injury in obesity and nonalcoholic fatty liver disease. *Liver Int*. 2014;34:e171-e179.
9. Savransky V, Reinke C, Jun J, et al. Chronic intermittent hypoxia and acetaminophen induce synergistic liver injury in mice. *Exp Physiol*. 2009;94:228-239.
10. Pestaner JP, Ishak KG, Mullick FG, Centeno JA. Ferrous sulfate toxicity: a review of autopsy findings. *Biol Trace Elem Res*. 1999;69:191-198.
11. Ramachandran R, Kakar S. Histological patterns in drug-induced liver disease. *J Clin Pathol*. 2009;62:481-492.
12. Lopez-Rocha E, Blancas L, Rodriguez-Mireles K, et al. Prevalence of DRESS syndrome. *Rev Alerg Mex*. 2014;61:14-23.
13. Ichai P, Laurent-Bellue A, Saliba F, et al. Acute liver failure/injury related to drug reaction with eosinophilia and systemic symptoms: outcomes and prognostic factors. *Transplantation*. 2017;101:1830-1837.
14. Cacoub P, Musette P, Descamps V, et al. The DRESS syndrome: a literature review. *Am J Med*. 2011;124:588-597.
15. Wadzinski J, Franks R, Roane D, Bayard M. Valproate-associated hyperammonemic encephalopathy. *J Am Board Fam Med*. 2007;20:499-502.
16. Nott L, Price TJ, Pittman K, Patterson K, Fletcher J. Hyperammonemia encephalopathy: an important cause of neurological deterioration following chemotherapy. *Leuk Lymphoma*. 2007;48:1702-1711.

17. Acikalin A, Disel NR, Direk EC, Ilginel MT, Sebe A, Bicakci S. A rare cause of postpartum coma: isolated hyperammonemia due to urea cycle disorder. *Am J Emerg Med.* 2015.

18. Belenky A, Igov I, Konstantino Y, et al. Endovascular diagnosis and intervention in patients with isolated hyperammonemia, with or without ascites, after liver transplantation. *J Vasc Interv Radiol.* 2009;20:259-263.

19. Cordano C, Traverso E, Calabro V, et al. Recurring hyperammonemic encephalopathy induced by bacteria usually not producing urease. *BMC Res Notes.* 2014;7:324.

20. Albersen M, Joniau S, Van Poppel H, Cuyle PJ, Knockaert DC, Meersseman W. Urea-splitting urinary tract infection contributing to hyperammonemic encephalopathy. *Nat Clin Pract Urol.* 2007;4:455-458.

21. Penniston KL, Tanumihardjo SA. The acute and chronic toxic effects of vitamin A. *Am J Clin Nutr.* 2006;83:191-201.

22. Levine PH, Delgado Y, Theise ND, West AB. Stellate-cell lipidosis in liver biopsy specimens. Recognition and significance. *Am J Clin Pathol.* 2003;119:254-258.

23. Geubel AP, De Galocsy C, Alves N, Rahier J, Dive C. Liver damage caused by therapeutic vitamin A administration: estimate of dose-related toxicity in 41 cases. *Gastroenterology.* 1991;100:1701-1709.

24. Miksad R, de Ledinghen V, McDougall C, Fiel I, Rosenberg H. Hepatic hydrothorax associated with vitamin a toxicity. *J Clin Gastroenterol.* 2002;34:275-279.

25. Wisell J, Boitnott J, Haas M, et al. Glycogen pseudoground glass change in hepatocytes. *Am J Surg Pathol.* 2006;30:1085-1090.

26. O'Shea AM, Wilson GJ, Ling SC, Minassian BA, Turnbull J, Cutz E. Lafora-like ground-glass inclusions in hepatocytes of pediatric patients: a report of two cases. *Pediatr Dev Pathol.* 2007;10:351-357.

27. Bejarano PA, Garcia MT, Rodriguez MM, Ruiz P, Tzakis AG. Liver glycogen bodies: ground-glass hepatocytes in transplanted patients. *Virchows Arch.* 2006;449:539-545.

28. Torbenson M, Thomas DL. Occult hepatitis B. *Lancet Infect Dis.* 2002;2:479-486.

29. Jezequel AM, Librari ML, Mosca P, Novelli G, Lorenzini L, Orlandi F. Changes induced in human liver by long-term anticonvulsant therapy Functional and ultrastructural data. *Liver.* 1984 4:307-317.

30. Farrell GC. Drugs and steatohepatitis. *Semin Liver Dis.* 2002;22:185-194.

31. Lewis JH, Ranard RC, Caruso A, et al. Amiodarone hepatotoxicity: prevalence and clinicopathologic correlations among 104 patients. *Hepatology.* 1989;9:679-685.

32. Kum LC, Chan WW, Hui HH, et al. Prevalence of amiodarone-related hepatotoxicity in 720 Chinese patients with or without baseline liver dysfunction. *Clin Cardiol.* 2006;29:295-299.

33. Lewis JH, Mullick F, Ishak KG, et al. Histopathologic analysis of suspected amiodarone hepatotoxicity. *Hum Pathol.* 1990;21:59-67.

34. Ryan P, Nanji S, Pollett A, et al. Chemotherapy-induced liver injury in metastatic colorectal cancer: semiquantitative histologic analysis of 334 resected liver specimens shows that vascular injury but not steatohepatitis is associated with preoperative chemotherapy. *Am J Surg Pathol.* 2010;34:784-791.

35. Vauthey JN, Pawlik TM, Ribero D, et al. Chemotherapy regimen predicts steatohepatitis and an increase in 90-day mortality after surgery for hepatic colorectal metastases. *J Clin Oncol.* 2006;24:2065-2072.

36. Pawlik TM, Olino K, Gleisner AL, Torbenson M, Schulick R, Choti MA. Preoperative chemotherapy for colorectal liver metastases: impact on hepatic histology and postoperative outcome. *J Gastrointest Surg.* 2007;11:860-868.

37. Zhao J, van Mierlo KMC, Gomez-Ramirez J, et al. Systematic review of the influence of chemotherapy-associated liver injury on outcome after partial hepatectomy for colorectal liver metastases. *Br J Surg.* 2017;104:990-1002.

38. Reasor MJ, Hastings KL, Ulrich RG. Drug-induced phospholipidosis: issues and future directions. *Expert Opin Drug Saf.* 2006;5:567-583.

39. Morris-Stiff G, White AD, Gomez D, et al. Nodular regenerative hyperplasia (NRH) complicating oxaliplatin chemotherapy in patients undergoing resection of colorectal liver metastases. *Eur J Surg Oncol.* 2014;40:1016-1020.

40. Pierard S, Coche JC, Lanthier P, et al. Severe hepatitis associated with the use of black cohosh: a report of two cases and an advice for caution. *Eur J Gastroenterol Hepatol.* 2009;21:941-945.

41. Franco DL, Kale S, Lam-Himlin DM, Harrison ME. Black cohosh hepatotoxicity with autoimmune hepatitis presentation. *Case Rep Gastroenterol*. 2017;11:23-28.

42. Fukumoto M. Radiation pathology: from thorotrast to the future beyond radioresistance. *Pathol Int*. 2014;64:251-262.

43. Takekawa S, Ueda Y, Hiramatsu Y, Komiyama K, Munechika H. History note: tragedy of Thorotrast. *Jpn J Radiol*. 2015;33:718-722.

44. Orlien SMS, Sandven I, Belay Berhe N, et al. Khat chewing increases the risk for developing chronic liver disease: a hospital-based case-control study. *Hepatology*. 2018.

45. Alhaddad OM, Elsabaawy MM, Rewisha EA, et al. Khat-induced liver injuries: a report of two cases. *Arab J Gastroenterol*. 2016;17:45-48.

46. Jenkins MG, Handslip R, Kumar M, et al. Reversible khat-induced hepatitis: two case reports and review of the literature. *Frontline Gastroenterol*. 2013;4:278-281.

47. Mahamoud HD, Muse SM, Roberts LR, Fischer PR, Torbenson MS, Fader T. Khat chewing and cirrhosis in Somaliland: case series. *Afr J Prim Health Care Fam Med*. 2016;8:e1-e4.

48. Peevers CG, Moorghen M, Collins PL, Gordon FH, McCune CA. Liver disease and cirrhosis because of Khat chewing in UK Somali men: a case series. *Liver Int*. 2010;30:1242-1243.

49. Bjornsson E, Talwalkar J, Treeprasertsuk S, et al. Drug-induced autoimmune hepatitis: clinical characteristics and prognosis. *Hepatology*. 2010;51:2040-2048.

50. Shalev O, Mosseri M, Ariel I, Stalnikowicz R. Methyldopa-induced immune hemolytic anemia and chronic active hepatitis. *Arch Intern Med*. 1983;143:592-593.

51. Islam S, Mekhloufi F, Paul JM, et al. Characteristics of clometacin-induced hepatitis with special reference to the presence of anti-actin cable antibodies. *Autoimmunity*. 1989;2:213-221.

FATTY LIVER DISEASE 6

CHAPTER OUTLINE

INTRODUCTION

Fatty liver disease is characterized by fat in hepatocytes that is visible by light microscopy. Oil red O stains will show small droplets of fat even in normal hepatocytes, but in fatty liver disease there is pathological accumulation that leads to visible fat by routine microscopic examination. The fat is divided into two broad categories based on the size of the fat droplets: macrovesicular (Fig. 6.1) and microvesicular (Fig. 6.2). In a nutshell, macrovesicular steatosis has medium- to large-sized droplets of fat, usually one per hepatocyte. In contrast, microvesicular steatosis has dozens of tiny droplets of fat per hepatocyte. This division of fat into microvesicular and macrovesicular is important because it reflects different forms of injury with different differentials. Macrovesicular steatosis is caused by dysregulation of lipid metabolism from various causes, while microvesicular steatosis is caused by mitochondrial toxins. Sometimes pathologists use the term mixed micro- and macrovesicular steatosis, but they should not. The term is wrong and can confuse clinicians and pathologists and patients. The reasons for the continued use of this term in pathology reports varies but includes not understanding basic liver pathology, a general obstinacy to following standard nomenclature, and probably a few others.

Almost every case of macrovesicular steatosis has smaller droplets of fat (Fig. 6.3), but this is simply part of the pattern of macrovesicular steatosis. Most cases of microvesicular steatosis will also have occasional droplets of macrovesicular steatosis, but this is simply part of the pattern of microvesicular steatosis (Fig. 6.4). In either situation, such cases should not be called mixed micro- and macrovesicular steatosis. Instead, if there is diffuse microvesicular steatosis with only occasional larger droplets of fat, call it microvesicular steatosis, while essentially all the other cases are macrovesicular steatosis.

There are a few unusual situations where the term intermediate droplet fat is used to describe fat droplets whose size is between micro- and macrovesicular steatosis—primarily implant or donor baseline biopsies obtained at the time of liver transplantation (Fig. 6.5). This term is largely used in research settings and is mentioned here only for the sake of completeness. Similar findings of intermediate droplet fat can be seen in hepatocytes adjacent to large areas of lobular necrosis, the most common example being acetaminophen toxicity.

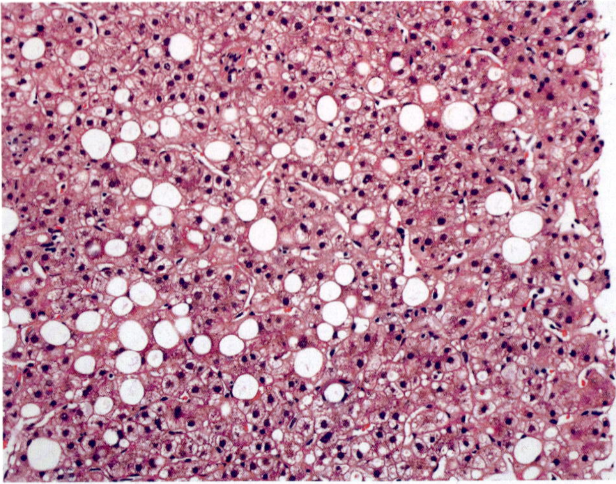

Figure 6.1. Macrovesicular steatosis. A typical pattern of macrovesicular steatosis. In each affected hepatocyte, a single large droplet of fat fills the cytoplasm and pushes the nucleus to the side.

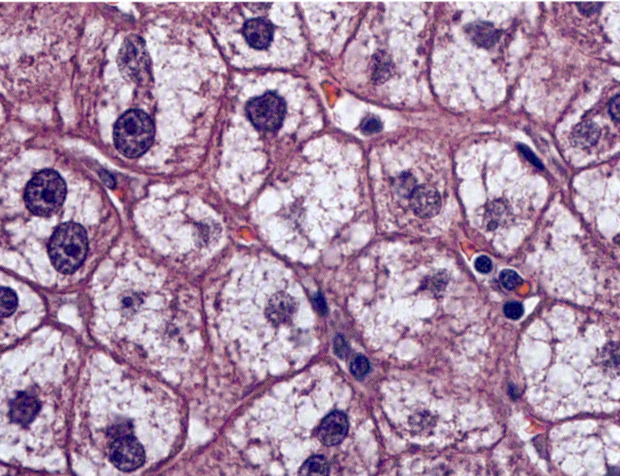

Figure 6.2. Microvesicular steatosis. The hepatocyte cytoplasm is filled with numerous tiny droplets that give it a foamy appearance.

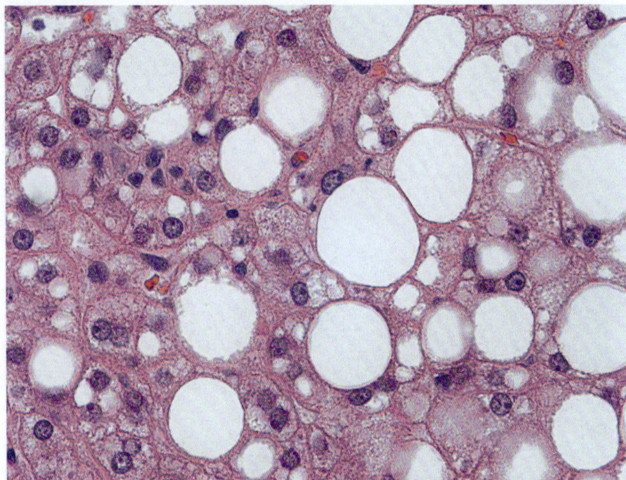

Figure 6.3. **Macrovesicular steatosis.** This image shows typical macrovesicular steatosis. You will readily see some smaller sized droplets of fat, but that is part of the pattern of macrovesicular steatosis. This should not be called mixed micro- and macrovesicular steatosis.

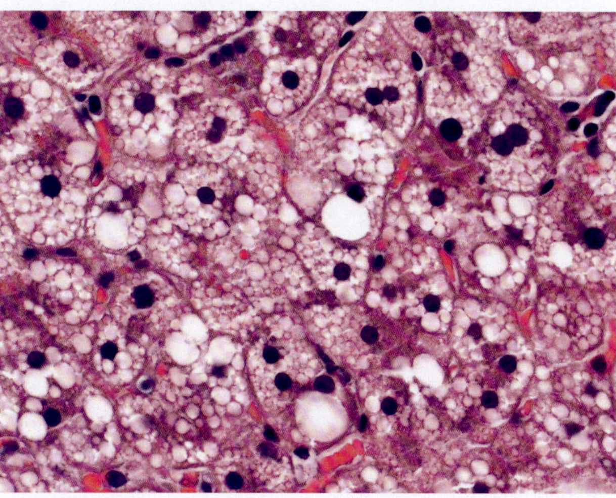

Figure 6.4. **Microvesicular steatosis.** Occasional droplets of macrovesicular steatosis are acceptable with the microvesicular pattern of steatosis as long as the microvesicular steatosis is diffuse and the dominant pattern.

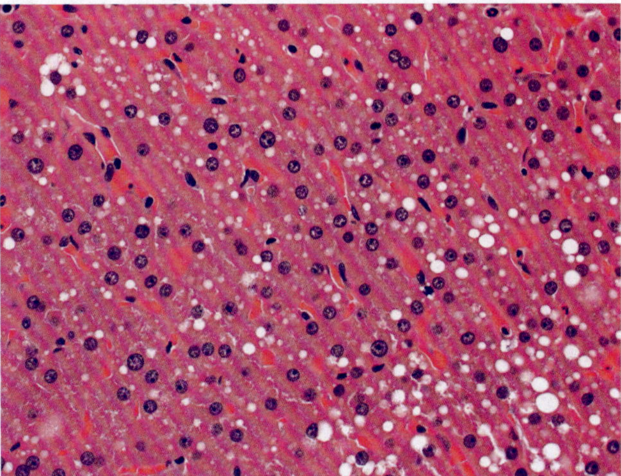

Figure 6.5. **Intermediate droplet steatosis.** This liver implant biopsy specimen shows occasionally droplets of intermediate-size fat and has no clinical significance. This pattern should not be called microvesicular steatosis.

NONALCOHOL FATTY LIVER DISEASE (NAFLD)

Nonalcohol fatty liver disease (NAFLD) is strongly associated with the metabolic syndrome, a constellation of hypertension, obesity, and insulin resistance. The term NAFLD includes both steatosis and steatohepatitis. For clinical purposes, a sharp distinction is made between steatosis and steatohepatitis, but in reality there is a gradient, as is true for most biological patterns.

ALL ABOUT THE FAT

The terms *fat* and *steatosis* are synonyms, with *fat* retaining its Anglo-Saxon heritage, and *steatosis* its Greek and New Latin roots. The two terms can be used interchangeably. Fat is required for diagnosing both steatosis and steatohepatitis, with a minimum cutoff of 5% or greater macrovesicular steatosis. Fat is graded as mild (5% to 33%), moderate (34% to 66%), or marked (>66%), while less than 5% fat is called minimal and in most cases has no clinical significance (Figs. 6.6–6.9). The fat grade is obtained by estimating the proportion

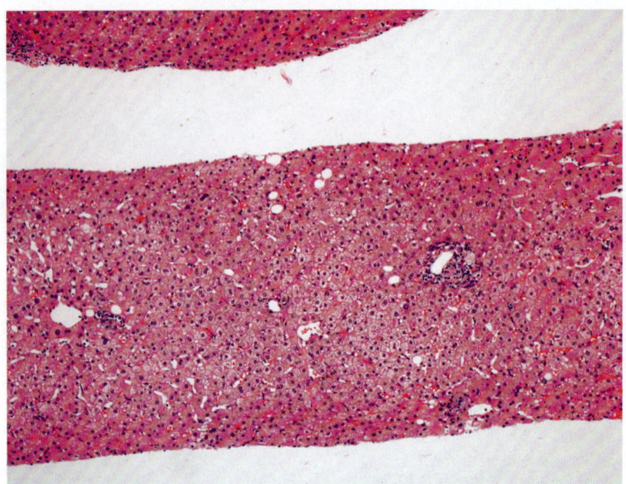

Figure 6.6. Minimal macrovesicular steatosis. There is minimal macrovesicular steatosis in this case, with less than 5% steatosis. Fat is best evaluated at a 10× or 20× lens.

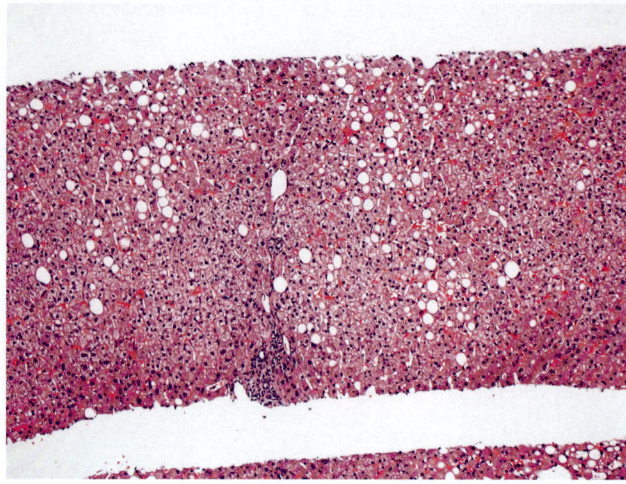

Figure 6.7. Mild macrovesicular steatosis. This biopsy shows about 10% macrovesicular steatosis.

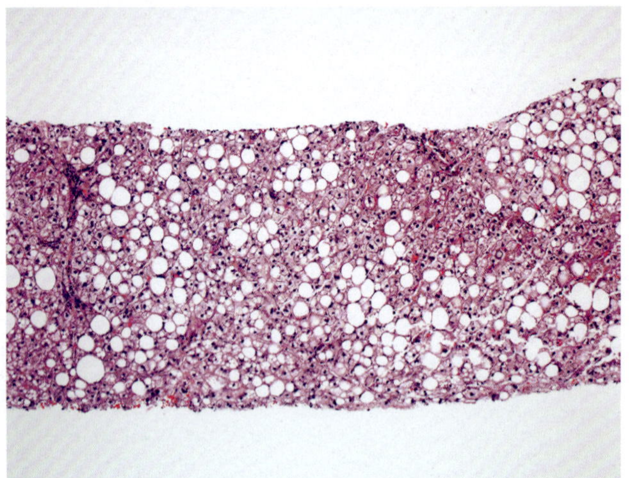

Figure 6.8. Moderate macrovesicular steatosis. This case shows an estimated 50% macrovesicular steatosis. Many of the hepatocytes also show glycogen accumulation, which gives the hepatocytes a clear cytoplasm, but this change should not be included with the steatosis estimate.

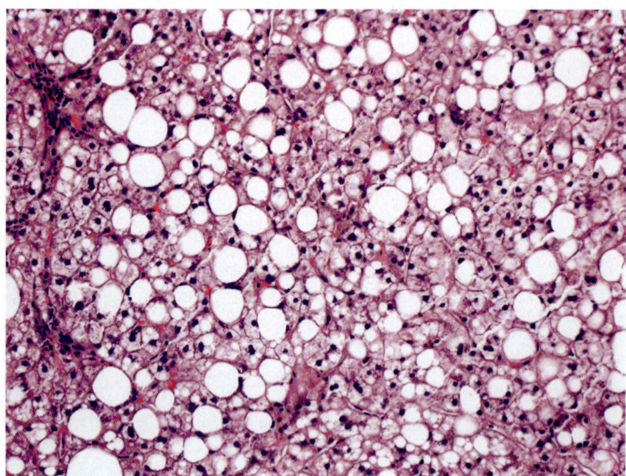

Figure 6.9. Marked macrovesicular steatosis. This wedge liver biopsy showed about 80% macrovesicular steatosis.

of hepatocytes with macrovesicular steatosis using a 10 or 20× lens. Average-out the percent of fat over the entire specimen. Remember this should be a skilled histological estimate, so try to do it accurately, but no one expects you to provide the exact percent of fat. In surgical pathology reports, a good approach is to estimate the percent fat to the nearest 10%, which works very well, conveying to clinicians and patients a clear sense of what the biopsy shows.

Some pathologists say they prefer to estimate the percent surface area of the lobules involved by fat and not the percent of hepatocytes with fat, a distinction that is erudite but of little clinical relevance, as the final result is about the same, well within the limits of estimating fat to the nearest 10%. There is one more point to consider when it comes to estimating fat—digital image analysis has consistently shown that the human eye tends to overestimate the percent of fat on histology slides,[1] tempting some pathologists into making mental adjustments to try and match a computer. Do not do this—stick to the methods of your fellow humans. The rise of the machines will come soon enough.

Fat can be found primarily in zone 3 (most common) or zone 1 or have an azonal or panacinar pattern. The zonal patterns of the fat are not clinically important, but for completeness are discussed here. When determining the zonal pattern of the fat, a useful approach is to ask what areas are *spared* of fat. For example, if the fat clearly is diminished to absent in zone 1, then this would be classified as a zone 3 pattern of fat (Fig. 6.10). The fat in adults with the metabolic syndrome commonly has zone 3 pattern. In kids with the metabolic syndrome, a zone 3 pattern is also the most common, but a zone 1 pattern can be encountered (Fig. 6.11).[2] In many cases, there is no clear zonal pattern, so the term azonal is used (Fig. 6.12). If there is so much fat that a zonal pattern cannot be discerned, the term panacinar is used (Fig. 6.13).

After the amount of fat is established, the next question is whether there is steatohepatitis. This distinction has clinical relevance because there is an increased rate of fibrosis progression for steatohepatitis compared with steatosis. One study found fibrosis progression occurred in both steatosis (39% of cases) and steatohepatitis (34% of cases), but steatosis progressed on average 1 stage in 14 years, while steatohepatitis 1 stage in 7 years.[3]

Overall, the greatest predictor of clinical outcomes is having some fibrosis on the index biopsy,[4,5] a general observation that is also true for other chronic inflammatory liver diseases such as chronic viral hepatitis.[6] Steatohepatitis (versus steatosis) does predict liver-related morbidity or mortality in univariate analysis but not in multivariate analysis when fibrosis is also factored in to the model.[4]

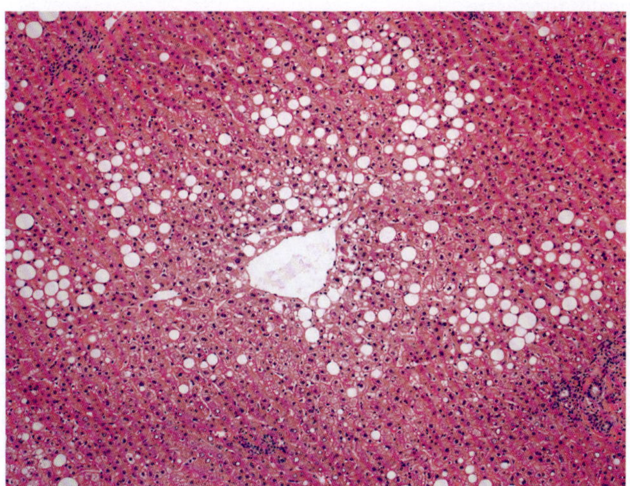

Figure 6.10. Macrovesicular steatosis, zone 3 pattern. There is more macrovesicular steatosis around the central vein, with the amount of fat diminishing in zone 2 and 1 hepatocytes.

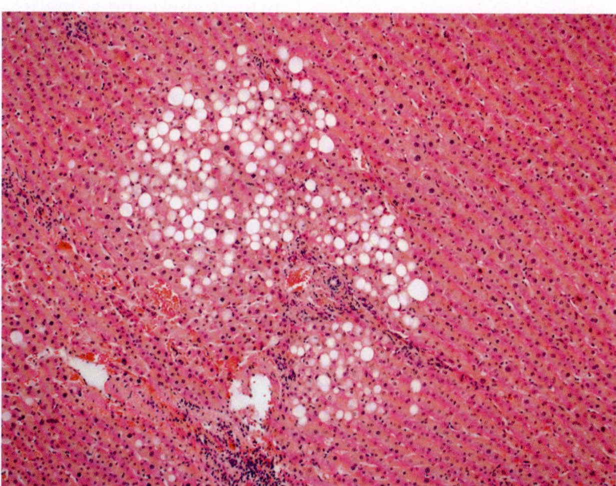

Figure 6.11. Macrovesicular steatosis, zone 1 pattern. The macrovesicular steatosis shows a clear zonal pattern, with the fat clustering around a portal tract.

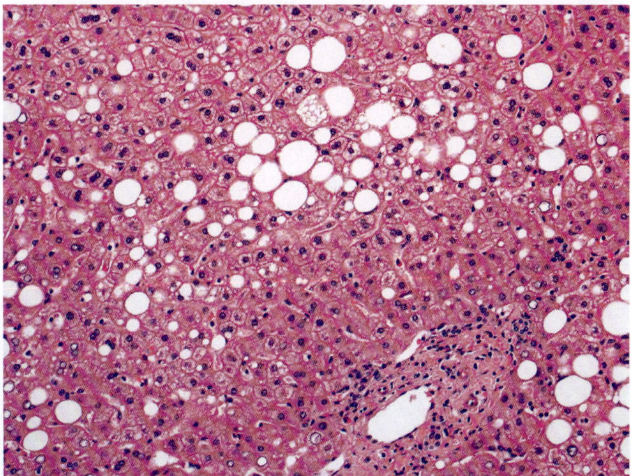

Figure 6.12. Macrovesicular steatosis, azonal pattern. The macrovesicular steatosis was not clearly accentuated in either zone 3 or zone 1 in this case.

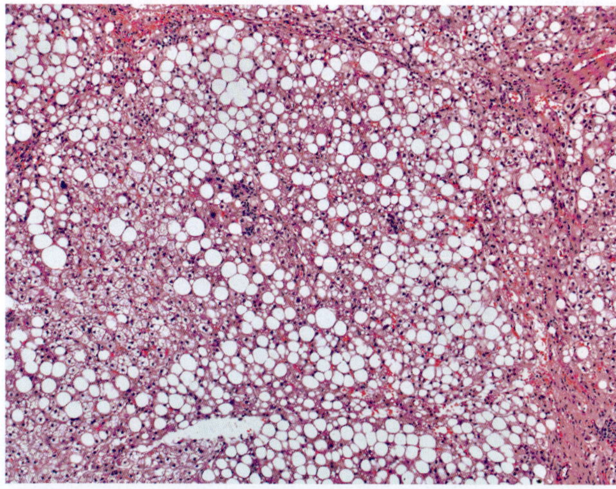

Figure 6.13. Macrovesicular steatosis, panacinar pattern. This wedge biopsy showed marked macrovesicular steatosis, with so much fat that any zonal pattern was obscured.

A second relevant observation is that a high percent of individuals can shift back and forth between steatosis and steatohepatitis throughout their disease course.[7] In other words, the disease categories of steatosis versus steatohepatitis are not permanent, or even semipermanent, but shift back and forth over time depending on factors that are largely unknown, but presumably reflect fluctuations in the patient's underlying metabolic syndrome.

All of this reminds us that the distinction between steatosis and steatohepatitis is important, but it is not any more important than the grade of activity in autoimmune hepatitis or grade of activity in viral hepatitis. With steatosis versus steatohepatitis, it is not like you are distinguishing between two separate diseases; instead, there is single disease that has a range of active injury, and the lower grades are called steatosis while the higher grades are called steatohepatitis. If the findings in a case are borderline for steatohepatitis, just say so in your report and accurately convey the amount of active injury you see.

HOW DO YOU GO FROM STEATOSIS TO STEATOHEPATITIS?

The distinction between steatosis and steatohepatitis rests on identifying active liver injury. The forms of active injury in steatohepatitis include ballooned hepatocytes, lobular inflammation, and acidophil bodies.[8] Portal chronic inflammation is also commonly present, usually mild and sometimes focally moderate.

Although active injury and fibrosis are scored separately, they are not completely independent. For example, portal inflammation and ballooned hepatocytes both correlate with fibrosis stage.[4]

BALLOON CELLS

Ballooned hepatocytes are a central feature of the steatohepatitis injury pattern.[8] The balloon cells should stand out from the background hepatocytes because they are enlarged and have a thin wispy cytoplasmic appearance, without fat, but often with Mallory hyaline (Figs. 6.14–6.16). Ballooned hepatocytes are often called balloon cells for short. Mallory hyaline can also be called Mallory–Denk bodies. When hunting for balloon cells, it is most productive to start in zone 3, especially in areas with fibrosis. The NAS system scores balloon cells as few or many, which admittedly is not the strictest scoring system, but it seems to work well enough in clinical practice. If they are easy to see at 20×, present in several fields, then that should be scored as many. If they are hard to find, present in only a few fields after careful hunting, then score the case as a few.

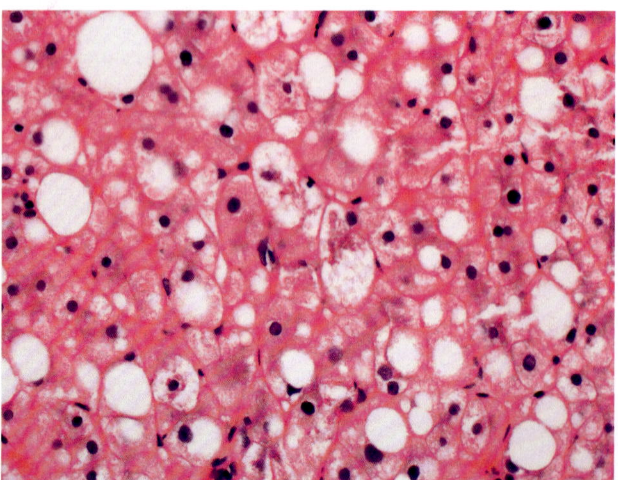

Figure 6.14. **Ballooned hepatocyte.** Several ballooned hepatocytes stand out because they are larger and more rounded than neighboring cells, with abundant rarified cytoplasm.

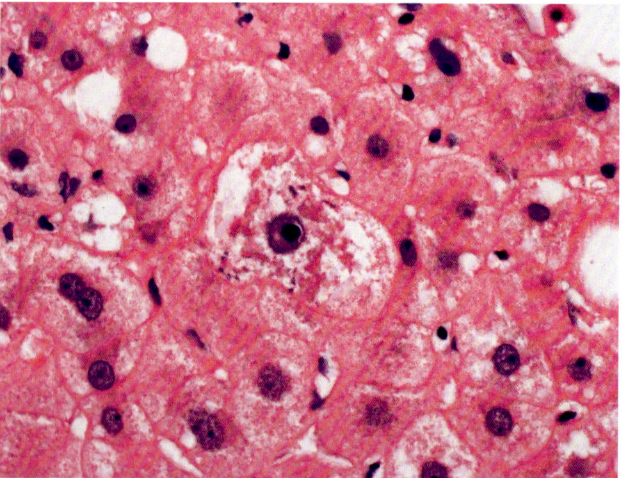

Figure 6.15. **Ballooned hepatocyte.** At high power, this ballooned hepatocyte has abundant Mallory hyaline—with a pink ropy appearance.

In some cases, the biopsy will show possible or equivocal ballooned hepatocytes (Figs. 6.17 and 6.18), but despite careful searching, no definite ballooned hepatocytes are identified. In this situation, you can be guided by other findings of active injury (lobular inflammation, apoptotic hepatocytes) to decide between steatosis and steatohepatitis. If there is convincing active injury but no ballooned hepatocytes, the best diagnosis is still steatohepatitis. Pericellular fibrosis is not used in this distinction, as the terms steatosis versus steatohepatitis indicates the grade of injury, while in contrast, pericellular fibrosis is a fibrosis stage that that can be seen with either.

Identification of a balloon cell for diagnostic purposes is based on H&E findings. In those balloon cells with Mallory hyaline, the Mallory hyaline can be highlighted with immunostains for ubiquitin (Fig. 6.19) or p62. The ballooned hepatocytes also tend to lose their expression of CK8 and 18.[9]

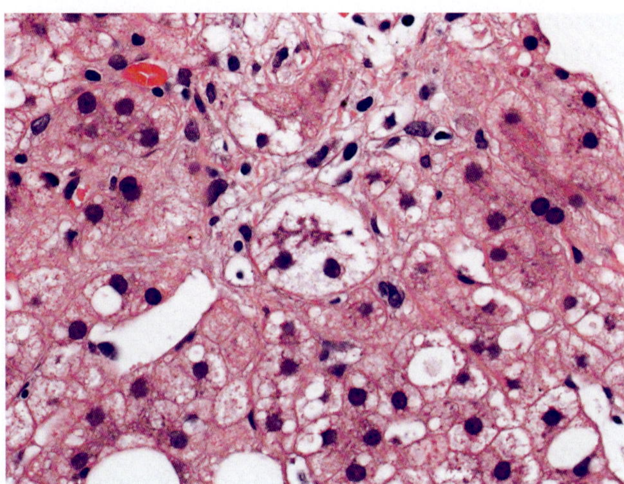

Figure 6.16. **Ballooned hepatocyte.** The balloon cell is many times bigger than neighboring hepatocytes and has Mallory hyaline.

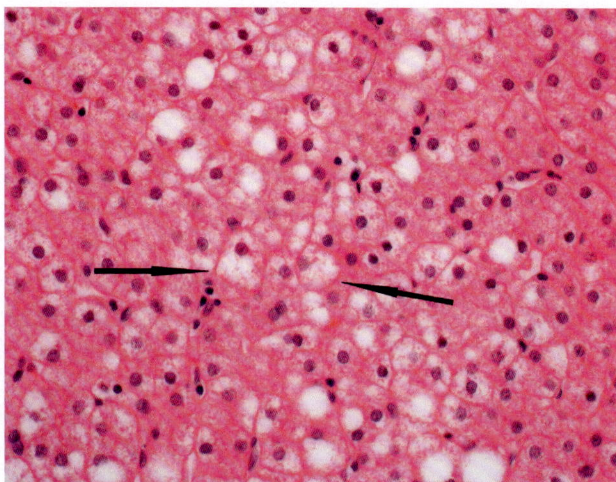

Figure 6.17. **Equivocal ballooned hepatocyte.** These possible balloon cells (arrows) are larger than neighboring cells and have somewhat clear cytoplasm, but I was not convinced. Are you? In cases with equivocal balloon cells, its best to keep on looking for more classic balloon cells and not score the equivocal ones.

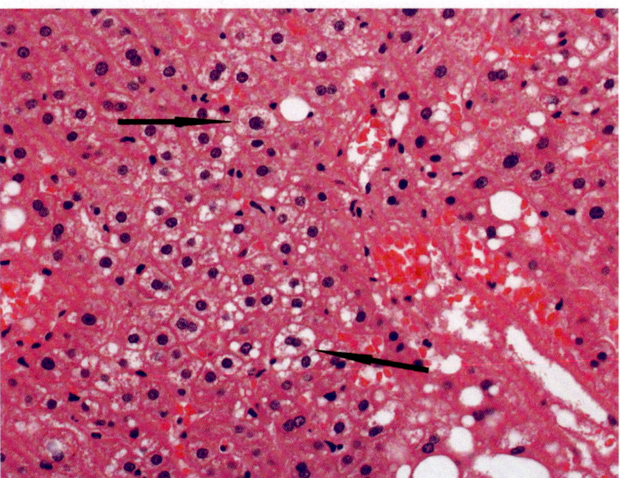

Figure 6.18. **Equivocal ballooned hepatocyte.** Another example of equivocal balloon cells. I would not score these as balloon cells. See also preceding image.

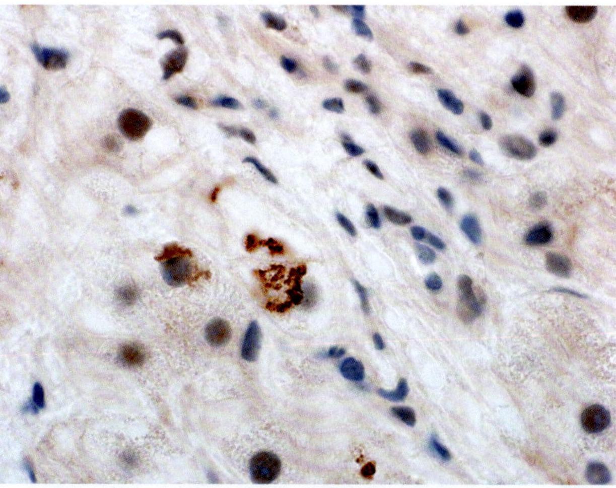

Figure 6.19. **Ballooned hepatocyte, ubiquitin immunostain.** The Mallory hyaline in this balloon cell is highlighted.

KEY FEATURES of Ballooned Hepatocytes

- They are not specific for fatty liver disease, but in the presence of fat, they are used as evidence of active injury.
- They are most commonly found in zone 3, particularly if there is zone 3 pericellular fibrosis.
- They are bigger than neighboring cells.
- They have rarified cytoplasm with thin wisps of pink cytoplasm.
- They do not have fat.
- They may have Mallory hyaline.
- They predict fibrosis progression in univariate but not multivariate analysis.[4]

LOBULAR INFLAMMATION

The lobular inflammation in steatohepatitis is predominately lymphocytic, with some admixed macrophages (Figs. 6.20 and 6.21). Lobular neutrophils can be present but are more common in alcoholic hepatitis (Fig. 6.22). The inflammation should be counted as the number of foci using a 20× lens. Acidophil bodies, even if seen without inflammatory cells, would also count as foci of inflammation. A reasonable approach is to count at least 5 representative fields and average them. Single lymphocytes in the sinusoids, or even a cluster of two, does not count as lobular inflammation (Fig. 6.23).

PORTAL INFLAMMATION

The portal inflammation in steatosis and steatohepatitis is usually mild, sometimes patchy moderate (Fig. 6.24), but hardly ever diffusely moderate and hardly ever marked. If there is diffuse moderate portal chronic inflammation or even focal marked portal inflammation, then other causes of chronic hepatitis, such as virus, drug, and autoimmune, should be carefully excluded. The inflammation is essentially always lymphocytic with occasional or rare plasma cells, eosinophils, and histiocytes. The frequency and amount of portal chronic inflammation tends to increase with fibrosis stage. In univariate analysis, portal inflammation is also associated with adverse clinical outcomes, but this association drops out when fibrosis stage is factored into the model.[4]

OTHER FINDINGS IN FATTY LIVER DISEASE

There are several additional findings in fatty liver disease that are common but not clinically important. Hepatocyte nuclei can show glycogenation (Fig. 6.25). The glycogenated

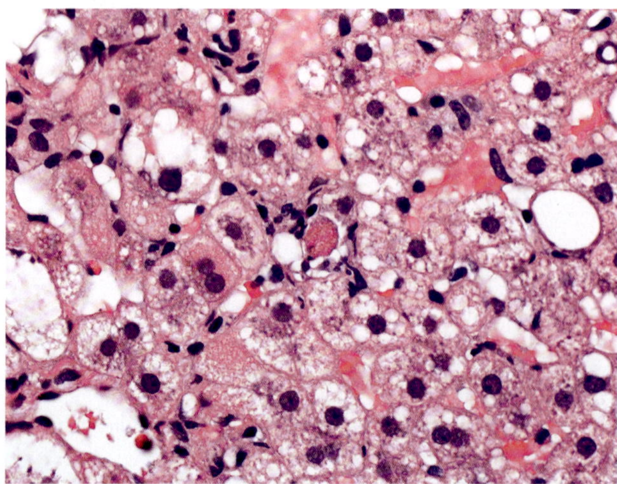

Figure 6.20. **Steatohepatitis, lobular inflammation.** The lobules show patchy lymphocytic inflammation and an acidophil body.

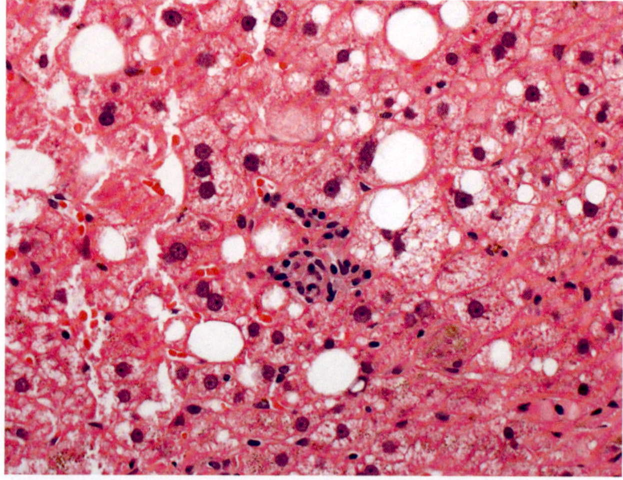

Figure 6.21. **Steatohepatitis, lobular inflammation.** There is mild lobular inflammation forming a small focus of lymphocytic and histiocytic inflammation.

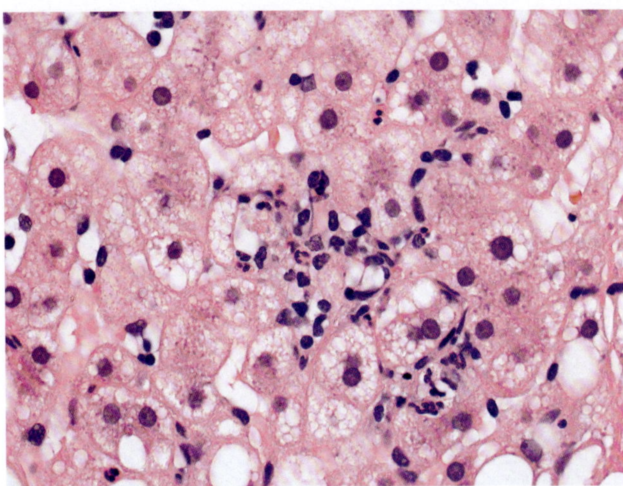

Figure 6.22. **Steatohepatitis, lobular inflammation, neutrophils.** The inflammation in this case of moderately active steatohepatitis was mostly lymphocytic, but occasional foci also had neutrophils.

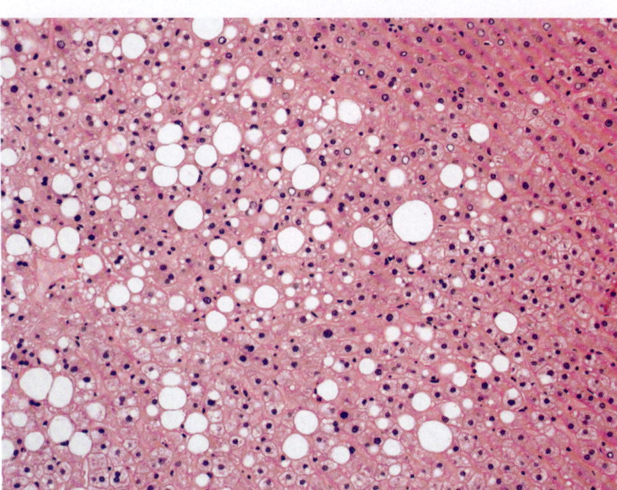

Figure 6.23. **Steatosis, no lobular inflammation.** There is no lobular inflammation in this biopsy with steatosis but not steatohepatitis.

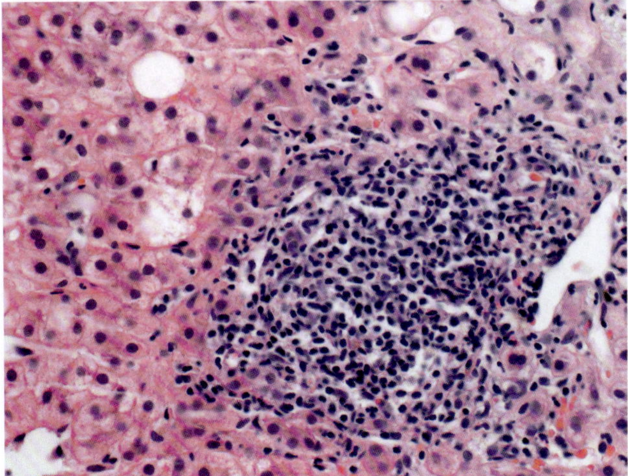

Figure 6.24. **Portal chronic inflammation.** There was patchy moderate portal chronic inflammation in this case of steatohepatitis with bridging fibrosis.

nuclei correlate, albeit not very strongly, with the presence of diabetes mellitus.[10,11] Megamitochondria are often present in hepatocytes (Fig. 6.26). Lipogranulomas are common and are usually found either in zone 3 or the portal tracts (Fig. 6.27). Although always fun to find, the term lipogranuloma can lead to confusion among the nonpathology community, and there is no need to include their presence in your pathology report. The lobules can show well-circumscribed foci of microvesicular steatosis (Figs. 6.28 and 6.29) in about 10% of cases. These foci are more common in cases of steatohepatitis and correlate with the grade of fat and the fibrosis stage,[12] but overall they have no strong clinical association that requires their presence or absence being included in the pathology report. Finally, the hepatic lobules can become arterialized with advanced fibrosis (Fig. 6.30). These arteries can even extend to the central veins, sometimes mimicking a portal tract that has lost a bile duct.[13]

Low-level elevations in serum ANA and ASMA titers are found in about 20% of patients with fatty liver disease who do not have autoimmune hepatitis, either clinically or histologically.[14,15] Rarely, titers can be as high as 1:640, without having evidence of autoimmune hepatitis.[15] However, some individuals will have autoimmune hepatitis, so biopsies can be very helpful.[16] Less commonly, AMA can be positive without evidence for primary biliary cirrhosis (Fig. 6.31). As one example, in one study the frequency of AMA positivity was just under 1% (4 of 607) in the setting of nonalcoholic and alcoholic fatty liver disease.[15]

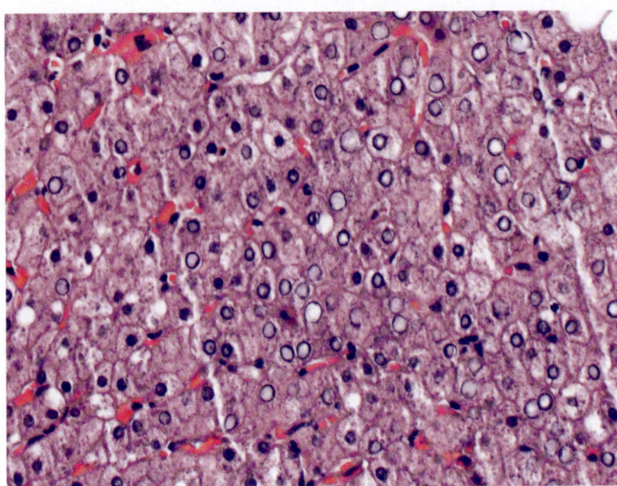

Figure 6.25. **Glycogenated nuclei.** A patch of hepatocytes show glycogenated nuclei. The nuclei are pale white with a rim of darker blue chromatin.

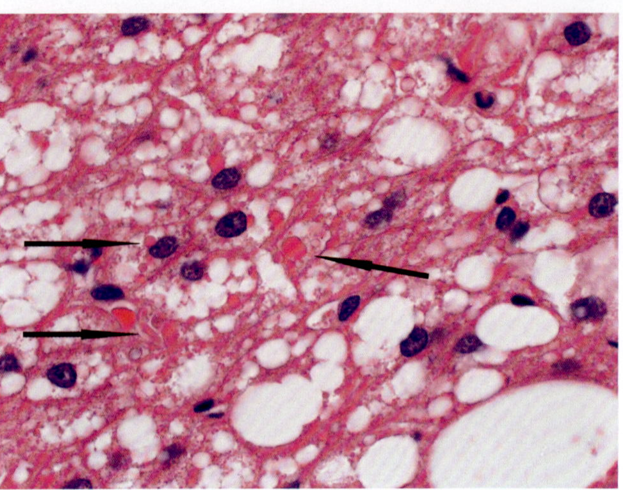

Figure 6.26. **Megamitochondria.** The megamitochondria appear as pink round to oval structures in the hepatocyte cytoplasm (arrows). Sometimes megamitochondria can be more needle-shaped.

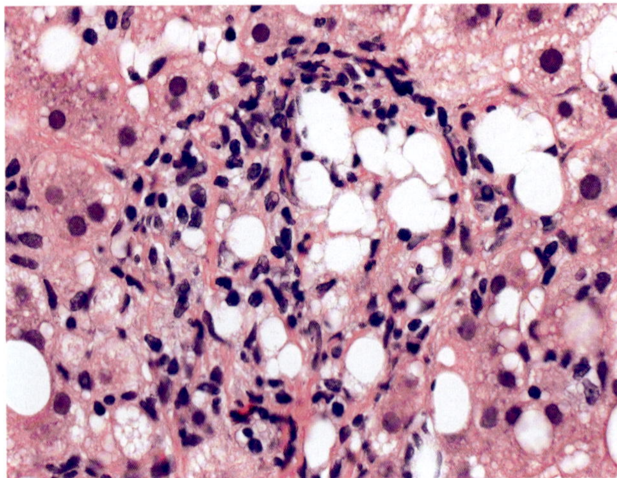

Figure 6.27. **Lipid granuloma.** This portal tract has an aggregate of lipid-laden macrophages with admixed lymphocytic inflammation and mild fibrosis.

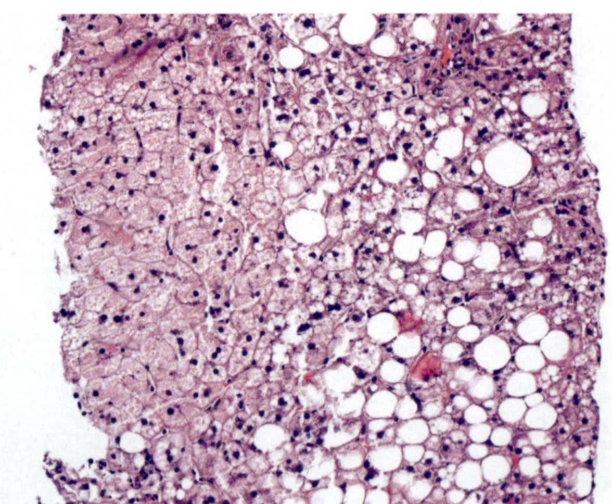

Figure 6.28. **Focus of microvesicular steatosis.** At the left edge of the biopsy, a distinctive patch of hepatocytes is present, without macrovesicular steatosis. On higher power (next image), the hepatocytes are filled with numerous tiny droplets of fat.

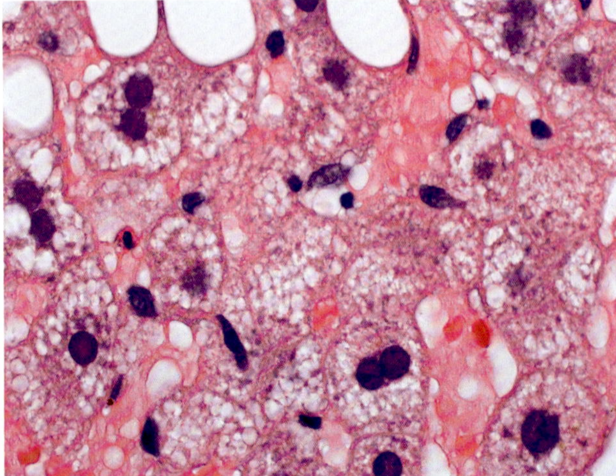

Figure 6.29. **Focus of microvesicular steatosis.** The foamy appearance of the cytoplasm results from numerous tiny droplets of fat (higher power view of prior image).

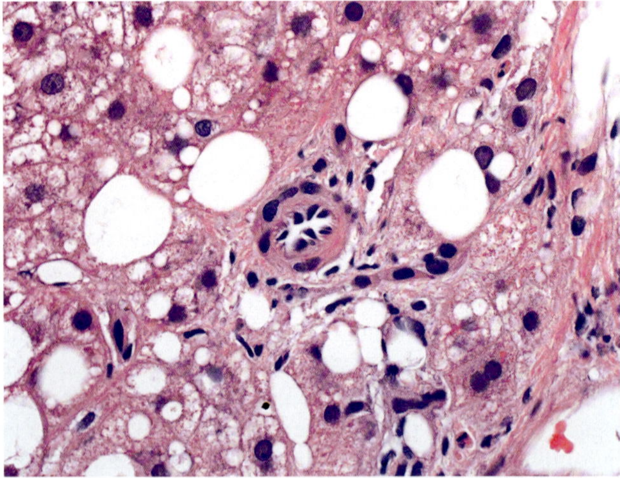

Figure 6.30. **Lobular artery.** A small lobular artery is seen in this case of steatohepatitis.

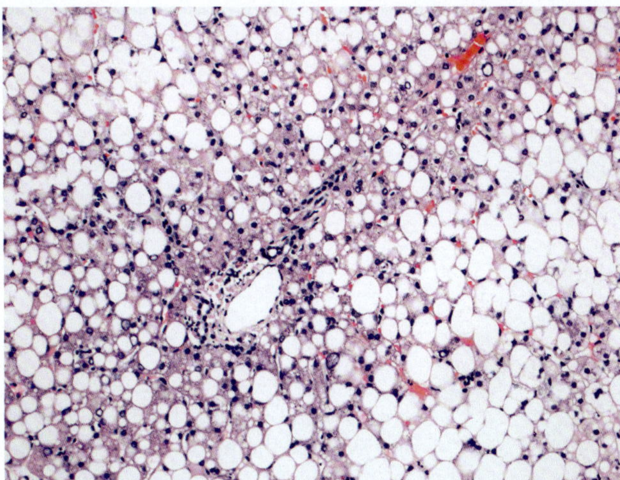

Figure 6.31. **Steatohepatitis with positive AMA.** In this case, the alkaline phosphatase and GGT showed minimal elevations, and the biopsy showed no evidence for biliary tract disease.

FORMAL GRADING AND STAGING

There are two major grading systems: NAS[8] and SAF[17] (Tables 6.1 and 6.2). They both use the same fibrosis staging system (Table 6.3). In terms of grading, both the NAS and SAF score the fat in the same way but have minor differences in the way inflammation and ballooned hepatocytes are scored (Tables 6.1 and 6.2). In the NAS, the lobular inflammation is scored on a scale of 0 to 3, while in the SAF, on a scale of 0 to 2. In both systems, the lobular inflammation should be scored using a 20× lens. The SAF also provides histological descriptions that are somewhat different for ballooned hepatocytes grade 1 versus 2 (Table 6.2), while in the NAS ballooned hepatocytes are scored only by their frequency.

The biggest difference in the two grading systems is how the individual components are reported. In the NAS, they are reported separately, but the scores for fat, lobular inflammation, and ballooned hepatocytes are also summed for a total grade. In the SAF system, the lobular inflammation and balloon cell scores are summed for an activity score (A), but the steatosis is reported out separately (S). For example, a case with 40% fat, moderate lobular hepatitis with rare balloon cells, and bridging fibrosis would be scored as S2 A3 F3, again with the fibrosis scored the same as the NAS system.

In the NAS system, the distinction of steatosis from steatohepatitis is made by the pathologist independent of the results of the scoring system, although of course there is a strong correlation between high scores and the likelihood of steatohepatitis.[8] In contrast, the SAF system has an interpretive graph where the scores are combined to distinguishing steatosis from steatohepatitis. In this approach, both balloon cells and lobular inflammation are required for a diagnosis of steatohepatitis. Thus, these patterns are classified as steatosis and not steatohepatitis in the SAF system: only fat, only fat plus balloon cells, or only fat plus lobular inflammation.

FAQ: Do you need to provide a formal grade and stage in cases of steatosis or steatohepatitis?

Answer: No. However, they can be very useful to convey what the biopsy shows. The NAS and SAF are both broadly similar and both perform very well in day to day clinical use.

DETERMINING ETIOLOGY

Many times the clinical findings are not available, and the pathologist does not know if the patient has the metabolic syndrome, alcohol use, or other risk factors. In this situation, the NAS grade and stage (or SAF if you prefer) can still be provided as shown below in the Sample Note.

TABLE 6.1: NAS Scoring System for Nonalcoholic Fatty Liver Disease, From the NASH-CRN Study Group.[8] After Scoring Each Component, Sum for a Maximum of 8 Points

Component	Finding	Notes
Fat (Macrovesicular Steatosis)		At least 5% fat needs to be present to qualify for fatty liver disease
1	6% to 33%	
2	34% to 66%	
3	67% to 100%	
Lobular Inflammation		Use a 20× lens, score at least 5 fields and average them
0	None	
1	<2 foci	
2	2 to 4 foci	
3	>4 foci	
Balloon Cells		Score only convincing balloon cells, not equivocal ones
0	None	
1	Few	One to a few
2	Many	Easily found, present in at least several fields

SAMPLE NOTE

Liver, needle biopsy: Mildly active steatohepatitis with bridging fibrosis. Please note.

Note: No clinical or laboratory information is available, other than that the patient has mildly elevated liver enzymes.

The biopsy is adequate for interpretation and shows mildly active steatohepatitis. There is moderate (approximately 40%) macrovesicular steatosis along with rare ballooned hepatocytes and mild patchy lobular inflammation. A trichrome stain shows bridging fibrosis. Iron and PASD stains are negative.

Clinical correlation will be needed to determine the cause of the fatty liver disease, but the histological differential includes primarily the metabolic syndrome and alcohol use. Drug effect and other rare genetic causes of fatty liver disease are also a possibility. The NAS grade and stage are provided below.

NAS Grade
Fat, 2

Lobular inflammation, 1

Ballooned hepatocytes, 1

Total NAS grade 4/8

NAS Stage
Bridging fibrosis, stage 3/4

TABLE 6.2: SAF Scoring System Scores the Steatosis (S), Activity (A), and Fibrosis (F) Separately[17]

Component	Finding	Notes
Steatosis, Macrovesicular		
0	(<5%)	
1	6% to 33%	
2	34% to 66%	
3	67% to 100%	
Lobular Inflammation		Use a 20× lens To get the final activity score, the lobular inflammation score and the ballooning score are added together
0	None	
1	≤2 foci per 20× field	
2	>2 foci per 20× field	
Balloon Cells		The balloon cell approach is different than that of the NAS, which does not consider the size of the balloon cells.
0	None	
1	Balloon cells show rounded contours with clear reticular cytoplasm. Their size is similar to normal hepatocytes. Typically few in number	
2	Cells are rounded, have clear cytoplasm, and are twice as large as normal hepatocytes. Typically many in number	

The final activity score is calculated by adding the lobular inflammation score and the ballooning score together. In contrast to the NAS system, the scores are not summed but instead reported out separately. For example, a case might be scored as S2 A2 F3, with the fibrosis scored the same as the NAS system.

ALCOHOL LIVER DISEASE

In general, alcoholic liver disease cannot be distinguished from metabolic syndrome–related liver disease in any given case. The pathologists' job is to identify the disease pattern and provide an assessment of the degree of active injury, degree of fibrosis, and presence of any additional disease process. Surgical pathology reports often provide a general differential for the fatty liver disease, but the etiology is determined by the clinical team and not by the histology. That being said, there are some findings that are more common in alcoholic liver disease, including numerous balloon cells with marked Malory hyaline (Figs. 6.32 and 6.33), diffuse lobular pericellular fibrosis (Fig. 6.34), neutrophilic lobular inflammation (Fig. 6.35), and lobular cholestasis (Fig. 6.36) that is not explained by drug effects, obstruction, or other causes.

TABLE 6.3: NAS Staging System for Nonalcoholic Fatty Liver Disease, From the NASH-CRN Study Group[8]

Fibrosis Stage	Histological Description	Comment
1a	Mild pericellular fibrosis	The pericellular fibrosis is seen only on trichrome stain
1b	Moderate pericellular fibrosis	The pericellular fibrosis is definitely evident on H&E stain
1c	Portal fibrosis only	No pericellular fibrosis
2	Both portal fibrosis and pericellular fibrosis	The portal fibrosis is usually mild. Any degree of portal plus pericellular fibrosis is stage 2
3	Bridging fibrosis	Any degree of bridging fibrosis
4	Cirrhosis	

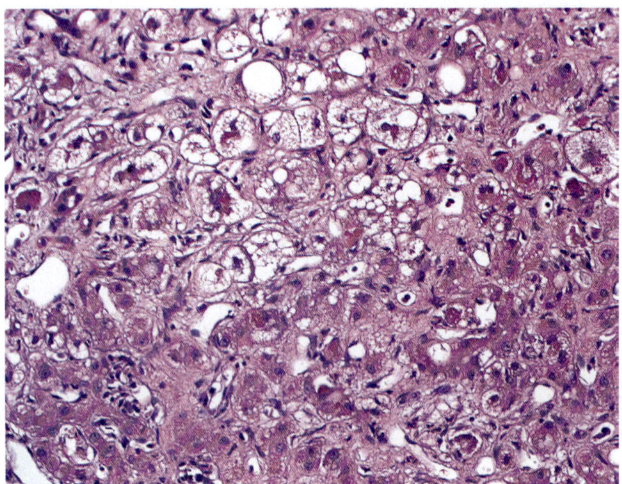

Figure 6.32. **Alcoholic liver disease, balloon cells.** Numerous ballooned hepatocytes are seen in the center of this image.

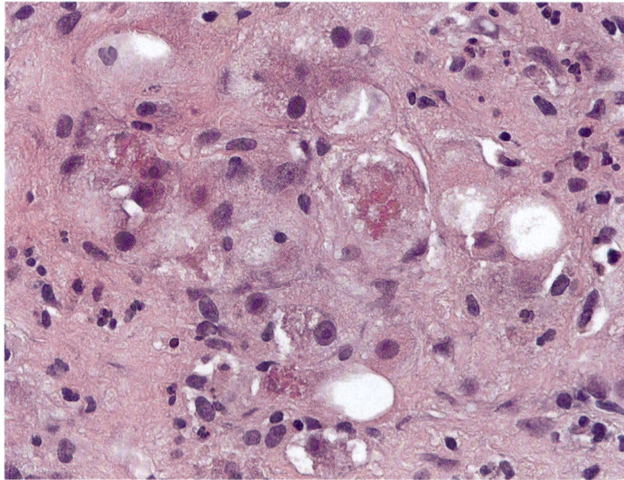

Figure 6.33. **Alcoholic liver disease, balloon cells.** The ballooned hepatocytes have abundant Mallory hyaline.

DRUG REACTIONS CAUSING FATTY LIVER DISEASE

Many different drugs can cause fatty liver disease. A few of the more common culprits are shown in Table 6.4. Amiodarone is one example that can cause steatohepatitis (Fig. 6.37). Often, there is much more striking balloon cells and Mallory hyaline than fat in cases of amiodarone toxicity. In many cases where drugs are associated with fatty liver disease, affected individuals also have the metabolic syndrome, or at least several elements thereof, and it is thought that the drugs play a synergistic effect with the metabolic syndrome in causing fatty liver disease.

Methotrexate is a well-known drug-related cause of fatty liver disease. As noted above, most affected individuals also have some elements of the metabolic syndrome.[18] Many years ago, baseline biopsies and follow-up biopsies were used to manage patients. That clinical approach has changed, and baseline biopsies are no longer part of management guidelines.[18,19] Instead, biopsies are typically performed when there are persistent elevations in liver enzymes, a drop in serum albumin, or a total cumulative

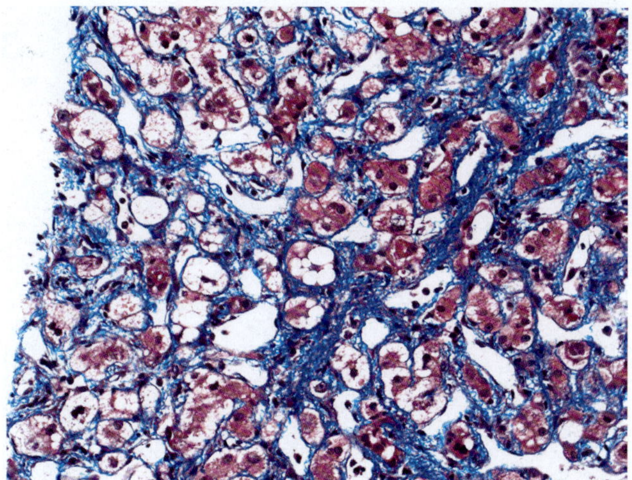

Figure 6.34. **Alcoholic liver disease, marked pericellular fibrosis, trichrome.** The lobules show diffuse, striking pericellular fibrosis. Not all cases of alcoholic liver disease will have this degree of pericellular fibrosis. This pattern of diffused marked pericellular fibrosis is unusual for ordinary fatty liver disease.

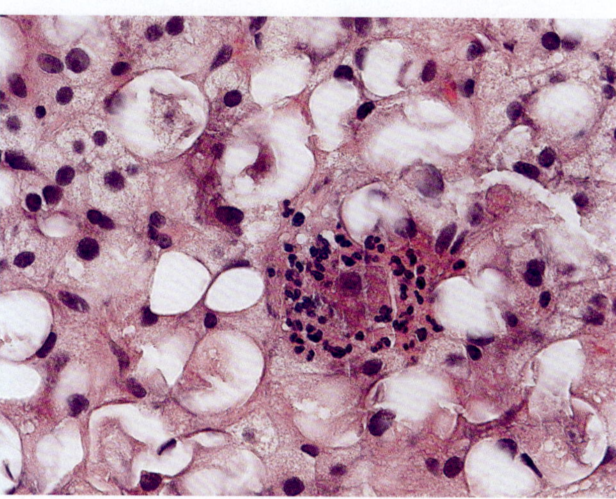

Figure 6.35. **Alcoholic liver disease, lobular neutrophils.** A cluster of neutrophils is seen surrounding a dying hepatocyte. Fat and balloon cells can be seen in the background.

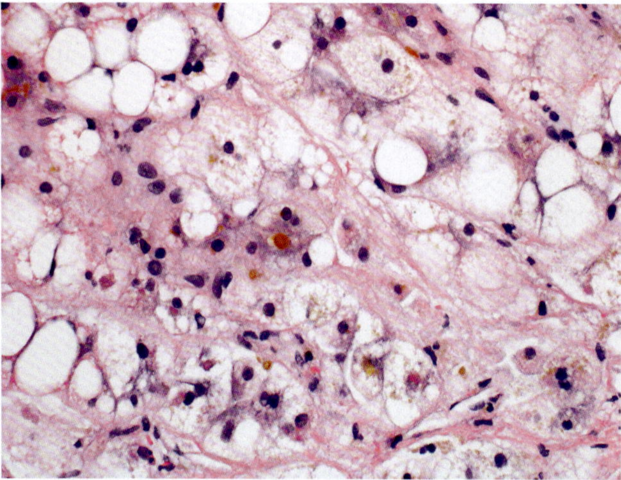

Figure 6.36. **Alcoholic liver disease, lobular cholestasis.** In this biopsy from a patient with a history of significant alcohol use, the liver shows moderately active steatohepatitis as well as moderate lobular cholestasis.

TABLE 6.4: Drugs That Can Cause Fatty Liver Disease

Drug	Comments
Amiodarone	
Glucocorticoids	
Irinotecan	Chemotherapeutic agent that is commonly used in colon cancer
Methotrexate	Used to treat rheumatological and dermatologic disorders
Oxaliplatin	Chemotherapeutic, commonly used in colon cancer
Perihexline	Antianginal agent
Tamoxifen	Estrogen receptor antagonist

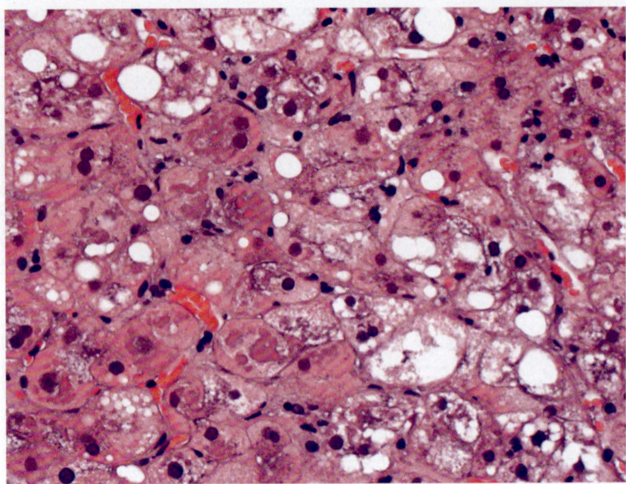

Figure 6.37. **Fatty liver disease from amiodarone.** The biopsy showed numerous ballooned hepatocytes with abundant Mallory hyaline and relative little steatosis.

dose of 4,000 mg. In many cases, patients are first screened by noninvasive testing for fibrosis and then proceed to liver biopsy only if the noninvasive test results are abnormal.

The histological findings typically show minimal or mild macrovesicular steatosis with disproportionately large amounts of balloon cells and abundant Mallory hyaline. There is a grading system for methotrexate injury, called the Roenigk scale,[20] but it suffers the drawback of combining grade and stage and overall tends to overestimate the degree of injury by giving high scores to cases with mild fibrosis.[18] Thus, currently the approach is largely that of ordinary fatty liver disease, and the pathologist indicates the amount of active injury (fat, balloon cells, inflammation) and provides a separate fibrosis stage.

OTHER RARE CAUSES OF MACROVESICULAR STEATOSIS

Fatty liver disease can also be caused by a large number of rare conditions (Table 6.5). The fatty liver disease in these settings can be steatosis (Fig. 6.38) or steatohepatitis (Fig. 6.39), although in my experience steatosis is more common. The changes can be histologically identical to those seen in the most common causes of fatty liver disease: metabolic syndrome, alcohol use, and drug effect.

MICROVESICULAR STEATOSIS

In this pattern of injury, there is diffuse microvesicular steatosis, generally with little or no inflammation (Fig. 6.40). Occasional larger droplets of fat are fine for the diagnosis. The etiologies all lead to direct mitochondrial injury (Table 6.6).

TABLE 6.5: Differential for Macrovesicular Steatosis in Cases Where the Metabolic Syndrome, Alcoholic Liver Disease, and Drug Effect Have all Been Excluded

Cause	Comment
Genetic Disease	
Cystic fibrosis[21,22]	
Lipodystrophies[2,23]	Can be genetic or acquired
Porphyria cutanea tarda[24]	
Weber–Christian disease[25,26]	
Wilson disease[27]	
Metabolic Conditions	
Diabetes mellitus	Even in patients who do not have the metabolic syndrome
Growth hormone deficiency[28]	
Hypothyroid disease[29]	
Elevated cortisol levels	
Malnutrition and Related	
Inflammation of the small bowel	Crohn disease, celiac disease, bacterial overgrowth
Jejunoilleal bypass surgery or extensive small bowel resection	
Malnutrition	Either marasmus or kwashiorkor
Portal vein thrombosis[11,30]	
Miscellaneous	
Volatile petrochemical products[31]	

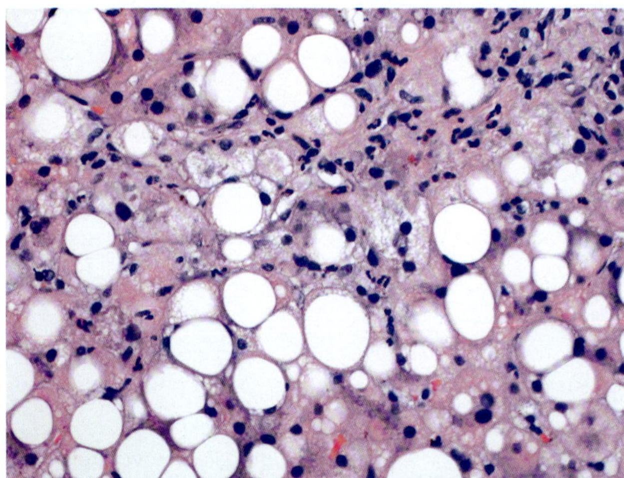

Figure 6.38. **Steatosis, elevated cortisol levels.** This person had elevated cortisol levels, and the liver biopsy showed steatohepatitis.

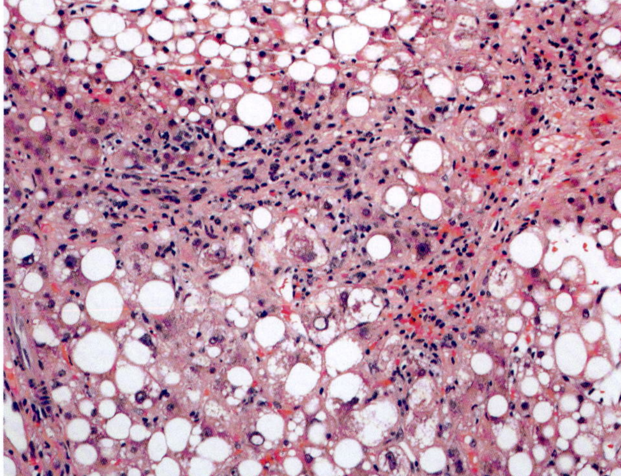

Figure 6.39. **Steatohepatitis, small bowel resection for neuroendocrine tumor.** After small bowel resection, steatohepatitis developed and was thought to result from bile acid malabsorption as a result of the surgery.

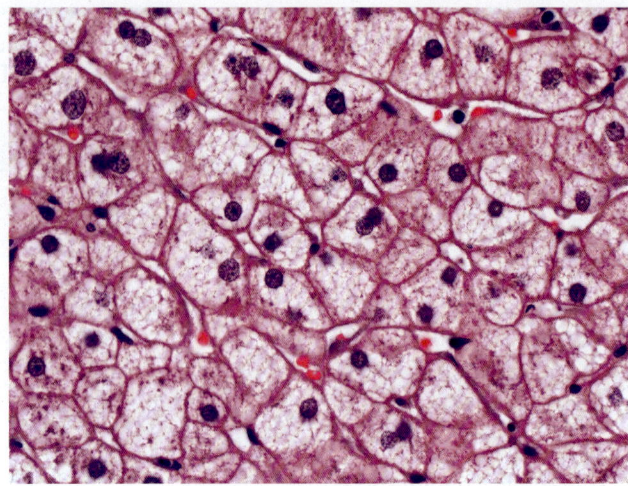

Figure 6.40. **Microvesicular steatosis.** Diffuse microvesicular steatosis is seen in this image, with each hepatocyte filled with numerous tiny droplets of fat.

TABLE 6.6: Differential for Microvesicular Steatosis

Cause	Note
Most Common Causes (All Are Still Rare)	
Drug/toxin	Examples include arsenic[32] and industrial solvents[33]
Acute fatty liver of pregnancy[34]	
Alcohol foamy degeneration[35]	
Genetic Diseases	
Alpers syndrome[36]	
Mitochondrial DNA depletion syndrome[37]	Navajo neuropathy is one example[38]
Ornithine transcarbamylase (OTC) deficiency[39,40]	
Wolman disease/cholesterol ester storage disease[41]	
Fatty acid oxidation disorders[42]	
Infection	
Superinfection of HDV on HBV[43,44]	Called Labrea hepatitis or Santa Marta hepatitis before recognition of HBV/HDV
Human herpes virus 6[45,46]	
Toxin of *Bacillus cereus*[47]	
Medication Effect	
Amiodarone[48,49]	
Nucleoside analogue reverse-transcriptase inhibitors used in treatment of human immunodeficiency virus (HIV) infection[50]	These drugs are now rarely used
Rye syndrome[51]	
Valproate[52]	

NEAR MISSES

CASE 1. A liver biopsy is performed in a 32-year-old man with mild obesity and mild but persistently elevated liver enzymes. The liver biopsy showed mild macrovesicular steatosis, with no evidence for steatohepatitis and no fibrosis. The iron stain showed moderate and fairly diffuse hepatocellular iron accumulation (Fig. 6.41). Subsequent evaluation determined the patient had homozygous C282Y mutations in the *HFE* gene.

This case illustrates the importance of looking for other disease processes beyond that of fatty liver disease. Patients often have histories consistent with fatty liver disease, the biopsy shows fatty liver disease, and it is easy to drop right into deciding between steatosis versus steatohepatitis, with subsequent grading of injury and staging of fibrosis. Do not forget to look for other concomitant disease processes. While patchy mild iron is not uncommon in ordinary fatty liver disease, the degree of iron accumulation in this case is too much for ordinary fatty liver disease, especially because there is no fibrosis.

Another example will illustrate this important point. A patient had all of the clinical features of the metabolic syndrome and underwent bariatric surgery, where a liver biopsy was also performed. The histological findings were that of steatohepatitis with minimal pericellular fibrosis but also showed moderate and diffuse portal chronic inflammation (Fig. 6.42), a pattern that is unusual for fatty liver disease. A note in the pathology report prompted additional laboratory testing, which revealed that the patient also had chronic hepatitis C.

CASE 2. A 45-year-old woman with the metabolic syndrome had mild and persistent elevations in her liver enzymes. Serology testing was negative for viral infections, ANA, and ASMA, but was positive for AMA. The biopsy showed marked macrovesicular steatosis (Fig. 6.43) with occasional ballooned hepatocytes, consistent with mildly active steatohepatitis. There was no fibrosis. The portal tracts showed minimal portal chronic inflammation, which was initially interpreted as consistent with an additional component of primary biliary cirrhosis because of the positive AMA. On rereview, the diagnosis was modified to steatohepatitis only.

Mild elevations in ANA and ASMA are fairly common in patients with fatty liver disease. AMA positivity is less common but can also be seen in about 1% of patients. In these settings, the positive serologies are usually nonspecific and do not correlate with other clinical or histological findings of autoimmune hepatitis or primary biliary cirrhosis. The approach in cases with fatty liver disease plus positive serologies is to require histological features of autoimmune hepatitis or primary biliary cirrhosis before making the additional diagnosis.

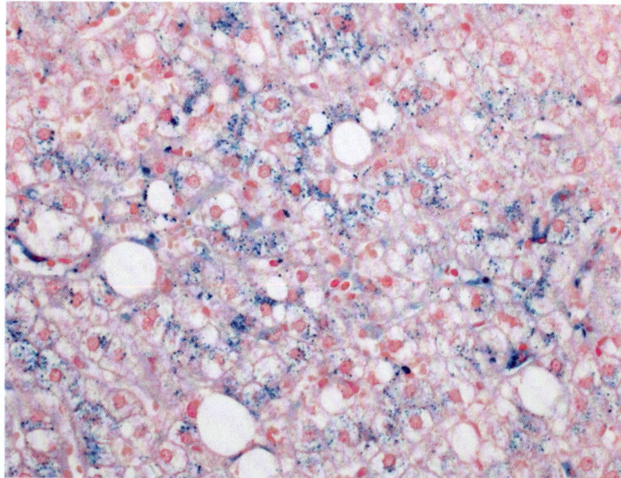

Figure 6.41. Near miss case 1, hemochromatosis in the setting of fatty liver disease. A Perls iron stain shows moderate diffuse hepatocellular iron accumulation.

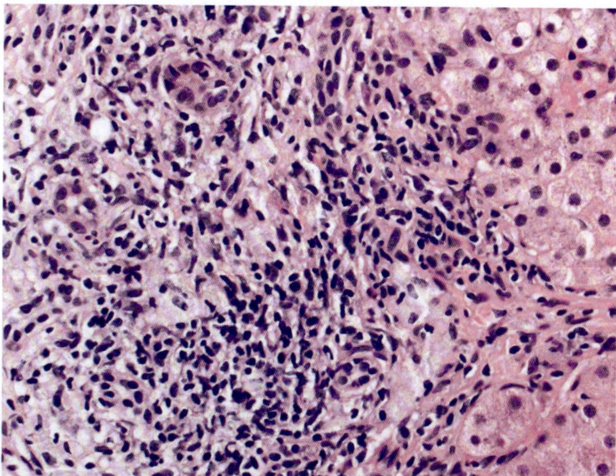

Figure 6.42. Near miss case 1, fatty liver disease with too much portal chronic inflammation. This case of fatty liver disease also had moderate portal chronic inflammation and ended up also having chronic hepatitis C.

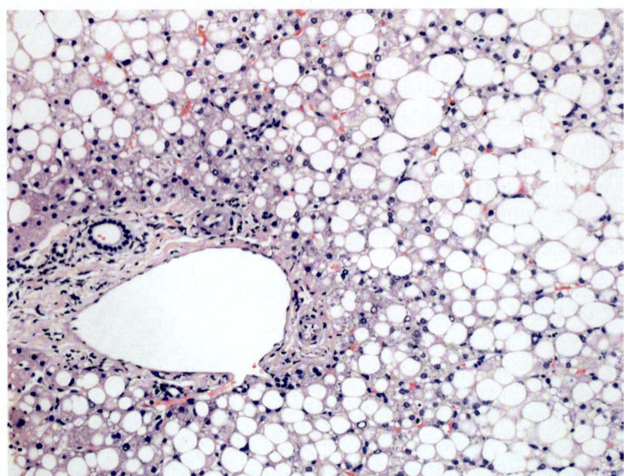

Figure 6.43. **Near miss case 2, steatohepatitis with mild AMA elevation.** The biopsy shows fatty liver disease, but no evidence for primary biliary cirrhosis.

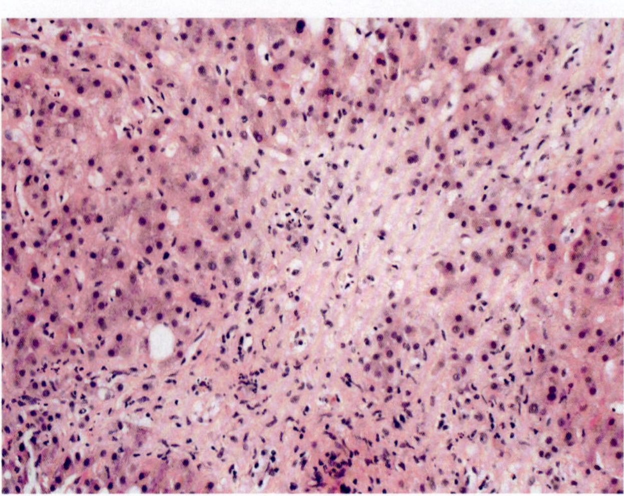

Figure 6.44. **Near miss case 3, steatohepatitis with zone 3 fibrosis.** There is marked zone 3 scarring.

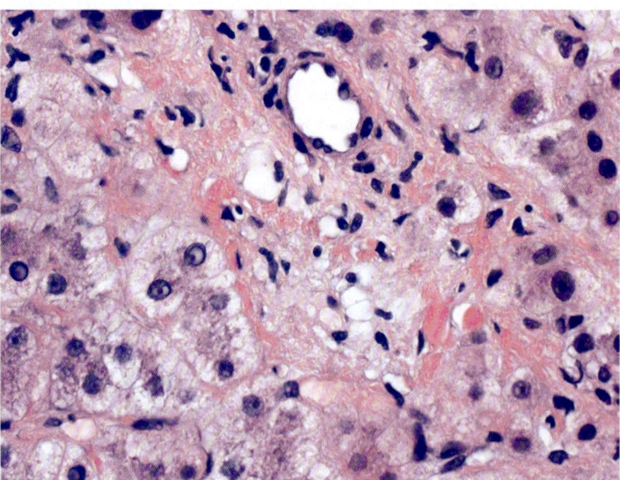

Figure 6.45. **Near miss case 3, steatohepatitis with arterioles growing into central veins.** The scarred zone 3 area shows an arteriole (upper mid part of image).

CASE 3. A patient with a past history of heavy alcohol consumption underwent a liver biopsy to determine the fibrosis stage and evaluate for active liver injury. There was minimal macrovesicular steatosis, but no evidence for active steatohepatitis. There was portal fibrosis and focal bridging fibrosis, but no evidence for established cirrhosis. The central veins were noted to be obliterated and/or fibrotic throughout much of the biopsy (Fig. 6.44), and a diagnosis of an additional component of possible veno-occlusive disease was considered. On review, the sclerosis of the central veins was noted to be part of the pathology of alcoholic hepatitis and did not indicate an additional disease process. In some cases of both nonalcoholic and alcoholic steatohepatitis (Fig. 6.45), the scarred zone 3 areas can induce ingrowth of small arterioles and suggest a portal tract without a duct.[13]

References

1. Hall AR, Dhillon AP, Green AC, et al. Hepatic steatosis estimated microscopically versus digital image analysis. *Liver Int*. 2013;33:926-935.
2. Africa JA, Behling CA, Brunt EM, et al; Nonalcoholic Steatohepatitis Clinical Research Network. In children with nonalcoholic fatty liver disease, zone 1 steatosis is associated with advanced fibrosis. *Clin Gastroenterol Hepatol*. 2018;16(3):438-446.e1.

3. Singh S, Allen AM, Wang Z, Prokop LJ, Murad MH, Loomba R. Fibrosis progression in nonalcoholic fatty liver vs nonalcoholic steatohepatitis: a systematic review and meta-analysis of paired-biopsy studies. *Clin Gastroenterol Hepatol*. 2015;13:643-654.e1-9; quiz e39-40.
4. Angulo P, Kleiner DE, Dam-Larsen S, et al. Liver fibrosis, but no other histologic features, is associated with long-term outcomes of patients with nonalcoholic fatty liver disease. *Gastroenterology*. 2015;149:389-397.e10.
5. Ekstedt M, Hagstrom H, Nasr P, et al. Fibrosis stage is the strongest predictor for disease-specific mortality in NAFLD after up to 33 years of follow-up. *Hepatology*. 2015;61:1547-1554.
6. Limketkai BN, Mehta SH, Sutcliffe CG, et al. Relationship of liver disease stage and antiviral therapy with liver-related events and death in adults coinfected with HIV/HCV. *JAMA*. 2012;308:370-378.
7. McPherson S, Hardy T, Henderson E, Burt AD, Day CP, Anstee QM. Evidence of NAFLD progression from steatosis to fibrosing-steatohepatitis using paired biopsies: implications for prognosis and clinical management. *J Hepatol*. 2015;62:1148-1155.
8. Kleiner DE, Brunt EM, Van Natta M, et al. Design and validation of a histological scoring system for nonalcoholic fatty liver disease. *Hepatology*. 2005;41:1313-1321.
9. Guy CD, Suzuki A, Burchette JL, et al. Costaining for keratins 8/18 plus ubiquitin improves detection of hepatocyte injury in nonalcoholic fatty liver disease. *Hum Pathol*. 2012;43:790-800.
10. Abraham S, Furth EE. Receiver operating characteristic analysis of glycogenated nuclei in liver biopsy specimens: quantitative evaluation of their relationship with diabetes and obesity. *Hum Pathol*. 1994;25:1063-1068.
11. Silverman JF, O'Brien KF, Long S, et al. Liver pathology in morbidly obese patients with and without diabetes. *Am J Gastroenterol*. 1990;85:1349-1355.
12. Tandra S, Yeh MM, Brunt EM, et al. Presence and significance of microvesicular steatosis in nonalcoholic fatty liver disease. *J Hepatol*. 2011;55:654-659.
13. Gill RM, Belt P, Wilson L, Bass NM, Ferrell LD. Centrizonal arteries and microvessels in nonalcoholic steatohepatitis. *Am J Surg Pathol*. 2011;35:1400-1404.
14. Loria P, Lonardo A, Leonardi F, et al. Non-organ-specific autoantibodies in nonalcoholic fatty liver disease: prevalence and correlates. *Dig Dis Sci*. 2003;48:2173-2181.
15. Ravi S, Shoreibah M, Raff E, et al. Autoimmune markers do not impact clinical presentation or natural history of steatohepatitis-related liver disease. *Dig Dis Sci*. 2015;60:3788-3793.
16. Adams LA, Lindor KD, Angulo P. The prevalence of autoantibodies and autoimmune hepatitis in patients with nonalcoholic fatty liver disease. *Am J Gastroenterol*. 2004;99:1316-1320.
17. Bedossa P, Poitou C, Veyrie N, et al. Histopathological algorithm and scoring system for evaluation of liver lesions in morbidly obese patients. *Hepatology*. 2012;56:1751-1759.
18. Shetty A, Cho W, Alazawi W, Syn WK. Methotrexate hepatotoxicity and the impact of nonalcoholic fatty liver disease. *Am J Med Sci*. 2017;354:172-181.
19. Kremer JM, Alarcon GS, Lightfoot RW Jr, et al. Methotrexate for rheumatoid arthritis. Suggested guidelines for monitoring liver toxicity. American College of Rheumatology. *Arthritis Rheum*. 1994;37:316-328.
20. Roenigk HH Jr, Auerbach R, Maibach HI, Weinstein GD. Methotrexate in psoriasis: revised guidelines. *J Am Acad Dermatol*. 1988;19:145-156.
21. Yap JY, O'Connor C, Mager DR, Taylor G, Roberts EA. Diagnostic challenges of nonalcoholic fatty liver disease (NAFLD) in children of normal weight. *Clin Res Hepatol Gastroenterol*. 2011;35:500-505.
22. Collardeau-Frachon S, Bouvier R, Le Gall C, et al. Unexpected diagnosis of cystic fibrosis at liver biopsy: a report of four pediatric cases. *Virchows Arch*. 2007;451:57-64.
23. Powell EE, Searle J, Mortimer R. Steatohepatitis associated with limb lipodystrophy. *Gastroenterology*. 1989;97:1022-1024.
24. Lefkowitch JH, Grossman ME. Hepatic pathology in porphyria cutanea tarda. *Liver*. 1983;3:19-29.
25. Kimura H, Kako M, Yo K, Oda T. Alcoholic hyalins (Mallory bodies) in a case of Weber-Christian disease: electron microscopic observations of liver involvement. *Gastroenterology*. 1980;78:807-812.
26. Wasserman JM, Thung SN, Berman R, Bodenheimer HC Jr, Sigal SH. Hepatic Weber-Christian disease. *Semin Liver Dis*. 2001;21:115-118.
27. Stattermayer AF, Traussnigg S, Dienes HP, et al. Hepatic steatosis in Wilson disease–role of copper and PNPLA3 mutations. *J Hepatol*. 2015;63:156-163.

28. Johannsson G, Bengtsson BA. Growth hormone and the metabolic syndrome. *J Endocrinol Invest*. 1999;22:41-46.

29. Chung GE, Kim D, Kim W, et al. Non-alcoholic fatty liver disease across the spectrum of hypothyroidism. *J Hepatol*. 2012;57:150-156.

30. Di Minno MN, Tufano A, Rusolillo A, Di Minno G, Tarantino G. High prevalence of nonalcoholic fatty liver in patients with idiopathic venous thromboembolism. *World J Gastroenterol*. 2010;16:6119-6122.

31. Cotrim HP, Andrade ZA, Parana R, Portugal M, Lyra LG, Freitas LA. Nonalcoholic steatohepatitis: a toxic liver disease in industrial workers. *Liver*. 1999;19:299-304.

32. Verheij J, Voortman J, van Nieuwkerk CM, Jarbandhan SV, Mulder CJ, Bloemena E. Hepatic morphopathologic findings of lead poisoning in a drug addict: a case report. *J Gastrointestin Liver Dis*. 2009;18:225-227.

33. Redlich CA, West AB, Fleming L, True LD, Cullen MR, Riely CA. Clinical and pathological characteristics of hepatotoxicity associated with occupational exposure to dimethylformamide. *Gastroenterology*. 1990;99:748-757.

34. Rolfes DB, Ishak KG. Acute fatty liver of pregnancy: a clinicopathologic study of 35 cases. *Hepatology*. 1985;5:1149-1158.

35. Uchida T, Kao H, Quispe-Sjogren M, Peters RL. Alcoholic foamy degeneration–a pattern of acute alcoholic injury of the liver. *Gastroenterology*. 1983;84:683-692.

36. Tesarova M, Mayr JA, Wenchich L, et al. Mitochondrial DNA depletion in Alpers syndrome. *Neuropediatrics*. 2004;35:217-223.

37. Mandel H, Hartman C, Berkowitz D, Elpeleg ON, Manov I, Iancu TC. The hepatic mitochondrial DNA depletion syndrome: ultrastructural changes in liver biopsies. *Hepatology*. 2001;34:776-784.

38. Holve S, Hu D, Shub M, Tyson RW, Sokol RJ. Liver disease in Navajo neuropathy. *J Pediatr*. 1999;135:482-493.

39. Capistrano-Estrada S, Marsden DL, Nyhan WL, Newbury RO, Krous HF, Tuchman M. Histopathological findings in a male with late-onset ornithine transcarbamylase deficiency. *Pediatr Pathol*. 1994;14:235-243.

40. Badizadegan K, Perez-Atayde AR. Focal glycogenosis of the liver in disorders of ureagenesis: its occurrence and diagnostic significance. *Hepatology*. 1997;26:365-373.

41. Hulkova H, Elleder M. Distinctive histopathological features that support a diagnosis of cholesterol ester storage disease in liver biopsy specimens. *Histopathology*. 2012;60:1107-1113.

42. Rinaldo P, Yoon HR, Yu C, Raymond K, Tiozzo C, Giordano G. Sudden and unexpected neonatal death: a protocol for the postmortem diagnosis of fatty acid oxidation disorders. *Semin Perinatol*. 1999;23:204-210.

43. Andrade ZA, Lesbordes JL, Ravisse P, et al. Fulminant hepatitis with microvesicular steatosis (a histologic comparison of cases occurring in Brazil–Labrea hepatitis–and in central Africa–Bangui hepatitis). *Rev Soc Bras Med Trop*. 1992;25:155-160.

44. Buitrago B, Popper H, Hadler SC, et al. Specific histologic features of Santa Marta hepatitis: a severe form of hepatitis delta-virus infection in northern South America. *Hepatology*. 1986;6:1285-1291.

45. Chang YL, Parker ME, Nuovo G, Miller JB. Human herpesvirus 6-related fulminant myocarditis and hepatitis in an immunocompetent adult with fatal outcome. *Hum Pathol*. 2009;40:740-745.

46. Aita K, Jin Y, Irie H, et al. Are there histopathologic characteristics particular to fulminant hepatic failure caused by human herpesvirus-6 infection? A case report and discussion. *Hum Pathol*. 2001;32:887-889.

47. Mahler H, Pasi A, Kramer JM, et al. Fulminant liver failure in association with the emetic toxin of Bacillus cereus. *N Engl J Med*. 1997;336:1142-1148.

48. Puli SR, Fraley MA, Puli V, Kuperman AB, Alpert MA. Hepatic cirrhosis caused by low-dose oral amiodarone therapy. *Am J Med Sci*. 2005;330:257-261.

49. Lewis JH, Mullick F, Ishak KG, et al. Histopathologic analysis of suspected amiodarone hepatotoxicity. *Hum Pathol*. 1990;21:59-67.

50. Coghlan ME, Sommadossi JP, Jhala NC, Many WJ, Saag MS, Johnson VA. Symptomatic lactic acidosis in hospitalized antiretroviral-treated patients with human immunodeficiency virus infection: a report of 12 cases. *Clin Infect Dis*. 2001;33:1914-1921.

51. Bove KE, McAdams AJ, Partin JC, Partin JS, Hug G, Schubert WK. The hepatic lesion in Reye's syndrome. *Gastroenterology*. 1975;69:685-697.

52. Scheffner D, Konig S, Rauterberg-Ruland I, Kochen W, Hofmann WJ, Unkelbach S. Fatal liver failure in 16 children with valproate therapy. *Epilepsia*. 1988;29:530-542.

7 AUTOIMMUNE HEPATITIS

CHAPTER OUTLINE

CLINICAL FINDINGS

Autoimmune hepatitis is a chronic liver disease where the immune system recognizes hepatocytes as "not self," leading to lymphocyte-mediated injury. Untreated disease has a high risk of progressing to cirrhosis and to liver failure. Most patients are young to middle-aged women, but individuals can present in the pediatric population, older population, or in men. At the time of diagnosis or during clinical follow-up, about 20% of patients will have additional autoimmune diseases involving other organs.[1]

About 70% of patients are diagnosed when they have signs or symptoms resulting from chronic liver disease, but a small subset present with fulminant or subfulminant acute liver failure. Another 25% of patients are identified incidentally during evaluations for other disease processes.

Once autoimmune hepatitis is diagnosed, steroid therapy leads to disease remission in about 75% of cases, with liver enzymes returning to normal within the first 6 months. Another 15% of individuals will respond, but more slowly, while 10% will be nonresponders, with worsening of liver enzymes while on therapy. When remission is obtained, other agents such as azathioprine are added, allowing reduction of the steroid dosages. In cases of nonresponse, it is helpful to rereview the biopsy for possible findings of additional disease processes, including overlap syndromes.

Your job as a pathologist is to examine the liver biopsy and determine if the findings are consistent with autoimmune hepatitis, suggest an alternative diagnosis when appropriate, suggest an overlap syndrome between autoimmune hepatitis plus another disease when appropriate, and determine the degree of fibrosis. The clinical team will establish the final diagnosis for the patient's liver disease by integrating the results of clinical findings, serology, and histology. The Autoimmune Hepatitis Group has published a formal scoring system to help with this process (Table 7.1). As can be seen, the pathologist's role is largely to determine if the findings are consistent with autoimmune hepatitis.

TABLE 7.1: International Autoimmune Hepatitis Group Criteria for Autoimmune Hepatitis[16]

Finding	Level of Positivity	Points Assigned	Notes
Autoantibodies			
All serological testing	Negative	0	
ANA or SMA	≥1:40	1	
ANA or SMA	≥1:80	2	2 points is the maximum for all Autoantibodies, even if the patient is positive for multiple autoantibodies
or LKM	≥1:40	2	
or SLA	Positive	2	
IgG	Less than upper limit of normal	0	
	>Upper normal limit	1	
	>1.10 times upper normal limit	2	

TABLE 7.1: International Autoimmune Hepatitis Group Criteria for Autoimmune Hepatitis[16] (Continued)

Finding	Level of Positivity	Points Assigned	Notes
Liver histology	Not compatible with AIH	0	Examples: fatty liver disease, vascular outflow disease, biliary obstruction, etc.
	Compatible with AIH	1	Hepatitic pattern of injury
	Typical of AIH	2	Hepatitic pattern of injury with interface activity and plasma cell–rich inflammation
Absence of viral hepatitis	Viral serology negative	2	
Interpretation	**≥7: definite AIH**		
	≥6: probable AIH		

AIH, autoimmune hepatitis; ANA, antinuclear antibodies; LKM, liver kidney microsomal antibodies; SLA, soluble liver antigen.

LABORATORY FINDINGS

AST and ALT levels are typically elevated more than 2× the upper limit of normal in autoimmune hepatitis, but enzyme levels can be much higher when there is moderate or greater hepatitis. GGT and alkaline phosphatase levels are also elevated, but typically less than 2× the upper limit of normal for alkaline phosphatase and 5× for GGT. If GGT or alkaline phosphatase levels are greater than this, patients are more likely to have an overlap syndrome with PBC or PSC.

Autoantibodies are detected in ~90% of individuals with autoimmune hepatitis.[2] Type 1 autoimmune hepatitis is defined by positive serology for antinuclear antibodies (ANA) and or anti–smooth muscle antibodies (ASMA). Soluble liver antigen (SLA) antibodies are present in about 30% of individuals. In contrast, type 2 autoimmune hepatitis is defined by positive serology for liver kidney microsomal antibodies (LKM-1) and or liver cytosol antibodies (LC1) (Table 7.2). Type 2 autoimmune hepatitis tends to have a more severe clinical course, although not all studies agree on this point. In most cases, the serology is either that of type

TABLE 7.2: Autoimmune Hepatitis Subtypes

Feature	Type 1	Type 2
Frequency	95%	5%
Autoantibodies[17]	ANA alone: 10% ASMA alone: 35% ANA and ASMA: 50% SLA: 30% negative for all: 10%	LKM and or LC1
Elevated serum IgG levels	>2× upper limit of normal in ~80%	>2× upper limit of normal in ~80%
Most common affected age-group	Teenage to adult	Pediatric and young adult
Histological findings	Hepatitic pattern with prominent plasma cells	Hepatitic pattern with prominent plasma cells
Progression to cirrhosis	45%	80%

ANA, antinuclear antibodies; LC1, liver cytosol antibodies; LKM, liver kidney microsomal antibodies; SLA, soluble liver antigen.

1 or type 2, but not both. In those rare cases that are positive for both type 1 and type 2 autoimmune hepatitis antibodies, the clinical course tends to follow type 2 autoimmune hepatitis. AMA titers are elevated in about 10% of individuals with autoimmune hepatitis, most who will not have an overlap syndrome between autoimmune hepatitis and PBC. Serum IgG are elevated in 80% of individuals at presentation and tend to normalize with remission. Serum IgM levels are elevated in 10% to 30% of cases, but to a lesser degree than IgG.

HISTOLOGICAL FINDINGS

CHECKLIST: Range of Histological Patterns in Autoimmune Hepatitis

- ☐ Fulminant hepatitis
- ☐ Acute hepatitis with moderate to marked lobular inflammation ± necrosis
- ☐ Nonspecific chronic hepatitis with mild portal and lobular inflammation and fibrosis
- ☐ Cirrhosis, usually with mild nonspecific inflammation

CHECKLIST: Typical Features of Untreated Autoimmune Hepatitis Presenting With Liver Disease (Excluding Fulminant Hepatitis and Incidentally Identified Cases)

- ☐ Hepatitic pattern usually with mild or greater lobular hepatitis
  - ○ Lobules may show regenerative rosettes
  - ○ Emperipolesis may be present
- ☐ Plasma cell–rich inflammation in portal tracts and lobules
  - ○ Interface activity usually moderate or greater
- ☐ Note: Incidentally identified cases, or those presenting with cirrhosis, usually have less inflammation, and plasma cells can be less prominent

OVERVIEW OF HISTOLOGICAL FINDINGS

The histological findings range from fulminant hepatitis to mild and nonspecific chronic hepatitis in a cirrhotic liver. The most common pattern in untreated cases shows mildly to moderately active lobular inflammation (Fig. 7.1) and mild to moderate portal chronic inflammation (Fig. 7.2) with interface activity (Fig. 7.3). Lymphoid aggregates are common in the portal tracts, present in about 2/3 of cases (Fig. 7.4), especially when there is at least moderate portal chronic inflammation. Mild bile duct lymphocytosis, without duct injury or destruction, is also common and does not have any strong clinical significance, being found in about 25% of cases (Fig. 7.5). The frequency varies considerably in the literature depending on the threshold of the authors for identifying bile duct lymphocytosis. Central vein or portal venulitis is also common, found in 10% to 20% of cases.[3]

INTERFACE ACTIVITY

Autoimmune hepatitis typically has interface activity (Figs. 7.6 and 7.7). In fact, interface activity is commonly listed in review articles, book chapters, and other pathology literature as being characteristic of autoimmune hepatitis. Although this statement is technically accurate, it can give the misleading impression that interface hepatitis is in some way specific for autoimmune hepatitis or has special diagnostic powers. But it does not. Interface hepatitis is present in acute and chronic hepatitis caused by any of the many different inflammatory diseases of the liver, including drug effects and viral hepatitis (Fig. 7.8), which of note tend to be the main clinical and histological differential for autoimmune hepatitis. For example,

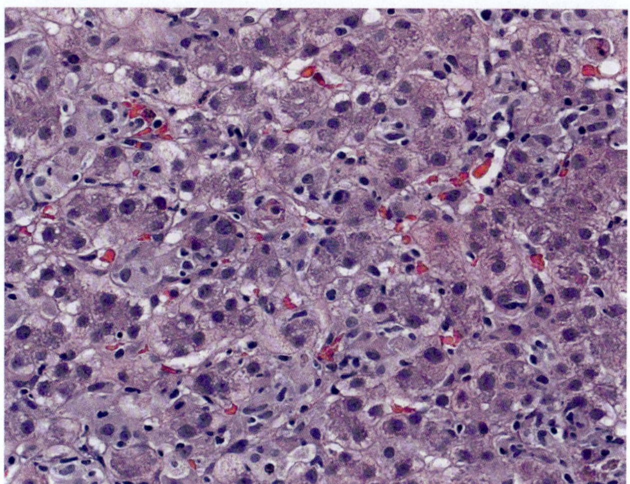

Figure 7.1. **Autoimmune hepatitis, lobular hepatitis.** Moderate lobular hepatitis is present.

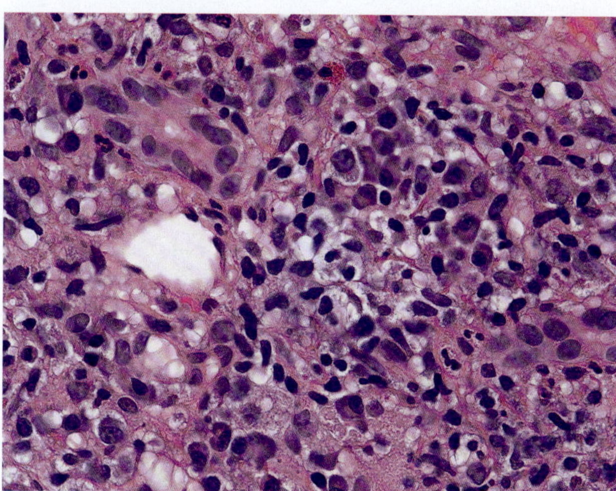

Figure 7.2. **Autoimmune hepatitis, portal inflammation.** Moderate portal chronic inflammation is seen. Note also the enrichment for plasma cells.

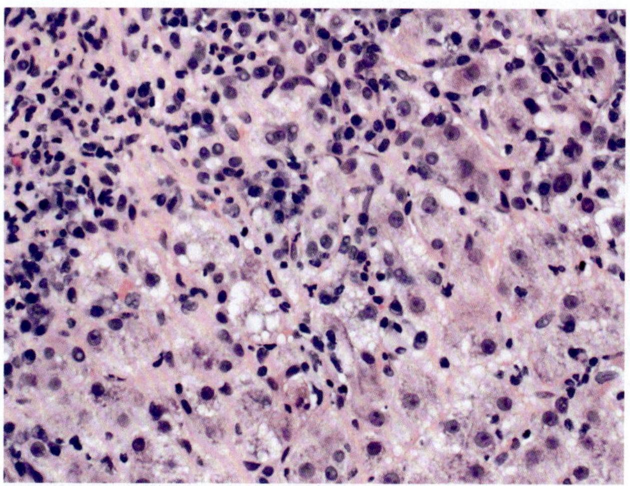

Figure 7.3. **Autoimmune hepatitis, interface activity.** Brisk interface activity obscures the normal sharp line between the portal tracts and lobules. The inflammation in the portal tract (top left of image) is lymphocytic with prominent plasma cells.

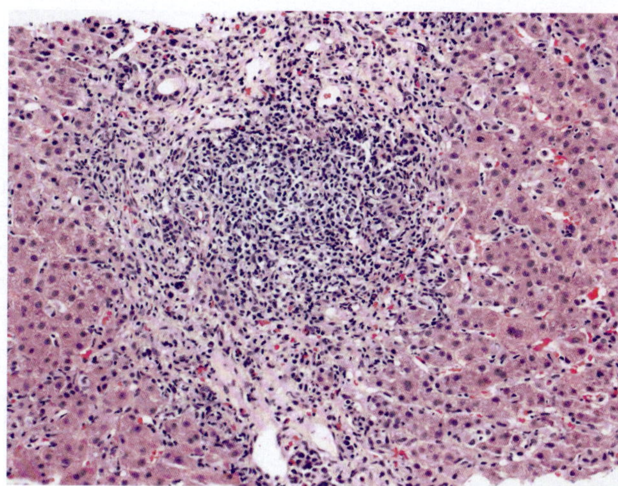

Figure 7.4. **Autoimmune hepatitis, lymphoid aggregates.** The portal tract also shows a lymphoid aggregate.

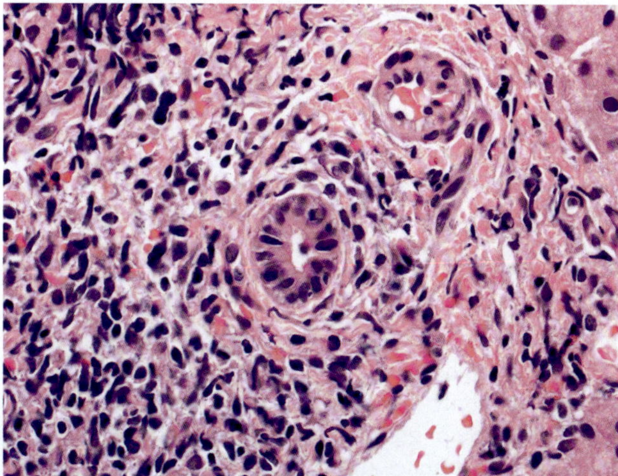

Figure 7.5. **Autoimmune hepatitis, duct lymphocytosis.** Mild bile duct lymphocytosis was present in multiple portal tracts but was not associated with duct injury or duct destruction.

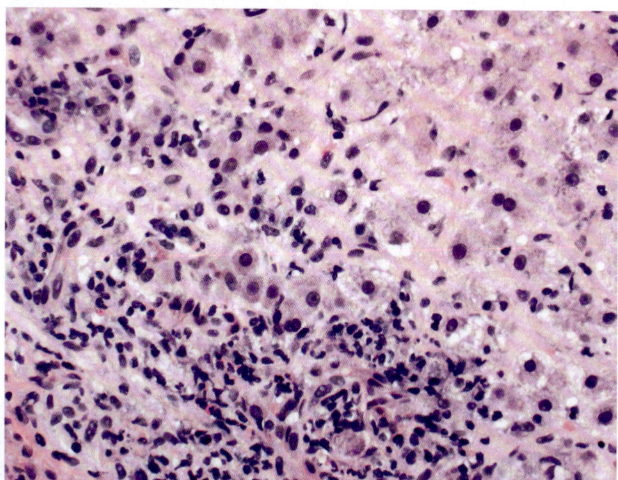

Figure 7.6. **Autoimmune hepatitis, interface activity.** Moderate interface activity is present, with lymphocytic inflammation of the hepatocytes immediately adjacent to the portal tract.

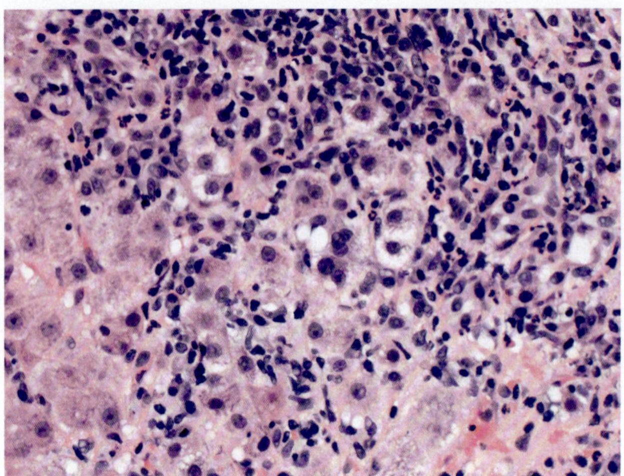

Figure 7.7. **Autoimmune hepatitis, interface activity.** The biopsy shows marked interface activity. The portal tract is in the upper right of the image.

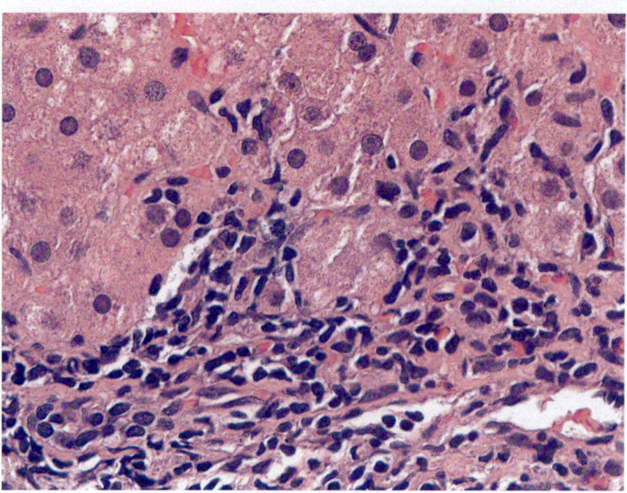

Figure 7.8. **Chronic hepatitis C, interface activity.** Moderate interface activity is present in this case of chronic hepatitis C.

one study found interface activity in 100% of hepatitic drug reactions.[4] Why all of the emphasis on interface activity then, on this particular finding in autoimmune hepatitis? There is no good reason really, other than that it has been repeated often enough in lectures, text books, and papers, to have taken on a life of its own.

A better way to incorporate interface activity into your understanding is this: (1) interface activity is commonly present in acute and chronic hepatitis from any cause when the pattern of injury is hepatitic; (2) untreated autoimmune hepatitis commonly has a hepatitic pattern, so you will find interface activity; and (3) if the primary pattern of injury is not hepatitic, the etiology is unlikely to be autoimmune hepatitis and you will not find significant interface activity.

PORTAL TRACT INFLAMMATION

The inflammation in the portal tracts (Figs. 7.9 and 7.10) is commonly plasma cell rich (~90% of cases).[4] Once again, this finding is not specific, as plasma cell–rich inflammation is also found in some drug reactions and in acute hepatitis A and B. Nonetheless, this finding is more common in autoimmune hepatitis than in other diseases, so can help support the diagnosis, remembering that in all cases the histological findings are never diagnostic per se, only supportive.

CHECKLIST: Other Causes of Plasma Cell–Rich Hepatitis

- □ Idiosyncratic drug reactions
- □ Acute viral hepatitis
  - ○ Hepatitis A or B is most common
- □ Wilson disease

LOBULAR CHANGES

The lobular inflammation is moderate (Fig. 7.11) in most untreated cases without advanced fibrosis. In asymptomatic patients identified incidentally, the lobular inflammation is more likely to be on the mild side (Fig. 7.12). When there is marked inflammation, zone 3 necrosis and/or bridging necrosis is commonly found (Fig. 7.13). Lobular plasma cells can be present, especially in cases of moderate or greater lobular inflammation (Fig. 7.14), generally paralleling the plasma cell–rich infiltrates in the portal tracts. Because of the active injury, the hepatocytes will often show small pseudoacini or rosettes (Fig. 7.15). This finding can be seen in any disease with significant hepatitis and/or with cholestasis, so it is not specific. For example, one study found rosettes in 40% of hepatitic drug reactions.[4]

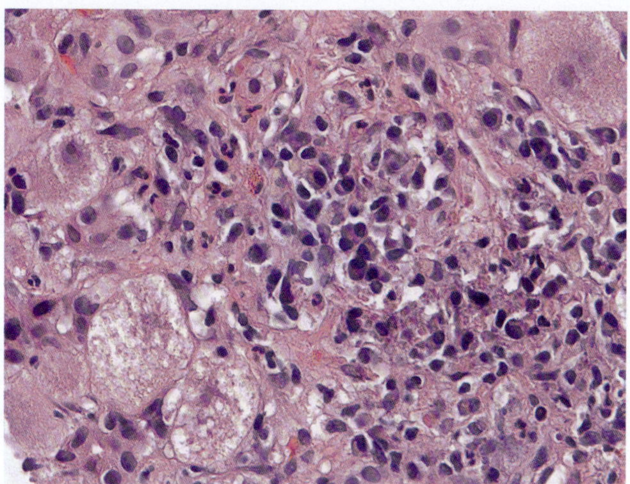

Figure 7.9. Autoimmune hepatitis, plasma cell–rich portal inflammation. Numerous plasma cells are present in the portal tracts.

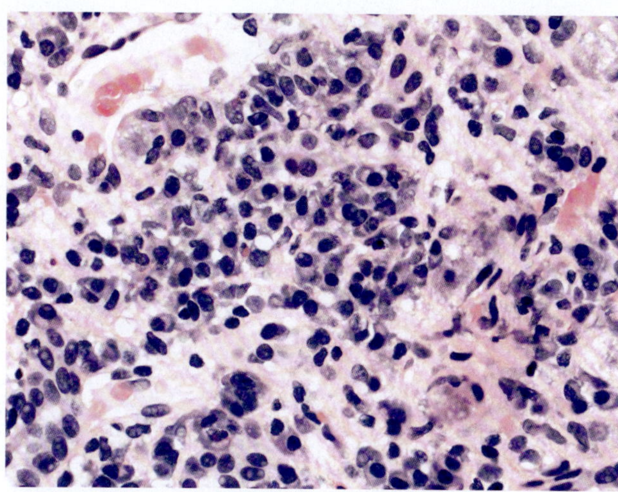

Figure 7.10. Autoimmune hepatitis, plasma cell–rich portal inflammation. Another example of plasma cell–rich portal inflammation. This finding is not entirely specific but is more common in autoimmune hepatitis.

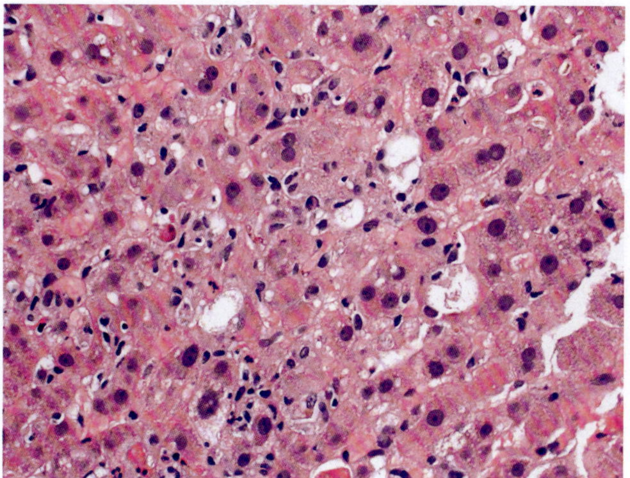

Figure 7.11. Autoimmune hepatitis, lobular hepatitis. There is moderate lobular hepatitis with lobular disarray, obscuring the normal trabecular architecture.

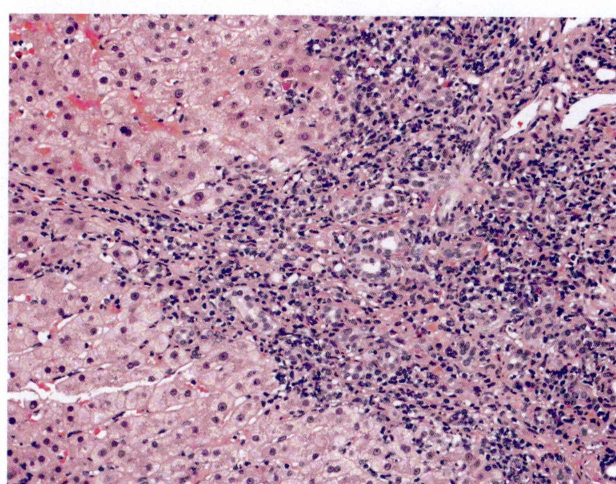

Figure 7.12. Autoimmune hepatitis, incidental identified disease. This case was incidentally identified when the liver looked nodular during cholecystectomy. The liver showed moderate portal chronic inflammation and minimal lobular activity.

In addition, some authors can see rosettes, and lots of them, in cases where other pathologists see none. Thus, use this finding with a grain of salt. Likewise, some authors report that hepatocyte emperipolesis of lymphocytes (Figs. 7.16 and 7.17) is a useful diagnostic finding for autoimmune hepatitis, although most pathologists who regularly use a microscope do not find this to be true, both because the finding is very dependent on who is looking through the microscope and because it is commonly found in other diseases, such as hepatic drug reactions.[4]

In a subset of cases, the lobular hepatitis can have a noticeable zone 3 accentuation (Fig. 7.18).[5] This finding is also common in drug effects and can be seen with acute viral hepatitis, so does not help identify the etiology. Several studies have suggested this pattern may represent an early form of autoimmune hepatitis, but this remains unclear, and the true significance of this pattern remains uncertain. Cases with a zone 3 predominant pattern often have less portal inflammation than other cases of autoimmune hepatitis.

In cases of moderate or greater hepatitis, the Kupffer cells commonly show a mild hyperplasia. In addition, the Kupffer cells can have small round cytoplasmic globules barely visible on H&E but highlighted by PASD (Figs 7.19 and 7.20). This finding appears to result from elevated gamma globin levels[6] but is not specific for autoimmune hepatitis. Similar

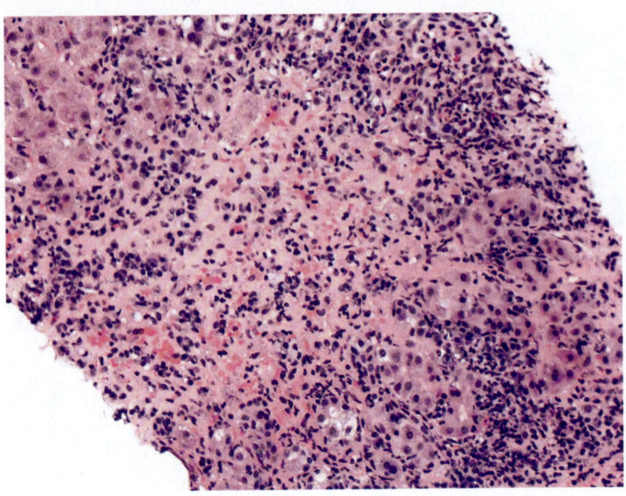

Figure 7.13. **Autoimmune hepatitis, lobular hepatitis.** Marked lobular hepatitis is seen, with zone 3 necrosis.

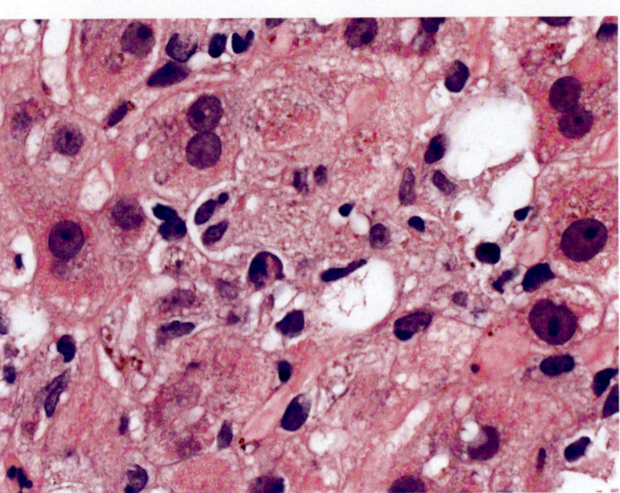

Figure 7.14. **Autoimmune hepatitis, lobular hepatitis.** Plasma cells can be found in the lobules. This finding parallels the plasma cell–rich inflammation found in the portal tracts and, while not entirely specific, also suggests autoimmune hepatitis.

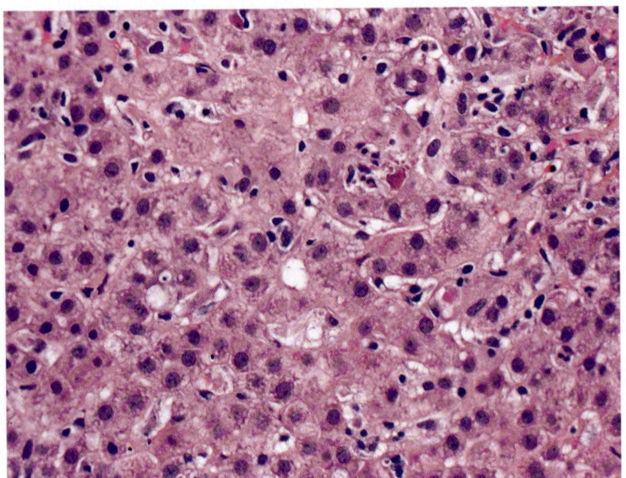

Figure 7.15. **Autoimmune hepatitis, lobular rosettes.** A rosette is seen in the center of the image, formed by the edges of a small group of hepatocytes.

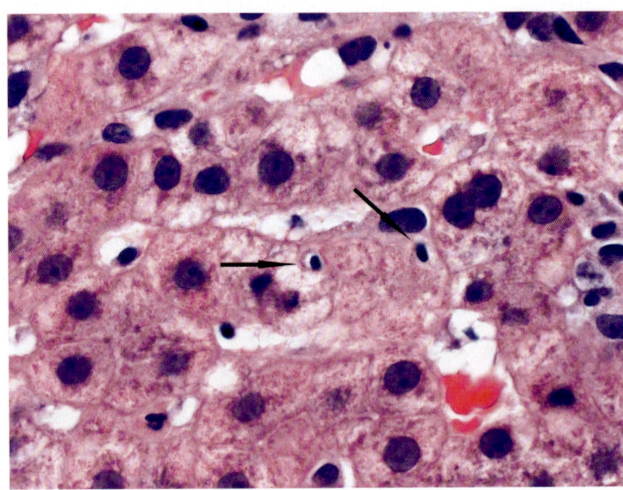

Figure 7.16. **Autoimmune hepatitis, emperipolesis (arrows).** Emperipolesis (lymphocytes or other cells/cellular debris inside hepatocytes) is well described in the literature but is often hard to reliably identify.

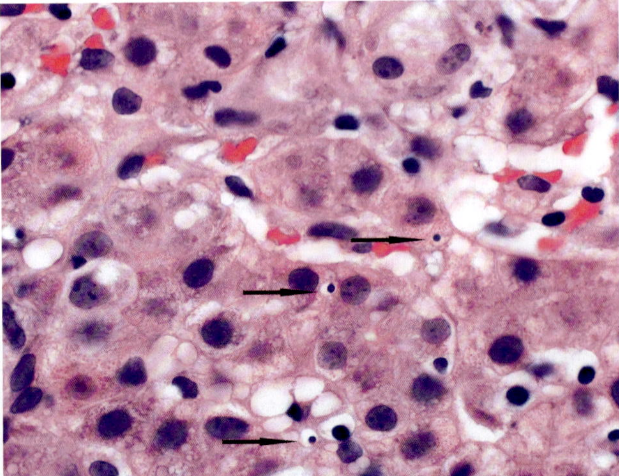

Figure 7.17. **Autoimmune hepatitis, emperipolesis (arrows).** Another example of emperipolesis. This finding is not specific and can also be seen in other causes of moderate to marked lobular hepatitis.

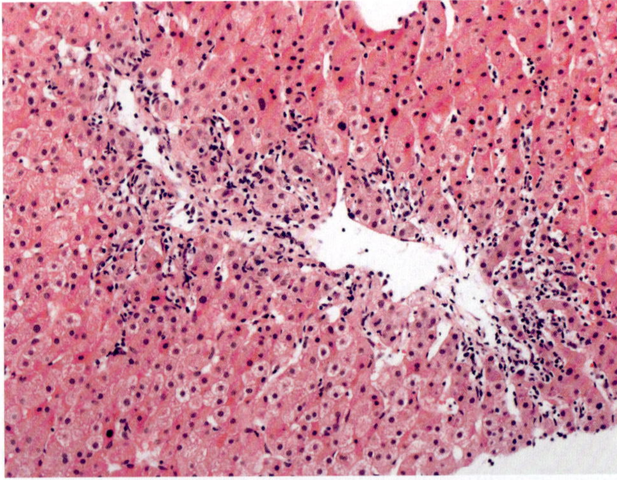

Figure 7.18. **Autoimmune hepatitis, zone 3 accentuation of hepatitis.** This case of autoimmune hepatitis showed a strong zone 3 pattern of inflammation with only mild portal chronic inflammation.

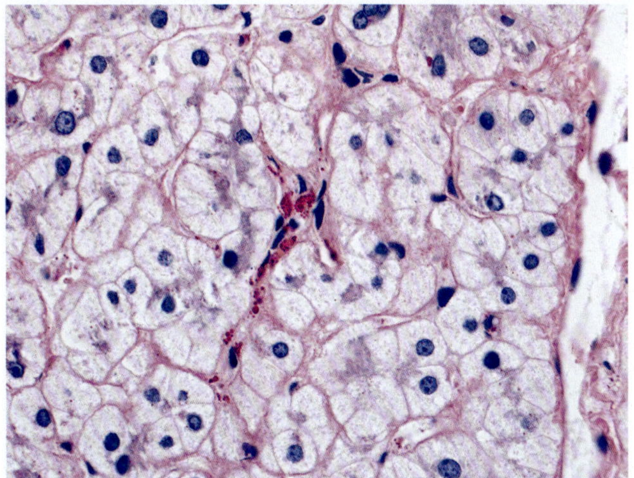

Figure 7.19. Autoimmune hepatitis, Kupffer cell globules, PASD. Kupffer cells have small globules that are highlighted in this PASD stain.

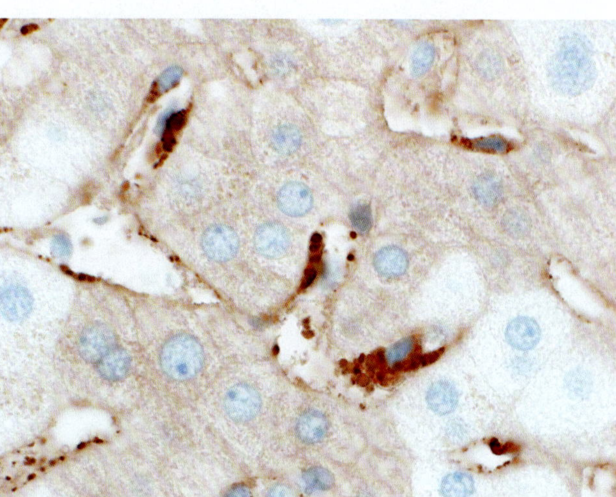

Figure 7.20. Autoimmune hepatitis, Kupffer cell globules, IgG. The globules stain positive for IgG.

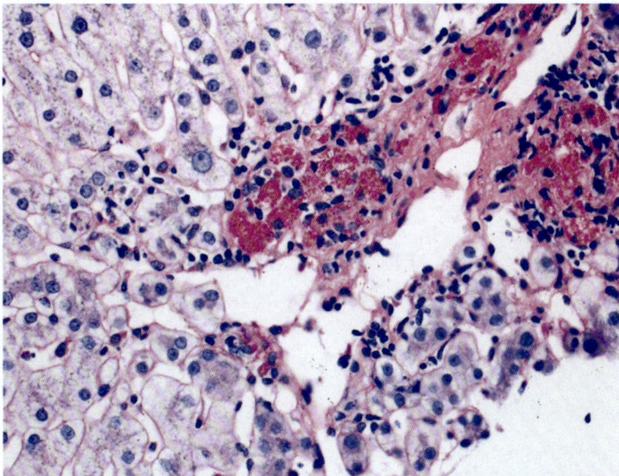

Figure 7.21. Drug reaction, Kupffer cell aggregates, PASD. In this drug reaction, there was a zone 3 pattern of hepatitis. A PASD stain shows clusters of Kupffer cells with cytoplasmic grunge but not the typical globules seen in autoimmune hepatitis.

changes can be seen in primary biliary cirrhosis and other diseases. Also, do not confuse this finding for the PASD positive, granular, cytoplasmic changes seen in ordinary Kupffer cell hyperplasia (Fig. 7.21), representing clean up from sites of lobular injury.

FULMINANT LIVER FAILURE

Fulminant liver failure is associated with massive liver necrosis. There can be residual portal tracts, sometimes with small rims of viable hepatocytes in zone 1 (Fig. 7.22), or patchier necrosis with areas of pancacinar necrosis alternating with areas of more preserved parenchyma. If enough time passes, the liver can develop regenerative nodules. The regenerative nodules can be several centimeters and can mimic tumors on imaging and on gross examination (Fig. 7.23).

In many cases of fulminant autoimmune hepatitis, the clinical and serological findings are typical and the overall diagnosis straightforward. However, in other cases, the clinical and serological findings are less clear. To help in this situation, a pattern of histological findings has been suggested as pointing to a diagnosis of autoimmune hepatitis when other causes have been clinically excluded and the serological testing for autoimmune hepatitis are equivocal. These findings including zone 3 accentuated residual inflammation, central perivenulitis, plasma cell–rich inflammation, and lymphoid aggregates in the portal tracts.[7]

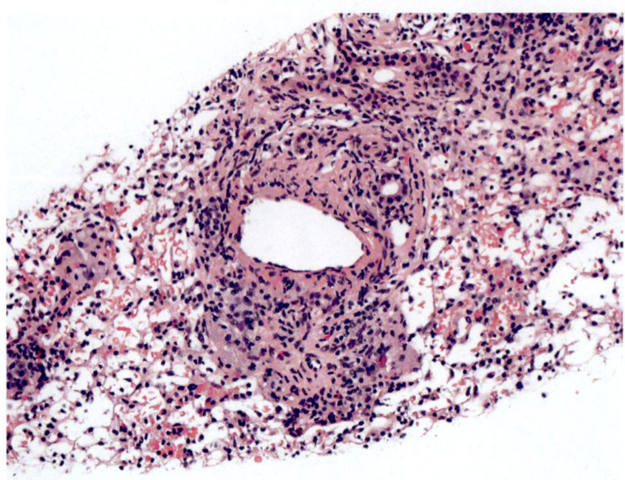

Figure 7.22. **Autoimmune hepatitis, panacinar necrosis.** There were almost no hepatocytes remaining in this biopsy of fulminant hepatitis.

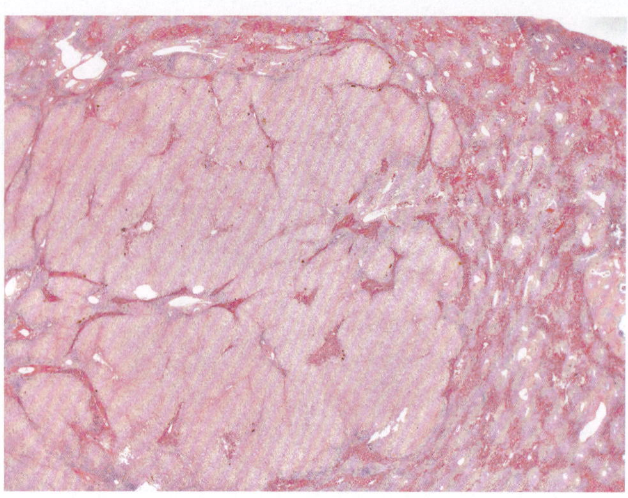

Figure 7.23. **Autoimmune hepatitis, subfulminant hepatitis.** A large regenerative nodule is seen in the background of massive liver necrosis.

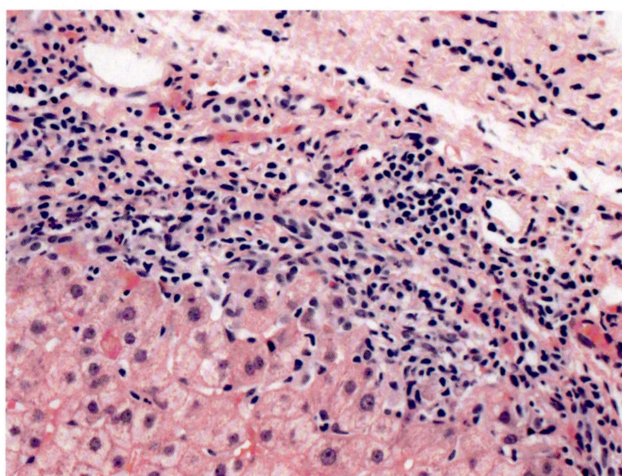

Figure 7.24. **Autoimmune hepatitis, "burned out."** This patient presented with cirrhosis. There was a mildly positive antinuclear antibodies (ANA) and anti–smooth muscle antibodies (ASMA) but no other clinical risk factors for cirrhosis. A biopsy showed patchy portal and septal chronic inflammation with mild interface activity and a mild plasma cell prominence.

CRYPTOGENIC CIRRHOSIS AND "BURNED OUT AUTOIMMUNE HEPATITIS"

Untreated autoimmune hepatitis can present with cirrhosis. In these cases, the inflammation is often largely abated or "burned out," leaving behind only mild nonspecific portal and septal lymphocytic inflammation. Interface activity can be a bit prominent in some of these cases (Fig. 7.24), but lobular hepatitis tends to be minimal to mild. The diagnosis of autoimmune hepatitis, as the cause of the cirrhosis can be suggested only after correlation with serological findings to confirm the presence of autoantibodies and after the exclusion of other causes of liver disease, in particularly fatty liver disease. In the young, less than 40 years of age, Wilson disease should also be clinically excluded.

AUTOIMMUNE HEPATITIS IN MEN

There are relative little data focused on autoimmune hepatitis in men. Clinically, men are less likely to have other autoimmune diseases.[8] Treatment is the same regardless of gender.[9] After treatment, men more likely to have clinical relapses.[8,10] The histological findings of autoimmune hepatitis have not been carefully examined in men. Anecdotally, the inflammatory patterns are broadly similar regardless of gender. Both commonly show plasma cell–rich inflammation, although in men plasma enrichment can be less striking.

IMMUNOHISTOCHEMICAL FINDINGS

In most cases, immunostains are not used to make a diagnosis of autoimmune hepatitis. The lymphocytic inflammation in the portal tracts and lobules is predominately activated T cells, and the lymphoid aggregates are composed in part by nodules of B lymphocytes, but these findings are not diagnostically useful. In some cases where you are struggling to differentiate autoimmune hepatitis from primary biliary cirrhosis, subtyping the plasma cells can be useful, as the portal tracts in autoimmune hepatitis typically have mostly IgG-positive plasma cells and only rare IgM-positive plasma cells, while in primary biliary cirrhosis the portal tracts typically have equal or greater numbers of IgM than IgG-positive plasma cells.[11–13] When using this approach, compare the same portal tract head to head on the different stains (Figs. 7.25 and 7.26). It is also helpful to do this for several different portal tracts, focusing on those portal tracts with the most plasma cells.

PEARLS & PITFALLS

- When using IgG and IgM immunostains, remember that their staining patterns are not entirely specific so they should be used in conjunction with other clinical and morphological findings.
- These stains are used to help distinguish autoimmune hepatitis (AIH) and PBC and have not been well enough studied to know if they play a role in diagnosing overlap syndromes.
- In most laboratories, these stains have significant background staining, but they are generally no problem to interpret anyway, if you focus on the brightly positive plasma cells.

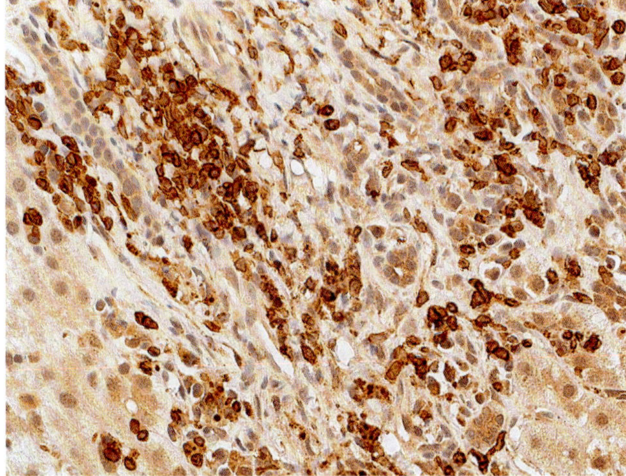

Figure 7.25. **Autoimmune hepatitis, IgG.** In this biopsy, the portal tracts contain mostly IgG-positive plasma cells with almost no IgM-positive plasma cells. There also is nonspecific background staining, but true positive cells are easy to identify.

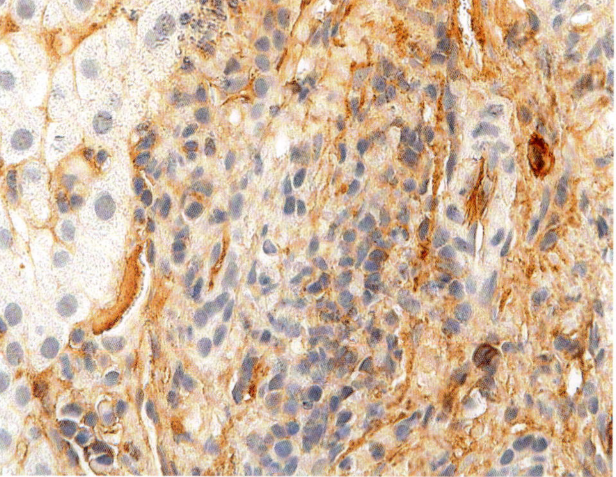

Figure 7.26. **Autoimmune hepatitis, IgM.** No positive plasma cells are seen. Note that background staining is a common finding, but truly positive cells have strong bright staining.

FIBROSIS STAGING

Fibrosis staging can be performed using descriptive terms (no fibrosis, portal fibrosis, bridging fibrosis, cirrhosis) or with formal staging systems such as the Ishak system or the Batts–Ludwig system. In cases of marked hepatitis, fibrosis evaluation can be particularly challenging because the marked portal inflammation can mimic portal fibrosis, bridging necrosis can mimic bridging fibrosis (Fig. 7.27), and marked bridging necrosis with panacinar collapse can mimic cirrhosis. In these cases, stage as accurately as you can and indicate in the report any caveats resulting from the marked hepatitis/necrosis.

Livers with marked hepatitis and extensive necrosis can (if there is enough time for the reparative process to begin) develop large regenerative nodules that resemble hepatocellular carcinoma on imaging and even on gross examination. These large nodules can sometimes prompt liver biopsies. Histologically, they are typical regenerative nodules with no cytological atypia. In addition, livers with subacute necrosis can have biopsies years later that show a distinctive pattern with some cores looking cirrhotic and others showing little or no fibrosis (Figs. 7.28 and 7.29).

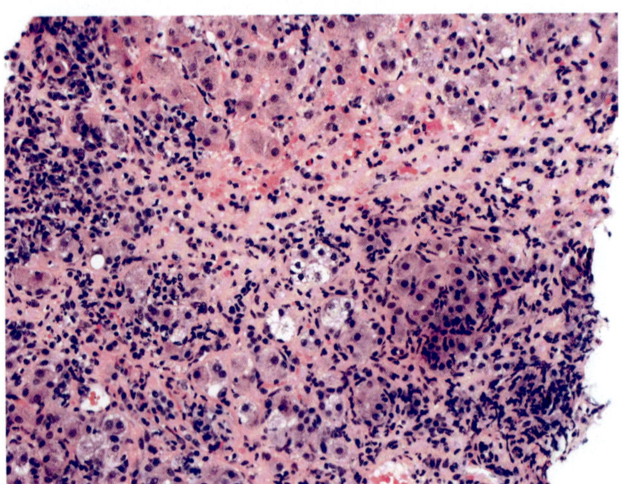

Figure 7.27. Autoimmune hepatitis, bridging necrosis. There is bridging necrosis in the center of this image, a finding that can be mistaken for bridging fibrosis on trichrome stains.

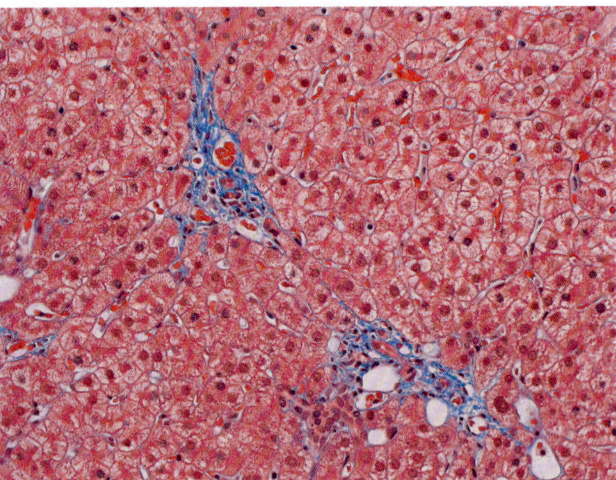

Figure 7.28. Autoimmune hepatitis, trichrome. This part of the biopsy showed no significant fibrosis.

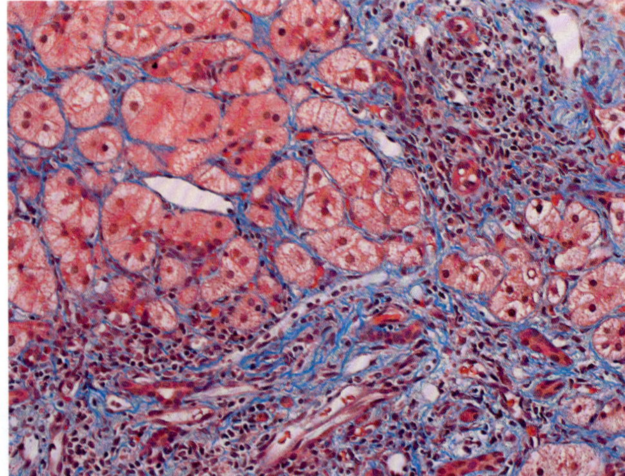

Figure 7.29. Autoimmune hepatitis, trichrome. This part of the biopsy showed changes of cirrhosis (same biopsy as shown above).

PEARLS & PITFALLS

Occasionally, pathologists and clinicians have the mistaken idea that at least some degree of fibrosis is needed for a confident diagnosis of autoimmune hepatitis, but this is not the case. The presence, or the absence, of fibrosis is independent of the diagnosis of autoimmune hepatitis.

PEDIATRIC AUTOIMMUNE HEPATITIS

The histological findings in pediatric autoimmune hepatitis are quite similar to those of adult autoimmune hepatitis, in regard to the portal and lobular hepatitis (Fig. 7.30). However, pediatric autoimmune hepatitis is also enriched for cases with more significant bile duct lymphocytosis and injury, as well as bile ductular proliferation (Fig. 7.31). Many of these cases will have imaging findings of primary sclerosing cholangitis either at the time of the biopsy or with clinical follow-up, even if there is no history of idiopathic inflammatory bowel disease at presentation. For this reason, children diagnosed with autoimmune hepatitis should also have their biliary tree examined by imaging. Wilson disease can also present with an autoimmune hepatitis like pattern of injury,[14,15] so should be excluded in all cases (Fig. 7.32).

Type 2 autoimmune hepatitis is enriched in children and is characterized by serum autoantibodies directed to anti-LKM and or anti-LC1 (Table 7.2). The histological findings are generally similar, with no distinguishing features from that of type 1 autoimmune hepatitis (Fig. 7.30).

OVERLAP SYNDROMES

CHECKLIST: Types of Overlap Syndromes

- ☐ Autoimmune hepatitis–PBC
- ☐ PBC–PSC (in theory at least; essentially not seen in clinical material)
- ☐ PSC–autoimmune hepatitis
- ☐ Autoimmune hepatitis–cholestatic liver disease not otherwise specified

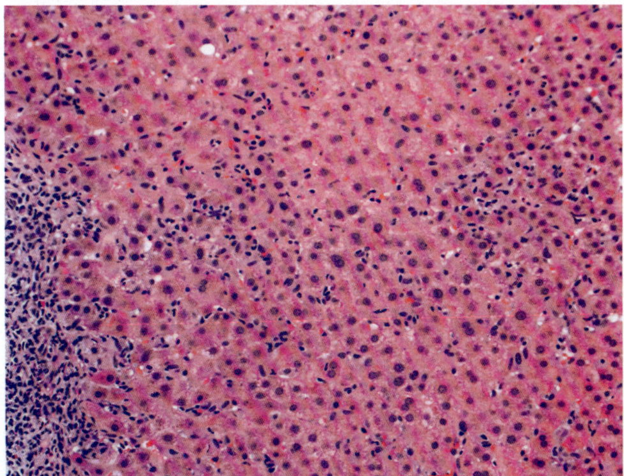

Figure 7.30. **Pediatric autoimmune hepatitis.** This case of pediatric hepatitis was strongly positive for liver kidney microsomal antibodies (LKM). The histology overall was typical for autoimmune hepatitis, with dense plasma cell–rich portal inflammation (left of image) and moderate lobular hepatitis.

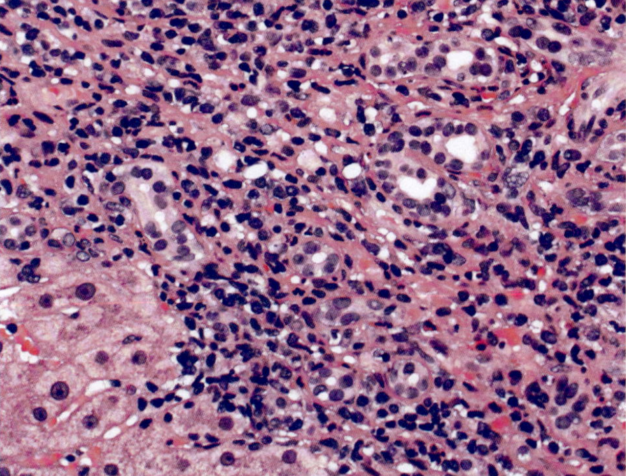

Figure 7.31. **Pediatric autoimmune hepatitis, bile ductular proliferation.** This case of autoimmune hepatitis also had patchy moderate bile ductular proliferation.

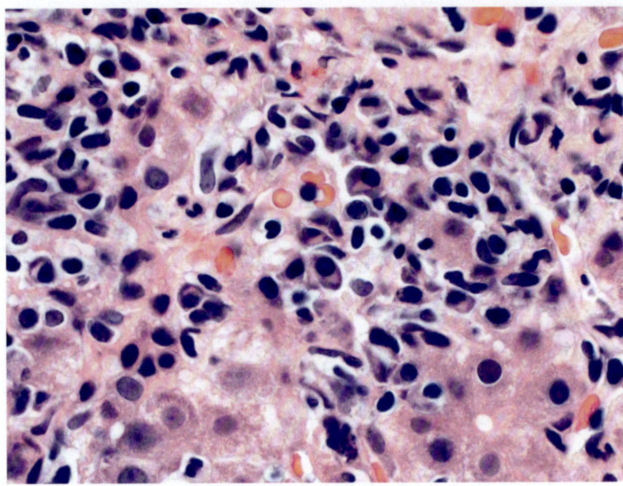

Figure 7.32. **Wilson disease mimicking autoimmune hepatitis.** This case of Wilson disease presented with a plasma cell–rich hepatitis that looked exactly like a typical autoimmune hepatitis.

Overlap syndromes between AIH and other inflammatory diseases of the liver are rare. In practice, the vast majority of overlap syndromes are either AIH–PBC or AIH–PSC, with the latter most commonly found in children and young adults. In surgical pathology specimens, the frequency of AIH–PBC overlap is about 1% to 5% of all autoimmune hepatitis cases. PBC–PSC overlap is essentially nonexistent.

AIH–PBC: OVERLAP BETWEEN AUTOIMMUNE HEPATITIS AND PRIMARY BILIARY CIRRHOSIS

The Paris system is designed to identify cases of autoimmune hepatitis–primary biliary cirrhosis overlap and is commonly used in research studies. This system is primarily based on serology and enzyme patterns but does incorporate a bit of histology (Table 7.3).

The pattern of autoimmune hepatitis–primary biliary cirrhosis overlap can also be suggested based on the histological findings. Both histological approaches and the Paris system generally agree in identifying cases as autoimmune hepatitis–primary biliary cirrhosis overlap, but there are many exceptions. In general, histologically identified cases all tend to fit within the Paris criteria, but not vice versa, indicating that the histology approach outlined herein tends to be more specific and less sensitive.

Despite the value of histology in identifying overlap syndromes, solid, reproducible histological definitions for overlap syndromes remain a challenge because of disease variability. For example, autoimmune hepatitis shows a spectrum of findings, including the common findings of mild bile duct lymphocytosis and patchy mild ductular proliferation, leading to challenges of deciding when the duct changes are enough to suggest an overlap syndrome. At the histological level, the most robust approach is to identify cases with typical

TABLE 7.3: Paris Criteria for Primary Biliary Cirrhosis–Autoimmune Hepatitis Overlap Syndrome[18]

Feature	Autoimmune Hepatitis Features (Two of Three Are Needed)	PBC (Two of Three Are Needed)
Liver enzymes	ALT ≥5 ULN	Alk. Phos. ≥2 ULN or GGT ≥5 ULN
Serology	IgG ≥2 ULN or positive ASMA	AMA positive
Histology	Interface hepatitis	Florid duct lesion

ASMA, anti–smooth muscle antibodies.

autoimmune hepatitis features but with too much duct injury for autoimmune hepatitis alone (Figs. 7.33–7.35) or cases of typical primary biliary cirrhosis with too much lobular hepatitis for primary biliary cirrhosis alone (Fig. 7.36). Admittedly, this useful rule benefits from seeing cases regularly, so is more useful in practices with high volumes of liver specimens.

Another approach is to consider an autoimmune hepatitis overlap syndrome when there are typical clinical and histological findings of autoimmune hepatitis, but with alkaline phosphatase levels >2× normal *plus* either a florid duct lesion or definite bile duct lymphocytic injury (not lymphocytosis alone). Finding established ductopenia and/or cholate stasis in a liver with autoimmune hepatitis, but without advanced fibrosis, would also strongly suggest an overlap syndrome (in a cirrhotic liver, these findings would be nonspecific). Copper and CK7 stains can be helpful in many cases when the liver is noncirrhotic liver, as periportal copper deposition suggests chronic cholestasis and CK7 is useful in highlight the ductular reaction, examining the portal tracts for ductopenia, and identifying intermediate hepatocytes (periportal hepatocytes that are CK7 positive).

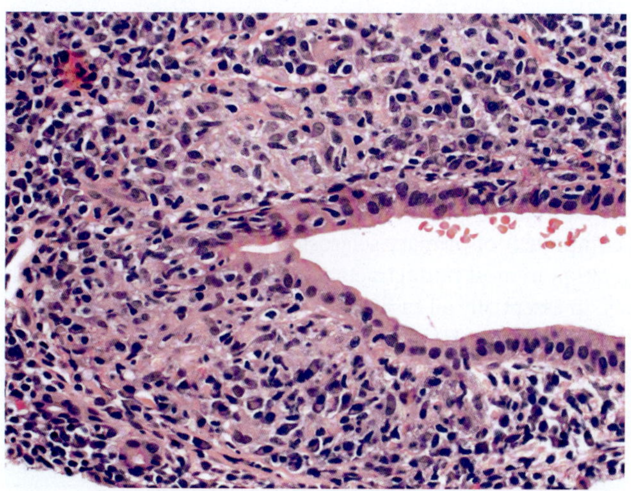

Figure 7.33. **Autoimmune hepatitis–primary biliary cirrhosis overlap syndrome.** This case showed predominately a hepatic pattern with moderate lobular hepatitis and plasma cell–rich portal inflammation and was positive for antinuclear antibodies (ANA) and anti–smooth muscle antibodies (ASMA). The biopsy also showed a single medium-sized bile duct with a florid bile duct lesion.

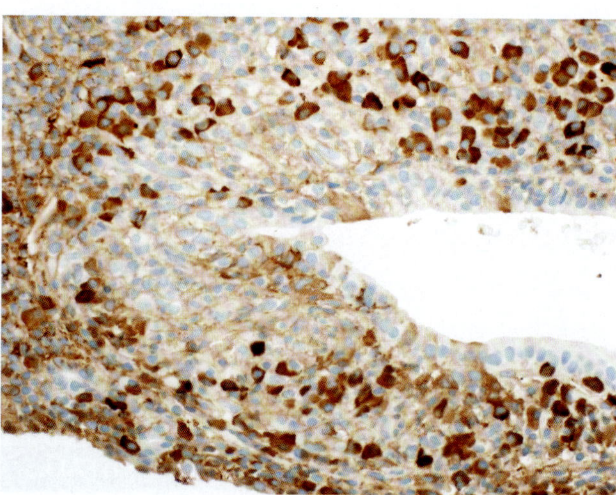

Figure 7.34. **Autoimmune hepatitis–primary biliary cirrhosis overlap syndrome, IgG.** An immunostain for IgG shows numerous positive plasma cells. Same field as Figure 7.33.

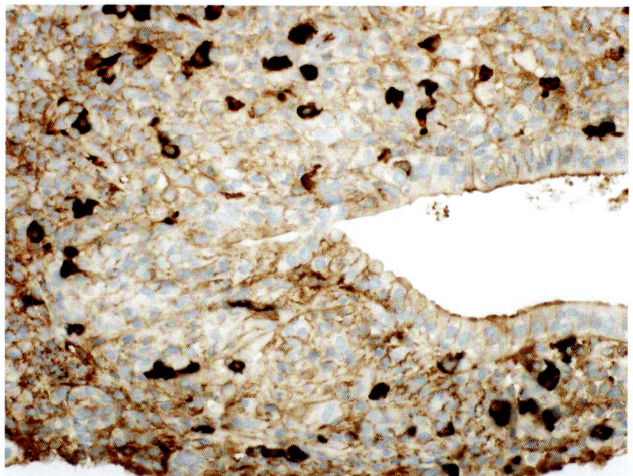

Figure 7.35. **Autoimmune hepatitis–primary biliary cirrhosis overlap syndrome, IgM.** An immunostain for IgM shows increased positive plasma cells, but not as numerous as IgG. Same field as Figures 7.33 and 7.34.

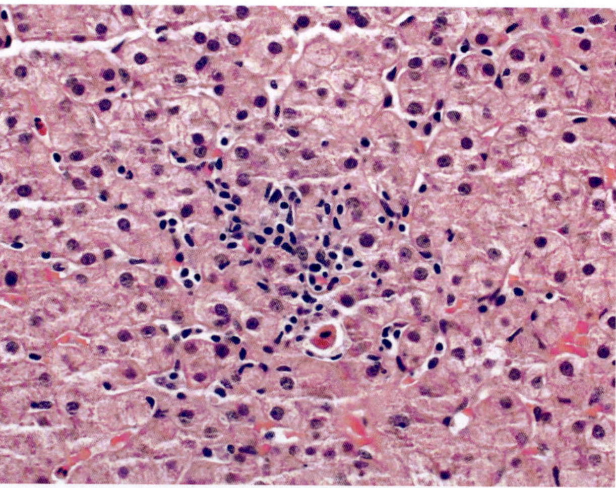

Figure 7.36. **Autoimmune hepatitis–primary biliary cirrhosis overlap syndrome.** In this case, the predominant findings were that of primary biliary cirrhosis, and there was a strongly positive AMA. In addition, there was patchy moderate lobular hepatitis.

Finally, a small percent of cases will show autoimmune hepatitis plus a definite cholestatic injury pattern, but one that does not fit for either primary biliary cirrhosis or primary sclerosing cholangitis. Some of these cases may be autoimmune hepatitis overlap with either AMA-negative primary biliary cirrhosis or small duct primary sclerosing cholangitis.

Interface activity is present in both autoimmune hepatitis and primary biliary cirrhosis and shows too much overlap to be very useful in most cases. Marked or diffuse interface activity is usually accompanied by a brisk lobular hepatitis, which tends to be more useful histologically in suggesting a component of autoimmune hepatitis. Granulomas are also not that helpful in isolation, being present in about 10% of autoimmune hepatitis cases.[3] However, granulomas plus active duct injury strongly suggest a component of primary biliary cirrhosis.

AIH–PSC: OVERLAP BETWEEN AUTOIMMUNE HEPATITIS AND PRIMARY SCLEROSING CHOLANGITIS

AIH–PSC overlap is primarily identified in children who present clinically and histologically with a hepatitic pattern of injury, and on follow-up develop an additional component of primary sclerosing cholangitis, often in the setting of ulcerative colitis or less commonly Crohn disease. For this reason, evaluation of the biliary tree and the colon is important in children diagnosed with autoimmune hepatitis. This clinical–histological pattern has been called autoimmune sclerosing cholangitis in the past.

When considering a possible diagnosis of autoimmune hepatitis–PSC overlap syndrome, a very useful guideline is consider whether there is more bile duct injury or ductular proliferation than is normal for autoimmune hepatitis. For example, cases of autoimmune hepatitis suggest an additional component of primary sclerosing cholangitis when there is at least mild bile ductular proliferation in most portal tracts or moderate or greater ductular proliferation in some portal tracts. In essentially all cases, the alkaline phosphatase levels are >2× normal, serving as a useful check to your H&E impression. Correlation with imaging of the extrahepatic biliary tree is important.

PEARLS & PITFALLS

Imaging of the biliary tree is most helpful for confirming an overlap syndrome between autoimmune hepatitis and PSC when there is no or mild liver fibrosis. Livers with advanced fibrosis or cirrhosis can have nonspecific distortion of the biliary tree on MRCP or ERCP, even if there is no primary sclerosing cholangitis.

NEAR MISSES

CASE 1. A 39-year-old man who has a history of ulcerative colitis developed new onset liver enzyme elevations, with AST of 110, ALT of 175, and alkaline phosphatase of 320. Liver enzyme testing performed 9 months earlier was normal. Imaging studies of the biliary tree were normal at presentation and viral serologies were negative. There was a mildly elevated ANA, and the biopsy was performed to rule out autoimmune hepatitis.

The liver biopsy looked almost normal, with no significant inflammation, no fatty change, and no evidence for biliary tract disease or autoimmune hepatitis. There was no fibrosis and no evidence for nodular regenerative hyperplasia. On careful examination, the stellate cells were noted to be mildly prominent (Fig. 7.37). Follow-up showed the patient was taking herbal supplements that were enriched for vitamin A.

Stellate cell hyperplasia is almost always a subtle finding and should be searched for in biopsies that look nearly normal. In liver biopsies with other active diseases, especially hepatitis and cholestatic liver diseases, Kupffer cell hyperplasia can closely mimic stellate cell hyperplasia. For this reason, a diagnosis of stellate cell hyperplasia in clinical cases is best made in biopsies that do not have significant Kupffer cell hyperplasia. In addition, a long exhausting study of any biopsy will often reveal a single or rare sinusoidal cell with some features of a stellate cell—this is insufficient for the diagnosis. In clinical cases of vitamin A toxicity, there is at least one definite hyperplastic stellate cell present in essentially

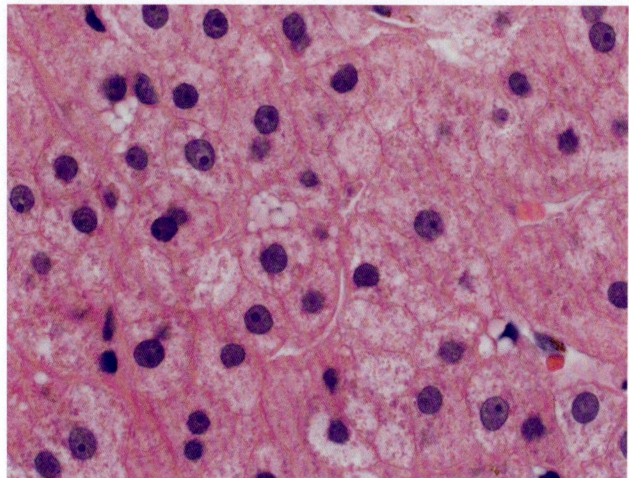

Figure 7.37. **Near miss case 1, stellate cell hyperplasia.** The hyperplastic stellate cells are visible in the sinusoids.

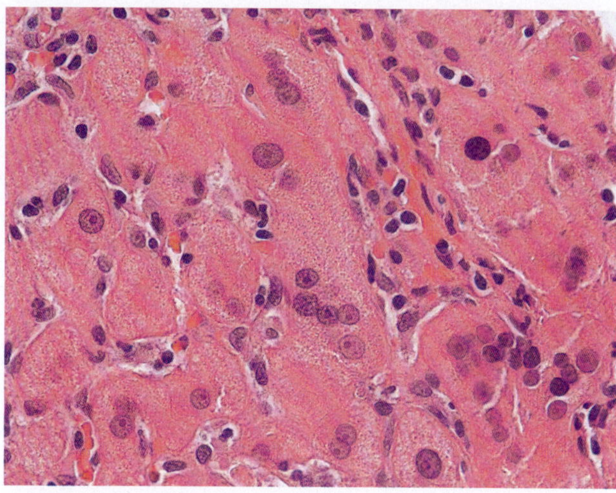

Figure 7.38. **Near miss case 2, giant cell hepatitis.** The hepatocytes are enlarged and multinucleated.

every high-power field. Another commonly used rule of thumb is that there are at least 10 picture-perfect hyperplastic stellate cells, even in a moderately sized biopsy, in cases with clinically relevant vitamin A toxicity.

CASE 2. A 43-year-old woman has a long standing history of mild liver enzyme elevations, with AST and ALT fluctuating between 1.5 and 2× ULN. Viral serology testing is negative. ANA, ASMA, and AMA are all weakly positive. Serum IgG and IgM are mildly elevated. Imaging of the liver is normal.

The case was received in consultation with a diagnosis of autoimmune hepatitis made by the referring pathologist. On review, the liver biopsy shows a giant cell hepatitis pattern (Fig. 7.38), with giant cell transformation of hepatocytes, mostly in a zone 3 distribution. There was mild Kupffer cell hyperplasia but only minimal lobular and portal inflammation.

The adult giant cell hepatitis pattern of injury was linked to autoimmune hepatitis in early studies because of mild elevations in autoimmune antibodies, as is also seen in this case. However, it is now clear from several decades of research that mild elevations of autoantibodies are nonspecific, especially if there is another pattern of liver injury. For example, mild ANA and/or ASMA elevations are seen in about 20% of individuals with steatohepatitis, who do not have autoimmune hepatitis. In addition, patients with a giant cell hepatitis pattern of injury typically do not meet clinical or histological criteria for autoimmune hepatitis. Thus, these cases currently are classified as a giant cell hepatitis pattern of injury, and not autoimmune hepatitis. The cause of giant cell hepatitis is currently unknown and probably multifactorial.

CASE 3. A 29-year-old woman with known chronic hepatitis C developed a sudden flare in liver enzymes. The patient's ANA was known to be positive at 1:160, so there was clinical concern for autoimmune hepatitis.

The biopsy shows a plasma cell–rich hepatitis with moderate portal chronic inflammation, moderate diffuse interface activity (Fig. 7.39) and moderate to marked lobular activity. The lobular inflammation was too much for typical chronic hepatitis C, suggesting an additional disease process. Before the histological findings could trick the pathologist (me) into suggesting a diagnosis of autoimmune hepatitis, additional test results came back indicating the patient had acute hepatitis B, with IgM antibodies and newly positive HBV DNA in the blood.

Most cases of plasma cell–rich hepatitis are autoimmune, but drug effects and acute viral infections can sometimes be plasma cell rich and closely mimic autoimmune hepatitis. Acute hepatitis A and acute hepatitis B are the most common viral causes, while drug effect causes include Clometacin, Minocycline, Methyldopa, and Nitrofurantoin. There are many others, but these seem to be the most common.

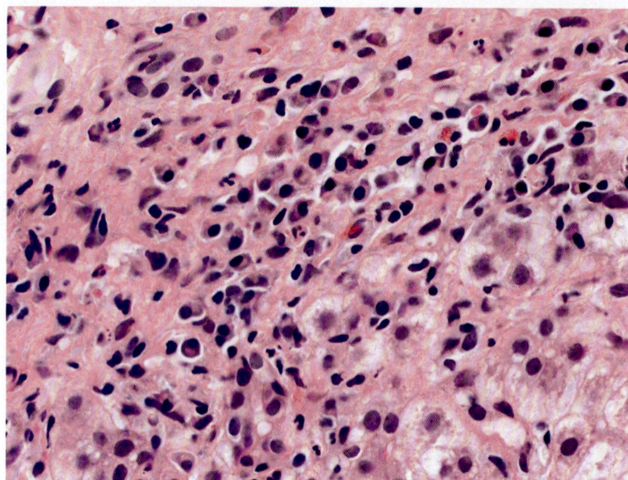

Figure 7.39. **Near miss case 3, acute hepatitis B superimposed on chronic hepatitis C.** This plasma cell–rich hepatitis resulted from acute hepatitis B.

References

1. Liberal R, Grant CR, Longhi MS, Mieli-Vergani G, Vergani D. Diagnostic criteria of autoimmune hepatitis. *Autoimmun Rev*. 2014;13:435-440.
2. Verma S, Torbenson M, Thuluvath PJ. The impact of ethnicity on the natural history of autoimmune hepatitis. *Hepatology*. 2007;46:1828-1835.
3. de Boer YS, van Nieuwkerk CM, Witte BI, Mulder CJ, Bouma G, Bloemena E. Assessment of the histopathological key features in autoimmune hepatitis. *Histopathology*. 2015;66:351-362.
4. Suzuki A, Brunt EM, Kleiner DE, et al. The use of liver biopsy evaluation in discrimination of idiopathic autoimmune hepatitis versus drug-induced liver injury. *Hepatology*. 2011;54:931-939.
5. Pratt DS, Fawaz KA, Rabson A, Dellelis R, Kaplan MM. A novel histological lesion in glucocorticoid-responsive chronic hepatitis. *Gastroenterology*. 1997;113:664-668.
6. Tucker SM, Jonas MM, Perez-Atayde AR. Hyaline droplets in Kupffer cells: a novel diagnostic clue for autoimmune hepatitis. *Am J Surg Pathol*. 2015;39:772-778.
7. Stravitz RT, Lefkowitch JH, Fontana RJ, et al. Autoimmune acute liver failure: proposed clinical and histological criteria. *Hepatology*. 2011;53:517-526.
8. Czaja AJ, Donaldson PT. Gender effects and synergisms with histocompatibility leukocyte antigens in type 1 autoimmune hepatitis. *Am J Gastroenterol*. 2002;97:2051-2057.
9. Czaja AJ, Bayraktar Y. Non-classical phenotypes of autoimmune hepatitis and advances in diagnosis and treatment. *World J Gastroenterol*. 2009;15:2314-2328.
10. Al-Chalabi T, Underhill JA, Portmann BC, McFarlane IG, Heneghan MA. Impact of gender on the long-term outcome and survival of patients with autoimmune hepatitis. *J Hepatol*. 2008;48:140-147.
11. Daniels JA, Torbenson M, Anders RA, Boitnott JK. Immunostaining of plasma cells in primary biliary cirrhosis. *Am J Clin Pathol*. 2009;131:243-249.
12. Cabibi D, Tarantino G, Barbaria F, Campione M, Craxi A, Di Marco V. Intrahepatic IgG/IgM plasma cells ratio helps in classifying autoimmune liver diseases. *Dig Liver Dis*. 2010;42:585-592.
13. Moreira RK, Revetta F, Koehler E, Washington MK. Diagnostic utility of IgG and IgM immunohistochemistry in autoimmune liver disease. *World J Gastroenterol*. 2010;16:453-457.
14. Roberts EA, Schilsky ML. A practice guideline on Wilson disease. *Hepatology*. 2003;37:1475-1492.
15. Milkiewicz P, Saksena S, Hubscher SG, Elias E. Wilson's disease with superimposed autoimmune features: report of two cases and review. *J Gastroenterol Hepatol*. 2000;15:570-574.
16. Hennes EM, Zeniya M, Czaja AJ, et al. Simplified criteria for the diagnosis of autoimmune hepatitis. *Hepatology*. 2008;48:169-176.
17. Bogdanos DP, Mieli-Vergani G, Vergani D. Autoantibodies and their antigens in autoimmune hepatitis. *Semin Liver Dis*. 2009;29:241-253.
18. Chazouilleres O, Wendum D, Serfaty L, Montembault S, Rosmorduc O, Poupon R. Primary biliary cirrhosis-autoimmune hepatitis overlap syndrome: clinical features and response to therapy. *Hepatology*. 1998;28:296-301.

CHOLESTATIC AND BILIARY TRACT DISEASE 8

CHAPTER OUTLINE

INTRODUCTION

The histological patterns in cholestatic liver disease range from bland lobular cholestasis, to acute obstruction, to chronic injury. Not surprisingly, individual cases can have mixed patterns, so the main focus should be on the predominant pattern of injury. In every case, it is important to correlate the histology with clinical findings, including imaging findings to rule out obstruction and serum liver enzyme levels to confirm a predominant elevation in alkaline phosphate. Imaging results of the biliary tree may not be available or not yet performed, in which case the pathology report can recommend its examination.

BLAND LOBULAR CHOLESTASIS PATTERN

CHECKLIST: Bland Lobular Cholestasis Pattern

Common Causes

- ☐ Drug effect (the most common cause overall in biopsy specimens)
- ☐ Decompensated cirrhosis
- ☐ Paraneoplastic syndrome
- ☐ Sepsis (rarely biopsied, but common at autopsy)
- ☐ Debilitating illnesses with multiorgan failure (rarely biopsied, but common at autopsy)

Rare Causes

- ☐ Thyroid disease, can be hypothyroid or hyperthyroid
- ☐ Bile salt deficiency diseases such as FIC, BSEP, or MDR3 deficiency
- ☐ Intrahepatic cholestasis of pregnancy
- ☐ Idiopathic ductopenia

The term *bland* is used to indicate that this pattern shows lobular cholestasis with little or no inflammation, necrosis, or bile duct changes. By way of contrast, the liver frequently shows cholestasis when there is marked inflammation or necrosis from many different causes, as the remaining hepatocytes are unable to adequately function to prevent cholestasis. In these cases, the cholestasis is a secondary finding and the findings are not classified as a bland lobular cholestasis pattern. In addition, in the bland cholestasis pattern, there should be no ductopenia and no evidence for biliary obstruction. If ductopenia or biliary obstruction is present, then they are considered the primary pattern of injury.

In the bland lobular cholestasis pattern, it does not matter if the bile is in the hepatocytes versus the canaliculi versus both (Fig. 8.1). Usually it is both. In severe and long-standing cases, there also can be cholangiolar cholestasis (Fig. 8.2). The differential for the bland lobular cholestasis pattern is primarily drug effect, paraneoplastic syndromes, or debilitating illnesses. Finally, livers with decompensated cirrhosis from any cause can become cholestatic when the liver reserve falls below physiological needs.

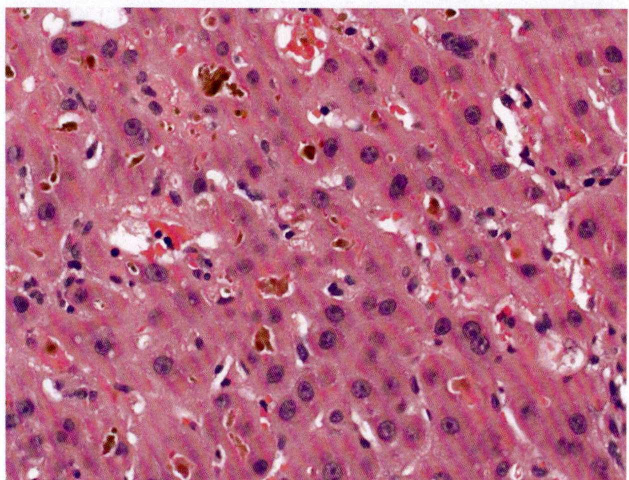

Figure 8.1. Bland lobular cholestasis. There is lobular cholestasis, primarily in the bile canaliculi.

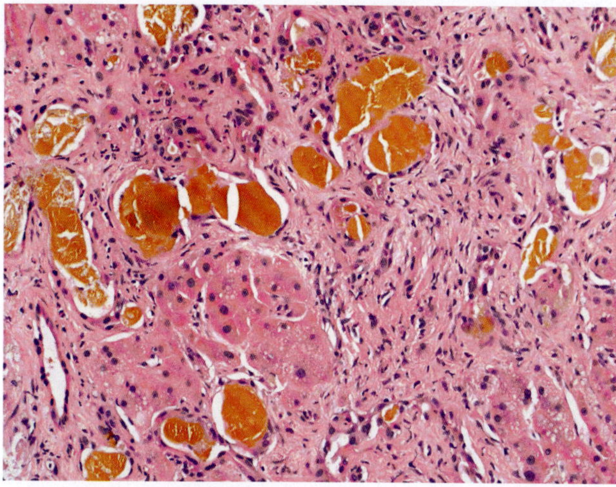

Figure 8.2. Cholangiolar cholestasis. The proliferating bile ductules had striking bile plugs in this case of decompensated liver cirrhosis. The lobules also showed marked cholestasis. The patient was not septic, and there was no biliary obstruction on imaging.

BILIARY CIRRHOSIS PATTERN

CHECKLIST: Biliary Cirrhosis Pattern

Not all features of this pattern will be present in any given case.

- □ Bile duct changes
  - ○ Ductopenia
  - ○ Periductal (onion-skin) fibrosis
  - ○ Fibro-obliterative duct lesions
  - ○ Bile duct duplication
- □ Hepatocyte changes
  - ○ Cholestasis
  - ○ Cholate stasis
  - ○ Copper deposition in zone 1 hepatocytes; not specific for biliary cirrhosis, but if absent, then biliary cirrhosis is unlikely
- □ Cirrhotic pattern
  - ○ Jigsaw pattern of cirrhotic nodules
  - ○ Halo sign

The biliary cirrhosis pattern is not specific for an etiology, but the basic pattern can be helpful in identify the general category of liver disease. Biliary cirrhosis commonly shows some degree of ductopenia (Fig. 8.3), cholate stasis (Fig. 8.4), and irregular cirrhotic nodules that resemble jigsaw pieces (Fig. 8.5). The hepatic arteries in the portal tracts can appear more prominent than usual. There can also be discrete foci of ghostly dead hepatocytes, called bile infarcts (Fig. 8.6). Bile infarcts can also be seen with severe acute biliary obstruction but are most common in severe long-standing cholestatic liver disease. In biliary cirrhosis, a copper stain will invariably show increased periportal and periseptal copper deposition (Fig. 8.7). In the setting of cirrhosis, copper deposition is not specific for etiology, but a negative copper stain makes it less likely that chronic cholestatic liver disease was the cause of the cirrhosis.

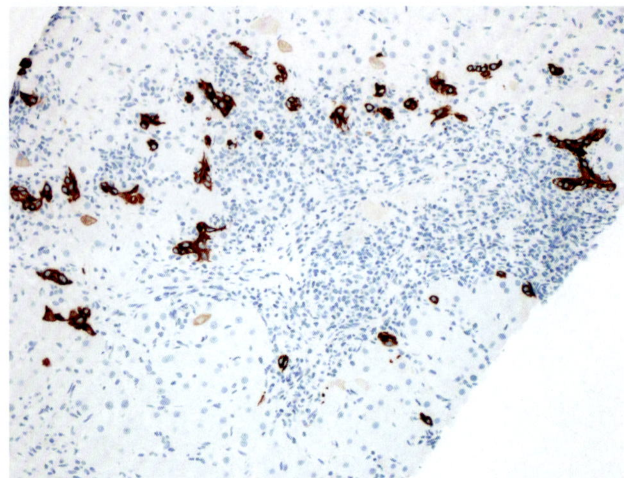

Figure 8.3. **Biliary cirrhosis pattern, ductopenia, CK7 stain.** The CK7 stain shows that the bile duct proper is missing and highlights proliferating bile ductules at the edge of the portal tract. The CK7 stain or other keratin stains are very helpful in evaluating for ductopenia.

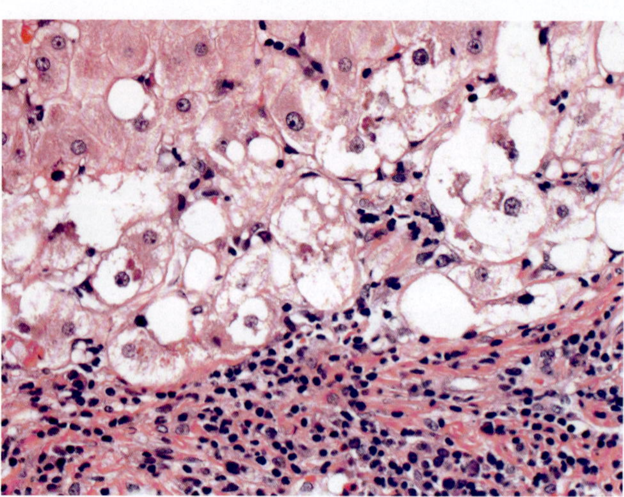

Figure 8.4. **Biliary cirrhosis pattern, cholate stasis.** This liver was biopsied to investigate clinically cryptogenic cirrhosis. The periportal hepatocytes show striking cholate stasis with marked ballooning and abundant Mallory hyaline. In most cases, the cholate stasis is not this striking.

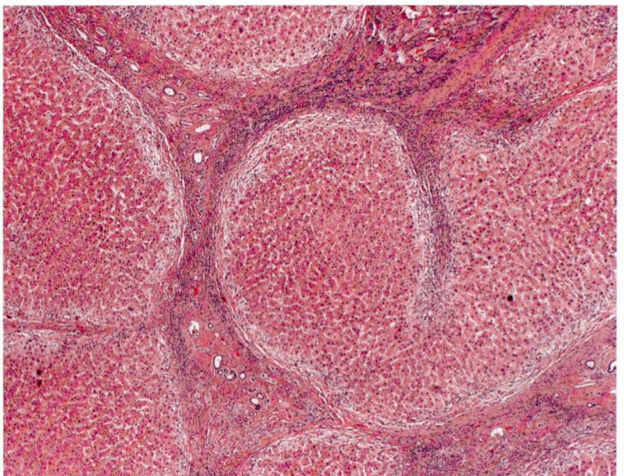

Figure 8.5. **Biliary cirrhosis pattern, jigsaw pattern of cirrhosis.** The cirrhotic nodules are a bit contorted, looking somewhat like a piece in a jigsaw puzzle. Note the rim of edema and cholates stasis at the edges of the cirrhotic nodules, a finding called a *halo sign*. This image is from a case of primary sclerosing cholangitis.

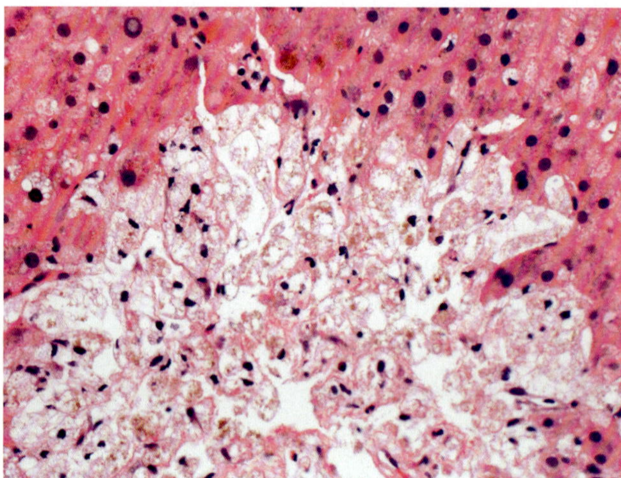

Figure 8.6. **Biliary cirrhosis pattern, bile infarct.** This biopsy showed a well-circumscribed area of bile-stained, pale, dead hepatocytes.

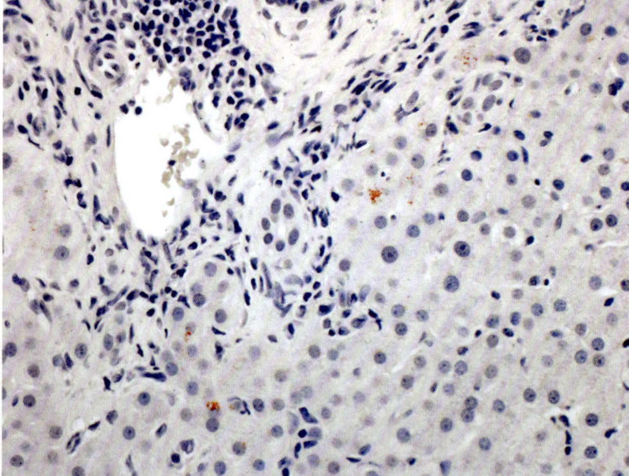

Figure 8.7. **Biliary cirrhosis pattern, copper stain.** A rhodanine copper stain shows focal periportal copper deposition.

BILIARY OBSTRUCTION PATTERN

CHECKLIST: Biliary Obstruction Pattern

- ☐ Liver enzymes
  - ○ Predominant alkaline phosphatase (>2X ULN) or gamma-glutamyltransferase (GGT) elevations (>5X ULN)
  - ○ Serum bilirubin is often elevated
- ☐ Early changes
  - ○ Bile ductular proliferation
  - ○ Mild and usually mixed inflammation, with primarily lymphocytes and neutrophils
  - ○ Portal edema, not very common, but seen in some cases of acute severe obstruction
- ☐ Long-term changes
  - ○ Bile ductular proliferation
  - ○ Bile duct duplication
  - ○ Ductopenia
  - ○ Periductal fibrosis
  - ○ Cholate stasis
  - ○ Biliary cirrhosis
- ☐ Special stains
  - ○ Periportal copper deposition
  - ○ CK7-positive intermediate hepatocytes

The main component of the biliary obstruction pattern is bile ductular proliferation (Figs. 8.8 and 8.9). The portal tracts will also show mild lymphocytic inflammation, and there are commonly neutrophils in close proximity to the proliferating bile ducts (Fig. 8.10). In early and severe obstruction, there can be portal edema (Fig. 8.11). In later disease, there can be bile duct duplication (Fig. 8.12) or ductopenia (Fig. 8.13). The lobules show minimal inflammation and mild reactive changes. Lobular cholestasis is not common in early acute obstruction but is more common with long-standing obstruction (Fig. 8.14). In early biliary obstruction, the portal tracts can look irregular and fibrotic because the portal tracts are expanded due to ductular proliferation, inflammation, and edema. However, the trichrome stain will lack the dense blue color of true fibrosis.

Biliary fibrosis from high-grade obstruction tends to develop more rapidly than fibrosis from chronic hepatitis. The fibrosis starts in the portal tracts and often shows irregular spiky portal fibrosis (Fig. 8.15). However, do not overcall fibrosis in acute obstruction, a common diagnostic pitfall because portal tracts are expanded by the bile ductular proliferation, inflammation, and edema (Figs. 8.16 and 8.17). Biliary cirrhosis is discussed above.

Several additional histological findings can also suggest chronic biliary tract disease. While none are specific for etiology, overall they are more common with chronic biliary tract disease. First, cholate stasis results from chronic exposure of the periportal hepatocytes to bile salts (Fig. 8.18). The hepatocytes become swollen and can have bits of Mallory hyaline (Fig. 8.19). Mild copper deposition is also common in cholate stasis.

Other findings include changes that result from chronic bile duct obstruction. These changes include bile duct duplication, periductal fibrosis, fibro-obliterative duct lesions, and ductopenia. With bile duct duplication, a small cluster of bile ducts is present in the portal tract, instead of the normal one or two bile duct profiles (Fig. 8.12). This finding is distinct from bile ductular proliferation, which also may be present. Bile duct duplication is probably the most subjective of the major findings that support a diagnosis of a biliary pattern of injury, but the finding can be helpful when it is decidedly present. Cases of

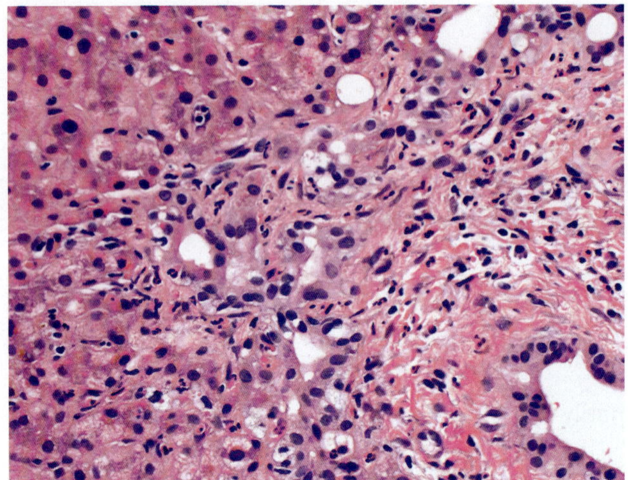

Figure 8.8. **Biliary obstruction pattern, bile ductular proliferation.** The proliferating bile ductules are evident at the periphery of the portal tract in this case of biliary obstruction.

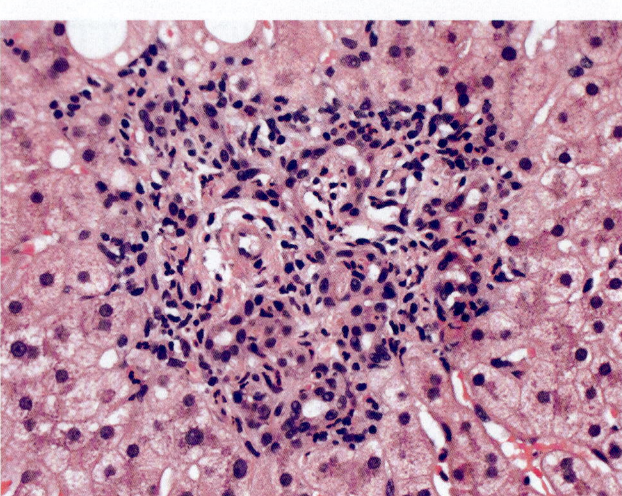

Figure 8.9. **Biliary obstruction pattern, bile ductular proliferation.** Another example of the biliary obstruction pattern of injury, with bile ductular proliferation and mild inflammation. This case resulted from biliary obstruction due to a pancreas tumor.

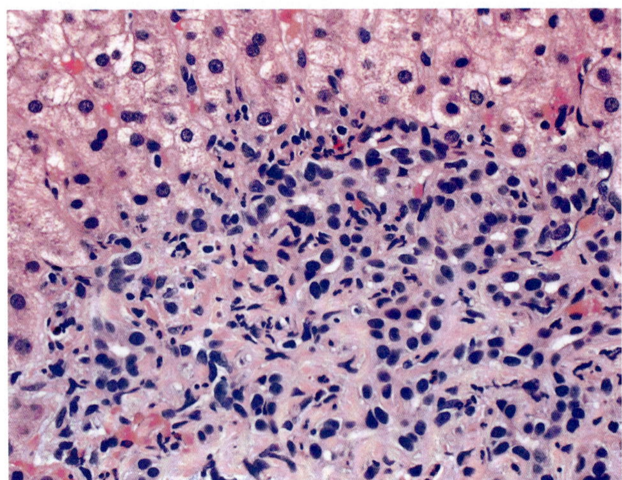

Figure 8.10. **Biliary obstruction pattern, mixed inflammation.** In addition to bile ductular proliferation, the portal tract also shows mild mixed inflammation (lymphocytes, neutrophils). Occasional eosinophils are also common in the portal inflammation.

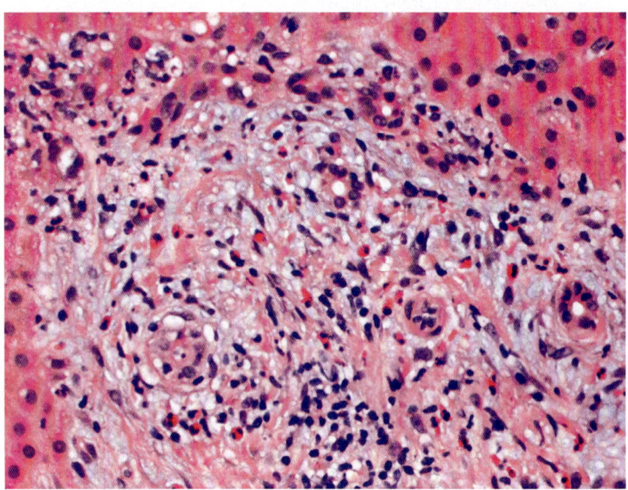

Figure 8.11. **Biliary obstruction pattern, portal edema.** In this case of acute obstruction, the portal tracts show edema that gives the stroma a bluish hue. The portal tract also shows bile ductular proliferation and mild inflammation with a mild prominence in eosinophils.

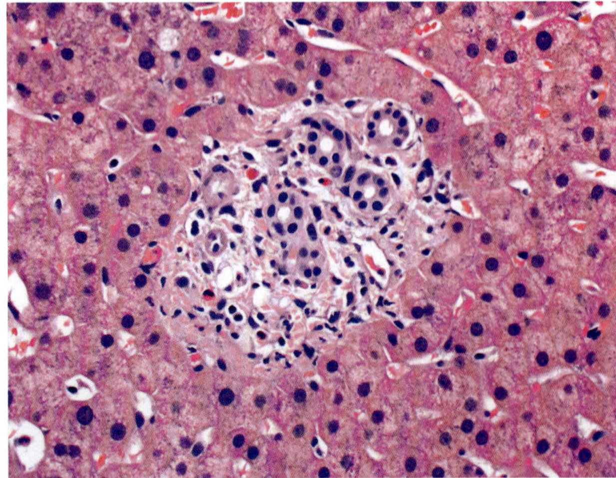

Figure 8.12. **Biliary obstruction pattern, bile duct duplication.** This portal tract shows a cluster of bile ducts.

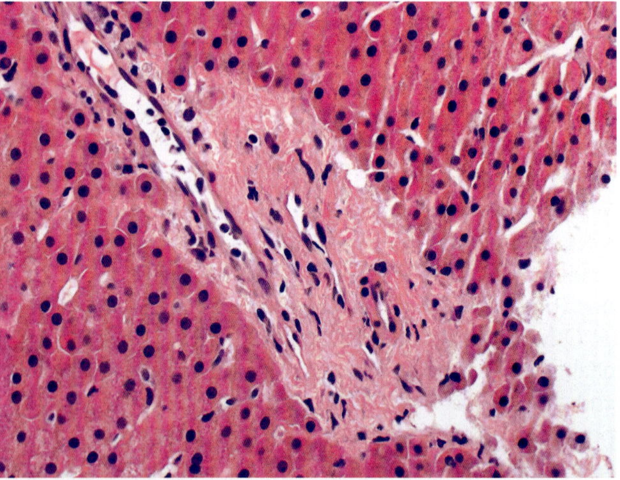

Figure 8.13. **Biliary obstruction pattern, ductopenia.** This allograft liver developed ductopenia after a long history of anastomotic strictures.

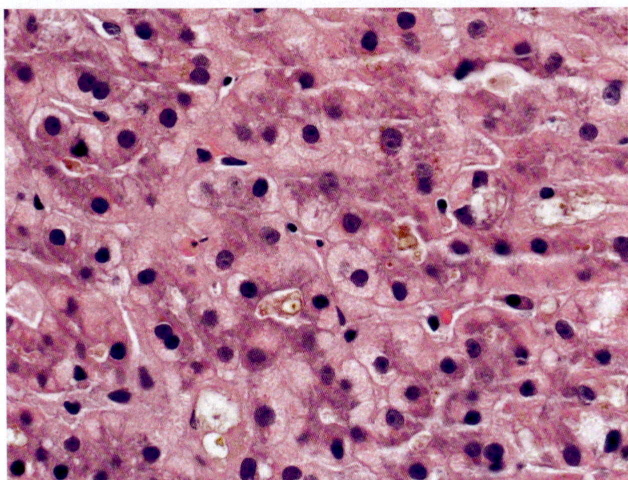

Figure 8.14. **Biliary obstruction pattern, lobular cholestasis.** The lobules show moderate cholestasis in this case of severe biliary tract obstruction.

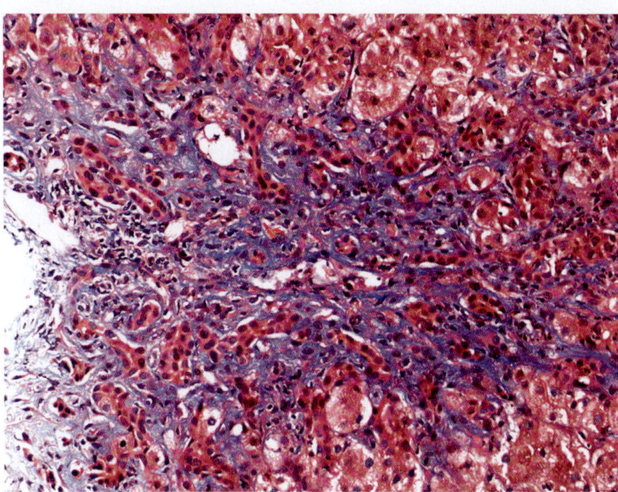

Figure 8.15. **Biliary obstruction pattern, portal fibrosis.** This case of obstructive biliary tract disease shows irregular portal fibrosis.

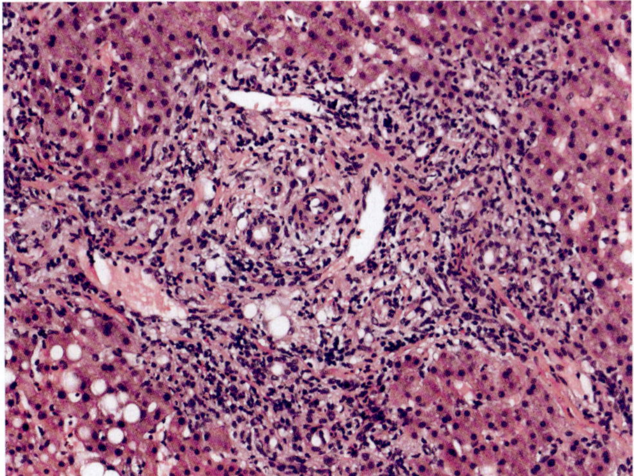

Figure 8.16. **Biliary obstruction pattern, portal expansion without fibrosis.** This portal tract is expanded by inflammation, edema, and a bile ductular proliferation, but shows no fibrosis (see next image)

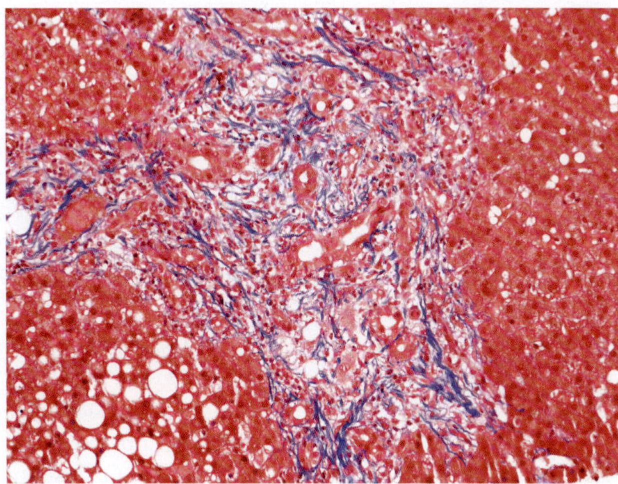

Figure 8.17. **Biliary obstruction pattern, portal expansion without fibrosis.** This trichrome stain shows no fibrosis

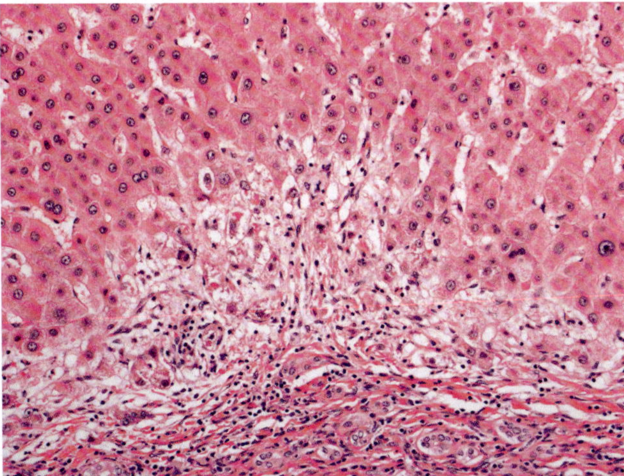

Figure 8.18. **Biliary obstruction pattern, cholate stasis.** The edge of the cirrhotic nodule looks paler because of edema and cholate stasis in the hepatocytes. Image from a case of primary sclerosing cholangitis.

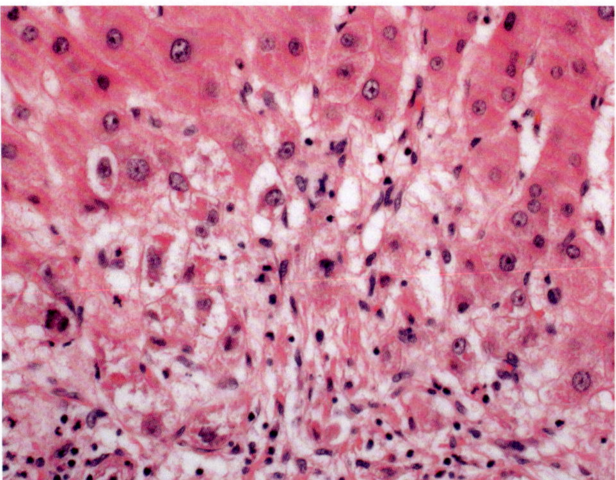

Figure 8.19. **Biliary obstruction pattern, cholate stasis.** At higher power magnification, the hepatocytes in cholate stasis appear ballooned and show Mallory hyaline. Image from a case of primary sclerosing cholangitis.

long-standing downstream biliary tract obstruction can develop onion-skinning fibrosis (Fig. 8.20) around bile ducts, which in time can lead to fibro-obliterative duct lesions (Fig. 8.21). Finally, ductopenia indicates chronic cholestatic liver disease. Ductopenia can result from all of the major cholestatic liver diseases such as primary sclerosing cholangitis and primary biliary cirrhosis. Usually, the liver also shows advanced fibrosis in these cases. In other cases, ductopenia can develop in nonfibrotic livers. Here, the differential is very long (Table 8.1), but the major etiologies to consider are drug effects and paraneoplastic syndromes. Pancreatic acinar cell metaplasia can be found in the hilum of the liver but is not specific for biliary tract disease.[1]

SPECIAL STAINS

There are two stains that can support a diagnosis of biliary tract disease: cytokeratin 7 and copper. They do not help determine the etiology of the biliary tract disease but provide strong support for the basic pattern of injury. Copper is normally excreted in bile, but with chronic cholestatic liver disease, the copper is not adequately excreted and gets deposited in the lysosomes of periportal hepatocytes (Figs. 8.22 and 8.23). Examine the copper stain carefully because the deposits can be very focal in early disease and/or in mild disease.

The cytokeratin 7 is helpful in several ways. First it can help identify bile duct loss. The formal definition for established ductopenia is that 50% or more of the portal tracts lack a bile duct. The portal tracts do not have to be complete to be included in the assessment of the bile ducts, but enough of the portal tract should be present so that a bile duct should have been seen, if present. Secondly, the cytokeratin 7 immunostain will highlight intermediate hepatocytes (Figs. 8.24 and 8.25). Intermediate hepatocytes are defined very simply: any hepatocyte that is CK7 positive. In chronic cholestatic liver disease, intermediate hepatocytes are present in zone 1. To be reasonably specific for chronic cholestatic liver disease, the intermediate hepatocytes should be more than rare. With biliary obstruction, intermediate hepatocytes are usually found as aggregates of cells or contiguous swaths of cells around many of the portal tracts, not as rare, isolated cells.

FAQ: Which stain is better for evaluating cholestasis, CK7 or copper?

Answer: The best approach is to use both stains. Detailed data have not been published on the results of CK7 and copper over time in biliary tract disease. Anecdotally, CK7 seems to highlight intermediate hepatocytes before there is copper deposition visible by copper stain. On the other hand, CK7 can show no or minimal intermediate hepatocytes once a stricture is dilated or otherwise treated, while the copper stain seems to be positive for longer.

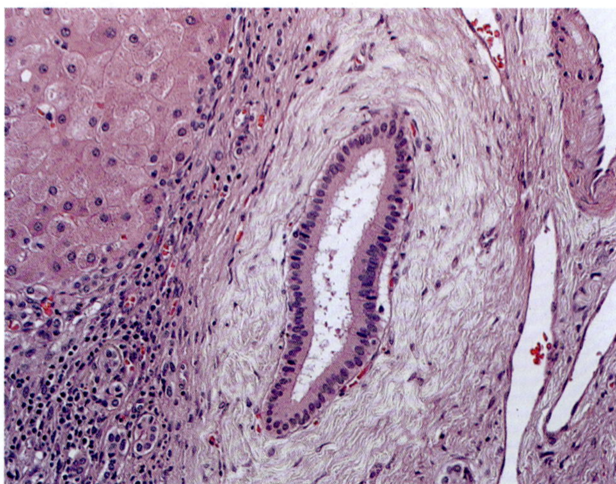

Figure 8.20. Biliary obstruction pattern, onion-skin fibrosis. This medium-sized portal tract shows concentric periductal fibrosis, from a case of primary sclerosing cholangitis.

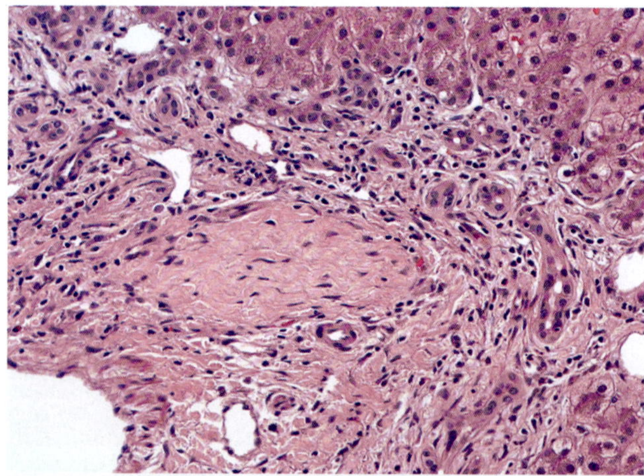

Figure 8.21. Biliary obstruction pattern, fibro-obliterative duct lesion. The portal tract has been replaced by a round fibrous scar.

TABLE 8.1: Differential for Ductopenia

Cause	Comment
Transplant Related	
Chronic rejection of liver allograft	
Mechanical problems after liver transplantation	Ischemic cholangiopathy and/or biliary anastomotic stricture
Graft vs. host disease	After bone marrow transplant
Chronic Biliary Tract Disease	
Primary sclerosing cholangitis	
Primary biliary cirrhosis	
Long-standing extrahepatic biliary tract obstruction	Etiologies include ischemic strictures, stones, recurrent pancreatitis, autoimmune pancreatitis, trauma, etc.
Secondary sclerosing cholangitis	Etiologies include portal biliopathy, mast cell cholangitis, intra-arterial chemotherapy, infection
Sarcoidosis	Thought to be a result of granulomas in the hilar lymph nodes that secondarily compress the bile ducts
ABCB4/MDR3 deficiency	In addition to ductopenia, cases can also have a fibrosing cholestatic pattern that resembles sclerosing cholangitis
Pediatric Liver Disease	
Paucity of intrahepatic bile ducts	
Neonatal giant cell hepatitis	Often subtle and does not reach full threshold of 50% of portal tracts with missing ducts
Biliary atresia	Not present in early disease, but more common with late disease and end-stage fibrosis
Paraneoplastic Syndrome	
Lymphoma	Hodgkin disease, peripheral T cell lymphoma
Drug/Medication	
Drug effect	Many different drugs
Total parenteral nutrition	Up to 25% of cases
Infection	
Acquired immunodeficiency syndrome (AIDS)	Thought to result from infection in most cases. Potential etiologies include Cryptosporidium, Microsporidium, cytomegalovirus, and Cyclospora
Recurrent pyogenic cholangitis	

CHECKLIST: Staining Patterns for CK7

- ☐ Zone 1 hepatocytes: chronic cholestatic injury
- ☐ Zone 3 hepatocytes: chronic venous outflow impairment
- ☐ Zone 3 hepatocytes without vascular disease: long-standing chronic lobular cholestasis, with or without bile duct disease—usually drugs, PFIC, or decompensated liver cirrhosis

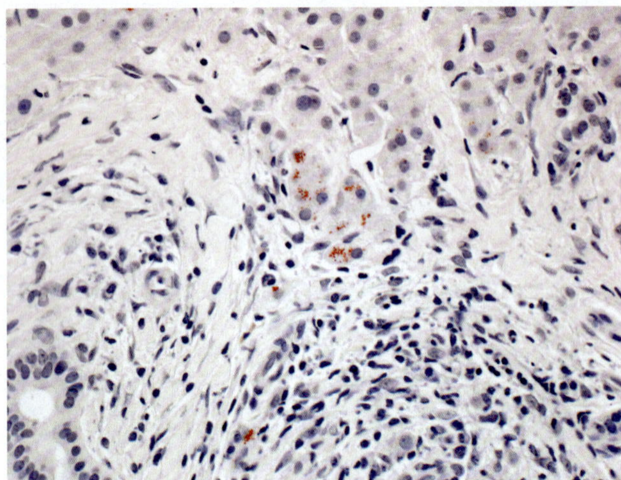

Figure 8.22. **Biliary obstruction pattern, copper stain.** A rhodanine copper stain shows focal periportal copper deposition. The copper deposition can be limited to one or two portal tracts in early disease, so you have to look carefully. A negative copper stain does not exclude biliary tract obstructive disease, especially if the stricture is early or has been successfully stented for a long time.

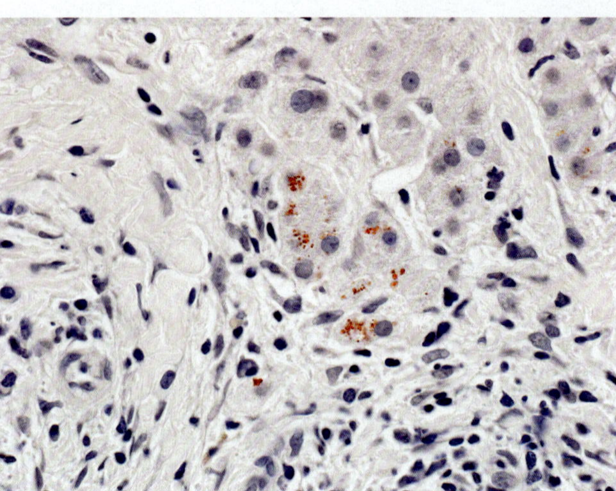

Figure 8.23. **Biliary obstruction pattern, copper stain.** At higher power, the copper has a distinctive red brown granular staining pattern. Sometimes lipofuschin can look somewhat similar, but it lacks the refractile staining quality of copper.

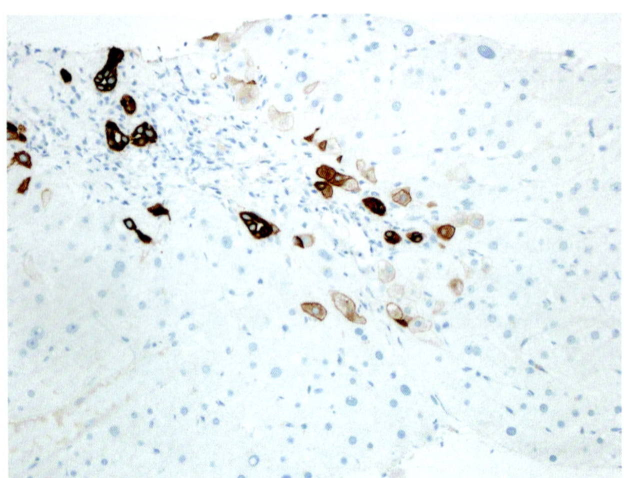

Figure 8.24. **Biliary obstruction pattern, CK7 immunostain.** Most of the portal tracts in this case had scattered CK7-positive intermediate hepatocytes. Proliferating bile ductules can also be seen; they stain darker than intermediate hepatocytes and are located at the interface of the portal tract and lobules.

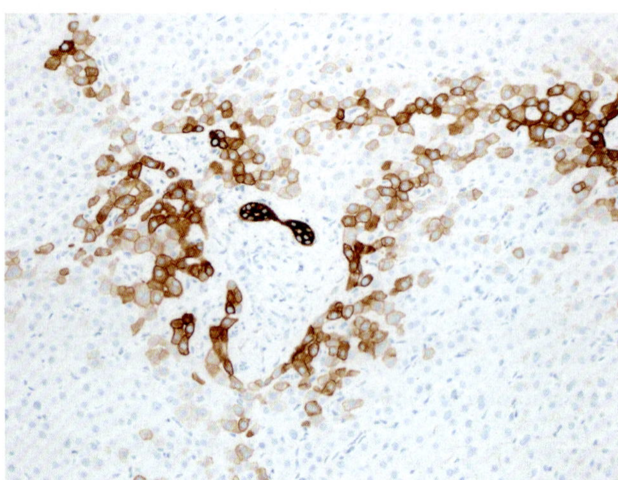

Figure 8.25. **Biliary obstruction pattern, CK7 immunostain.** Another example of intermediate hepatocytes.

DISEASES THAT CAN MIMIC BILIARY OBSTRUCTION

There are two main disease patterns that can mimic biliary obstruction because they have mild or greater bile ductular proliferation. Almost any disease can have minimal ductular proliferation, but more significant ductular proliferation is seen when there is marked lobular hepatitis or necrosis. For example, acute viral hepatitis can sometimes mimic biliary obstruction.[2] In this setting, the presence of moderate or marked lobular inflammation will clarify that hepatitis is the main pattern of injury. The second pattern of injury that can mimic biliary obstruction is chronic vascular outflow disease. In this setting, the sinusoidal dilatation and congestion will clarify that vascular outflow disease is the main pattern of injury.

ASCENDING CHOLANGITIS

Ascending cholangitis results from bacterial infections of the biliary tree. Most individuals will have a preexisting biliary obstruction from stones, strictures, or mass lesions. Most cases are diagnosed based on clinical findings such as abdominal pain, fever, and jaundice, and liver biopsies are only rarely performed. When a biopsy is obtained, the histological findings show the underlying changes of obstruction plus the superimposed infection. The superimposed infection leads to variably dilated bile ducts with thin attenuated epithelium and abundant intraluminal neutrophils (Fig. 8.26). An ordinary bile ductular proliferation can have neutrophilic inflammation, but in cases of ascending cholangitis, the neutrophils are in the lumen of the bile duct proper.

PRIMARY SCLEROSING CHOLANGITIS

CHECKLIST: Primary Sclerosing Cholangitis (PSC)

- ☐ Male:female ratio about 5:1
- ☐ 70% will have ulcerative colitis at the time of or after the diagnosis of PSC
- ☐ 10% will have Crohn disease at the time of or after the diagnosis of PSC
- ☐ Serology: pANCA (not very sensitive or specific); 50% seronegative
- ☐ Histology: biliary obstruction pattern
- ☐ Small duct PSC: 5% of all PSC cases; defined as changes of PSC in liver biopsy but with normal or near normal extrahepatic biliary tree
- ☐ Major clinical complications: cholangiocarcinoma, biliary cirrhosis

Primary sclerosing cholangitis results from strictures of the extrahepatic and intrahepatic biliary tree. On needle biopsy specimens, primary sclerosing cholangitis is a portal-based disease with bile ductular proliferation (Fig. 8.27) and generally minimal to mild portal inflammation (Fig. 8.28) composed of admixed neutrophils, lymphocytes, and rare plasma cells. Bile duct lymphocytosis can be seen, but primarily in larger bile ducts of the liver hilum. In addition, the larger hilar bile ducts are often dilated and have a thick cuff of plasma cell–rich inflammation (Fig. 8.29). The lumens can be filled with neutrophils when there is superimposed infectious cholangitis. In peripheral needle biopsies, bile duct lymphocytosis is usually absent to minimal and essentially never striking.

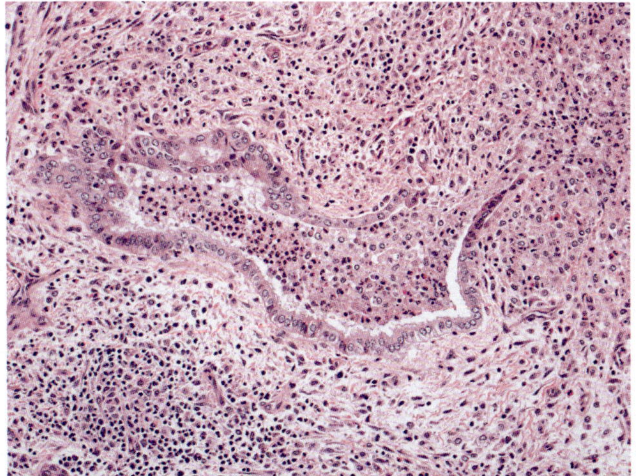

Figure 8.26. **Ascending cholangitis.** The bile duct is dilated and filled with neutrophils.

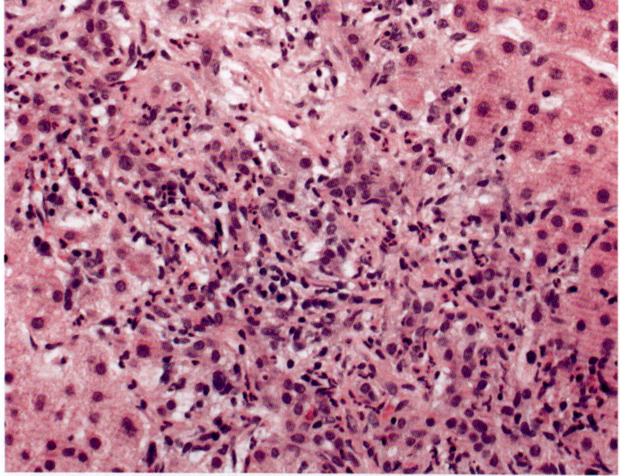

Figure 8.27. **Primary sclerosing cholangitis, bile ductular proliferation.** The portal tract shows a brisk bile ductular proliferation with mixed inflammation.

There is little or no lobular inflammation in primary sclerosing cholangitis. Lobular cholestasis is usually absent at first clinical presentation. Fatty liver disease is rare in patients with primary sclerosing cholangitis, even if they have the metabolic syndrome.[3]

In time, the small- and medium-sized bile ducts can show bile duct duplication, onion-skinning fibrosis, fibro-obliterative duct lesions, and ductopenia. Onion-skinning fibrosis is defined as concentric and often laminated fibrosis around a bile duct, which also typically shows attenuated epithelium (Fig. 8.30). Fibro-obliterative duct lesions are scars that replace the bile duct with a distinctive round plug of fibrosis (Fig. 8.31). They are most commonly found in medium-sized bile ducts.[4]

The histological findings in primary sclerosing cholangitis are essentially identical to those of biliary obstruction, which makes perfect sense, as primary sclerosing cholangitis leads to strictures of the biliary tree. There are no findings pathognomonic for primary sclerosing cholangitis, and no findings can be used to separate this disease from other causes of chronic biliary obstruction, including onion-skinning fibrosis and fibro-obliterative duct lesions, both of which can be seen in other biliary tract obstructive diseases such as ischemic strictures, chronic hepatolithiasis,[5] sarcoidosis with obstructive features,[6] segmental cholangiectasia,[7] and MDR3 deficiency in adults.[8] Primary biliary cirrhosis can rarely show focal equivocal onion-skinning fibrosis, usually in small-sized bile ducts.[9] Fibro-obliterative duct lesions are not seen in primary biliary cirrhosis.

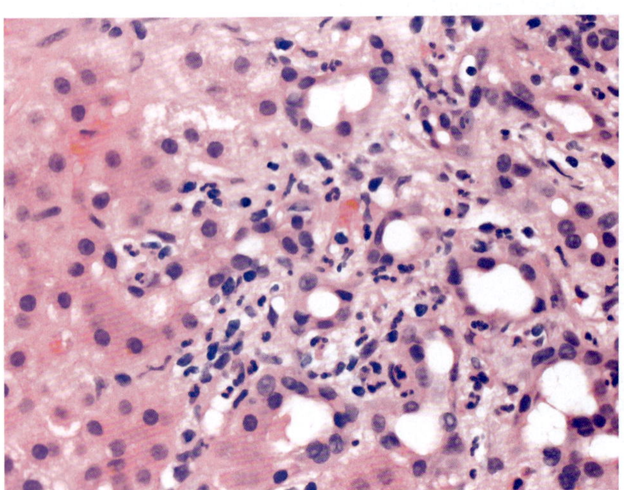

Figure 8.28. **Primary sclerosing cholangitis, portal inflammation.** At higher power the portal inflammation in this portal tract is predominately neutrophils. Admixed lymphocytes are also seen.

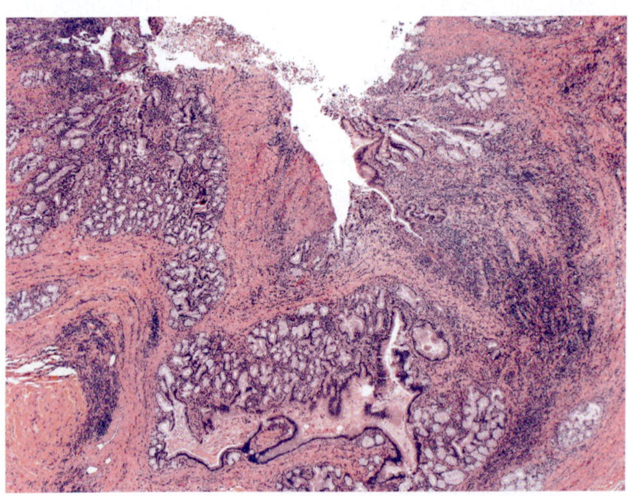

Figure 8.29. **Primary sclerosing cholangitis, hilar-sized bile ducts.** This section from the liver hilum shows dense inflammation around the bile duct and the peribiliary glands.

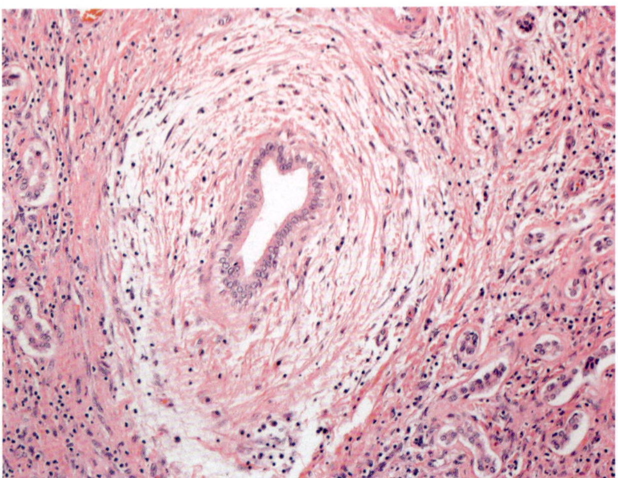

Figure 8.30. **Primary sclerosing cholangitis, onion-skin fibrosis.** The bile duct shows concentric somewhat edematous fibrosis.

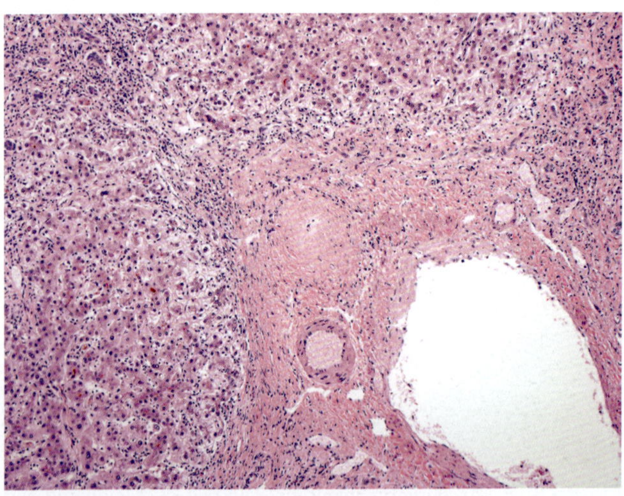

Figure 8.31. **Primary sclerosing cholangitis, fibro-obliterative duct lesion.** The bile duct has been replaced by a round fibrosis scar.

SMALL DUCT PRIMARY SCLEROSING CHOLANGITIS

The histology in small duct primary sclerosing cholangitis is the same as it is for typical primary sclerosing cholangitis. The only difference is the imaging, which shows normal or nearly normal extrahepatic bile ducts. This disease pattern is rare, making up 5% of all primary sclerosing cholangitis cases.

PRIMARY BILIARY CIRRHOSIS

CHECKLIST: Primary Biliary Cirrhosis, AKA Primary Biliary Cholangitis

- ☐ Male: female ratio is about 1:8
- ☐ No association with inflammatory bowel disease
- ☐ Serology: Antimitochondrial antibody (AMA) M2 positive in 95%; 5% AMA negative
- ☐ Serology: 10% also are positive for ANA and/or ASMA but the vast majority will have no autoimmune hepatitis
- ☐ Histology: Patchy but usually moderate portal inflammation with bile duct lymphocytosis and injury; florid duct lesions (50%), epithelioid granulomas in the lobules (20%) or portal tracts (40%)
- ☐ Risk factor for biliary cirrhosis

A NEW NAME?

A self-appointed committee of medical terminology activists has worked hard to rename *primary biliary cirrhosis* as *primary biliary cholangitis*, criticizing the old name as being inaccurate because cirrhosis is not inevitable and choosing to substitute for it a new name that is sufficiently bland and redundant (is there another form of cholangitis besides biliary?) that only a committee could have chosen it. While neither term is perfect, at least the first term was not silly from the outset, as the disease was first recognized largely in patients with advanced fibrosis.

CLINICAL AND LABORATORY FINDINGS

Typical patients with primary biliary cirrhosis are middle-aged women with alkaline phosphatase–predominant liver enzyme elevations and a positive antimitochondrial antibody (M2 subtype). This clinical pattern, as well as the histological findings, are distinct from primary sclerosing cholangitis and autoimmune hepatitis (Table 8.2). On biopsy, there are no significant differences in the histology findings between AMA-positive and AMA-negative primary biliary cirrhosis.

FAQ: What does the "M2" mean, in the test AMA M2 subtype?

Answer: Historically, testing for AMAs was performed using indirect immunofluorescence, where the patient's serum was applied to tissue sections of rat stomach/kidney. This method detects a number of different AMA antibodies, which are called M1 through M9. It turns out that the M2 subtype is most specific for primary biliary cirrhosis.

What is the target of the M2 subtype? Studies have shown that the antigen is located on the inner mitochondrial membranes and appears be mostly directed at the E2 subunit of pyruvate dehydrogenase complex and 2-oxoglutarate dehydrogenase complex.

Currently, most laboratories test for AMA using ELISA and not indirect immunofluorescence.

TABLE 8.2: A Comparison of Primary Biliary Cirrhosis, Primary Sclerosing Cholangitis, and Autoimmune Hepatitis

Findings	PBC	PSC	AIH
Gender (F:M)	Female 8:1 male	Female 1:5 Male	Female 9:1 Male
Liver enzyme elevations	Alk phos predominant	Alk phos predominant	AST/ALT predominant
Serological pattern	AMA (antimitochondrial antibody) 10% seronegative	pANCA (not very sensitive or specific) 50% seronegative	ANA, ASMA (type 1) LKM (type 2) 20% seronegative
Clinical associations	Sjogren syndrome, thyroid dysfunction, systemic sclerosis[36]	Inflammatory bowel disease (80%); PSC > Crohn disease	Other autoimmune conditions (40%)
Major histological patterns in untreated cases	Early: portal-based inflammation with duct injury Late: biliary cirrhosis, ductopenia, cholate stasis	Early: biliary obstruction pattern with bile ductular proliferation Late: biliary cirrhosis, ductopenia, cholate stasis	Plasma cell–rich inflammation with portal and lobular chronic inflammation Late: "burned out" cirrhosis
Other important findings	Florid duct lesion, granulomas	Fibro-obliterative duct lesion	
Plasma cells	Often plasma cell rich; IgM positive plasma cells are equal or greater than IgG	Not prominent in peripheral needle biopsies; can be prominent in hilum around large inflamed bile ducts	Prominent in 80% of cases; IgG > IgM
Cirrhotic pattern	Biliary pattern of cirrhosis	Biliary pattern of cirrhosis	Often nondescript cirrhosis with minimal to mild inflammation

HISTOLOGY FINDINGS

Histologically, primary biliary cirrhosis is a portal-based disease, with patchy moderate portal chronic inflammation (Fig. 8.32). There is inflammation and destruction of bile ducts, in particular the medium-sized bile ducts, also called *septal bile ducts*. The larger hilar ducts are generally intact and without much active injury. There can be mild patchy bile ductular proliferation in the smallest portal tracts when the septal-sized bile ducts downstream of them are injured and obstructed.

The portal inflammation is predominately lymphocytic and often shows a strong enrichment for plasma cells (Fig. 8.33). Interface activity is common in portal tracts with moderate or greater inflammation, but primary biliary cirrhosis lacks the significant lobular hepatitis seen in untreated autoimmune hepatitis. There can be rare scattered foci of mild lobular inflammation in primary biliary cirrhosis, often with a zone 3 predominance, but not much more lobular hepatitis than that (Fig. 8.34).

The medium-sized bile ducts are targeted by immune-mediated destruction and show reactive changes and a loose granulomatous inflammatory response. The constellation of an injured duct associated with a loose granulomatous inflammation is called a florid duct lesion (Figs. 8.35 and 8.36). Florid duct lesions are found in about 50% of biopsies.[10]

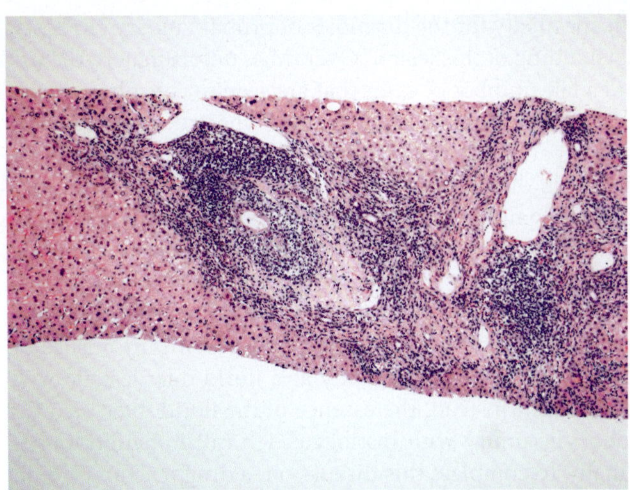

Figure 8.32. **Primary biliary cirrhosis, moderate portal chronic inflammation.** At low power, the inflammation is predominately portal, with little to no lobular inflammation.

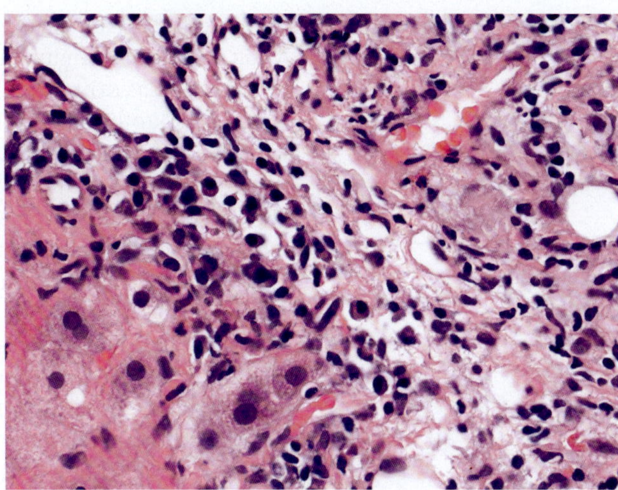

Figure 8.33. **Primary biliary cirrhosis, plasma cell–rich portal chronic inflammation.** At high power, numerous plasma cells are present.

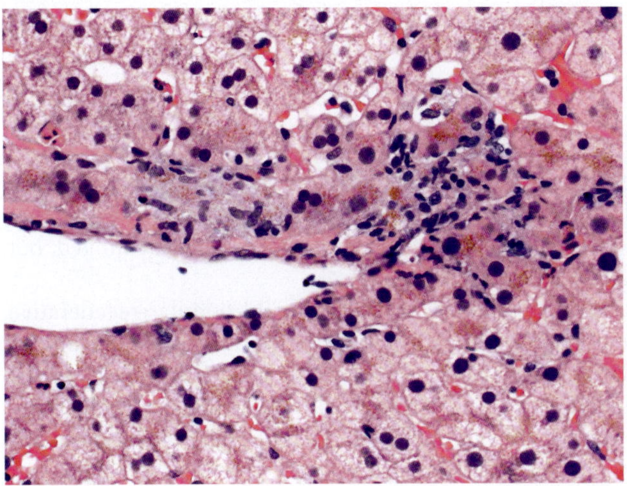

Figure 8.34. **Primary biliary cirrhosis, lobular inflammation.** This case of primary biliary cirrhosis shows occasional foci of lobular inflammation in zone 3.

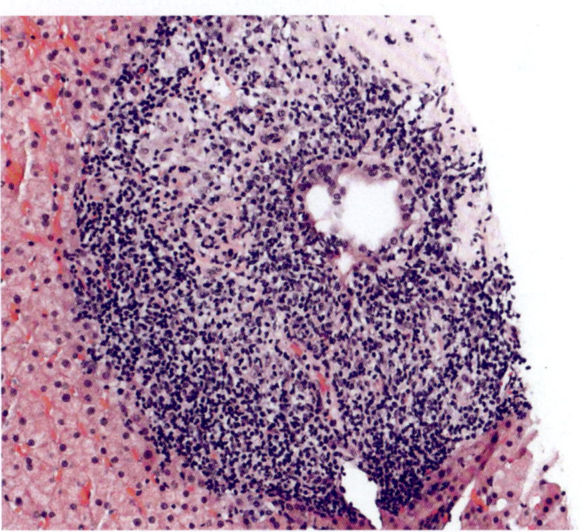

Figure 8.35. **Primary biliary cirrhosis, florid duct lesion.** There is dense lymphohistiocytic inflammation surround an injured bile duct.

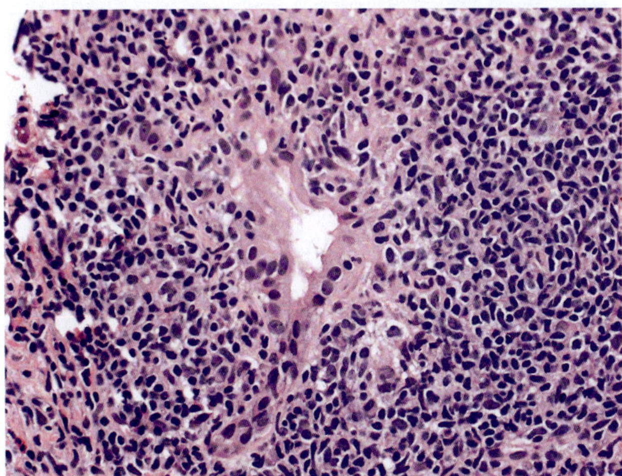

Figure 8.36. **Primary biliary cirrhosis, florid duct lesion.** Another example showing duct-centric inflammation with bile duct injury. The inflammation is predominately lymphocytic but histiocytes are also seen.

Florid duct lesions have high specificity for the diagnosis of primary biliary cirrhosis, if you stick to the original understanding of this lesion. Over time, unfortunately, the use of this term has drifted a bit and a fair number of cases that are seen in consultation and are reported to have a florid duct lesion, do not. In most cases where this term is used wrongly, the biopsies instead shows patchy, mild, and nonspecific bile duct lymphocytosis, which does not qualify for a florid duct lesion (Fig. 8.37). Another frequent misuse of this term is when there is bile duct lymphocytosis in the setting of downstream biliary tract obstructive disease, especially when the portal tract shows edematous changes. The portal inflammation in these cases can have increased numbers of macrophages, and mild bile duct lymphocytosis is common. In such cases, the prominent ductular reaction will clarify the diagnosis as being biliary tract obstruction. A third misuse of this term: a portal granuloma (Fig. 8.38) does not qualify as a florid duct lesion, even if it happens to be close to the bile duct. Instead, the essence of the florid duct lesion is significant duct-centered lymphocytic injury with histiocyte-rich inflammation immediately around the bile duct. Finally, to complete this discussion, a drug reaction should still be excluded in cases with florid duct lesions, as similar lesions can rarely be seen in drug reactions.

When florid duct lesions are absent (about ½ of cases), you can still diagnose primary biliary cirrhosis when there is a portal-based inflammation with cholestatic injury. In early or mild disease, the features of cholestatic injury are best seen with CK7 and copper stains. Epithelioid, noncaseating and usually small-sized granulomas can be present in both the portal tracts (~40% of cases)[10] and the lobules (~20% of cases)[9,10] (Figs. 8.38 and 8.39). Granulomas per se are neither sensitive nor specific for primary biliary cirrhosis but can help support the diagnosis in the setting of other typical features.

Ductopenia can develop over time, especially with more advanced fibrosis. A rare subset of individuals with primary biliary cirrhosis have been described who have early ductopenia, despite having no fibrosis (Fig. 8.40).[11] Data on this subset of patients are limited, but they appear to have a more aggressive clinical course.

Other findings in primary biliary cirrhosis can include mild nodular regenerative hyperplasia,[12] mildly prominent eosinophils in a few of the portal tracts, and patchy mild lobular inflammation that often has a zone 3 accentuation. Lobular cholestasis visible on the H&E is rare unless there is advanced fibrosis. If present outside this setting, significant lobular cholestasis suggests the original diagnosis is wrong or there is a superimposed injury.

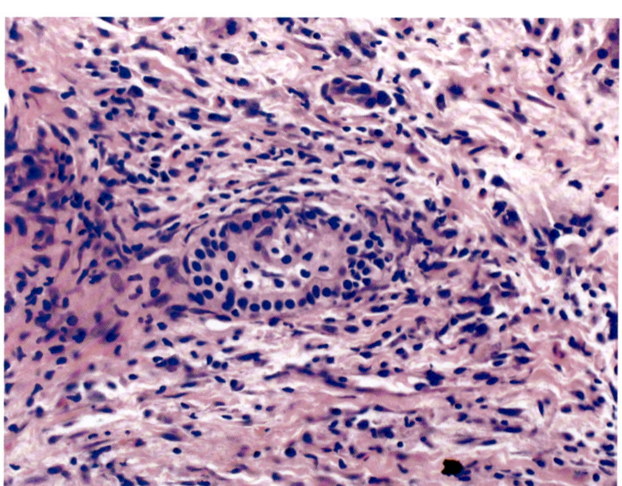

Figure 8.37. Drug reaction with duct injury. This antibiotic related drug reaction somewhat mimics a florid duct lesion, with portal inflammation and duct injury.

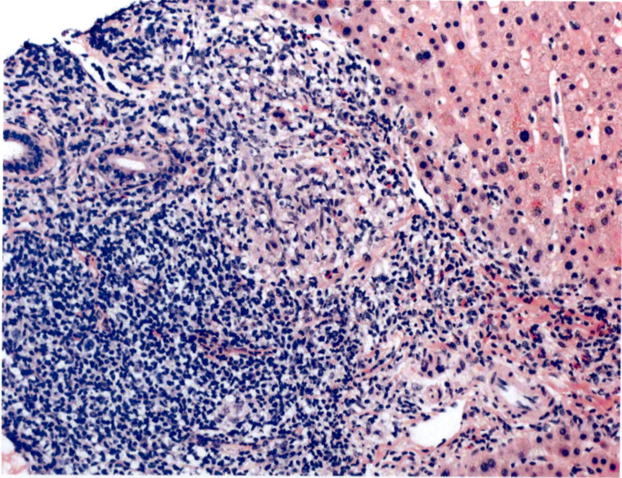

Figure 8.38. Primary biliary cirrhosis, granuloma. An epithelioid granuloma is present in this portal tract. There is no florid duct lesion in this image.

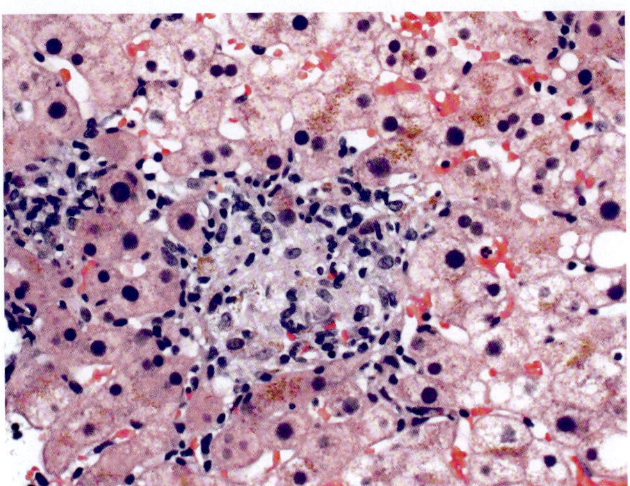

Figure 8.39. **Primary biliary cirrhosis, lobular granuloma.** A small epithelioid granuloma is seen in a case of primary biliary cirrhosis.

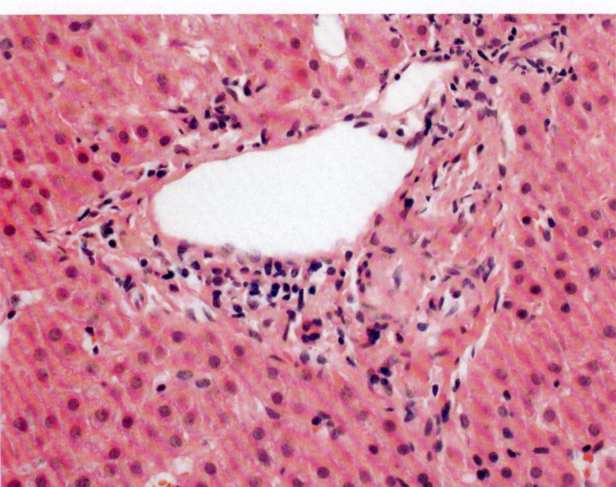

Figure 8.40. **Primary biliary cirrhosis, early ductopenia pattern.** There was no fibrosis in this case, but the portal tracts showed extensive bile duct loss.

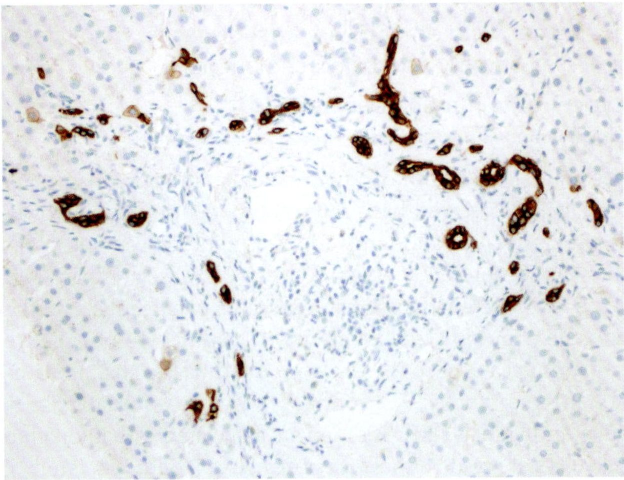

Figure 8.41. **Idiopathic ductopenia, CK7.** The ductules at the periphery of the portal tract are highlighted by the CK7, but the bile duct itself is missing.

IDIOPATHIC DUCTOPENIA

CHECKLIST: Idiopathic Ductopenia

- ☐ By definition, all known causes of ductopenia need to be excluded, including PSC, PBC, extrahepatic biliary obstruction, and bile salt deficiency disease, such as FIC, BSEP, and MDR3 deficiency
- ☐ Etiology: The differential list is long, but includes mostly drugs and paraneoplastic syndromes
- ☐ Histology: Loss of bile ducts, lobules may be deeply cholestatic, fibrosis varies from none to cirrhosis

The diagnosis of idiopathic ductopenia means there is definite bile duct loss (Fig. 8.41), but the cause is not identified despite histological and clinical evaluation. This of course means that we, the pathologists, will not make the final diagnosis of idiopathic ductopenia in most cases, as many possible etiologies have to be excluded by our clinical colleagues before a case is appropriately labeled as idiopathic (Table 8.1). However, pathologists do make the diagnosis of ductopenia, and there can be histological findings that can guide the subsequent clinical evaluation for etiology. Ductopenia in the setting of advanced fibrosis or cirrhosis suggests primary biliary cirrhosis, primary sclerosing cholangitis, other causes of biliary obstruction, or bile salt deficiencies—which can sometimes present in adults, particularly MDR3 defiency.[13,14] Ductopenia without fibrosis suggests a paraneoplastic effect or drug effect, although many cases remain idiopathic despite full clinical and histological evaluation.

IGG4 SCLEROSING DISEASE

CHECKLIST: IgG4 Sclerosing Disease

- ☐ Three main patterns can be seen on peripheral needle biopsies: mild nonspecific portal inflammation; sclerosing cholangitis; inflammatory pseudotumor
- ☐ Usually men in 50 to 70 years' age range
- ☐ Serum IgG4 levels elevated; levels >135 mg/dL supports IgG4 disease
- ☐ Increased number of IgG4-positive plasma cells in the portal tracts
- ☐ IgG4 liver disease can show overlap with other biliary tract diseases, which need to be excluded first, in particular primary sclerosing cholangitis
- ☐ Strongly associated with type 1 autoimmune pancreatitis

IgG4 sclerosing disease is a systemic disease with organ-specific manifestations. Overall, 60% of individuals with systemic IgG4 disease will have some component of liver involvement.[15] IgG4 disease has a male predominance and tends to affect middle-aged and older individuals, with a mean age at first clinical presentation in the mid-60s.[16] Greater than 90% of IgG4 disease involving the liver is associated with type I autoimmune pancreatitis, and the pancreatic disease usually leads to the clinical presentation, which can include obstructive jaundice and/or a pancreatic mass. Some cases also present with hilar masses that are concerning for cholangiocarcinoma on imaging studies.[17] In contrast, most cases of primary sclerosing cholangitis present in younger individuals (20s, 30s) and are associated with idiopathic inflammatory bowel disease, while clinical presentation with obstructive jaundice is rare.[16,18] Both diseases have strictures of the intrahepatic and extrahepatic biliary tree, but the strictures are steroid responsive only in IgG4 disease and not in primary sclerosing cholangitis.

There are three main histological patterns of injury seen in the liver with IgG4 disease and a rare fourth pattern. In all of them, correlation with serum IgG4 levels is important (levels >135 mg/dL supports IgG4 disease). Imaging of the biliary tree shows variable degrees of intrahepatic and extrahepatic biliary strictures.[16] The additional presence of a pancreatic mass can strongly suggest IgG4 sclerosing disease.

On peripheral needle biopsy, one of the more common patterns is mild nonspecific portal and lobular inflammation, with no findings to indicate IgG4 disease, including a lack of increased IgG4-positive plasma cells. In these cases, the diagnosis is based on findings in other organs as well as clinical and serological findings.

A second common pattern on needle biopsy is that of obstructive biliary tract disease, with patchy bile ductular proliferation and mild to focally moderate portal chronic inflammation. With this pattern of injury, the changes can represent a combination of IgG4 disease directly involving the liver as well as secondary obstructive type changes resulting from bile duct obstruction at the level of the pancreas and/or larger branches of the bile duct. In this pattern, the portal inflammation can be plasma cell rich and increased IgG4 positive plasma cells might be seen, in particular if a medium- or larger sized bile duct is sampled. Neutrophils are often present when there is a bile ductular proliferation. Rarely, the inflammation, edema, and fibrosis in the larger portal tracts can form small nodules, sometimes with storiform fibrosis or phlebitis. Other common findings include mild lobular cholestasis.

For cases of IgG4 disease with a chronic biliary tract disease pattern of injury, the histological differential includes primary sclerosing cholangitis, in large part because in both cases the histology findings can be dominated by a biliary obstruction pattern (Fig. 8.42).

Both diseases can have bile duct duplication, periductal fibrosis, periportal copper deposition, and CK7-positive intermediated hepatocytes.[16,18] However, primary sclerosing cholangitis presents at a younger age, usually in the teens or 20s, generally does not present with biliary obstruction, and is strongly associated with inflammatory bowel disease. In contrast, IgG4 sclerosing cholangitis affects older men (usually in 50s and 60s), presents with obstructive clinical disease in about 75% of cases,[16,18] and is strongly associated with type 1 autoimmune pancreatitis. Histologically, both diseases can have onion-skinning fibrosis and bile duct duplication.[16,18] However, established ductopenia, fibro-obliterative duct lesions, or advanced fibrosis would all strongly favor primary sclerosing cholangitis. IgG4 immunostains can be helpful but need to be correlated with the clinical and histological findings, especially because 20% of otherwise typical cases of primary sclerosing cholangitis can have >10 positive IgG4 plasma cells in the larger hilar portal tracts, mimicking IgG4 disease.[19]

The third major pattern is that of a mass lesion.[20] On imaging, the mass lesions can suggest cholangiocarcinoma or other malignancies. The mass lesions are portal based in most cases and are composed of edematous and irregular fibroinflammatory nodules (Fig. 8.43). Histologically, the mass lesions look essentially like an inflammatory pseudotumor but also have prominent IgG4 positive plasma cells. Depending on sampling, phlebitis and/or storiform fibrosis can be found and sometimes be prominent.

A final and very rare pattern shows an overall hepatitic pattern that is in keeping with autoimmune hepatis but has prominent IgG4-positive plasma cells in the portal tracts. These individuals tend to be treated and respond like ordinary autoimmune hepatitis.[21]

IGG4 IMMUNOHISTOCHEMISTRY

Immunostains for IgG4 disease (Fig. 8.44) should always be interpreted in the context of clinical and serological findings, as well as the overall pattern of histological injury. A common guideline is that the presence of 10 or more IgG4-positive plasma cells per high-power field supports a diagnosis of IgG4 disease on needle biopsy (50 or more on resection specimens). However, at least 1/3 of cases of IgG4 sclerosing cholangitis will have less than 10 IgG4-positive plasma cells on peripheral needle biopsy, underscoring the need to correlate results with other findings. In many of these cases, the lack of IgG4-positive plasma cells on needle biopsy reflects the size of the sampled portal tracts, as medium- and larger sized portal tracts are more likely to be enriched with IgG4-positive plasma cells but these can be missed on peripheral needle biopsies. Immunostains for IgG4 disease are sensitive but not entirely specific, even when larger portal tracts are sampled. For example, about 20% of explanted livers for primary sclerosing cholangitis are associated with mildly elevated serum IgG4 levels and show large hilar bile ducts with chronic plasma cell–rich inflammation containing greater than 10 positive plasma cells per high-power field.[19] Thus, we end up where we usually do, where the best final diagnosis is achieved by combining the histological observations with the results of clinical, imaging, and laboratory findings.

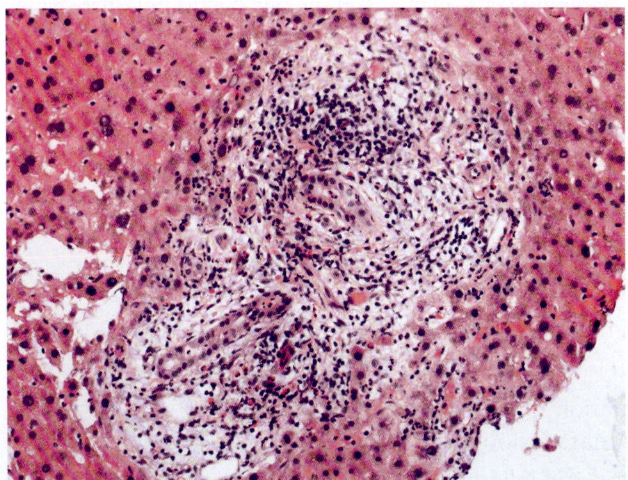

Figure 8.42. **IgG 4 disease.** The portal tracts show mild bile ductular proliferation with edema and mild mixed portal inflammation.

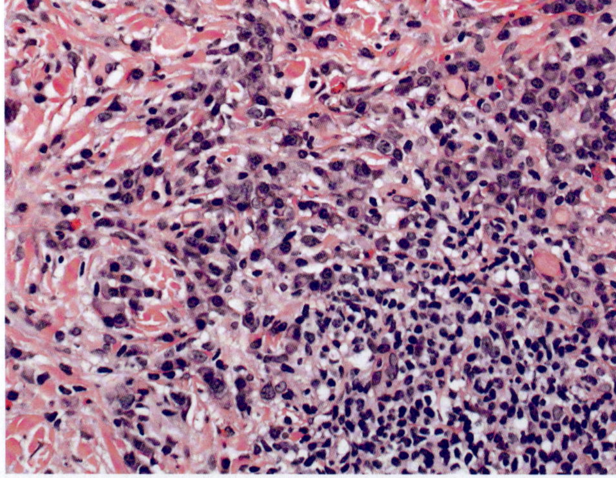

Figure 8.43. **IgG 4 disease.** A small fibroinflammatory nodule was biopsied and shows fibrosis with plasma cell–rich inflammation.

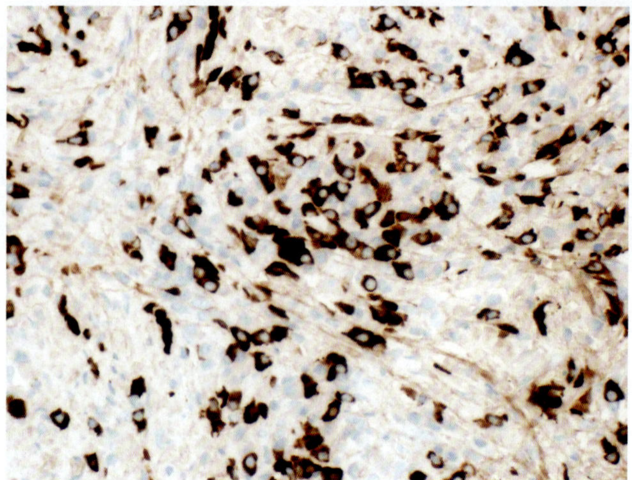

Figure 8.44. **IgG 4 disease, IgG4 immunostain.** Numerous IgG4 positive plasma cells are seen (same case as above). A common criteria used is greater than 10 per high-power field. However, the immunostain data have to be interpreted in the context of the H&E findings.

In general, a final diagnosis of IgG4-related liver disease requires compatible clinical and imaging findings, elevated serum IgG4 levels, compatible histology, and steroid responsiveness of the liver disease. The biliary strictures generally show some improvement within 4 to 6 weeks of starting the steroid therapy.

SCLEROSING CHOLANGITIS ASSOCIATED WITH TYPE 2 AUTOIMMUNE PANCREATITIS

Type 2 autoimmune pancreatitis can also be associated with liver disease. Most cases occur in children. Because of the rarity of type 2 autoimmune pancreatitis, the histological changes in the liver are less well described than in type 1 autoimmune pancreatitis (IgG4-associated disease). The histological changes in type 2 autoimmune pancreatitis can include an obstructive pattern of injury, resulting from obstruction at the level of the inflamed pancreas. In addition, the bile ducts can have what is called a *granulocytic epithelial lesion*, with neutrophilic inflammation within the bile duct proper, often associated with epithelial injury.[22] Granulocytic lesions tend to be very patchy, affecting only a minority of portal tracts in most cases.[22,23] In terms of the differential diagnosis, there is no increase in serum IgG4 and immunostains for IgG4 are within normal limits. Moreover, the neutrophils are not as numerous as they are in ascending cholangitis, and the bile duct is not dilated.

SEGMENTAL CHOLANGIECTASIA

CHECKLIST: Segmental Cholangiectasia

- ☐ Risk factors are mostly unknown but
  - ○ biliary stones are commonly present
  - ○ may be more common in Asia
- ☐ Imaging: Segmental dilatation of intrahepatic bile ducts; often mimics a cholangiocarcinoma or other mass lesion
- ☐ Histology: Cystically dilated and inflamed biliary system restricted mostly to one segment of the liver

This disease appears to result from recurrent infections of the biliary tree, isolated to a segment of the liver, while the rest of the liver is unaffected. The etiology is not entirely clear but appears to result from intrahepatic biliary stones (Fig. 8.45), which are found in most cases, leading to focal biliary obstruction and recurrent bacterial infections. The bile ducts in the affected segment of the liver are dilated into cystlike structures (Fig. 8.46) and have acute and chronic inflammation with fibrotic walls (Fig. 8.47).[7] The dilated ducts often have a thickened cuff of dense hyalinized fibrosis (Fig. 8.47). These changes can lead to a masslike lesion that suggests cholangiocarcinoma or a cystic biliary neoplasm by imaging studies.[7]

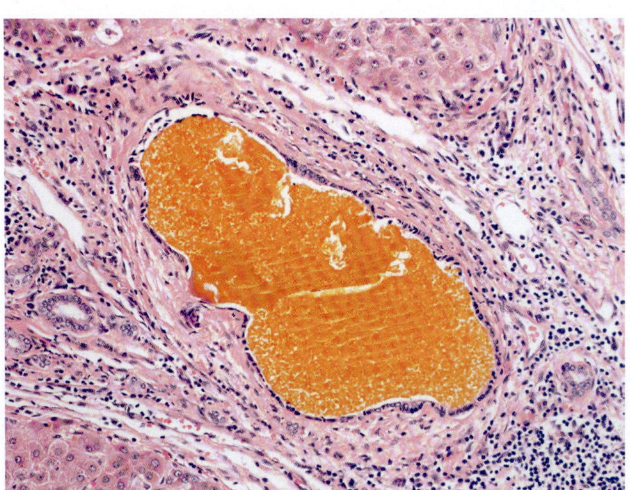

Figure 8.45. **Intrahepatic stone.** This liver had numerous intrahepatic stones.

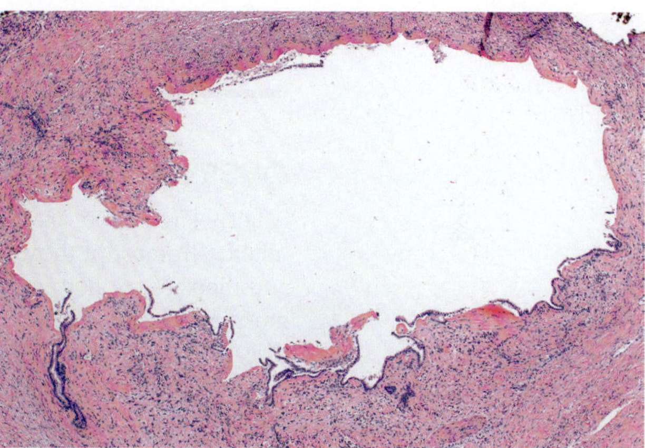

Figure 8.46. **Segmental cholangiectasia.** The bile duct is markedly dilated.

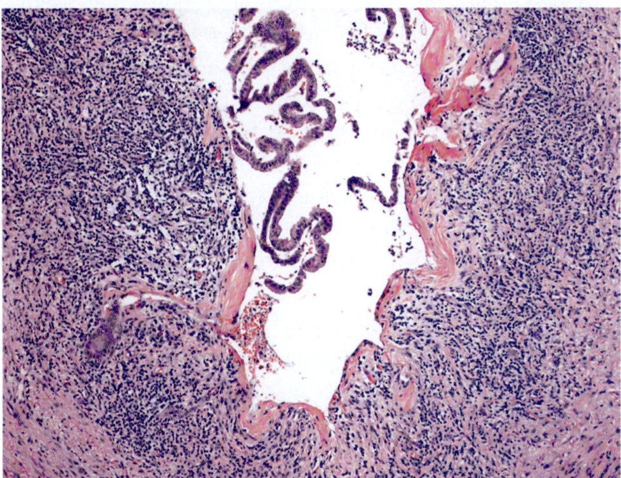

Figure 8.47. **Segmental cholangiectasia.** This bile duct is cuffed by a rind of marked inflammation. There is a thickened hyalinized layer of subepithelial collagen.

PEDIATRIC CHOLESTATIC LIVER DISEASE

CHECKLIST: Pediatric Cholestatic Liver Disease

- ☐ Various genetic diseases. This category includes a large number of diseases that present in infancy such as alpha-1-antitrypsin deficiency, Niemann–Pick disease type C, Aageneas syndrome, North American Indian familial cholestasis (also called North American Indian childhood cirrhosis), the Zellweger syndrome
- ☐ Bile salt deficiency: ATPB81 deficiency, ABCB11 deficiency, ABCB4 deficiency
- ☐ Biliary atresia
- ☐ Paucity of intrahepatic bile ducts
- ☐ Neonatal giant cell hepatitis
- ☐ Sepsis
- ☐ Total parenteral nutrition

OVERVIEW

A fairly large list of pediatric diseases can present with a cholestatic pattern of injury in infancy. In most of these cases, the diagnosis is made by clinical and serological findings, and biopsies are not part of the routine management. These diseases include various and mostly very rare genetic conditions such as alpha-1-antitrypsin deficiency, Niemann–Pick disease type C, hypopituitarism, Aageneas syndrome, North American Indian familial cholestasis, and the Zellweger syndrome.

Alpha-1-antitrypsin deficiency can rarely present in infancy with a cholestatic pattern of liver enzyme elevations. Almost all cases result from ZZ disease, and in most cases, the diagnosis is made by finding low levels of serum alpha-1-antitrypsin protein and confirmed by Pi testing or genetic testing. Biopsies are not necessary but can show a number of different cholestatic patterns including a bland lobular cholestasis pattern, neonatal giant cell hepatitis pattern, or paucity of intrahepatic bile ducts pattern. The globules of alpha-1-antitrypsin are absent or very rare in the first 4 months of life, so PASD stains can be negative or only equivocally positive. Likewise, Niemann–Pick disease type C can present clinically with cholestatic liver disease, but biopsies in infants can lack the abnormal Kupffer cells typical of Niemann–Pick disease type C. Instead, the biopsies in Niemann–Pick disease type C can show a bland lobular cholestatic pattern or have findings that suggest biliary obstruction. Other causes of pediatric cholestatic liver disease are evident from clinical findings, including sepsis and total parenteral nutrition.

Biopsies in any of the many causes of pediatric cholestatic liver disease will show lobular cholestasis, relatively little inflammation, abundant extramedullary hematopoiesis, and mild patchy giant cell transformation of hepatocytes. Total parenteral nutrition also frequently has early ductopenia.[24]

When liver biopsies are performed, the clinical causes above have usually been excluded and the goal is to evaluate for biliary atresia, paucity of intrahepatic bile ducts, or neonatal giant cell hepatitis.

BILIARY ATRESIA

Biliary atresia results from atresia of the extrahepatic bile ducts. Infants typically present within 1 to 6 weeks of birth with jaundice, pruritus, and failure to thrive. Pale stools and dark urine are common. Serum studies show elevated levels of alkaline phosphatase, GGT, and conjugated bilirubin. About 20% of individuals will have other organ structural anomalies, the most common being spleen abnormalities such as no spleen or multiple spleens. Other findings may include structural abnormalities of the heart, intestine, or pancreas.

The etiology is not known but might be immune mediated, at least in part, as the duct remnants are typically inflamed. The location of the atresia varies in different cases, but the vast majority of cases have atresia of the right and left hepatic ducts as they exit the liver. Imaging studies can be helpful but do not always have the resolution to make the diagnosis.

HIDA scans typically show failure to secrete bile, but this imaging finding is not specific, as it can also be observed with neonatal giant cell hepatitis and with paucity of intrahepatic bile ducts. However, with rare exceptions, an HIDA scan that shows biliary excretion would help rule out biliary atresia.

Biliary atresia is treated by a Kasai procedure whenever possible, where bile is restored by removing the extrahepatic biliary tree and sewing a loop of small bowel to the liver hilum, which allows bile to ooze out of the small but patent bile ducts in the hilum. The Kasai procedure is generally not curative but serves as an important bridge to liver transplantation.

The pattern of injury in biliary atresia is basically that of obstruction (Figs. 8.48 and 8.49), regardless of the location of the atretic section of the bile duct. The portal tracts show bile ductular proliferation and portal fibrosis as the primary pattern of injury. As a caveat, biopsies very early in the course of the disease can show minimal ductular proliferation, with lobular cholestasis as the predominant injury pattern, but biopsies in this very early stage are rare. As another finding, the portal arteries often have thicker walls than normal because of muscular hyperplasia. Cases diagnosed later in life often have ductopenia (Fig. 8.50). Lobular cholestasis can range from absent to marked (Fig. 8.51). Focal giant cell transformation of hepatocytes is common (Fig. 8.52). Extramedullary hematopoiesis can be prominent and can superficially resemble hepatitis, but the lobules show minimal or absent true inflammation.

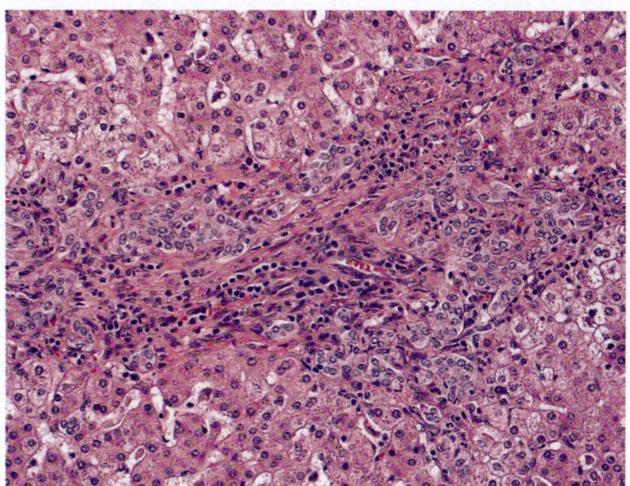

Figure 8.48. **Biliary atresia.** The portal tracts show marked bile ductular proliferation with minimal inflammation.

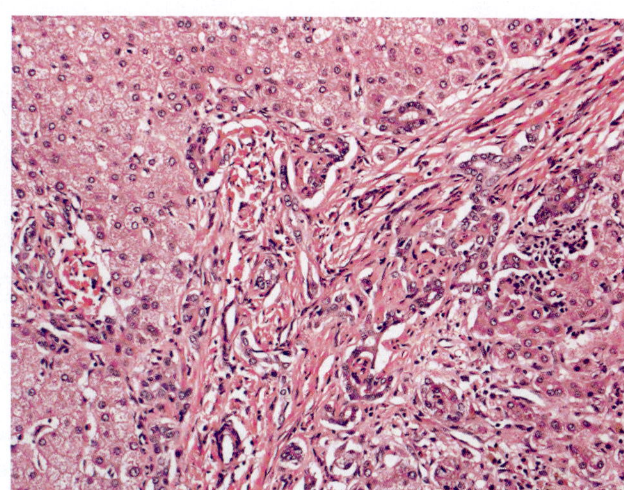

Figure 8.49. **Biliary atresia.** Another example of biliary atresia showing the typical pattern of portal fibrosis and bile ductular proliferation.

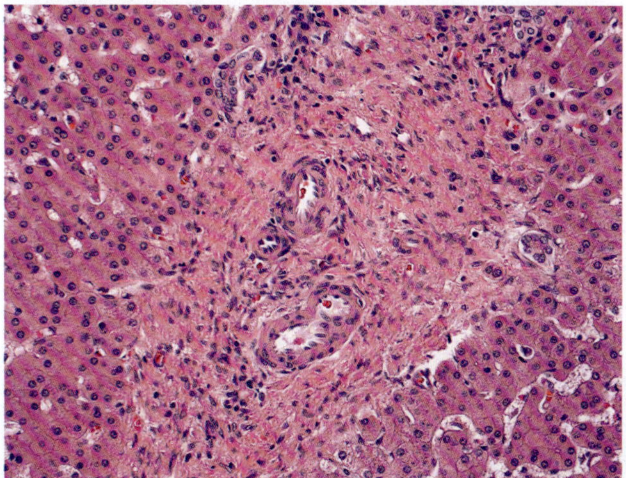

Figure 8.50. **Biliary atresia.** In this case, there was early ductopenia. Very mild bile ductular proliferation can still be seen at the periphery.

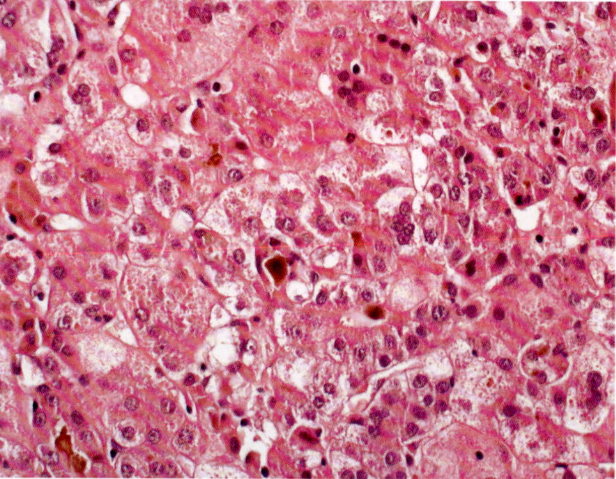

Figure 8.51. **Biliary atresia, lobular cholestasis.** There is diffuse moderate lobular cholestasis in this wedge biopsy obtained at the time of a Kasai procedure.

The diagnosis is made on H&E, but immunostains can sometimes be useful adjuncts. CK7 will show numerous intermediate hepatocytes, highlight the ductular proliferation, and will show no ductopenia in early disease. A CD56 can sometimes be helpful, as the bile ductules will be strongly positive in biliary atresia but are negative or show focal minimal staining in other nonobstructive pediatric cholestatic liver diseases.[25] A trichrome stain shows at least portal fibrosis in most cases, except for the very early ones. Bridging fibrosis or cirrhosis has a worse prognosis.

Neonatal alpha-1-antitrypsin deficiency can present with similar clinical (and histological) findings to biliary atresia, so should be excluded by laboratory testing in all cases. PASD stains are not helpful, as the hepatocyte globules are frequently absent in infants less than 4 to 6 month of age. The other major disease considerations in the differential for biliary atresia are shown in Table 8.3.

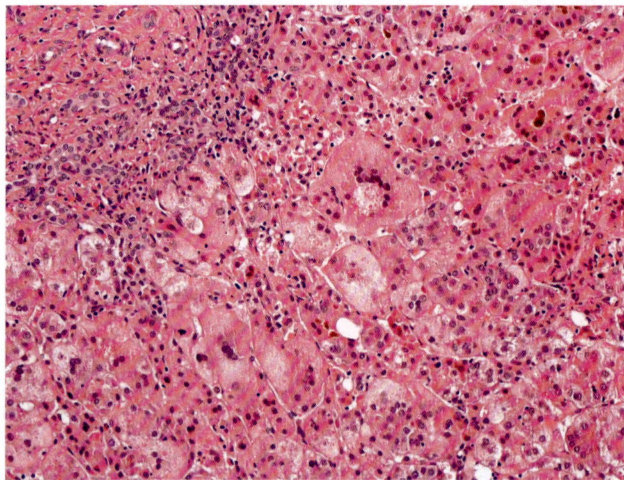

Figure 8.52. **Biliary atresia, focal giant cells.** This case of biliary atresia showed scattered giant transformation of hepatocytes.

TABLE 8.3: Major Categories of Pediatric Cholestatic Liver Diseases

Finding	Biliary Atresia	Neonatal Giant Cell Hepatitis	Paucity of Intrahepatic Bile Ducts
Major pattern of injury	Extrahepatic biliary obstruction	Giant cell transformation of hepatocytes plus cholestasis	Loss of bile ducts
Bile ductular proliferation	Prominent	Mild in 25% of cases	Minimal or absent
Ductular cholestasis	Can be seen	Rare	Absent
Giant cell transformation of hepatocytes	About 20% of cases, mild	All cases, range from mild to marked	Minimal or absent
Lobular cholestasis	Common	Common	None to mild at presentation
Portal fibrosis	Common	Rare	None to mild at presentation

NEONATAL GIANT CELL HEPATITIS

This pattern of injury shows a striking giant cell transformation of hepatocytes. Infants present with elevated conjugated bilirubin levels but have normal imaging studies of the extrahepatic bile ducts. There are numerous potential causes. Overall, a cause is found in about ½ of cases, the most common being pituitary abnormalities with lack of growth hormone production, infections such as CMV or echovirus, or immune system dysregulation. Moreover, a subset of other pediatric cholestatic liver diseases can present initially with a pattern of neonatal giant cell hepatitis, with the full clinical and histological findings of the disease developing only later. These include rare cases of biliary atresia, Alagille syndrome, and bile salt deficiencies. Other genetic diseases such as cystic fibrosis and alpha-1-antitrypsin deficiency can also first present with a neonatal giant cell hepatitis pattern of injury.

The most striking finding at low power is the numerous multinucleated hepatocytes (Fig. 8.53). These hepatocytes are large with amphophilic to eosinophilic cytoplasm and have between 4 and 10 hepatocytes. The percent of affected hepatocytes varies between 5% and 90% but tends to be around 40%. The transformed hepatocytes mostly cluster in zone 3, but some cases will have an azonal or zone 1 pattern. To date, no correlation with etiology and zonation has been recognized. The lobules often show mild to moderate cholestasis (Fig. 8.54). Minimal focal bile ductular proliferation is acceptable, but the biopsy findings should not suggest biliary obstruction. Extramedullary hematopoiesis is common, but lobular inflammation is generally absent or minimal.

Fibrosis is typically absent or minimal/equivocal. More advanced fibrosis can be seen, but most of these cases will end up not being idiopathic neonatal giant cell hepatitis after full workup and tend to be enriched for biliary atresia and other cholestatic liver diseases such as bile salt deficiencies.

PAUCITY OF INTRAHEPATIC BILE DUCTS

Paucity of intrahepatic bile ducts is an important pattern of injury that, like neonatal giant cell hepatitis, can be associated with different causes. Similar to patients with biliary atresia and neonatal giant cell hepatitis, patients with paucity of intrahepatic bile ducts present within weeks to months after birth with jaundice, elevated conjugated bilirubin levels, and pale stools. Alagille syndrome represents a subset of cases of paucity of intrahepatic bile ducts that is caused by JAG1 mutations. Affected patients also commonly have hypothyroidism, pancreas insufficiency, and various anatomical abnormalities including butterfly vertebrae and cardiovascular structural defects.

Regardless of the cause, the major findings in cases of paucity of intrahepatic bile ducts are within the portal tracts, which show bile ducts that are atrophic or absent (Fig. 8.55). Some of the portal tracts can show a mild bile ductular proliferation, but the overall

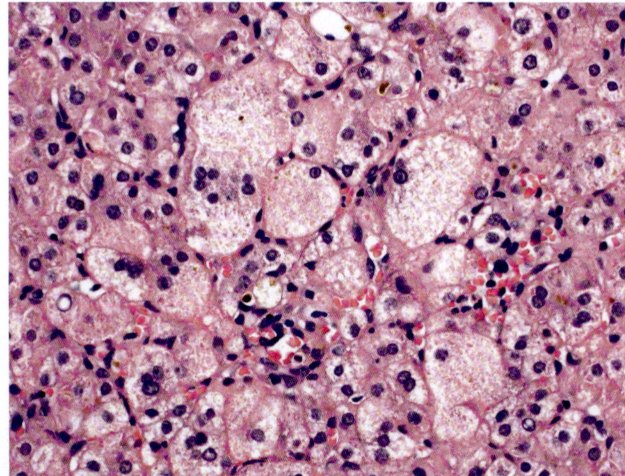

Figure 8.53. Neonatal giant cell hepatitis. The lobules show cholestasis and striking giant cell transformation. This is one of the rare cases where a definite cause was identified: hepatitis B.

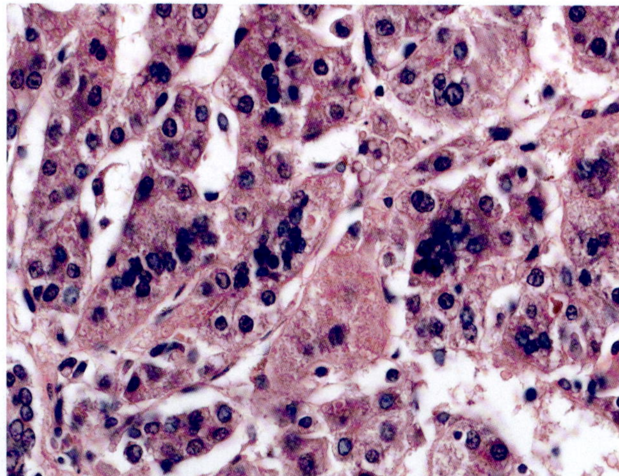

Figure 8.54. Neonatal giant cell hepatitis. In this idiopathic case, the giant cell transformation of hepatocyte was striking. The lobular cholestasis was relative mild, and there was no significant lobular inflammation.

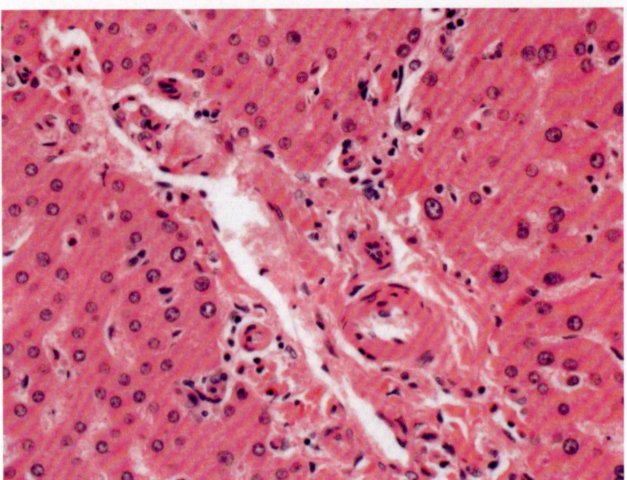

Figure 8.55. **Paucity of intrahepatic bile ducts.** In this case, there was only mild cholestasis, but almost all of the smaller branches of the portal tracts were missing their bile ducts.

pattern of injury should not suggest obstruction. A CK7 immunostain is helpful to evaluate the bile duct loss and will also show intermediate hepatocytes. The bile duct loss is primarily in the smaller portal tracts, and medium- and larger sized portal tracts will often still have bile ducts visible on H&E, sometimes with mild lymphocytic inflammation. The bile duct loss is patchy in the early phases of the disease and may not be evident on a small biopsy. The portal tracts in general can show mild nonspecific inflammation, and the lobules may show minimal inflammation, but the overall pattern of injury is typically not hepatitic. Mild to moderate lobular cholestasis is common, especially in later disease, often with patchy hepatocyte giant cell transformation. The lobules also commonly show extramedullary hematopoiesis. Fibrosis is unusual when patients first present with liver disease, and if present suggests other diagnoses, such as biliary atresia or other forms of obstruction. However, fibrosis has been reported in biopsies with long-standing ductopenia, especially with Alagille syndrome.

BILE SALT DEFICIENCY DISEASES

CHECKLIST: Inherited Bile Salt Deficiency Diseases

- ☐ ***ATP8B1* mutation, FIC deficiency.** Formerly called BRIC1 or PFIC 1 depending on clinical course. Also called Byler disease and Greenland familial cholestasis in some of the first descriptions of the disease
- ☐ ***ABCB11* mutation, BSEP deficiency.** Formerly called BRIC2 or PFIC2 depending on clinical course. Early literature also referred to this disease as Byler syndrome
- ☐ ***ABCB4* deficiency, MDR3 deficiency**

Note: BRIC = benign recurrent intrahepatic cholestasis; PFIC = progressive familial intrahepatic cholestasis.

The most common genetic cholestatic liver diseases are a group of diseases called *familial intrahepatic cholestatic liver disease*. The term *intrahepatic* served to distinguish this group of diseases from biliary atresia, which results from extrahepatic atresia of the bile ducts. All have an autosomal recessive pattern of inheritance. Before the underlying genetic causes were known, they were classified by their clinical course into either benign recurrent intrahepatic cholestasis or progressive familial intrahepatic cholestasis. Now, however, the diseases are classified by their underlying mutation, although the older terms are still commonly used, so are also shown in the checklist. Heterozygous mutations predispose to other diseases, notably gallstones at young age and intrahepatic cholestasis of pregnancy. Of note, about 1/3 of cases with a clinical coarse of progressive familial intrahepatic cholestasis have an unknown genetic basis,[26] which will hopefully rapidly change given the now widespread availability of whole genome sequencing.

FIC1 deficiency also has extrahepatic manifestations because the protein is important for the normal function of other organs, such as the lungs and pancreas and ear tubes. An elevated risk of hepatocellular carcinoma and of cholangiocarcinoma has been identified for BSEP deficiency but not for FIC1 or MDR3 deficiency.

SERUM FINDINGS

All cases of familial intrahepatic cholestasis have elevated serum conjugated bilirubin levels. Other patterns in laboratory findings have strong correlations with underlying genetic mutations. Although not entirely specific, the broad patterns can help classify the disease (Table 8.4). For example, elevated serum GGT levels favor MDR3 deficiency; low albumin levels are more common with FIC deficiency, while an elevated serum AFP level favors BSEP deficiency.[27] The AST and ALT levels are also typically elevated in all cases, usually in the mild range. Somewhat higher levels of ALT (5× or more of normal) is seen more commonly with BSEP deficiency.

HISTOLOGICAL FINDINGS

Biopsies in all of the bile salt deficiencies show a cholestatic pattern of injury. The H&E findings do not reliably distinguish between the specific subtypes, but there are some broad correlations between histology and genetic changes that can help classify disease. These correlates are most evident in early biopsies. As the diseases progress, they can all lead to a biliary pattern of cirrhosis that is largely similar by light microscopy. For those cases without an identified genetic mutation, the degree of fibrosis on index liver biopsy can help predict prognosis.

FIC1 deficiency tends to show a bland lobular cholestasis pattern of injury with the bile predominately located in the canaliculi (Fig. 8.56). The hepatocytes often look smaller than normal. Giant cell transformation of hepatocytes is relatively rare and inflammation is generally absent or minimal. There have been no well-developed immunostains for identifying this disease. Electron microscopy shows the typical Bylers bile—a coarse granular bile located in dilated bile canaliculi. Of note, the characteristic electron microscopy findings are not as evident and can be absent in formalin-fixed paraffin-embedded tissues. Interestingly, after liver transplantation, the allograft liver can develop steatohepatitis with progression to cirrhosis.[28,29] This is thought to reflect defects in bile acid reabsorption at the intestinal level.

In BSEP deficiency, biopsies tend to show a neonatal giant cell hepatitis pattern (Fig. 8.57). In addition, mild lobular hepatitis can sometime be seen, a finding typically absent in FIC1 and MDR3 deficiency. In comparison to idiopathic neonatal giant cell hepatitis, BSEP deficiency tends to have more lobular inflammation and somewhat less giant cell transformation, but there can be significant histological overlap. Obstructive changes are not seen, but a subset of cases will show mild ductopenia. BSEP deficiency is also more likely than the other causes to have advanced fibrosis before the age of 1 year. Elevated risks for hepatocellular carcinoma and cholangiocarcinoma are well documented. Immunostains for BSEP show reduced or absent protein expression, but a normal staining pattern can sometimes be observed when mutations lead to normal levels of BSEP protein but with reduced or absent protein function.

Patients with MDR3 deficiency can present in infancy or as adults. An important laboratory clue is that the serum GGT levels are elevated, in contrast to FIC1 and BSEP deficiency. In early disease, MDR3 deficiency leads to a cholestatic pattern of injury that often has bile ductular proliferation, mimicking downstream biliary tract obstruction (Fig. 8.58). The cholestasis tends to be more hepatocellular than canalicular, in contrast to FIC1 deficiency.

TABLE 8.4: Summary of Key Clinical, Laboratory, and Pathology Findings in Diseases of Bile Salt Deficiency

Finding	*ATP8B1* (FIC) Deficiency	*ABCB11* (BSEP) Deficiency	*ABCB4* (MDR3) Deficiency
Serum			
Bilirubin	Elevated conjugated bilirubin	Elevated conjugated bilirubin	Elevated conjugated bilirubin
GGT	Normal or low	Normal or low	Elevated
ALT	Mild elevations	Mild to moderate elevations	Mild elevations
AFP	Normal	Elevated	Normal
Cholesterol	Elevated, occasionally	Elevated, frequently	Normal
Albumin	Low	Normal	Normal
Main Pathology Findings			
Light microscopy	Bland lobular cholestasis	Neonatal giant cell hepatitis Lobular cholestasis Subset with paucity of intrahepatic ducts	Lobular cholestasis Bile ductular proliferation
Advanced fibrosis/cirrhosis in first year of life	No	Yes	No
Electron microscopy	Course granular bile	Amorphous to filamentous bile	Cholesterol crystals in bile (not always seen)
Immunohistochemistry	No well-developed stains	Reduction or loss of BSEP	Reduction or loss of MDR3
Additional Clinical Findings			
Extrahepatic findings	Diarrhea, pancreatic disease, hearing loss	None	None
Risk for cholelithiasis	None reported to date	Yes	Yes
Risk of hepatocellular and cholangiocarcinoma	None reported to date	Yes	Rare reports

GGT, gamma-glutamyltransferase.

When advanced fibrosis is present, the histological findings are nonspecific. In fact, some cases of cryptogenic cirrhosis in adults have been linked to heterozygous *ABCB4* mutations.[8] Cholesterol crystals in the bile can be seen by electron microscopy and rarely on H&E.[8]

The interpretation of immunostains for MDR3 is similar to that of BSEP, with reduced or absent staining strongly supporting a diagnosis of MDR3 deficiency, while a normal MDR3 staining pattern does not completely exclude MDR3 deficiency.

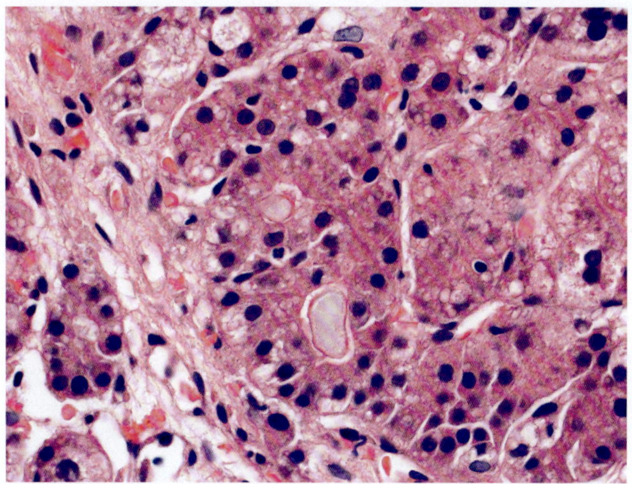

Figure 8.56. **FIC1 deficiency.** The lobules show dilated canaliculi with bile plugs and little or no inflammation.

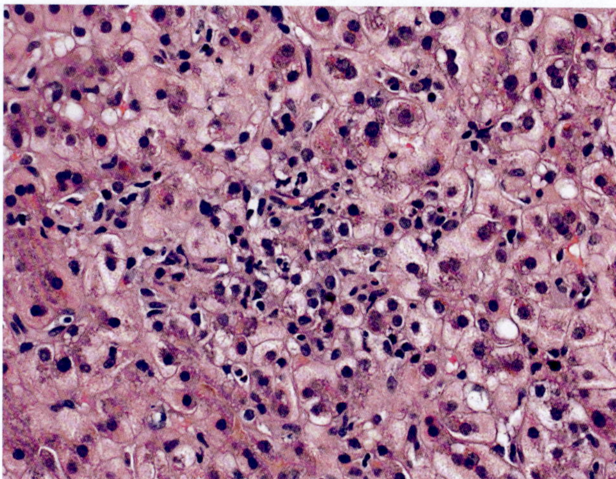

Figure 8.57. **BSEP deficiency.** The liver showed moderate cholestasis and mild patchy lobular inflammation. Focal minimal giant cell transformation was present (not shown).

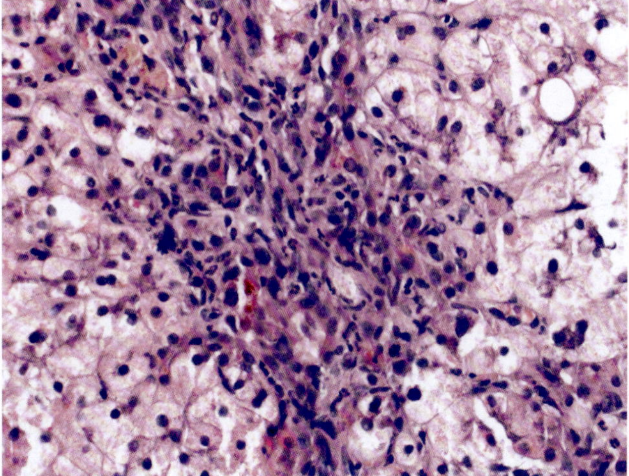

Figure 8.58. **MDR3 deficiency.** The portal tract shows an obstructive type pattern with mild bile ductular proliferation and mild mixed inflammation.

INHERITED DEFECTS IN BILIRUBIN METABOLISM

This group of inherited defects in bilirubin metabolism are very different clinically and histologically from the group of bile salt deficiencies. There are five main genetic diseases of biliary metabolism, all of which are autosomal recessive: Rotor syndrome, Dubin–Johnson syndrome, Gilbert syndrome, and Criggler–Najjar syndrome types I and II (Table 8.5).

Mutations in the *UGT1A1* gene lead to Crigler–Najjar syndromes I and II as well as Gilbert syndrome. The resulting clinical syndrome reflects the degree of residual gene activity. Crigler–Najjar syndrome type 1 has the least gene residual gene activity and presents with persistent jaundice developing in the first few days of life (Fig. 8.59). If untreated, there can be serious neurological complications. Treatment is largely focused on aggressive phototherapy to reduce the levels of unconjugated bilirubin in the blood. In contrast, Crigler–Najjar syndrome type II usually presents later in life and typically can be managed with phenobarbital therapy to lower bilirubin levels. Patients with Gilbert syndrome are clinically asymptomatic but can have episodes of jaundice when they are placed under stress from fasting, illnesses such as infections, or a drug reaction. Likewise, individuals with the Rotor syndrome and Dubin–Johnson syndrome are generally asymptomatic but can become jaundiced when placed under stress.

TABLE 8.5: The Five Major Inherited Defects in Bilirubin Metabolism

Disease	Gene	Bilirubin Elevations	Key Clinical and Histological Findings
Crigler–Najjar syndrome type I	UGT1A1	Unconjugated	Present with jaundice in first week of life. Biopsy with bland lobular cholestasis pattern
Crigler–Najjar syndrome type II	UGT1A1	Unconjugated	Present in later childhood/teen age years with cholestasis Biopsy with bland lobular cholestasis pattern
Gilbert's syndrome	UGT1A1	Unconjugated	Episodes of jaundice, otherwise asymptomatic Bland lobular cholestasis pattern of injury if biopsied during an episode of jaundice
Rotor syndrome	SLCO1B1 SLCO1B3	Conjugated	Episodes of jaundice, otherwise asymptomatic Bland lobular cholestasis pattern of injury if biopsied during an episode of jaundice Lipfouschin prominent in about ¼ of cases
Dubin–Johnson syndrome	ABCC2	Conjugated	Episodes of jaundice, otherwise asymptomatic Bland lobular cholestasis pattern of injury if biopsied during an episode of jaundice. Dense brown, granular lipofuschin pigment in hepatocytes.

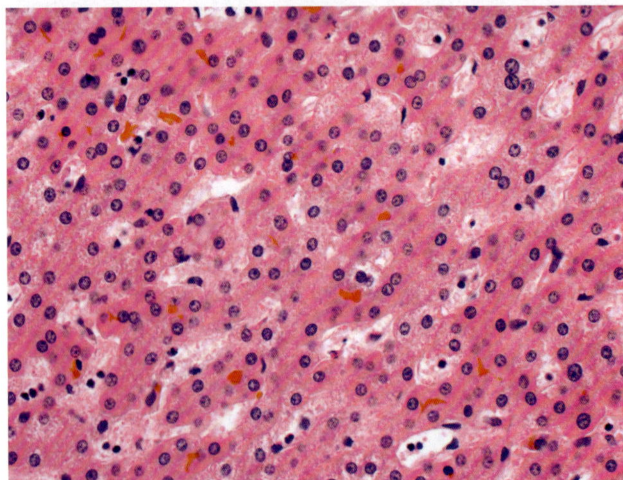

Figure 8.59. **Crigler–Najjar syndrome type 1.** The lobules show moderate cholestasis with no inflammation.

Biopsies are not very common for any of these conditions, but the findings generally show a bland lobular cholestasis pattern when the patient is cholestatic. There is minimal or absent lobular inflammation and absent to mild patchy portal chronic inflammation. There is no evidence for biliary obstruction. Lipofuscin is also common, in particular with Gilbert syndrome (Fig. 8.60)[26,30] and Dubin–Johnson syndrome (Fig. 8.61).[31] The lipofuschin pigment in the Dubin–Johnson syndrome can be courser and more deeply brown than

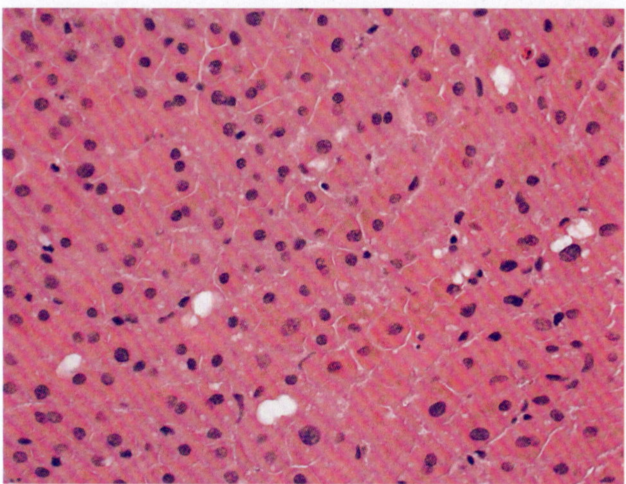

Figure 8.60. **Gilbert syndrome.** The lobules show abundant lipofuschin.

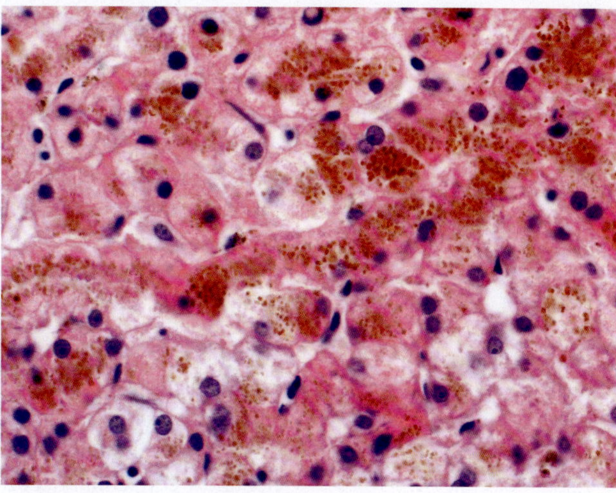

Figure 8.61. **Dubin–Johnson syndrome.** The lobules show dense granular lipofuschin accumulation.

ordinary lipofuscin pigment, but the finding is often not sufficiently distinct from ordinary lipofuscin to distinguish the two. Both tend to have a zone 3 distribution and be heavier in individual hepatocytes immediately around the bile canaliculi. Dubin–Johnson syndrome can rarely present with a neonatal cholestatic pattern.[32]

CYSTIC BILIARY DISEASES AND BILE DUCT MALFORMATIONS

CHECKLIST: Cystic Biliary Diseases and Bile Duct Malformations

- ☐ Congenital hepatic fibrosis
- ☐ Caroli syndrome/disease
- ☐ Autosomal recessive polycystic kidney disease
- ☐ Autosomal dominant polycystic liver disease

CONGENITAL HEPATIC FIBROSIS/AUTOSOMAL RECESSIVE POLYCYSTIC KIDNEY AND LIVER DISEASE

Congenital hepatic fibrosis is an inherited malformation disease of the bile ducts. The kidneys are also involved in most cases, as part of autosomal recessive polycystic kidney disease. Thus, congenital hepatic fibrosis is considered to be the liver manifestation of autosomal recessive polycystic kidney disease in most cases. In rare cases, the changes of congenital hepatic fibrosis are isolated to the liver, with no evidence for renal involvement.

The disease most commonly presents in children and young adults as renal disease. Most cases result from autosomal recessive mutations in the *PKHD1* gene, which encodes the protein fibrocystin, which is important for the normal development of tubules in the kidney and bile ducts in the liver. Different mutations in the *PKHD1* gene tend to correlate with clinical presentation, which have been classified as perinatal (many of whom die shortly after birth), neonatal, infantile, juvenile (age 1 to 5 years mostly), and postjuvenile/adult. Clinical findings are largely that of renal and/or liver disease. A larger number of cases have also been reported with congenital abnormalities in other organs.

Histological examination of the liver shows abnormal bile ducts at the edge of the portal tracts. The bile ducts form an interanastomosing mesh at the periphery, are often mildly dilated, and sometimes can have bile plugs (Fig. 8.62). In very young individuals, the malformed ducts at the periphery of the portal tracts may have a red granular material instead of bile (Fig. 8.63). The typical bile ducts that should be located in the center of the portal tracts are often absent or rare in younger individuals. In some cases there can be a superimposed ascending cholangitis pattern. Portal veins are often atrophic and sometimes, especially with advancing fibrosis, appear to be absent.

The bile duct malformations are present at birth, but fibrosis can take time develop. Fibrosis can progress to cirrhosis, but the rate of progression is highly variable, even within the same family. Well-formed regenerative nodules are not always present in cirrhotic livers, but the diagnosis of cirrhosis can be made when there is extensive bridging that leads to parenchymal nodularity. The nodularity sometimes has a jigsawlike quality at low power.

CAROLI SYNDROME/CAROLI DISEASE

The original definition of Caroli disease was an autosomal recessive disease with macroscopic cysts in the hilum of the liver connected to the biliary tree, with a background liver that did not show congenital hepatic fibrosis. The grossly identified cystic lesions are not true cysts, but instead are fusiform dilatations of the biliary tree. On microscopic examination, they are lined by biliary epithelium and often show significant acute and chronic inflammation with a fibrotic wall. In contrast, the term *Caroli syndrome* was used for cases with similar macroscopic cysts and histological findings, but in the setting of a background liver that showed congenital hepatic fibrosis. Historically, it was felt that Caroli syndrome was an autosomal recessive disease and part of the autosomal recessive polycystic kidney disease spectrum, while Caroli disease resulted from sporadic mutations. However, not all findings fit into these patterns and current evidence suggests both Caroli syndrome, and Caroli disease are part of the autosomal recessive polycystic kidney disease spectrum, at least in most cases.[33]

AUTOSOMAL DOMINANT POLYCYSTIC KIDNEY AND LIVER DISEASE

Autosomal dominant polycystic kidney and liver disease is caused by mutations in *PKD1* or *PKD2*. In addition to cystic renal disease, cystic liver disease is found in about 75% of patients. Other abnormalities are commonly present in other organs, including ovarian cysts, colonic diverticula, and cardiac valve defects. There are rare cases of polycystic liver disease without renal involvement, which result from mutations in other genes, especially *PCLD*. The findings in the liver are essentially the same as with liver disease in *PKD1* or *PKD2* mutations.

The liver is often massively enlarged by numerous macroscopically visible cysts. Liver involvement is usually diffuse, but rarely there can be involvement of just one lobe of the liver, usually the left lobe. The liver cysts range in size from sub centimeter to >10 cm and are unilocular. They are filled with a thin clear or yellow fluid and do not connect to the bile ducts. The cysts are lined by biliary epithelium and have a thin connective tissue wall (Fig. 8.64). The biliary epithelium shows no atypia (Fig. 8.65) but can be reactive when there is cyst hemorrhage or inflammation. Older cysts with hemorrhage can show involution and fibrosis, with loss of the biliary epithelium (Fig. 8.66). When there is a superimposed infection, the cysts become inflamed and the walls fibrotic.

Von Meyenburg complexes are also found in the background liver (Fig. 8.67) and in some cases appear to be precursors to the larger cysts. The Von Meyenburg complexes in polycystic liver disease look the same as sporadic Von Meyenburg complexes—dilated interanastomosing bile duct structures in a fibrous stroma. Also of note, sporadic Von Meyenburg complexes are often multiple, so multifocality in isolation does not indicate the patient has polycystic liver disease. In contrast, a large proportion of portal tracts will be affected in the setting of polycystic kidney and liver disease.

SOLITARY BILE DUCT CYSTS

Solitary bile duct cysts can also develop in the liver. They are lined by typical biliary epithelium with a thin supporting stroma. Most cysts are asymptomatic unless they become large or become superinfected. Rare cases of tumors arising within the cysts have been reported, including neuroendocrine tumors, adenocarcinoma, and squamous cell carcinoma. When treatment is needed they are either resected (especially if imaging findings raise a concern for malignancy arising within the cyst) or treated by fenestration or sclerotherapy.

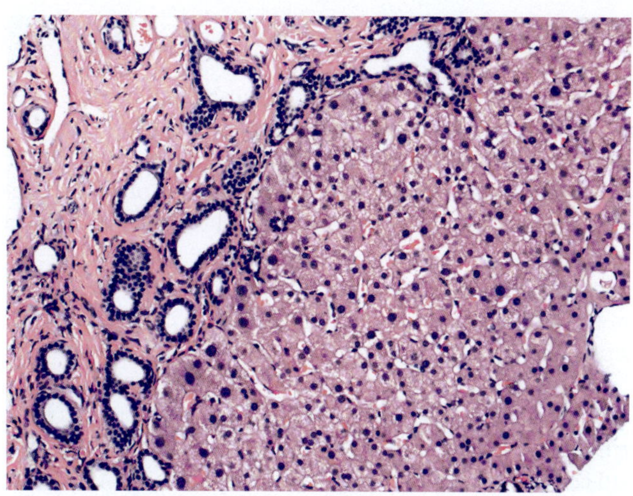

Figure 8.62. **Congenital hepatic fibrosis.** There is a proliferation of mildly dilated ductules at the periphery of this cirrhotic nodule.

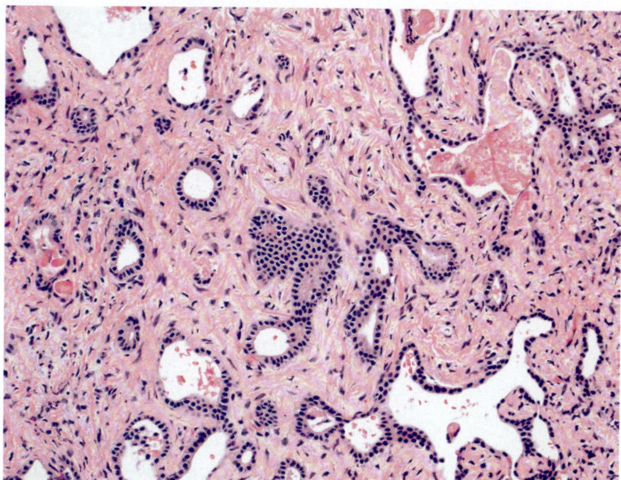

Figure 8.63. **Congenital hepatic fibrosis.** The dilated bile ducts contain red, granular material (upper right of image)

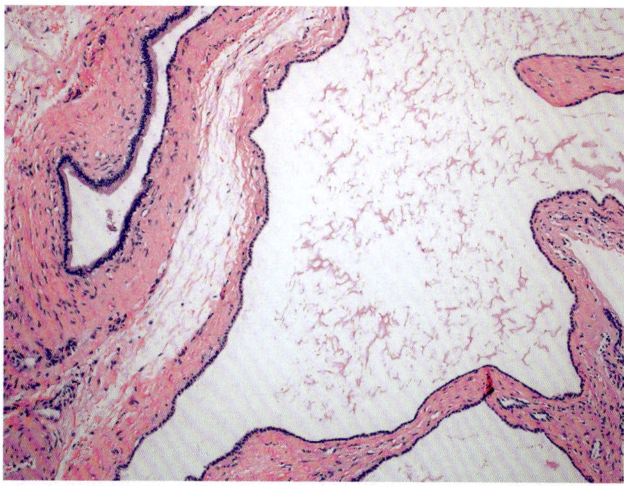

Figure 8.64. **Autosomal dominant polycystic liver disease.** Large dilated biliary cysts are seen.

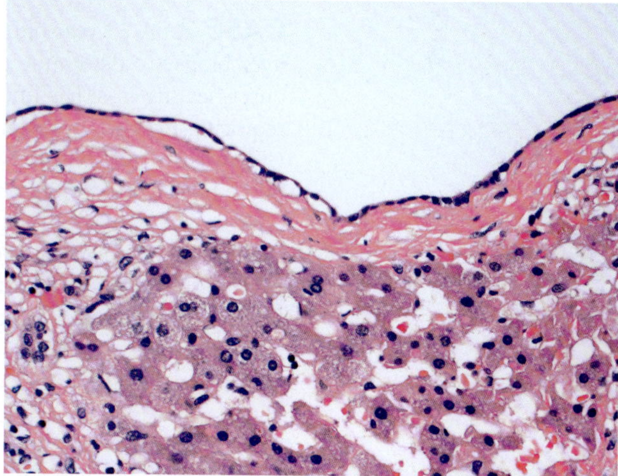

Figure 8.65. **Autosomal dominant polycystic liver disease.** The biliary epithelium is cytologically bland.

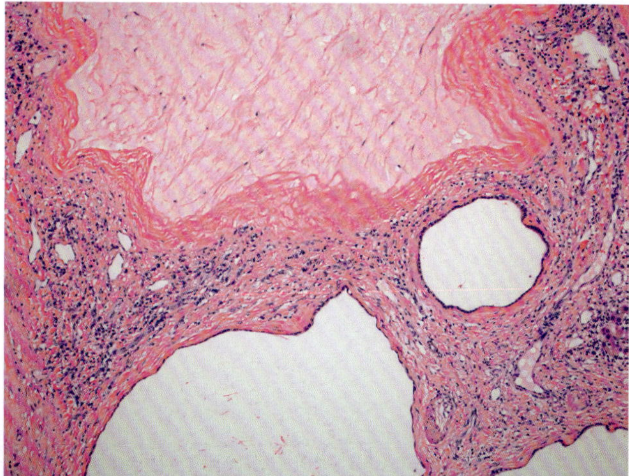

Figure 8.66. **Autosomal dominant polycystic liver disease.** Biliary cysts often become hemorrhagic and can become obliterated/fibrotic (top of image).

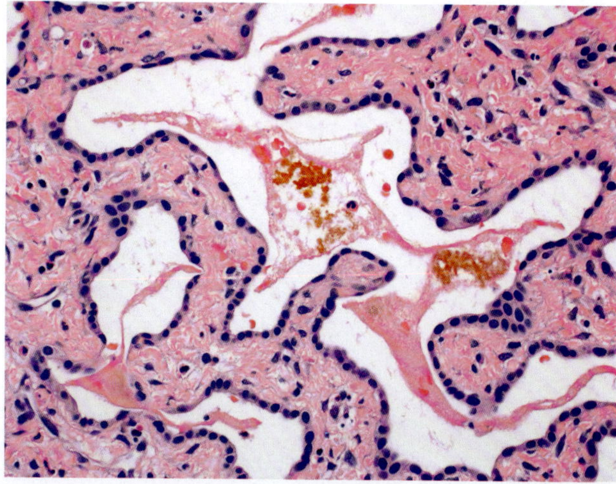

Figure 8.67. **Von Meyenberg complex.** This Von Myenberg complex arose in the setting of autosomal dominant polycystic liver disease. It shows dilated, interanastomosing bile ducts with inspissated bile.

NEAR MISSES

CASE 1. A 65-year-old man was known to have end-stage cirrhosis from chronic hepatitis C. His liver function status was gradually deteriorating, with increasing bilirubin and episodes of hyperammoniaemia. Imaging showed a possible mass, which was targeted for biopsy. The case was signed out as negative for neoplasm but with changes of sepsis (Fig. 8.68). The patient was not septic clinically, so the clinical team asked for the specimen to be sent out in consultation for rereview.

The biopsy was negative for tumor and showed established cirrhosis with cholestatic changes, including bile plugs in the bile ductules. This pattern has been called *cholangitis lenta* and has been linked to sepsis by several studies. However, many patients with this pattern of injury are not septic, such as illustrated by the current case. This pattern can also be seen in livers with long-standing cholestasis from any cause, which seems to the most likely explanation for the current case. Debilitated patients with decompensated liver disease, from any cause that leads to cholestasis, are at increased risk for sepsis and this likely explains why the cholangitis lenta pattern has been linked to sepsis—both can have similar underlying risk factors. Nonetheless, the cholangitis lenta pattern should not be considered to be a sepsis pattern per se. In fact, the most common histological findings with sepsis are nonspecific hepatitis and fatty change, sometimes with lobular cholestasis.

CASE 2. A 23-year-old man with cirrhosis by clinical and imaging findings underwent liver biopsy to determine possible etiologies. The young man also had a history of early onset hearing loss. His uncle had cryptogenic cirrhosis with cholestatic pattern of injury, requiring liver transplantation at young age. Alkaline phosphatase levels were elevated, GGT was low, and bilirubin was 6. Viral and autoimmune serologies were negative. Imaging of the biliary tree and liver vasculature were normal.

The biopsy showed established cirrhosis with no significant inflammation or fatty change. The lobules showed moderate cholestasis (Fig. 8.69). The bile was located in the bile canaliculi. There was no bile duct loss and no fibro-obliterative duct lesions or other findings to suggest chronic obstructive biliary tract disease. PASD and iron stains were negative.

The case was initially dictated as showing nonspecific findings with cirrhosis and cholestasis. However, while thinking about the case and reexamining the slides, the constellation of histological findings (while nonspecific in isolation) plus the history of young age, hearing loss, low GGT levels, and unexplained cholestatic cirrhosis in an Uncle, all came together to suggest testing for bile salt deficiencies. Testing for known mutations was

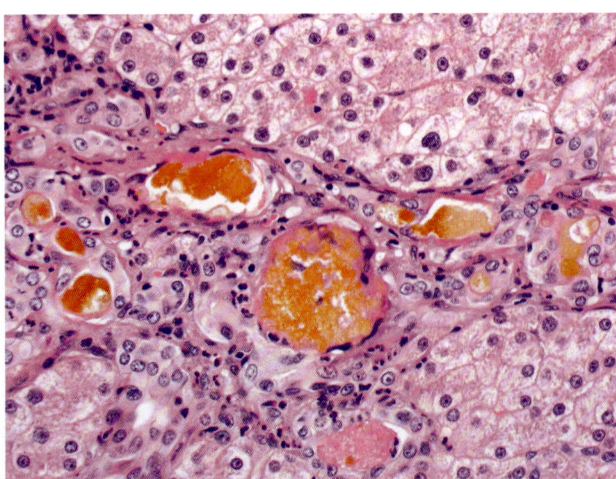

Figure 8.68. **Near miss case 1, cholangiolar cholestasis pattern.** This cholangiolar cholestasis pattern is not specific for sepsis but is commonly seen in persons with debilitating illnesses and prolonged cholestasis.

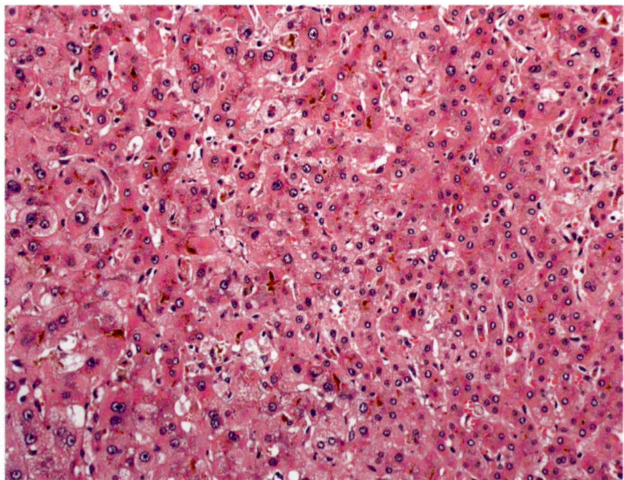

Figure 8.69. **Near miss case 2, bile salt deficiency.** There is lobular cholestasis in a young man with a family history of cholestatic liver disease.

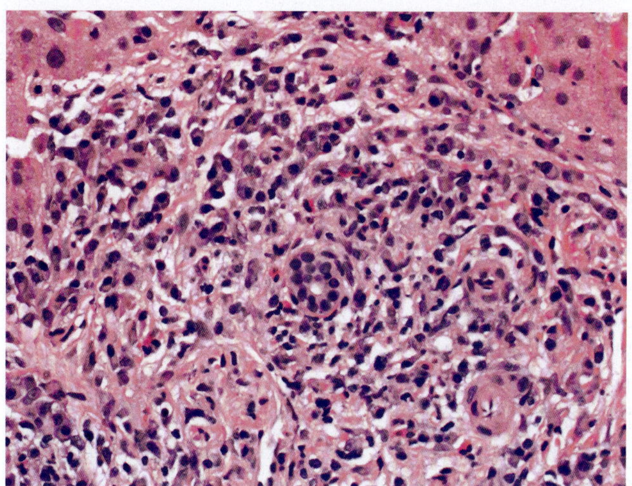

Figure 8.70. Near miss case 3, IgG4 disease. There is plasma cell–rich portal inflammation.

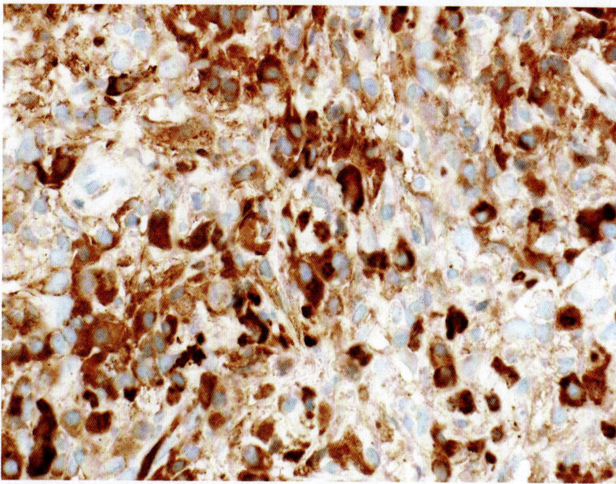

Figure 8.71. Near miss case 3, IgG4 disease. Numerous IgG4-positive plasma cells are present.

negative, but about 1/3 of patients with genetic bile salt deficiencies have an unknown genetic basis, so the findings overall were still considered a probable case of genetic bile salt deficiency.

CASE 3. A 62-year-old man was previously in normal health but presented with jaundice and clinical findings of biliary obstruction. An ultrasound showed a normal gallbladder but possible biliary strictures. The electronic medical record indicated the patient had been taking no medications prior to clinical presentation, including herbal supplements. Imaging of the biliary tree and pancreas were suboptimal due to artifacts, but a biopsy was obtained at the same time.

The biopsy showed moderate portal chronic inflammation that was plasma cell rich (Fig. 8.70). There was mild interface activity, mild bile ductular proliferation, and minimal lobular hepatitis. There was no fibrosis. The plasma cell–rich portal inflammation raised the possibility of autoimmune hepatitis, but serologies were negative and there was only minimal lobular inflammation. The observation that the inflammation was predominately portal based, plus the plasma cell–rich inflammation, also suggested the possibility of primary biliary cirrhosis. AMA testing had not been performed. However, in thinking about the case, there was no real bile duct injury. In addition, patients with primary biliary cirrhosis do not typically present with clinical obstruction. One other idea was then brought to mind—IgG4 disease. Before the stain was back, the patient had been reimaged, showing a pancreas mass and biliary strictures. The IgG4 stain came back next and was strongly positive, consistent with IgG4 disease (Fig. 8.71). Subsequent serological testing showed an elevated level of serum IgG4, and the patient responded well to steroid therapy.

References

1. Kuo FY, Swanson PE, Yeh MM. Pancreatic acinar tissue in liver explants: a morphologic and immunohistochemical study. *Am J Surg Pathol*. 2009;33:66-71.
2. Johnson K, Kotiesh A, Boitnott JK, Torbenson M. Histology of symptomatic acute hepatitis C infection in immunocompetent adults. *Am J Surg Pathol*. 2007;31:1754-1758.
3. Bosch DE, Yeh MM. Primary sclerosing cholangitis is protective against non-alcoholic fatty liver disease in inflammatory bowel disease. *Hum Pathol*. 2017.
4. Harrison RF, Hubscher SG. The spectrum of bile duct lesions in end-stage primary sclerosing cholangitis. *Histopathology*. 1991;19:321-327.
5. Nakanuma Y, Yamaguchi K, Ohta G, Terada T. Pathologic features of hepatolithiasis in Japan. *Hum Pathol*. 1988;19:1181-1186.
6. Nakanuma Y, Kouda W, Harada K, Hiramatsu K. Hepatic sarcoidosis with vanishing bile duct syndrome, cirrhosis, and portal phlebosclerosis. Report of an autopsy case. *J Clin Gastroenterol*. 2001;32:181-184.

7. Zhao L, Hosseini M, Wilcox R, et al. Segmental cholangiectasia clinically worrisome for cholangiocarcinoma: comparison with recurrent pyogenic cholangitis. *Hum Pathol*. 2015;46:426-433.
8. Wendum D, Barbu V, Rosmorduc O, Arrive L, Flejou JF, Poupon R. Aspects of liver pathology in adult patients with MDR3/ABCB4 gene mutations. *Virchows Arch*. 2012;460:291-298.
9. Drebber U, Mueller JJ, Klein E, et al. Liver biopsy in primary biliary cirrhosis: clinicopathological data and stage. *Pathol Int*. 2009;59:546-554.
10. Degott C, Zafrani ES, Callard P, Balkau B, Poupon RE, Poupon R. Histopathological study of primary biliary cirrhosis and the effect of ursodeoxycholic acid treatment on histology progression. *Hepatology*. 1999;29:1007-1012.
11. Vleggaar FP, van Buuren HR, Zondervan PE, ten Kate FJ, Hop WC. Jaundice in non-cirrhotic primary biliary cirrhosis: the premature ductopenic variant. *Gut*. 2001;49:276-281.
12. Colina F, Pinedo F, Solis JA, Moreno D, Nevado M. Nodular regenerative hyperplasia of the liver in early histological stages of primary biliary cirrhosis. *Gastroenterology*. 1992;102:1319-1324.
13. Degiorgio D, Crosignani A, Colombo C, et al. ABCB4 mutations in adult patients with cholestatic liver disease: impact and phenotypic expression. *J Gastroenterol*. 2016;51:271-280.
14. Oliveira HM, Pereira C, Santos Silva E, Pinto-Basto J, Pessegueiro Miranda H. Elevation of gamma-glutamyl transferase in adult: Should we think about progressive familiar intrahepatic cholestasis? *Dig Liver Dis*. 2016;48:203-205.
15. Zen Y, Kawakami H, Kim JH. IgG4-related sclerosing cholangitis: all we need to know. *J Gastroenterol*. 2016;51:295-312.
16. Deshpande V, Sainani NI, Chung RT, et al. IgG4-associated cholangitis: a comparative histological and immunophenotypic study with primary sclerosing cholangitis on liver biopsy material. *Mod Pathol*. 2009;22:1287-1295.
17. Lin J, Cummings OW, Greenson JK, et al. IgG4-related sclerosing cholangitis in the absence of autoimmune pancreatitis mimicking extrahepatic cholangiocarcinoma. *Scand J Gastroenterol*. 2015;50:447-453.
18. Nishino T, Oyama H, Hashimoto E, et al. Clinicopathological differentiation between sclerosing cholangitis with autoimmune pancreatitis and primary sclerosing cholangitis. *J Gastroenterol*. 2007;42:550-559.
19. Zhang L, Lewis JT, Abraham SC, et al. IgG4+ plasma cell infiltrates in liver explants with primary sclerosing cholangitis. *Am J Surg Pathol*. 2010;34:88-94.
20. Chen JH, Deshpande V. IgG4-related disease and the liver. *Gastroenterol Clin North Am*. 2017;46:195-216.
21. Canivet CM, Anty R, Patouraux S, et al. Immunoglobulin G4-associated autoimmune hepatitis may be found in Western countries. *Dig Liver Dis*. 2016;48:302-308.
22. Zen Y, Grammatikopoulos T, Heneghan MA, Vergani D, Mieli-Vergani G, Portmann BC. Sclerosing cholangitis with granulocytic epithelial lesion: a benign form of sclerosing cholangiopathy. *Am J Surg Pathol*. 2012;36:1555-1561.
23. Grammatikopoulos T, Zen Y, Portmann B, et al. Steroid-responsive autoimmune sclerosing cholangitis with liver granulocytic epithelial lesions. *J Pediatr Gastroenterol Nutr*. 2013;56:e3-e4.
24. Naini BV, Lassman CR. Total parenteral nutrition therapy and liver injury: a histopathologic study with clinical correlation. *Hum Pathol*. 2012;43:826-833.
25. Torbenson M, Wang J, Abraham S, Maitra A, Boitnott J. Bile ducts and ductules are positive for CD56 (N-CAM) in most cases of extrahepatic biliary atresia. *Am J Surg Pathol*. 2003;27:1454-1457.
26. Morotti RA, Suchy FJ, Magid MS. Progressive familial intrahepatic cholestasis (PFIC) type 1, 2, and 3: a review of the liver pathology findings. *Semin Liver Dis*. 2011;31:3-10.
27. Davit-Spraul A, Fabre M, Branchereau S, et al. ATP8B1 and ABCB11 analysis in 62 children with normal gamma-glutamyl transferase progressive familial intrahepatic cholestasis (PFIC): phenotypic differences between PFIC1 and PFIC2 and natural history. *Hepatology*. 2010;51:1645-1655.
28. Lykavieris P, van Mil S, Cresteil D, et al. Progressive familial intrahepatic cholestasis type 1 and extrahepatic features: no catch-up of stature growth, exacerbation of diarrhea, and appearance of liver steatosis after liver transplantation. *J Hepatol*. 2003;39:447-452.
29. Miyagawa-Hayashino A, Egawa H, Yorifuji T, et al. Allograft steatohepatitis in progressive familial intrahepatic cholestasis type 1 after living donor liver transplantation. *Liver Transpl*. 2009;15:610-618.

30. Dawson J, Carr-Locke DL, Talbot IC, Rosenthal FD. Gilbert's syndrome: evidence of morphological heterogeneity. *Gut*. 1979;20:848-853.

31. Rastogi A, Krishnani N, Pandey R. Dubin-Johnson syndrome–a clinicopathologic study of twenty cases. *Indian J Pathol Microbiol*. 2006;49:500-504.

32. Regev RH, Stolar O, Raz A, Dolfin T. Treatment of severe cholestasis in neonatal Dubin-Johnson syndrome with ursodeoxycholic acid. *J Perinat Med*. 2002;30:185-187.

33. Gunay-Aygun M. Liver and kidney disease in ciliopathies. *Am J Med Genet C Semin Med Genet*. 2009;151C:296-306.

34. Hindupur S, Yeung M, Shroff P, Fritz J, Kirmani N. Vanishing bile duct syndrome in a patient with advanced AIDS. *HIV Med*. 2007;8:70-72.

35. Aldeen T, Davies S. Vanishing bile duct syndrome in a patient with advanced AIDS. *HIV Med*. 2007; 8: 70-72. 573-574.

36. Chalifoux SL, Konyn PG, Choi G, Saab S. Extrahepatic manifestations of primary biliary cholangitis. *Gut Liver*. 2017;11:771-780.

9 VASCULAR DISEASE

CHAPTER OUTLINE

GENERAL HISTOLOGIAL PATTERNS

CHECKLIST: Broad Patterns in Vascular Disease

- ☐ Portal vein disease, acute
  - ○ Mild: macrovesicular steatosis
  - ○ Severe; ischemic necrosis if there is severe hypotension
- ☐ Portal vein disease, chronic
  - ○ Hepatoportal sclerosis
    - ■ Portal vein atrophy/fibrosis
    - ■ Portal vein herniation
  - ○ Nodular regenerative hyperplasia
- ☐ Hepatic artery disease, acute
  - ○ Mild or intermittent arterial disease: mild nonspecific changes with increased hepatic apoptosis and mitosis
  - ○ Severe arterial disease: ischemic necrosis, usually occurs with reduced portal vein blood flow
- ☐ Hepatic artery disease, chronic
  - ○ Bile ductular proliferation as a result of ischemic biliary strictures
  - ○ Ductopenia due to chronic biliary ischemia
- ☐ Sinusoidal obstructive disease
  - ○ Sinusoidal congestion, dilatation
  - ○ Occlusion of terminal central veins (not always present)
  - ○ Perivenular/pericellular fibrosis with long-standing disease
- ☐ Vascular outflow disease
  - ○ Sinusoidal congestion, dilatation
  - ○ Occlusion/thrombosis of larger central veins
  - ○ Reactive bile ductular proliferation in portal tracts, usually mild
  - ○ Perivenular/pericellular fibrosis with long-standing disease
- ☐ Peliosis hepatitis
- ☐ Various pseudotumors and tumors

In most clinical cases where hepatic disease is caused by vascular flow changes, the diagnosis is made by clinical and imaging findings, so the vascular patterns of injury are relatively uncommon in biopsy specimens. The most common clinical scenarios where vascular diseases are encountered in medical liver biopsies are (1) biopsies to rule out veno-occlusive disease (also known as sinusoidal obstructive syndrome) after chemotherapy, (2) biopsies to investigate unexplained portal hypertension, which can show changes of hepatoportal sclerosis, and (3) biopsies to determine fibrosis stage in individuals with known congestive hepatopathy from cardiac disease.

PATTERNS OF INJURY WITH PORTAL VEIN DISEASE

CHECKLIST: Portal Vein Disease

- ☐ Portal vein disease, acute
  - ○ Macrovesicular steatosis
  - ○ Ischemic necrosis if there is severe hypotension

- ☐ Portal vein disease, chronic
  - ○ Hepatoportal sclerosis
    - ■ Portal vein atrophy/fibrosis
    - ■ Muscular hypertrophy of portal vein wall
    - ■ Portal vein herniation
  - ○ Nodular regenerative hyperplasia

ACUTE PORTAL VEIN DISEASE

The patterns of injury with portal vein disease depend on the severity of the reduction in portal vein flow and on the duration of reduced blood flow. Severe acute hypotension can lead to ischemic necrosis. The necrosis can have a zone 3 pattern or a panacinar pattern in more severe cases. Acute but less severe portal vein thrombosis can present with macrovesicular steatosis and increased lobular apoptosis.[1]

CHRONIC PORTAL VEIN DISEASE

CHECKLIST: Causes of Noncirrhotic Portal Hypertension

- ☐ Prehepatic
  - ○ Portal vein thrombosis
  - ○ Portal vein strictures
- ☐ Hepatic
  - ○ Schistosomiasis
  - ○ Sarcoidosis
  - ○ Nodular regenerative hyperplasia
  - ○ Idiopathic portal hypertension (shows a hepatoportosclerosis pattern of injury)
  - ○ Peliosis hepatis
  - ○ Veno-occlusive disease
- ☐ Hepatic vein thrombosis
- ☐ Idiopathic

Thrombosis of the extrahepatic portal vein can lead to portal hypertension, splenomegaly, and ascites, an important cause of *noncirrhotic portal hypertension*. In a large autopsy-based study, the prevalence in the general population was found to be 1%,[2] but the frequency is much higher in certain patient populations, such as those with cirrhosis or hepatobiliary malignancy. There are many known causes of extrahepatic portal vein thrombosis, but approximately 15% of cases remain idiopathic.[2] Inherited prothrombotic disorders are important predisposing conditions, including factor V Leiden mutations. The most common noninherited risk factors identified are the following, with patients often having more than one of these risk factors: cirrhosis (30%), hypercoagulable conditions such as pregnancy or use of oral contraceptives (30%), primary and metastatic liver malignancies (25%), structural abnormalities from prior surgery or perinatal injury of the umbilical vein, usually from canalization (25%), myeloproliferative disorders (15%), or intraabdominal inflammatory diseases that directly involve the portal vein (e.g., pancreatitis, diverticulitis, etc.) (15%).[3] There are increasingly compelling data that fatty liver disease may also be an independent risk factor for portal vein thrombosis.[4]

The most common pattern of injury associated with chronic portal vein disease is called *hepatoportal sclerosis*. With this pattern of injury, the portal veins can show varying degrees of abnormalities including portal vein herniation (Fig. 9.1), portal vein atrophy (Fig. 9.2), muscularization of the portal vein wall (Fig. 9.3), portal vein loss, and portal vein fibrosis. In some cases where the small branches of the portal veins are obliterated, the larger portal veins can be dilated (Fig. 9.4). These abnormalities are often very subtle and can be easily overlooked.

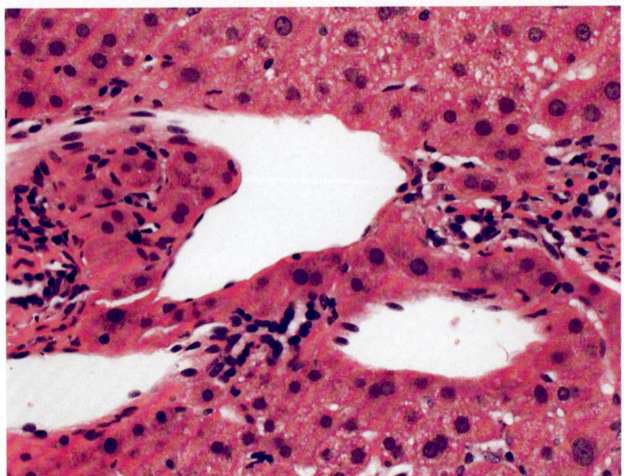

Figure 9.1. **Hepatoportal sclerosis, portal vein herniation.** The portal vein appears to herniate out into the lobule. In normal portal tracts, the portal vein is entirely enveloped by the fibrous tissue in the portal tract.

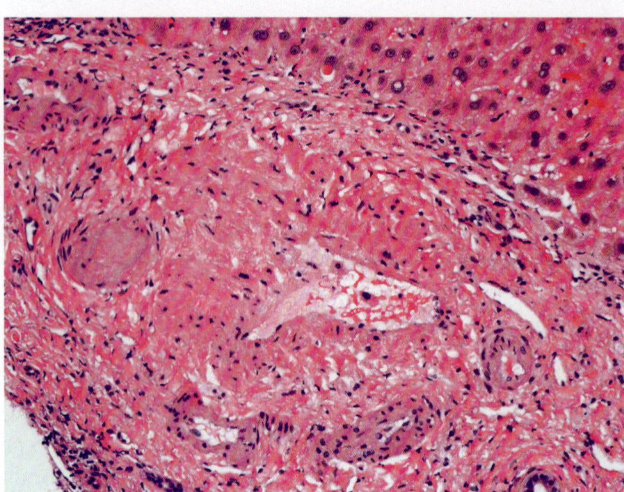

Figure 9.2. **Hepatoportal sclerosis, portal vein atrophy.** The portal vein is smaller (atrophic) than it should be in comparison to the overall size of the portal tract. It also shows thickening of the muscular wall.

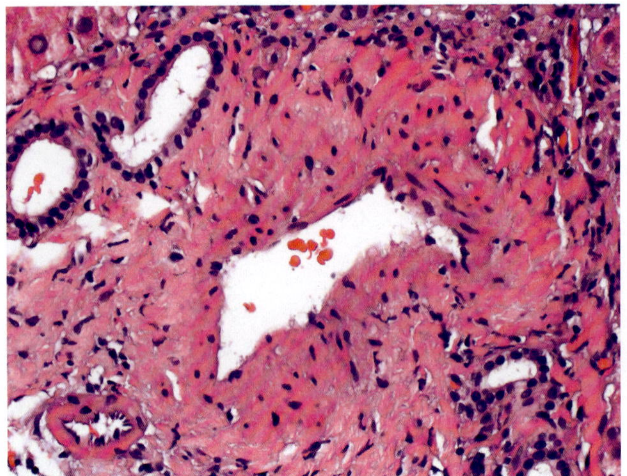

Figure 9.3. **Hepatoportal sclerosis, portal vein wall muscularization.** This small portal vein has developed a thick muscular coat. Portal veins in the largest portal tracts will normally have a muscular coat, but not the medium-sized and smaller portal veins. This finding can also be seen in some cirrhotic livers.

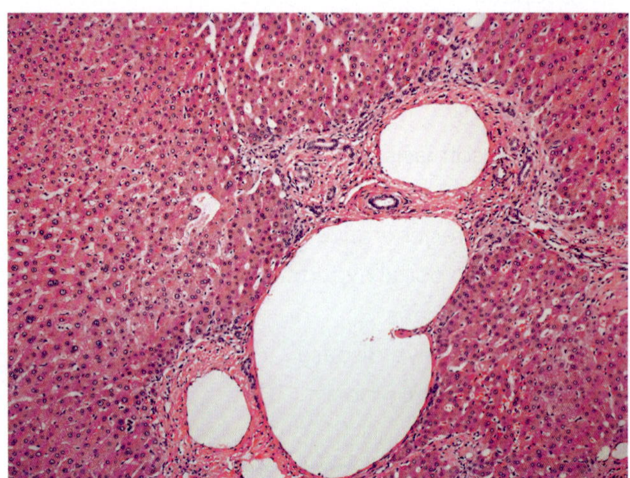

Figure 9.4. **Hepatoportal sclerosis, portal vein dilatation.** In this case, the medium-sized portal veins were markedly dilated because the smaller branches were obliterated.

On the other hand, because the findings are so subtle, they can be nonspecific and easily overcalled, so it is helpful to see relevant changes in multiple portal tracts to ensure that they are a reproducible finding. The different components of the hepatoportal sclerosis pattern can coexist, but overall portal vein herniation seems to be an earlier lesion. In some cases, the biopsy can show remotely thrombosed and recannulated veins, often with striking muscularization of the vein wall (Fig. 9.5). In general, the medium-sized portal veins are the best place to identify muscular hypertrophy, while the small branches of the portal veins are the first to show atrophy/loss.

In addition to portal vein changes, chronic portal vein disease can lead to nodular regenerative hyperplasia, with parenchymal nodularity caused by nodules of ordinary-sized hepatocytes surrounded by thinner, more atrophic hepatocytes. A reticulin stain will highlight the changes in plate thickness. There should be no more than mild portal fibrosis for a diagnosis of nodular regenerative hyperplasia. This pattern of nodular regenerative hyperplasia is not specific for vascular disease but can help support the diagnosis when present. It can be seen with or without other findings of hepatoportal sclerosis.

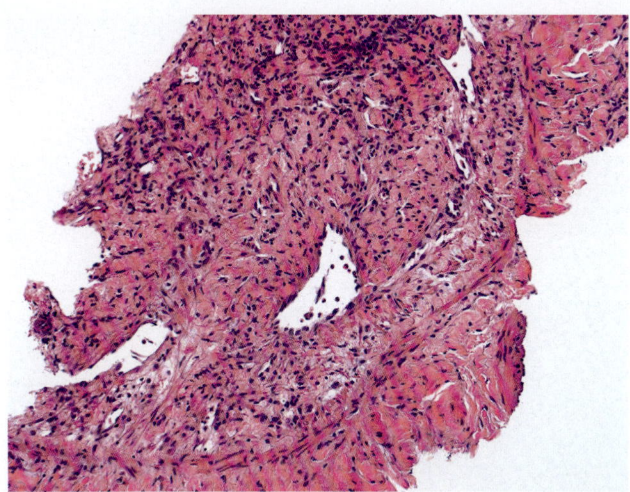

Figure 9.5. **Thrombus portal vein.** This needle biopsy showed a portal vein with a remote thrombosis. Finding a portal vein thrombus on biopsies is rare because of sampling, even with portal vein thrombotic disease.

Finally, portal vein thrombi can lead to strictures of the extrahepatic bile ducts, a finding called portal biliopathy.[5] Portal biliopathy results when collaterals that develop to go around the thrombosed portal vein compress the extrahepatic bile ducts, leading to biliary obstruction.

PATTERNS OF INJURY WITH HEPATIC ARTERY DISEASE

Hepatic artery disease is less common than portal vein disease, but also can result from thrombi or vasculitis. In the setting of liver transplantation, anastomotic strictures can also develop, with varying degrees of vascular flow impairment. In the native liver (nontransplanted liver), the portal vein carries sufficient blood flow that it can compensate for loss of the extrahepatic arterial blood supply in most cases.

Arterial thrombosis of the intrahepatic arteries can lead to focal, well-defined hepatic infarcts, usually with a subcapsular location, although such lesions can also be caused by intrahepatic portal vein thrombosis. Causes of arterial thrombosis include atherosclerosis or other causes of emboli, thrombosis resulting from a hypercoagulable state, or iatrogenic injury of the hepatic artery (usually the right hepatic artery after laparoscopic cholecystectomy).

In the allograft liver, hepatic artery thrombosis leads to an early pattern of injury characterized by increases in both hepatocyte apoptosis and hepatocyte mitosis.[6,7] There is typically little or no inflammation and no other major findings. If the arterial blood flow is severe and the portal vein blood flow is insufficient to compensate, then patchy areas of lobular and panacinar necrosis can develop (Fig. 9.6). Because the bile ducts obtain most of their blood supply from the hepatic arteries, in severe cases, the lack of adequate hepatic artery blood flow will lead to chronic biliary tract disease, with bile duct strictures and loss.

In the nontransplant setting, arteritis is almost always part of a systemic vasculitis, such as polyarteritis nodosa. The arteries will show varying degrees of mixed inflammation with lymphocytes, plasma cells, and neutrophils (Fig. 9.7). The arteries can also show fibrinoid necrosis (Fig. 9.8). This pattern of fibrinoid necrosis should not be mistaken for arterial hyalinization, which is associated with systemic hypertension and diabetes mellitus (Fig. 9.9).

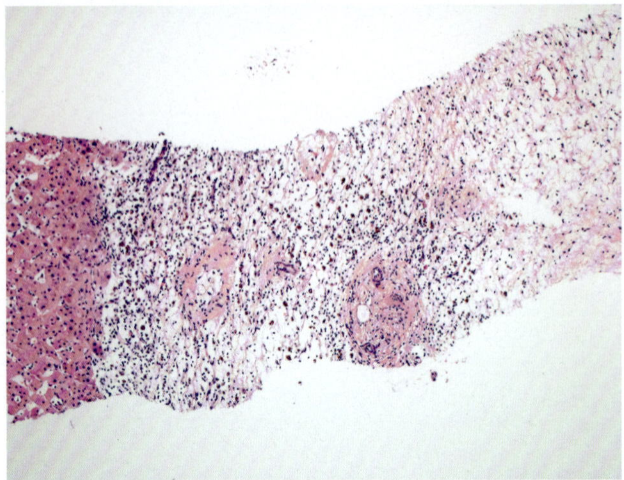

Figure 9.6. Hepatic artery disease, malignant hypertension. Ischemia from malignant hypertension led to patchy areas of well-delineated hepatocyte dropout. Residual portal tracts and central veins are evident within the area of hepatocyte loss.

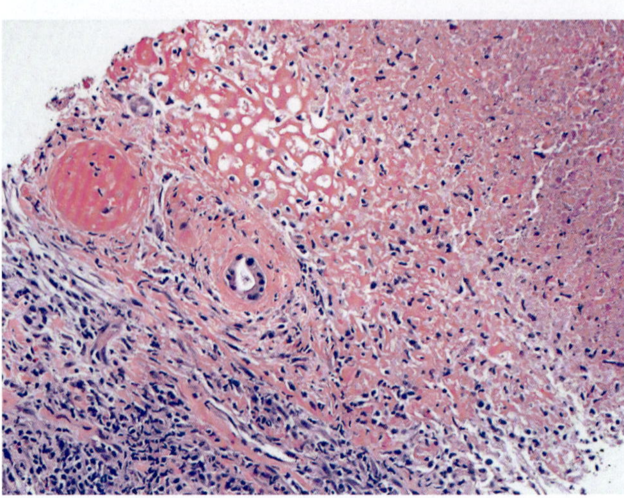

Figure 9.7. Polyarteritis nodosa. The portal tract shows fibrinoid necrosis of the hepatic artery adjacent to a focus of parenchymal necrosis (upper right corner of image).

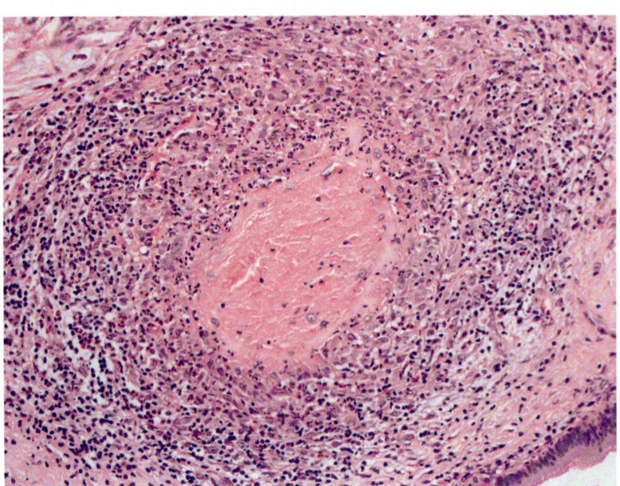

Figure 9.8. Polyarteritis nodosa. The necrotic artery is surrounded by mixed inflammation.

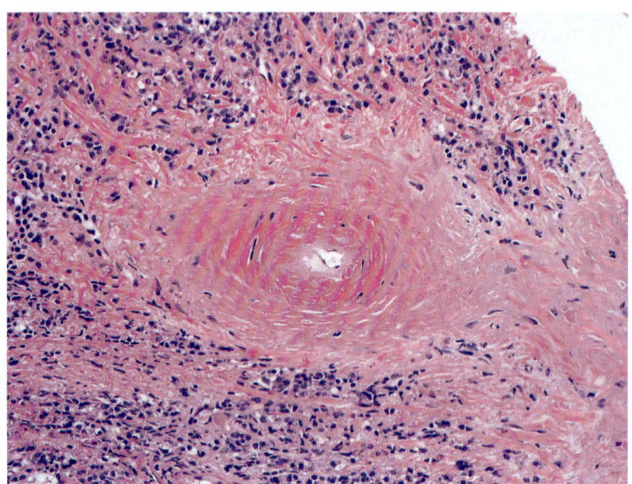

Figure 9.9. Arterial hyalinization. The artery shows striking hyalinization in the setting of hypertension and diabetes mellitus. This finding should not be mistaken for fibrinoid necrosis.

SINUSOIDALINUSOIDAL DISEASE

VENO-OCCLUSIVE DISEASE

CHECKLIST: Causes of Veno-Occlusive Disease/Sinusoidal Obstructive Syndrome

- ☐ Cancer chemotherapy
  - ○ Oxaliplatin is one example
- ☐ Radiation therapy
- ☐ Bone marrow transplant
- ☐ Herbal teas/remedies

Sinusoidal occlusion results from anything that impedes blood flow through the sinusoids, including vascular and nonvascular causes. The most common nonvascular cause is sinusoidal fibrosis, but less common causes include amyloid, hepatocyte swelling from glycogen accumulation in the setting of glycogenic hepatopathy,[8] and tumor infiltration.

The most common vascular cause is veno-occlusive disease, which also called *sinusoidal obstructive syndrome*.

The process of renaming an established disease is usually driven by disease name activists who feel strongly about correcting important historical wrongs to save people from confusion. To do so, old diseases are given new names. Thus, the term *veno-occlusive disease* was deemed unworthy and renamed *sinusoidal obstruction syndrome*. It is the same disease, just a new name. Which term should you use? It is really up to you. Both terms will be used intermittently in this section, to try to keep everyone happy.

Veno-occlusive disease is caused by endothelial injury and typically affects the endothelial cells lining the sinusoids and the terminal central veins. The most common injuries are toxins such as chemotherapy, radiation therapy, or inflammatory injury, commonly from drugs or herbal remedies. It is hard to confidently and directly see the injured endothelial cells on H&E, so the diagnosis is made by observing the secondary changes. These secondary changes include varying combinations of these four findings: (1) sinusoidal dilatation, usually mild and patchy (Fig. 9.10); (2) central vein occlusion by fibrin thrombi and or fibrosis; (3) pericellular and or zone 3 fibrosis (Fig. 9.11); and (4) nodular regenerative hyperplasia (Fig. 9.12). Not all of these features will be present in any given biopsy, but typically at least two of the four will be found.

The sinusoidal dilatation is usually mild but can be moderate and often shows a clear zone 3 pattern. The changes are not as dramatic as seen in most cases of vascular outflow disease affecting the major veins, such as Budd–Chiari or congestive hepatopathy from cardiac disease. Of course, equivocal mild patchy sinusoidal dilatation is fairly common in many different biopsies (Fig. 9.13), even those biopsies that are essentially normal, so the changes should be clearly above baseline to be diagnostically useful.

The central veins can show occlusion/fibrosis in about 2/3 of cases. Earlier lesions can show rare fibrin thrombi, while later lesions tend to show fibrotic occlusions. Cases of the veno-occlusive disease resulting from drug reactions or herbal remedies often have mild lymphocytic inflammation around the injured central vein (Fig. 9.14). In time, perivenular and zone 3 perisinusodal fibrosis can develop.

The zone 3 hepatocytes can also show atrophy, and this can sometimes lead to a nodular regenerative hyperplasia pattern of injury. For the diagnosis of nodular regenerative hyperplasia, there should be a reasonably evident nodularity on low-power H&E examination and not simply some mild atrophy of hepatocytes in zone 3 or focal mild changes on reticulin. A reticulin stain is helpful for confirming the parenchymal nodularity but should not be over interpreted. Other than these changes, the lobules generally show only mild nonspecific findings, with little or no inflammation and occasionally a few acidophil bodies. Lobular cholestasis is usually absent or mild.

The portal tracts show mild nonspecific changes, typically with mild chronic inflammation and occasionally with a very mild and focal ductular reaction.

PEARLS & PITFALLS

- Milder changes of sinusoidal obstructive syndrome tend to merge imperceptibly with nonspecific reactive changes, so it is important to make sure that changes you see are clearly above background. If at least two of the key histological findings are present and if there is a compatible history, then the diagnosis is confidently rendered. If only one of the key histological findings are present, then terms such as *suggestive of sinusoidal obstructive syndrome* can be helpful.
    - Key histological findings: Sinusoidal dilatation/congestion that is above background changes; nodular regenerative hyperplasia; occlusion of terminal branches of the central veins; and pericellular/perivenular fibrosis (seen only in long-standing cases).
- Wedge biopsies of the liver often show artifactual sinusoidal dilatation that results from the use of cautery. Most cases such show no zonal pattern to the dilatation, but a zone 3 pattern can be seen. The changes tend to be present at a uniform distance from the edge of the biopsy and extend around the entire biopsy. Moreover, the red blood cells in the dilated sinusoids are typically destroyed by the cautery leaving behind an amorphous gray material.

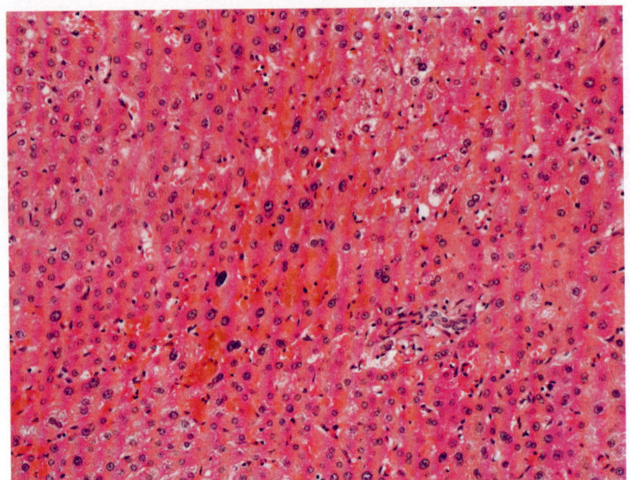

Figure 9.10. **Veno-occlusive disease/sinusoidal obstruction syndrome, sinusoidal dilatation.** There is mild zone 3 sinusoidal congestion in this case of chemotherapy-associated sinusoidal obstruction syndrome.

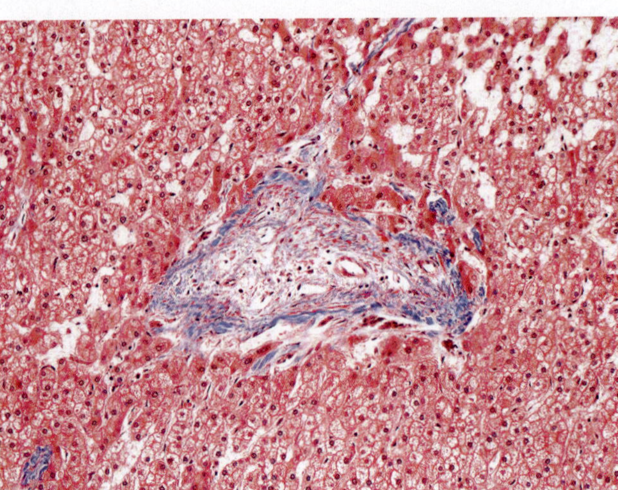

Figure 9.11. **Veno-occlusive disease/sinusoidal obstruction syndrome, zone 3 fibrosis.** There is early fibrous occlusion of the central vein.

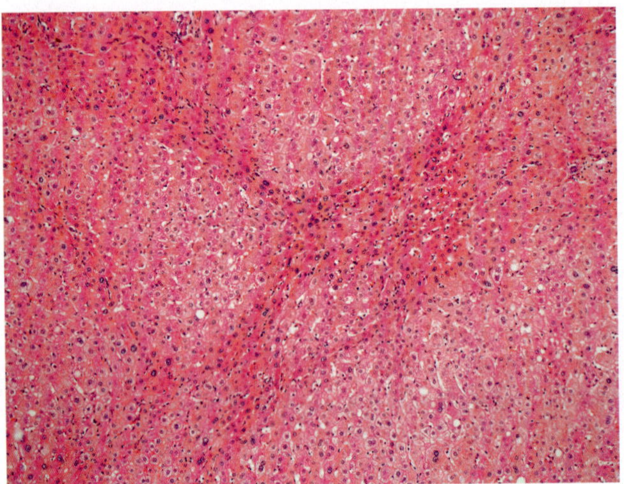

Figure 9.12. **Veno-occlusive disease/sinusoidal obstruction syndrome, nodular regenerative hyperplasia.** The liver parenchyma shows a distinct nodularity at low power, despite the lack of fibrosis. This case was caused by chemotherapy and was associated with other findings of the sinusoidal obstruction syndrome.

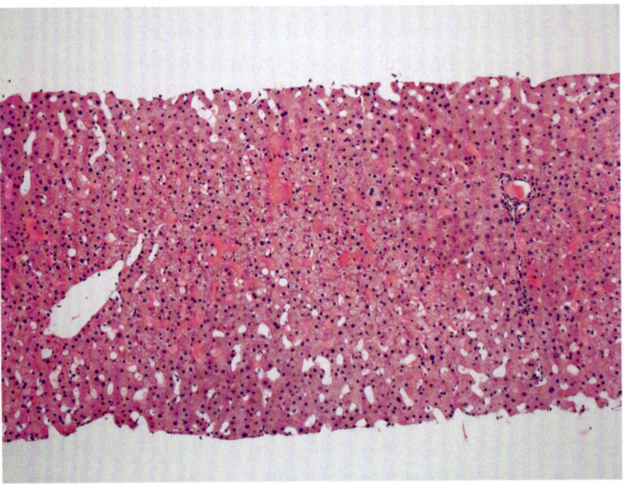

Figure 9.13. **Nonspecific sinusoidal dilatation.** There is mild nonspecific sinusoidal dilatation in this case, but overall this degree of sinusoidal changes is within normal limits.

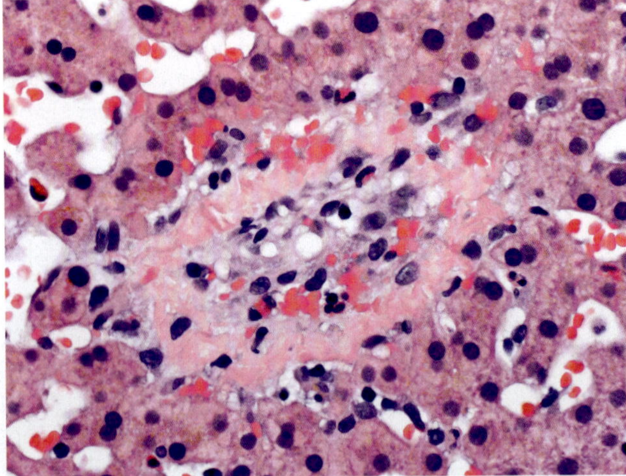

Figure 9.14. **Veno-occlusive disease.** This case of veno-occlusive disease resulted from a herbal remedy.

SICKLE CELL DISEASE

Sickle cell trait results from heterozygosity for hemoglobin S (normal allele is hemoglobin A). Sickle cell trait is usually clinically asymptomatic, but rare exertion-related deaths are well documented.[9] The histological findings in asymptomatic sickle cell trait are that of sickled red cells in the liver sinusoids. The findings can be subtle, but when sickled cells are specifically looked for, they can be reproducibly identified with high sensitivity and specificity.[10]

Sickle cell disease (homozygous SS disease) can manifest with significant liver disease but is only rarely biopsied and then mostly to obtain liver tissue for quantitative iron analysis. Because patients with sickle cell disease also have an increased risk for cholelithiasis, biopsies are also common at the time of cholecystectomy. In most cases, liver biopsies show congested and dilated sinusoids (Fig. 9.15) along with pericellular fibrosis.[11,12] Sickled red blood cells as well erythrophagocytosis can be found in most cases (Fig. 9.16).[13,14] There can be ischemic zone 3 necrosis in cases of sickle cell crises.

Biopsies also show Kupffer cell and hepatocellular iron accumulation that range from mild to marked. Fibrosis can develop, with about 10% to 20% of individuals progressing to cirrhosis.[15,16] Finally, other findings may be present reflecting concomitant disease processes, such as a biliary obstruction patterns owing to biliary stones or chronic hepatitis in cases with chronic hepatitis C or B.[12,13,17]

Biopsy specimens are not obtained during sickle cell crises, but in addition to the findings described above, the liver can show a range of findings from bland cholestasis to an ischemic pattern of necrosis. Acute hepatic sequestration results from sequestration of sickled red blood cells in dilated and congested hepatic sinusoids and is accompanied by a marked drop in the hematocrit.

VASCULAR OUTFLOW DISEASE

CHECKLIST: Causes of Vascular Outflow Disease

- □ Budd–Chiari with thrombosis of hepatic veins or vena cava
  - ○ Causes include inherited thrombotic disorders, polythemia vera, oral contraception, recent pregnancy, systemic inflammatory disorders such as inflammatory bowel disease, or sarcoidosis
- □ Right-sided heart disease
- □ Compression of hepatic veins or vena cava from adjacent mass lesions

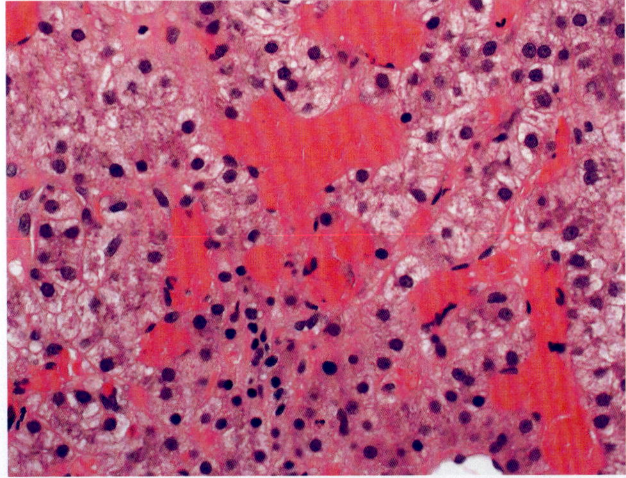

Figure 9.15. **Sickle cell disease.** The biopsy shows congested and dilated sinusoids.

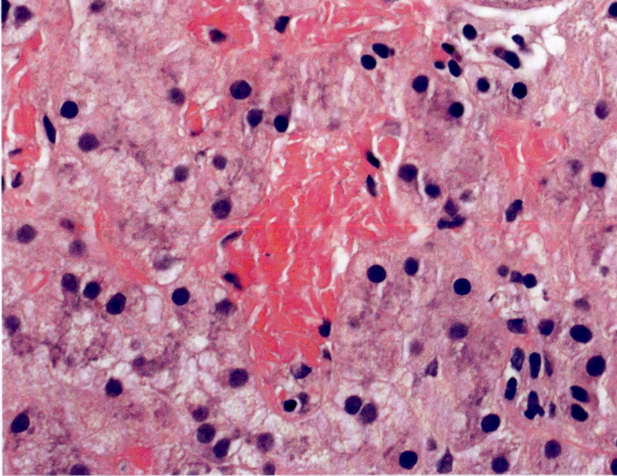

Figure 9.16. **Sickle cell disease.** Sickled red blood cells as well erythrophagocytosis are seen.

Other Causes of Sinusoidal Dilation and Congestion Unrelated to Hepatic Vein Disease

- Drug effects such as estrogen, androgen, and azathioprine
- Veno-occlusive disease
- Sickle cell anemia
- Hemophagocytosis syndrome
- Autoimmune diseases
  - Many different ones, such as rheumatoid arthritis, Castleman disease, sarcoidosis
- Paraneoplastic syndromes
  - Renal cell carcinoma
  - Hodgkin lymphoma
- Systemic infections
  - Examples include tuberculosis, human immunodeficiency virus (HIV) infection, and brucellosis
  - Not always clear if it is a result of infection, comorbid conditions, or a drug effect

Vascular outflow disease can result from multiple different causes, but the histological findings all look about the same. The disease pattern is centered on the zone 3 region of the lobules and shows variable sinusoidal dilation, congestion, hepatocyte atrophy, and/or hepatocyte dropout (Figs. 9.17–9.19). In rare cases, the zone 3 hepatocytes can also develop round cytoplasmic inclusions (Fig. 9.20). With acute obstruction, it is often stated that extravasated red blood cells are prominent in the space of Disse, which can be true it seems, but confidently identify this finding requires an eye of faith in most cases.

In many cases, the portal tracts can also show a mild bile ductular proliferation, which can mimic biliary obstruction.[18] The diagnosis of vascular outflow disease is H&E based, but CK7 will highlight intermediate hepatocytes in the zone 3 region and can be helpful when findings are subtle (Figs. 9.21 and 9.22).[19] With long-standing disease, there can be fibrosis of the central veins and pericellular fibrosis in the zone 3 hepatocytes (Fig. 9.23). With advanced fibrosis or cirrhosis, the sinusoidal dilation can become less pronounced and in some cases not evident at all. There still will be significant zone 3 fibrosis.

Some of the changes seen in vascular outflow disease are also present in veno-occlusive disease, in particular the sinusoidal dilatation and congestion. However, in vascular outflow disease, the sinusoidal dilatation and congestion tends to be much more prominent. Zone 3 fibrosis is also more prominent in cases of vascular outflow disease. In addition, the clinical history and imaging findings will help sort out the proper diagnosis (e.g., history of chemotherapy, heart disease, hepatic vein thrombosis, etc.).

There is a spectrum of histological changes in vascular outflow disease, depending on the disease's severity and duration. When the pattern of vascular outflow disease is well developed, the diagnosis is straightforward. However, in many cases, the findings can be considerably more subtle. Sinusoidal dilation and congestion is the most sensitive histological findings, but when mild is also very nonspecific (Fig. 9.24). The specificity improves when there is at least moderate sinusoidal dilation, but not all cases will show this degree of sinusoidal dilation, even with legitimate cases of outflow disease. Thus, other findings, such as zone 3 fibrosis or atrophy of zone 3 hepatocytes, can help distinguish real outflow disease from nonspecific changes. Trichrome and reticulin stains can help confirm these changes.

Fibrosis staging can be performed with a staging system specifically designed for vascular outflow disease.[20] In this system, stage 1 is any central vein fibrosis. Stage 2 is defined as portal fibrosis plus zone 3 fibrosis and is further subdivided into 2A, where the central vein fibrosis is more prominent, and stage 2B, where there is at least moderate portal fibrosis and the portal fibrosis is more prominent than the zone 3 fibrosis. Stage 3 fibrosis is defined as bridging fibrosis. Stage 4 is cirrhosis.

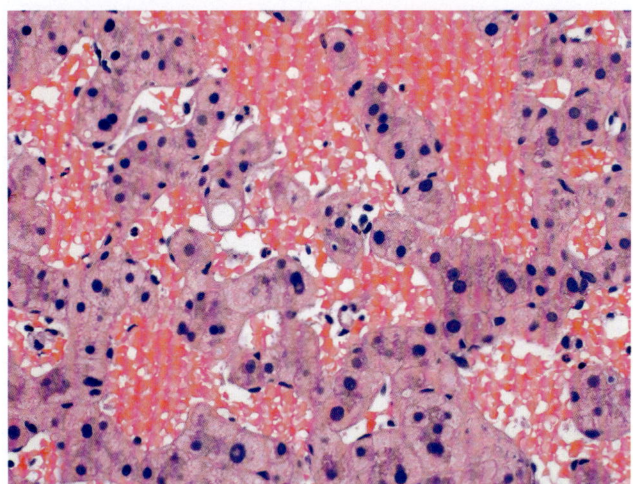

Figure 9.17. **Vascular outflow disease, zone 3 congestion.** This case of congestive heart failure shows marked diffuse sinusoidal dilatation.

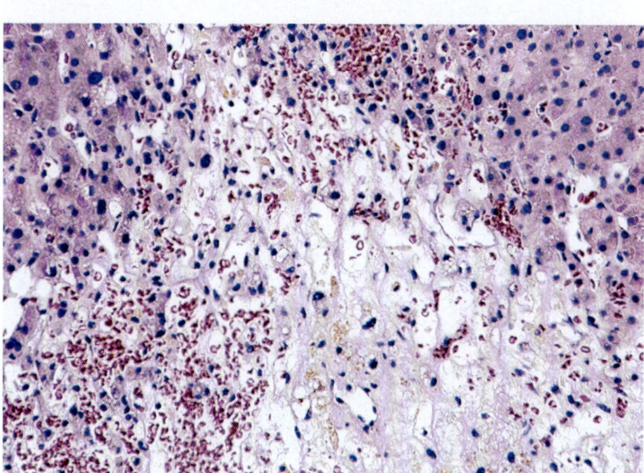

Figure 9.18. **Vascular outflow disease, zone 3 hepatocyte dropout.** In this case of Budd–Chiari syndrome, the zone 3 hepatocytes show significant dropout, leaving behind loose, edematous, and often hemorrhagic connective tissue.

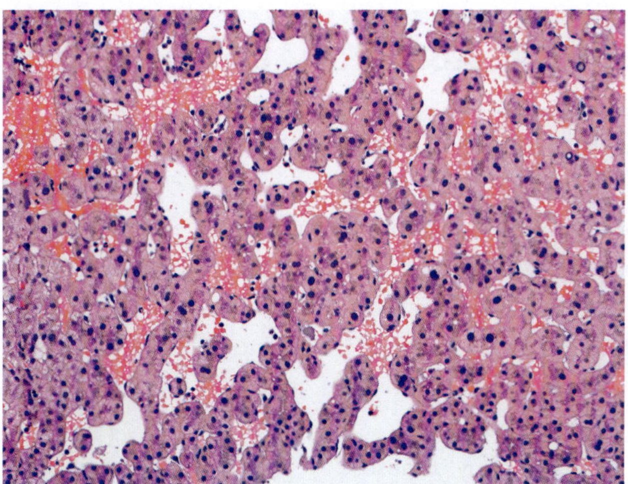

Figure 9.19. **Vascular outflow disease.** The lobules show moderate to marked sinusoidal dilatation and congestion with hepatocyte atrophy.

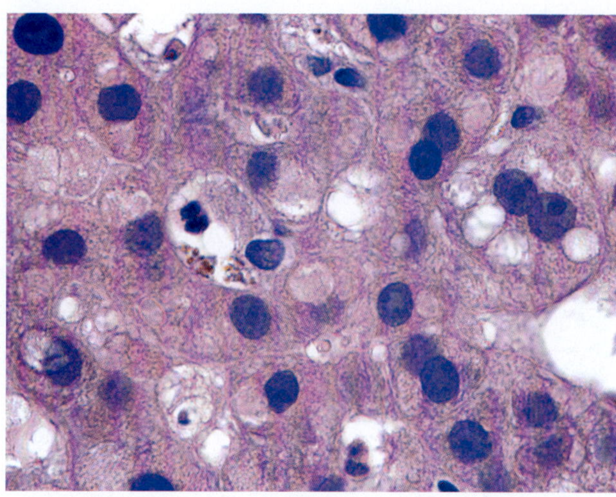

Figure 9.20. **Hepatocyte inclusions in vascular outflow disease.** This is an uncommon finding, but the zone 3 hepatocytes can sometimes develop round cytoplasmic inclusions.

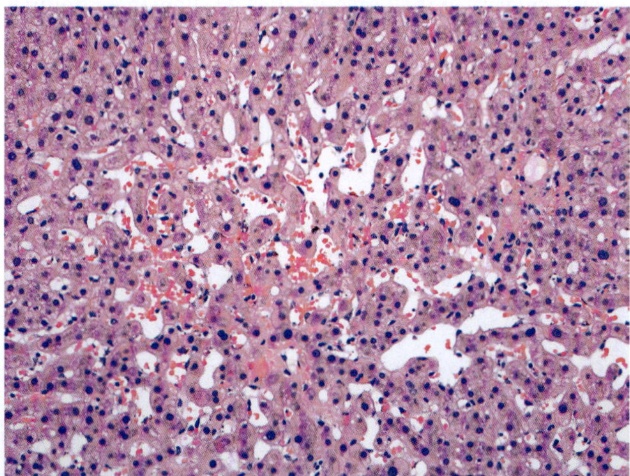

Figure 9.21. **Vascular outflow disease.** The lobules show mild sinusoidal dilatation.

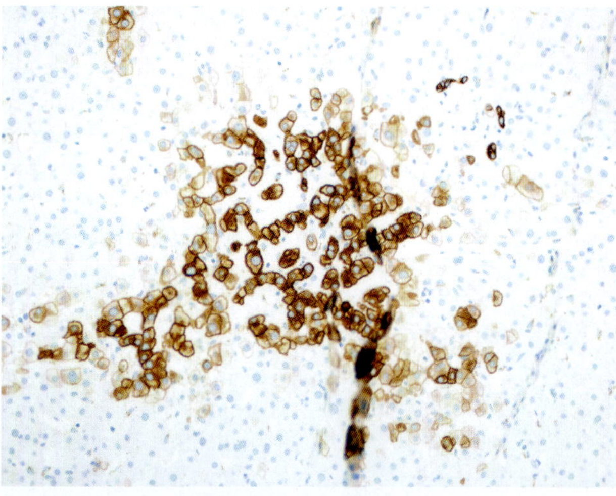

Figure 9.22. **Vascular outflow disease, CK7 immunostain.** A CK7 immunostain highlights the zone 3 hepatocytes. Same case and field as Figure 9.21.

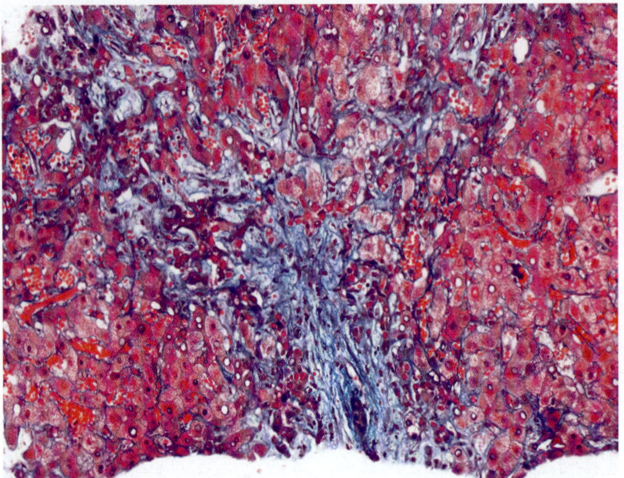

Figure 9.23. **Vascular outflow disease, trichrome.** There is pericellular fibrosis in zone 3, as well fibrosis of the central vein itself.

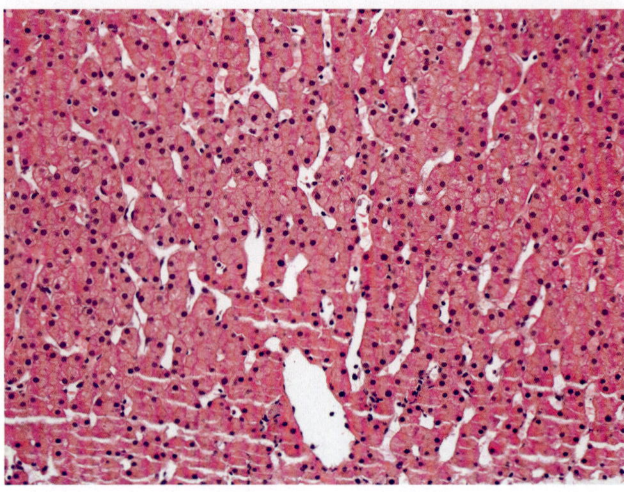

Figure 9.24. **Nonspecific sinusoidal dilatation.** There is some sinusoidal dilation in this image, but it is within normal limits. There was no evidence for vascular outflow disease of any sort in this case.

CONGENITAL/GENETIC ABNORMALITIES

CHECKLIST: Congenital/Genetic abnormalities in Hepatic Blood Flow

- ☐ Portal vein disease
  - ○ Abernethy syndrome with congenitally absent portal vein
  - ○ VATER syndrome with absent or atrophic portal veins
  - ○ Turner syndrome with atrophic or absent portal veins
    - ■ Steatosis or steatohepatitis is also a common finding
- ☐ Telangiectasia
  - ○ Hereditary hemorrhagic telangiectasia
- ☐ Hereditary lymphedema such as Milroy disease

There are many congenital or genetic abnormalities that are associated with abnormal liver vascular changes, mostly with atrophy or absence of the portal veins. The genetic conditions that lead to portal vein atrophy or absence all share the same pattern of injury. Although the individual components will vary in their severity, they all show these findings to varying degrees: absent or atrophic portal veins, abnormal arterialization of the portal tracts and lobules, patchy bile ductular proliferations that resemble downstream biliary tract disease,[21,22] nodular regenerative hyperplasia, and a propensity to develop focal nodular hyperplasia.[21,23] Fibrosis tends to be mild or absent. Hepatocellular carcinomas can also develop, even in noncirrhotic livers.

HEREDITARY HEMORRHAGIC TELANGIECTASIA

Hereditary hemorrhagic telangiectasia (HHT) is a rare autosomal dominant genetic disorder that leads to abnormally formed blood vessels (telangiectasias) in various organs including the liver. The disease is also known as the Osler–Weber–Rendu syndrome and is caused by various mutations (in genes *ENG*, *ACVRL1*, *MADH4*, and others that are unknown) that disrupt the TGF-beta signaling pathway. Liver disease is found on imaging studies in 54% of patients.[24] The ALK1 mutations are most likely to have symptomatic liver disease.[25]

There are two basic vascular lesions found when there is liver involvement: arteriovenous malformations (AVM) and telangiectasias. Both can be present in any given case, and lesions can be single or multiple. Overall, AVMs are the most common liver lesion (seen in 50% to 75% of cases) followed by telangiectasias (50%).[26,27]

The AVMs can be either grossly visible lesions or microscopic lesions. Grossly visible lesions are most likely to be targeted by biopsies, while the background parenchyma in resection or transplant specimens often show microscopic foci. The AVMs show clusters of larger caliber vessels with abnormal wall thickening (Fig. 9.25). Smaller lesions often have a visible remnant of a portal tract. Larger lesions show areas of fibrosis, hemorrhage, and hemosiderin-laden macrophages. The surrounding hepatic parenchyma can show a focal nodular hyperplasia. Overall, focal nodular hyperplasias are seen in 5% of all individuals with HHT.[26]

The telangiectasias are composed of focal collections of dilated, interanastomosing, and thin-walled vessels (Fig. 9.26). The telangiectasias often appear infiltrative around their edges but do not show cytological atypia. The smaller telangiectasias clearly arise in portal tracts. Telangiectasias can be gross or microscopic findings.

Other common changes include patchy sinusoidal dilatation and nodular regeneration.[28,29] Ischemic cholangiopathy has also been described in several studies.[29,30]

HEREDITARY LYMPHEDEMA

Hereditary lymphedema is a family of rare diseases that lead to abnormal structure or function of the lymphatics. There are many different mutations and different inheritance patterns, including, autosomal recessive, autosomal dominant, and X linked. The disease penetrance ranges from low to high. Most of the mutations impair the function of the VEGFR3 pathway or the RAS pathway, leading to either structurally intact lymphatics with functional impairment, where lymph is poorly absorbed at the "blind end loop" start point of lymphatics, or structurally disorganized lymphatics, including valves that do not function.

Individuals can present as infants (type I). Examples include Milroy disease and Norwegian lymphedema cholestasis syndrome. Cholestasis is seen in many of these cases. Depending on the mutations, the clinical findings can resolve, often within the first year of life, though there can be persistent findings into teen age and adult years. Individuals can also present around puberty (type II), for example Meige disease, or as an adult (lymphedema tarda).

Overall, the degree of lymphedema varies considerably but can include peripheral subcutaneous lymphedema, chylous ascites, and less commonly pleural or pericardial effusions. The lymphedema can involve the arms, face, trunk, and legs, but in milder cases tends to show disease primarily in the lower extremities. Treatment is never curative but includes compression therapies and lymphatic drainage.

The histological findings in the liver have not been described to date, but they are likely to be variable from case to case, given the large number of mutations, clinical syndromes, and varying disease penetrance. Nonetheless, they cluster into cases with structural

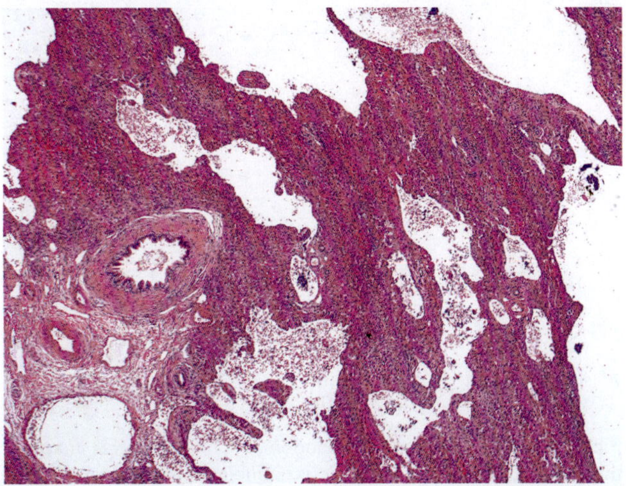

Figure 9.25. Hereditary hemorrhagic telangiectasia, arteriovenous malformation. At low power, a tangle of venous structures distort the hepatic architecture.

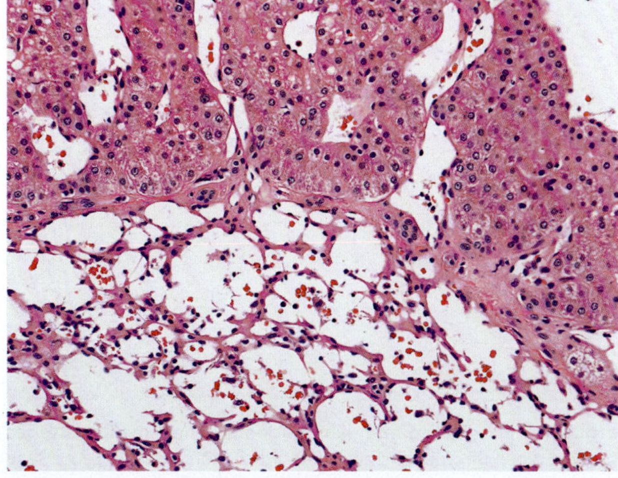

Figure 9.26. Telangiectasias. A tangle of thin-walled dilated vessels is seen.

abnormalities involving the liver microvasculature or into cases with a general vascular outflow disease pattern of injury. The structural changes can include varying combinations of dilated arteries, sometimes with what appears to be lymph in the arteries (Fig. 9.27), and reactive arterial endothelium, which sometimes gives the endothelial cells an epithelioid morphology (Fig. 9.28). In some cases, it can be hard to tell exactly what is artery, vein, or abnormal lymphatic on the H&E. There can be glomeruloid-like malformations in the arterial lumens (Figs. 9.29 and 9.30) along with small thrombi. In cases with a vascular outflow pattern of injury, the lobules show sinusoidal dilatation and congestion (Fig. 9.31). The portal tracts often show a mild bile ductular proliferation (Fig. 9.32). In addition, lobular cholestasis can be prominent in some conditions, such as Aagenaes syndrome (lymphedema cholestasis syndrome 1).

Other findings can mask the true nature of the disease. For example, in one case, the dilated lymphatics in the hilum obstructed the bile ducts leading to a secondary sclerosing cholangitis.[31] Fibrosis is variable, and cirrhosis has been reported.[32]

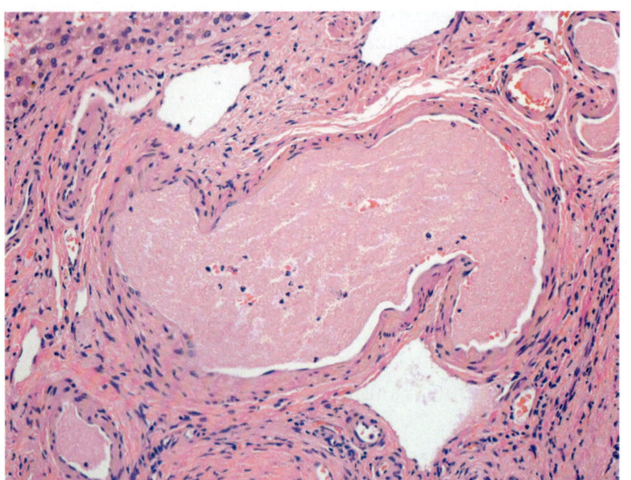

Figure 9.27. **Hereditary lymphedema.** This case of adult-onset disease showed dilated arteries that sometimes had lymphlike material within their lumens.

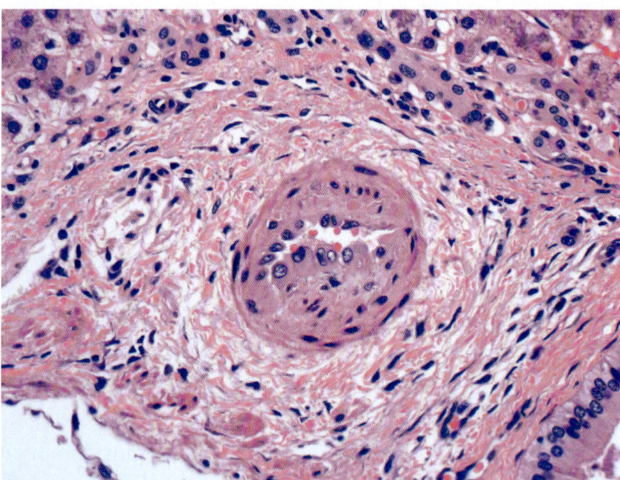

Figure 9.28. **Hereditary lymphedema.** The endothelial cells in some of the arteries have an unusual epithelioid morphology.

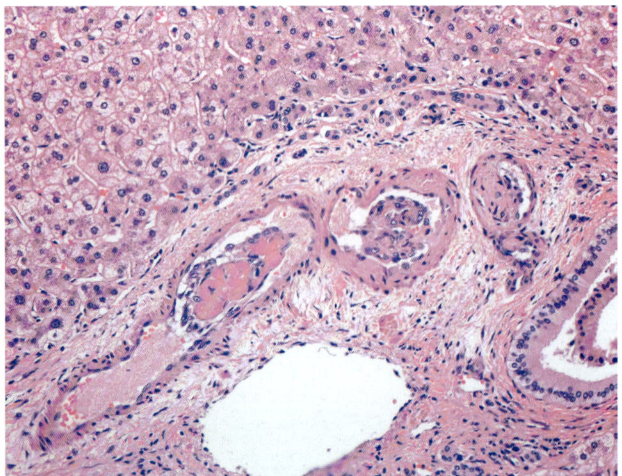

Figure 9.29. **Hereditary lymphedema.** The smaller arteries showed small thrombi and glomeruloid clusters of cells. Same case as Figure 9.28.

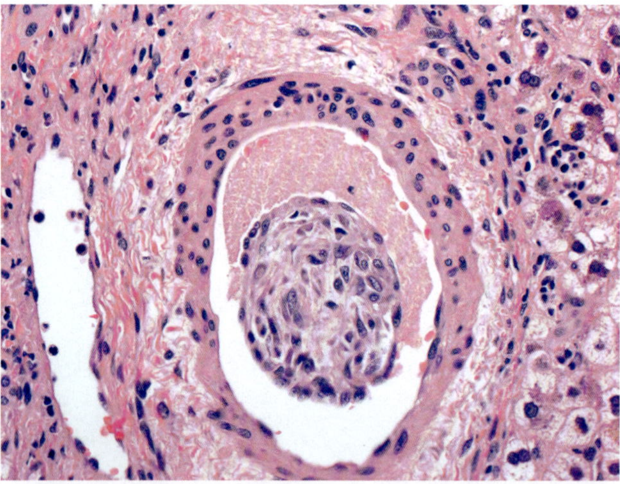

Figure 9.30. **Hereditary lymphedema.** A higher power image of the glomeruloid-like malformations. Same case as Figure 9.28.

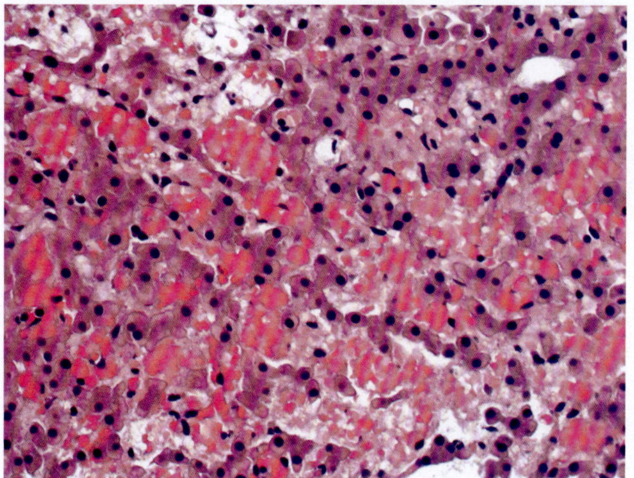

Figure 9.31. **Hereditary lymphedema.** This case of Milroy syndrome showed patchy lobular congestion that was somewhat irregular in distribution but overall showed a zone 3 predominance.

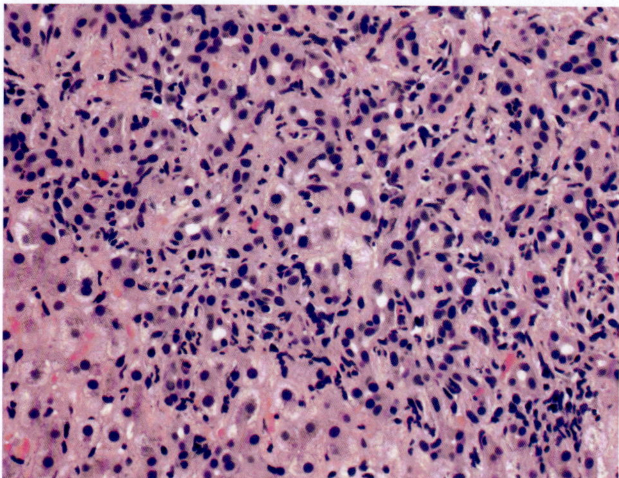

Figure 9.32. **Hereditary lymphedema.** This case of Milroy syndrome (same case as Fig. 9.31) also showed moderate patchy bile ductular proliferation.

NODULAR REGENERATIVE HYPERPLASIA

CHECKLIST: Nodular Regenerative Hyperplasia (NRH)

- ☐ Typical enzyme pattern is disproportionate elevations in alkaline phosphatase
- ☐ Often is associated with portal hypertension
- ☐ Gross examination (e.g., at surgery) can suggest cirrhosis
- ☐ Histology shows a vague parenchymal nodularity at low power
  - ○ There should be no more than mild fibrosis (portal fibrosis or less)
  - ○ The nodularity should be caused by areas of atrophic hepatocytes alternating with normal or larger sized hepatocytes.
- ☐ Other findings can include subtle portal vein abnormalities

Pitfall

- ☐ Common mimic of NRH: variation in glycogen content can give a vague nodularity at low power. Usually the glycogen is accentuated in zones 3. This finding is most common in individuals with diabetes mellitus.

Nodular regenerative hyperplasia has many different clinical associations, but they mostly fall into the categories of autoimmune conditions, vascular flow changes in the setting of portal vein thrombosis, drug effect, lymphoma, and/or leukemia, or after liver transplantation.[33–35] The liver can look grossly cirrhotic when seen at surgery or autopsy. However, sections of the liver show no significant fibrosis, but instead a vague but diffuse parenchymal nodularity (Fig. 9.33). These changes are most evident at low-power examination and can often be highlighted by a reticulin stain (Fig. 9.34). A reticulin stain can show a fair amount of nonspecific changes (Fig. 9.35), so the nodularity should be evident on H&E, enhanced by reticulin, and diffuse in the specimen. Nodular regenerative hyperplasia can be an isolated histological finding or it can be observed in the setting of other histological abnormities such as hepatoportal sclerosis, so the biopsy should also be carefully examined for other changes. The parenchymal nodularity results from small atrophic hepatocytes, usually located in zone 3, that alternate with the normal-sized to slightly enlarged hepatocytes.

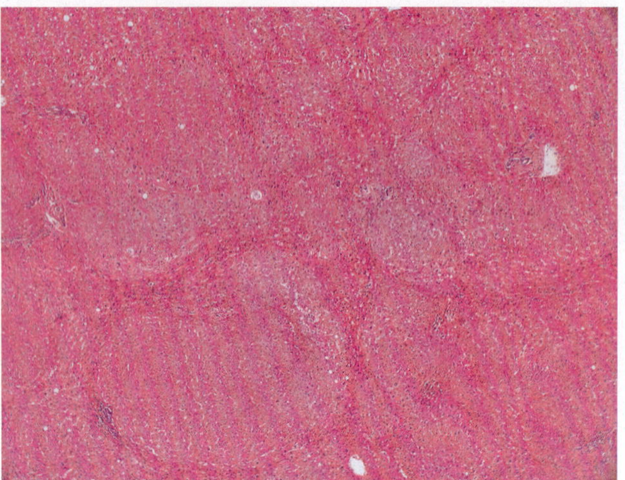

Figure 9.33. **Nodular regenerative hyperplasia.** The hepatic parenchyma shows distinctive nodularity at low power, but there is no fibrosis.

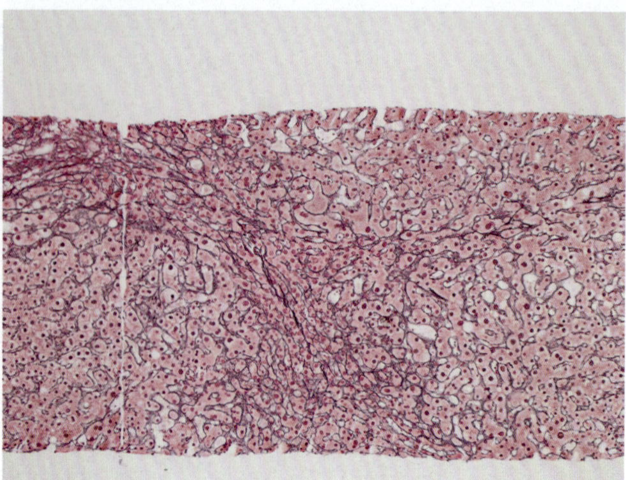

Figure 9.34. **Nodular regenerative hyperplasia, reticulin stain.** The reticulin stain highlights parenchymal nodularity without fibrosis.

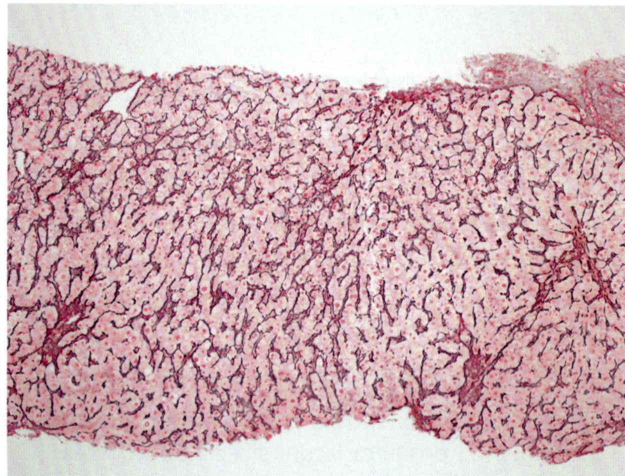

Figure 9.35. **Reticulin stain with nonspecific changes.** The reticulin stain show mild nonspecific changes in this case. On the reticulin stain, there was one focus (this image) that had an area with smaller hepatocytes (center of image) but there was no parenchymal nodularity on H&E and this focal reticulin finding was considered insufficient for a diagnosis of nodular regenerative hyperplasia.

PELIOSIS HEPATITIS

CHECKLIST: Causes of Peliosis Hepatitis

- □ Debilitating illness, examples include
  - ○ Tuberculosis, leprosy
  - ○ Acquired immunodeficiency syndrome (AIDS) (can be *Bartonella* related)
  - ○ Cancer (most commonly lymphoma/leukemia)
  - ○ Light chain deposition disease
- □ Malnutrition
- □ Medications, examples include
  - ○ Oral contraceptives
  - ○ Androgens
  - ○ Azathioprine

Peliosis hepatitis is defined by cystlike spaces filled with blood in the hepatic lobules (Fig. 9.36). These cystlike spaces range in size from 1 mm to several cm and have no endothelial lining (Fig. 9.37), although long-standing cysts can start to endothelialize. In general, they do not have a clear anatomic distribution and can be focal or more diffusely distributed in the liver. The peliotic, cystic areas may have blood or serum within them, as well as areas of thrombosis. The background liver typically shows no significant inflammation, unless there is another underlying disease such as chronic viral hepatitis. The livers are noncirrhotic, and there is no evidence for generalized vascular inflow or outflow disease.

Peliosis hepatitis is often an incidental finding, but clinical associations include portal hypertension[36,37] and cyst rupture with intraperitoneal hemorrhage (very rare).[38] In addition to the liver, peliotic changes can be found in other organs, most commonly the spleen, bone marrow, and lymph nodes.[39] Rarely other organs can be involved including the gastrointestinal (GI) tract, adrenals, and kidney.[39]

SEGMENTAL ATROPHY AND NODULAR ELASTOSIS

Segmental atrophy is a benign pseudotumor of the liver that has several different sequential stages of histological findings.[40] Nodular elastosis is a later stage and overall the most distinctive stage.

These lesions present as clinical masses and range in size from 1 to 10 cm.[40] While the etiology is not precisely known, they seem to result from a local thrombosis of a vessel feeding a smaller subsegment of the liver, which leads to ischemic parenchymal collapses with a loss of hepatocytes, exuberant bile ductular proliferation, and mild mixed inflammation (Fig. 9.38). Entrapped bile ducts can become cystically dilated (Fig. 9.39). In some cases, these retention type biliary cysts can dominate the histology, at least focally, and suggest other types of cystic biliary tract disease. In time, the inflammation and ductular proliferation diminishes and are gradually replaced by a distinctive matrix composed of elastic and reticulin fibers. The matrix is quite striking in the nodular elastosis stage, with the mass lesion composed mostly of extracellular matrix and a few scattered islands of ordinary looking hepatocytes (Fig. 9.40). The extracellular matrix can be highlighted by reticulin (Fig. 9.41) and elastic stains such as the VVG (Fig. 9.42). The elastosis commonly extends to and involves the liver capsule.

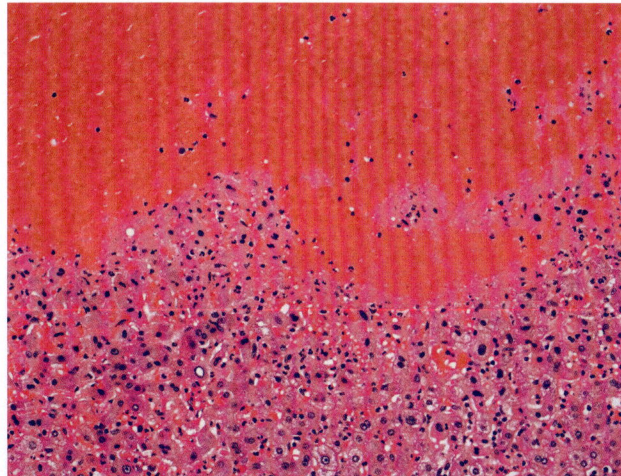

Figure 9.36. **Peliosis hepatis.** This liver has large irregular cystic spaces filled with blood and was associated with chronic debilitating illness.

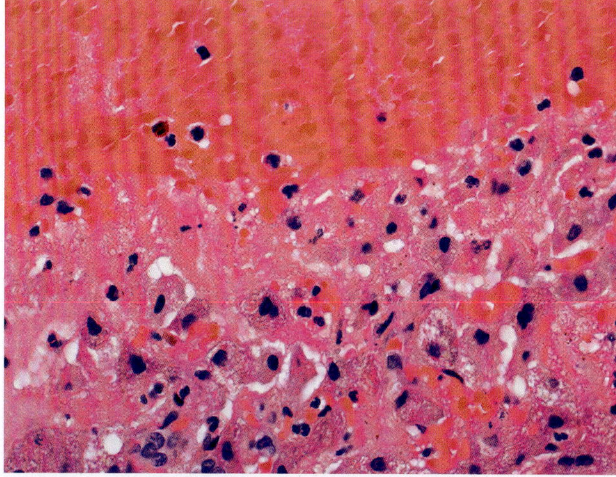

Figure 9.37. **Peliosis hepatis.** At high power, the cystic spaces show no endothelial lining. Same case as preceding image

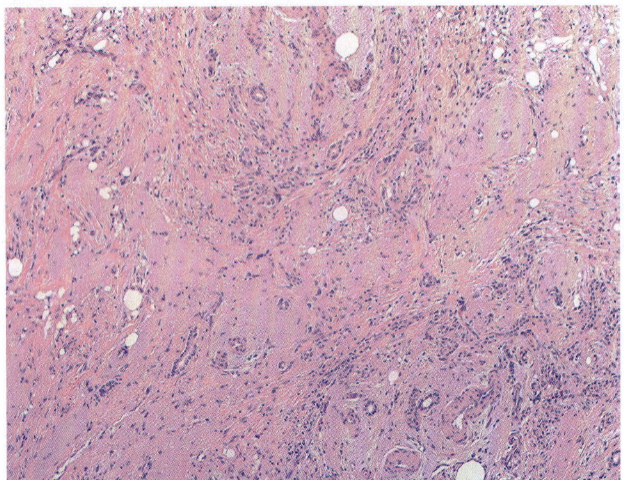

Figure 9.38. **Segmental atrophy, early stage with parenchymal collapse.** At low power, there is widespread parenchymal collapse. Much of the inflammation and ductular proliferation have abated and early elastotic changes are present.

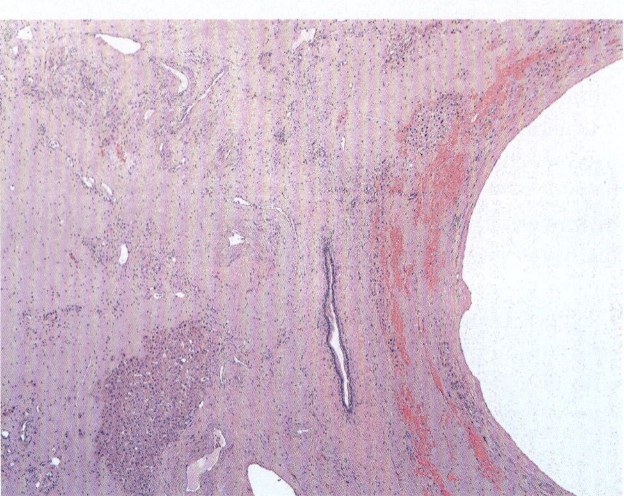

Figure 9.39. **Segmental atrophy, retention biliary cyst.** A biliary cyst is seen in the right side of this image. This lesion has well developed elastosis, as seen on the right side of the image.

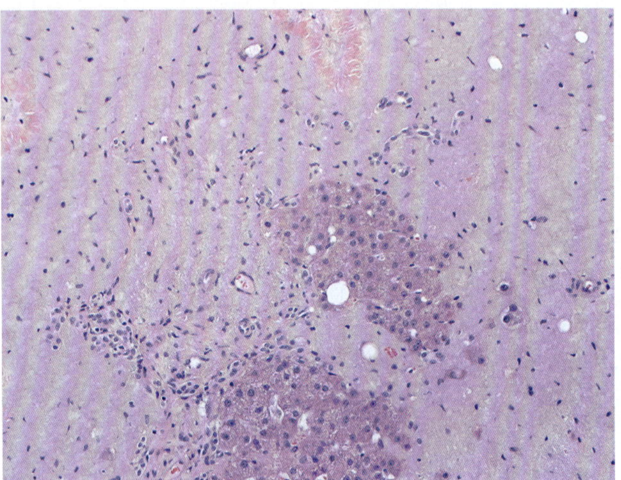

Figure 9.40. **Segmental atrophy, nodular elastosis stage.** The distinctive elastotic matrix surrounds a few islands of otherwise unremarkable hepatocytes.

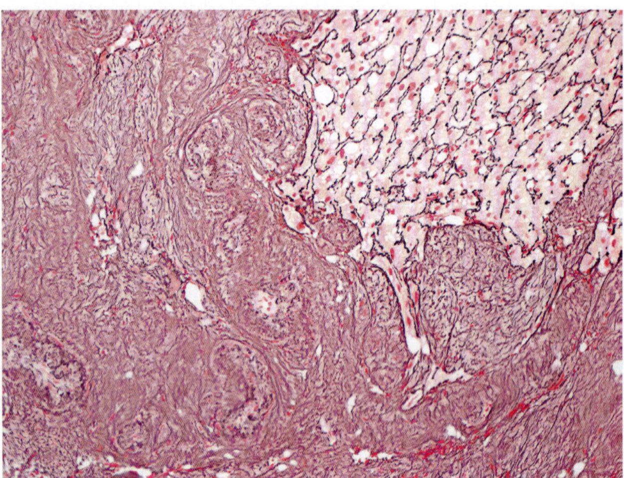

Figure 9.41. **Segmental atrophy, nodular elastosis stage, reticulin stain.** The matrix also has numerous reticulin fibers.

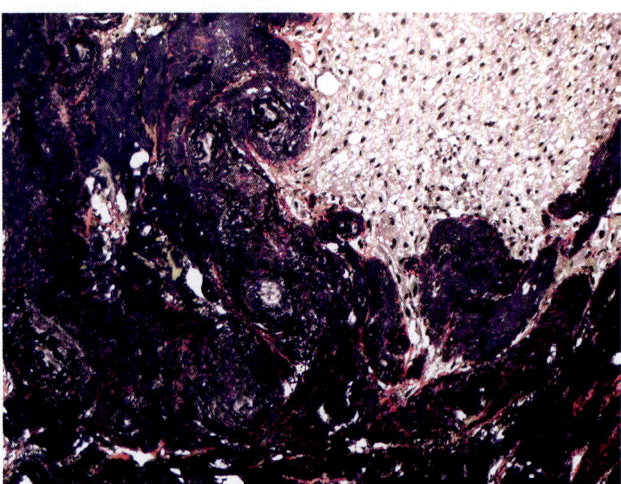

Figure 9.42. **Segmental atrophy, nodular elastosis stage, VVG.** The abundant elastic fibers in the matrix stain deeply black. An island of hepatocytes in the upper right corner can also be seen. Same case as Figure 9.41.

At low-power examination, there are scattered short, plump, spindle cells in the matrix. These spindled cells are sparse and show no atypia and no mitoses (Fig. 9.43). On vimentin stain, these cells show a distinctive morphology that resembles a dendritic cell (Fig. 9.44). Thrombosed vessels are almost always seen in resected specimens but may not be sampled in biopsy specimens (Fig. 9.45). Over time, the elastosis can gradually be replaced by fibrosis, leaving behind a distinctive round scar, often containing small islands of ordinary looking hepatocytes. Occasionally, the scar will develop small calcifications.

It remains unclear why these lesions develop. Most cases of subcapsular vascular insults that knock out a segment of a liver go through similar stages of parenchymal loss, ductular proliferation, and inflammation, but then proceed directly on to scaring, without developing a pseudotumor or the distinctive elastosis pattern of injury. This mystery awaits further studies.

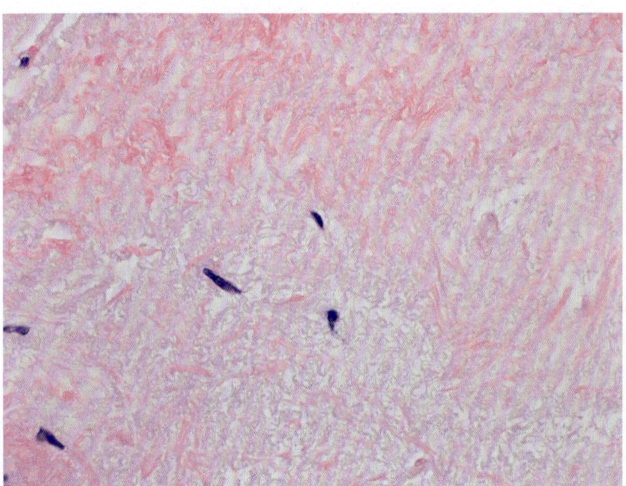

Figure 9.43. **Segmental atrophy, nodular elastosis stage.** The matrix has plump, stubby spindle cells

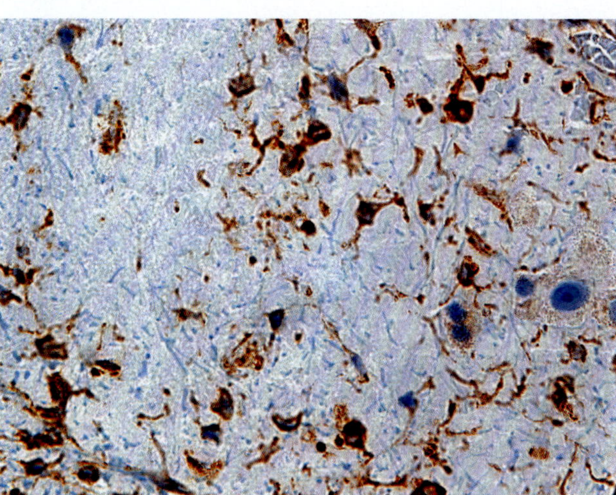

Figure 9.44. **Segmental atrophy, nodular elastosis stage, vimentin.** The cells in the matrix have a dendritic morphology.

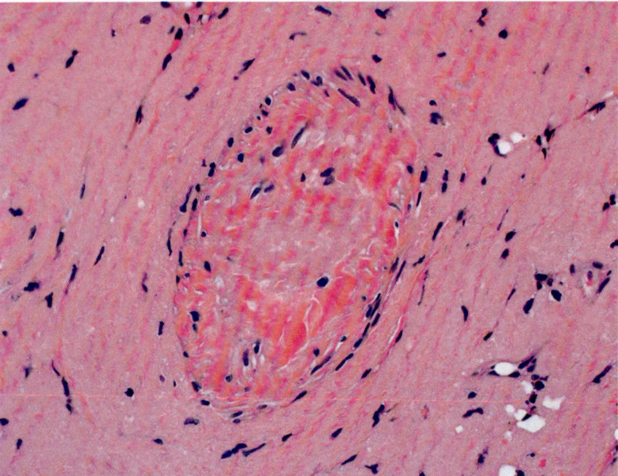

Figure 9.45. **Segmental atrophy, thrombosed vessels.** A vessel shows thrombosis.

TUMORS ASSOCIATED WITH VASCULAR DISEASE

CHECKLIST: Tumors That Can Develop in Livers With Chronic Vascular Flow Abnormalities

- ☐ Focal nodular hyperplasia
- ☐ Hepatic adenoma
- ☐ Macroregenerative nodules
- ☐ Hepatocellular carcinoma
- ☐ Hepatocellular pseudotumor

Almost all of the benign and malignant types of hepatic tumors can develop in livers with long-standing vascular inflow or outflow abnormalities, even if the liver is noncirrhotic. Focal nodular hyperplasias develop with vascular in flow disease (e.g., Abernathy syndrome),[21,23] intrahepatic shunts (e.g., hereditary hemorrhagic telangiectasia),[26] and vascular outflow disease (e.g., Budd–Chiari syndrome or chronic congestive liver disease).[41–43] In all of these settings, the diagnosis of focal nodular hyperplasia is made in the usual way, as they look and stain like sporadic lesions. Hepatic adenomas[44,45] and hepatocellular carcinomas[46,47] have also been described in livers with abnormal hepatic blood inflow (e.g., Abernathy syndrome) or abnormal blood outflow (e.g., Budd–Chiari). In all of these tumors, the diagnosis is made in the usual way.

Finally, a rare benign lesion occurs in noncirrhotic livers and is called a *hepatocellular pseudotumor*. This pseudotumor does not fit well into typical categories of macroregenerative nodules or focal nodular hyperplasia. On imaging, these lesions show an ill-defined mass with abnormal areas of hyperperfusion. Biopsies show a vaguely nodular parenchyma with sinusoidal dilatation, and depending on sampling, often show a thrombosed vessel, usually a portal vein, which presumably led to the parenchymal changes (Figs. 9.46 and 9.47).

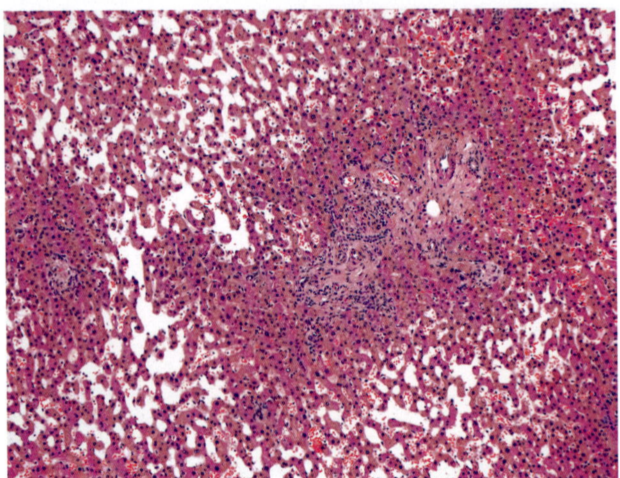

Figure 9.46. **Hepatocellular pseudotumor.** Imaging showed an ill-defined lesion with vascular flow changes. Biopsies were benign but showed no definite tumor. A resection showed a grossly ill-defined lesion and sections showed patchy sinusoidal dilatation, some areas of vague parenchymal nodularity, with increased arterioles and a ductular proliferation in the portal tracts.

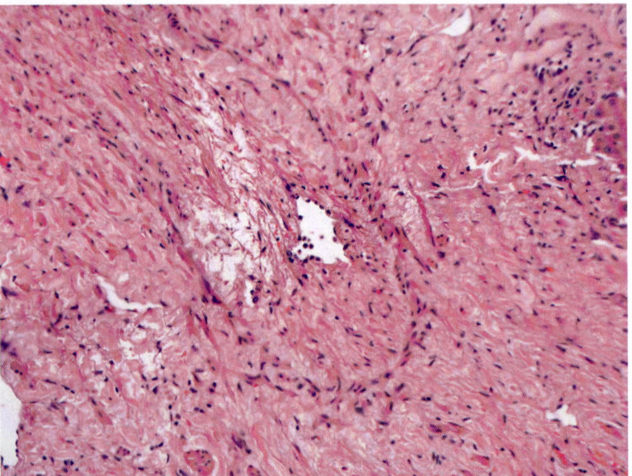

Figure 9.47. **Hepatocellular pseudotumor.** The larger branches of the portal tracts in this hepatic pseudotumor showed remote fibrotic thrombi.

NEAR MISSES

CASE 1. A 53-year-old woman underwent resection of a hepatocellular carcinoma. A separate vascular lesion was noted on imaging and was resected. The hepatocellular carcinoma was straightforward to diagnose, but the resected vascular lesion was harder to classify. The referring pathologist had a differential diagnosis of hemangioma versus angiosarcoma but noted that neither diagnosis seemed to be a very good fit.

On review, the vascular lesion dissected through the hepatic parenchyma in an unusual pattern. Large hemangiomas can have infiltrative borders, but this lesion did not show a central large hemangioma with infiltrative borders but instead was more diffusely infiltrative (Fig. 9.48). The vascular channels were more angular and less well formed than typical hemangiomas. On the other hand, there was no parenchymal destruction and no cytological atypia to suggest an angiosarcoma. Overall, the findings suggested a vascular malformation, either sporadic or syndromic. Follow-up information was received that the patient had a clinical diagnosis of hereditary hemorrhagic telangiectasia.

This case illustrates several important points. First, clinical history simplifies many otherwise-challenging cases. Secondly, the referring pathologist did an excellent job of realizing that the vascular lesion did not fit very well for either a hemangioma or an angiosarcoma. It can be tempting to force difficult cases into categories with which we are familiar and can be challenging to recognize when we do not recognize the true nature of a lesion. However, this comes with time and experience, which teaches both the central core of disease patterns as well as their outer boundaries.

CASE 2. A 63-year-old woman had intermittent elevations in liver enzymes, predominately alkaline phosphatase. Recent testing showed an AST of 42, ALT of 53, and alkaline phosphatase of 310. The patient was taking no medications, viral serologies were negative, BMI was normal, while ANA was positive at 1:160. The biopsy was submitted for review because it was histologically almost normal.

On review, the biopsy showed no inflammation, no granulomas, no biliary tract disease, and no sinusoidal infiltrative processes. It was indeed almost normal. However, the central veins and zone 3 sinusoids showed mild, equivocal dilatation (Fig. 9.49). The finding was diffuse, but there was no atrophy of the zone 3 hepatocytes. To follow-up, a CK7 stain was preformed and showed intermediate hepatocytes in zone 3 (Fig. 9.50). Taken together, the findings were enough to raise the possibility of vascular outflow disease. Subsequent clinical evaluation showed mild congestive heart failure.

Vascular diseases can be very subtle on biopsy specimens, and when mild, the findings can be insufficient to fully establish the correct diagnosis. Nonetheless, the biopsy findings are still clinically very helpful in ruling out relevant diseases and in suggesting how to

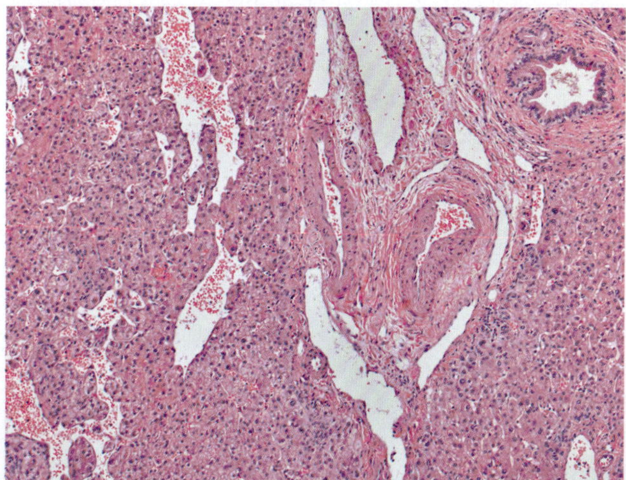

Figure 9.48. **Near miss case 1, hereditary hemorrhagic telangiectasia.** The biopsy shows irregular vascular channels dissecting through the parenchyma.

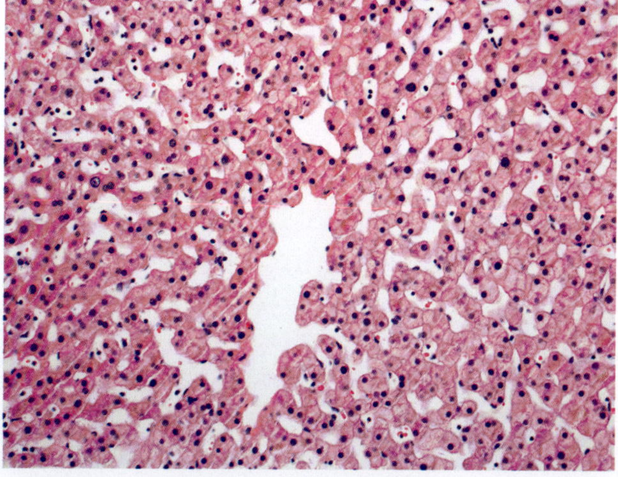

Figure 9.49. **Near miss case 2, subtle vascular outflow disease.** The biopsy shows equivocal mild sinusoidal dilatation.

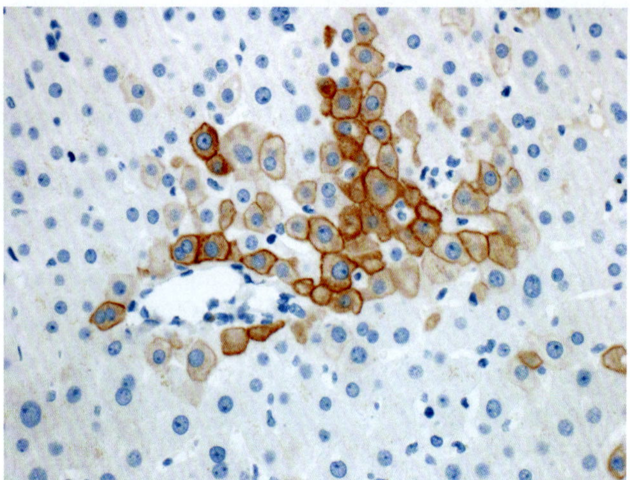

Figure 9.50. Near miss case 2, subtle vascular outflow disease. A CK7 is positive in the zone 3 hepatocytes.

further work up the patient. In the case reviewed here, the biopsy was helpful in ruling out disease patterns that commonly have a disproportionate elevation in alkaline phosphatase: biliary tract disease, sinusoidal infiltrative disease, and granulomas. The biopsy findings, while subtle and not definitive, were also helpful in identifying the correct disease pattern, one that also commonly has a disproportionate elevation in alkaline phosphatase: vascular outflow disease.

References

1. Zahmatkeshan M, Geramizadeh B, Eshraghian A, et al. De novo fatty liver due to vascular complications after liver transplantation. *Transpl Proc*. 2011;43:615-617.
2. Ogren M, Bergqvist D, Bjorck M, Acosta S, Eriksson H, Sternby NH. Portal vein thrombosis: prevalence, patient characteristics and lifetime risk: a population study based on 23,796 consecutive autopsies. *World J Gastroenterol*. 2006;12:2115-2119.
3. Janssen HL, Wijnhoud A, Haagsma EB, et al. Extrahepatic portal vein thrombosis: aetiology and determinants of survival. *Gut*. 2001;49:720-724.
4. Ghabril M, Agarwal S, Lacerda M, Chalasani N, Kwo P, Tector AJ. Portal vein thrombosis is a risk factor for poor early outcomes after liver transplantation: analysis of risk factors and outcomes for portal vein thrombosis in waitlisted patients. *Transplantation*. 2016;100:126-133.
5. Khuroo MS, Rather AA, Khuroo NS, Khuroo MS. Portal biliopathy. *World J Gastroenterol*. 2016;22:7973-7982.
6. Gollackner B, Sedivy R, Rockenschaub S, et al. Increased apoptosis of hepatocytes in vascular occlusion after orthotopic liver transplantation. *Transpl Int*. 2000;13:49-53.
7. Liu TC, Nguyen TT, Torbenson MS. Concurrent increase in mitosis and apoptosis: a histological pattern of hepatic arterial flow abnormalities in post-transplant liver biopsies. *Mod Pathol*. 2012.
8. Torbenson M, Chen YY, Brunt E, et al. Glycogenic hepatopathy: an underrecognized hepatic complication of diabetes mellitus. *Am J Surg Pathol*. 2006;30:508-513.
9. Hughes RL, Feig J. Sickle cell trait-related exertional deaths: observations at autopsy and review of the literature. *Mil Med*. 2015;180:e929-e932.
10. Thogmartin JR, Wilson CI, Palma NA, Ignacio SS, Pellan WA. Histological diagnosis of sickle cell trait: a blinded analysis. *Am J Forensic Med Pathol*. 2009;30:36-39.
11. Charlotte F, Bachir D, Nenert M, et al. Vascular lesions of the liver in sickle cell disease. A clinicopathological study in 26 living patients. *Arch Pathol Lab Med*. 1995;119:46-52.
12. Gurkan E, Ergun Y, Zorludemir S, Baslamisli F, Kocak R. Liver involvement in sickle cell disease. *Turk J Gastroenterol*. 2005;16:194-198.
13. Omata M, Johnson CS, Tong M, Tatter D. Pathological spectrum of liver diseases in sickle cell disease. *Dig Dis Sci*. 1986;31:247-256.

14. Maher MM, Mansour AH. Study of chronic hepatopathy in patients with sickle cell disease. *Gastroenterol Res*. 2009;2:338-343.

15. Darbari DS, Kple-Faget P, Kwagyan J, Rana S, Gordeuk VR, Castro O. Circumstances of death in adult sickle cell disease patients. *Am J Hematol*. 2006;81:858-863.

16. Perronne V, Roberts-Harewood M, Bachir D, et al. Patterns of mortality in sickle cell disease in adults in France and England. *Hematol J*. 2002;3:56-60.

17. Traina F, Jorge SG, Yamanaka A, de Meirelles LR, Costa FF, Saad ST. Chronic liver abnormalities in sickle cell disease: a clinicopathological study in 70 living patients. *Acta Haematol*. 2007;118:129-135.

18. Kakar S, Batts KP, Poterucha JJ, Burgart LJ. Histologic changes mimicking biliary disease in liver biopsies with venous outflow impairment. *Mod Pathol*. 2004;17:874-878.

19. Pai RK, Hart JA. Aberrant expression of cytokeratin 7 in perivenular hepatocytes correlates with a cholestatic chemistry profile in patients with heart failure. *Mod Pathol*. 2010;23:1650-1656.

20. Dai DF, Swanson PE, Krieger EV, Liou IW, Carithers RL, Yeh MM. Congestive hepatic fibrosis score: a novel histologic assessment of clinical severity. *Mod Pathol*. 2014;27:1552-1558.

21. Lisovsky M, Konstas AA, Misdraji J. Congenital extrahepatic portosystemic shunts (Abernethy malformation): a histopathologic evaluation. *Am J Surg Pathol*. 2011;35:1381-1390.

22. Chawla A, Kahn E, Becker J, et al. Focal nodular hyperplasia of the liver and hypercholesterolemia in a child with VACTERL syndrome. *J Pediatr Gastroenterol Nutr*. 1993;17:434-437.

23. Osorio MJ, Bonow A, Bond GJ, et al. Abernethy malformation complicated by hepatopulmonary syndrome and a liver mass successfully treated by liver transplantation. *Pediatr Transpl*. 2011;15:E149-E151.

24. Singh S, Swanson KL, Hathcock MA, et al. Identifying the presence of clinically significant hepatic involvement in hereditary haemorrhagic telangiectasia using a simple clinical scoring index. *J Hepatol*. 2014;61:124-131.

25. Lesca G, Olivieri C, Burnichon N, et al. Genotype-phenotype correlations in hereditary hemorrhagic telangiectasia: data from the French-Italian HHT network. *Genet Med*. 2007;9:14-22.

26. Scardapane A, Ficco M, Sabba C, et al. Hepatic nodular regenerative lesions in patients with hereditary haemorrhagic telangiectasia: computed tomography and magnetic resonance findings. *Radiol Med*. 2013;118:1-13.

27. Giordano P, Lenato GM, Suppressa P, et al. Hereditary hemorrhagic telangiectasia: arteriovenous malformations in children. *J Pediatr*. 2013;163:179-186 e1-e3.

28. Blewitt RW, Brown CM, Wyatt JI. The pathology of acute hepatic disintegration in hereditary haemorrhagic telangiectasia. *Histopathology*. 2003;42:265-269.

29. Brenard R, Chapaux X, Deltenre P, et al. Large spectrum of liver vascular lesions including high prevalence of focal nodular hyperplasia in patients with hereditary haemorrhagic telangiectasia: the Belgian Registry based on 30 patients. *Eur J Gastroenterol Hepatol*. 2010;22:1253-1259.

30. Mavrakis A, Demetris A, Ochoa ER, Rabinovitz M. Hereditary hemorrhagic telangiectasia of the liver complicated by ischemic bile duct necrosis and sepsis: case report and review of the literature. *Dig Dis Sci*. 2010;55:2113-2117.

31. Viveiros A, Reiterer M, Schaefer B, et al. CCBE1 mutation causing sclerosing cholangitis: Expanding the spectrum of lymphedema-cholestasis syndrome. *Hepatology*. 2017;66:286-288.

32. Drivdal M, Trydal T, Hagve TA, Bergstad I, Aagenaes O. Prognosis, with evaluation of general biochemistry, of liver disease in lymphoedema cholestasis syndrome 1 (LCS1/Aagenaes syndrome). *Scand J Gastroenterol*. 2006;41:465-471.

33. Hubscher SG. What is the long-term outcome of the liver allograft? *J Hepatol*. 2011;55:702-717.

34. Devarbhavi H, Abraham S, Kamath PS. Significance of nodular regenerative hyperplasia occurring de novo following liver transplantation. *Liver Transpl*. 2007;13:1552-1556.

35. Gane E, Portmann B, Saxena R, Wong P, Ramage J, Williams R. Nodular regenerative hyperplasia of the liver graft after liver transplantation. *Hepatology*. 1994;20:88-94.

36. Berzigotti A, Magalotti D, Zappoli P, Rossi C, Callea F, Zoli M. Peliosis hepatis as an early histological finding in idiopathic portal hypertension: a case report. *World J Gastroenterol*. 2006;12:3612-3615.

37. Yu CY, Chang LC, Chen LW, et al. Peliosis hepatis complicated by portal hypertension following renal transplantation. *World J Gastroenterol*. 2014;20:2420-2425.

38. Biswas S, Gogna S, Patel P. A fatal case of intra-abdominal hemorrhage following diagnostic blind percutaneous liver biopsy in a patient with peliosis hepatis. *Gastroenterol Res*. 2017;10:318-321.

39. Tsokos M, Erbersdobler A. Pathology of peliosis. *Forensic Sci Int*. 2005;149:25-33.
40. Singhi AD, Maklouf HR, Mehrotra AK, et al. Segmental atrophy of the liver: a distinctive pseudotumor of the liver with variable histologic appearances. *Am J Surg Pathol*. 2011;35:364-371.
41. Cazals-Hatem D, Vilgrain V, Genin P, et al. Arterial and portal circulation and parenchymal changes in Budd-Chiari syndrome: a study in 17 explanted livers. *Hepatology*. 2003;37:510-519.
42. Ibarrola C, Castellano VM, Colina F. Focal hyperplastic hepatocellular nodules in hepatic venous outflow obstruction: a clinicopathological study of four patients and 24 nodules. *Histopathology*. 2004;44:172-179.
43. Choi JY, Lee HC, Yim JH, et al. Focal nodular hyperplasia or focal nodular hyperplasia-like lesions of the liver: a special emphasis on diagnosis. *J Gastroenterol Hepatol*. 2011;26:1004-1009.
44. Sempoux C, Paradis V, Komuta M, et al. Hepatocellular nodules expressing markers of hepatocellular adenomas in Budd-Chiari syndrome and other rare hepatic vascular disorders. *J Hepatol*. 2015;63:1173-1180.
45. Chira RI, Calauz A, Manole S, Valean S, Mircea PA. Unusual discovery after an examination for abdominal pain: Abernethy 1b malformation and liver adenomatosis. A case report. *J Gastrointestin Liver Dis*. 2017;26:85-88.
46. Sakr M, Abdelhakam SM, Dabbous H, et al. Characteristics of hepatocellular carcinoma in Egyptian patients with primary Budd-Chiari syndrome. *Liver Int*. 2017;37:415-422.
47. Park H, Yoon JY, Park KH, et al. Hepatocellular carcinoma in Budd-Chiari syndrome: a single center experience with long-term follow-up in South Korea. *World J Gastroenterol*. 2012;18:1946-1952.

SYSTEMIC DISEASES INVOLVING THE LIVER 10

CHAPTER OUTLINE

AMYLOID

Amyloid in the liver is almost always part of systemic amyloid disease, although sometimes liver disease can be the primary clinical presentation. Amyloid deposits in the liver look about the same as they do anywhere else in the body, and like everywhere else, the H&E findings can range from subtle to obvious. There are many different types of amyloid, and almost all of them have been reported in the liver. The most common form of amyloid in the liver is related to plasma cell dyscrasias. The amyloid deposits are typically massive and found in the lobules and portal tracts (Figs. 10.1 and 10.2). The lobular amyloid deposits often lead to significant hepatocyte atrophy. Rare forms can show deposition only in the hepatic arteries (Fig. 10.3). Mass lesions can also rarely occur, called *amyloidomas* (Fig. 10.4).

A positive Congo red stain is necessary to make the diagnosis of amyloidosis. On light microscopy, the amyloid deposits show a distinctive orange-red color, called *congophilia* (Figs. 10.5 and 10.6). On polarization, the amyloid shows birefringence (Fig. 10.7), but you may need to turn off the lights in your room and turn off your routine microscope filters to optimally see the birefringence. While the birefringence is commonly described

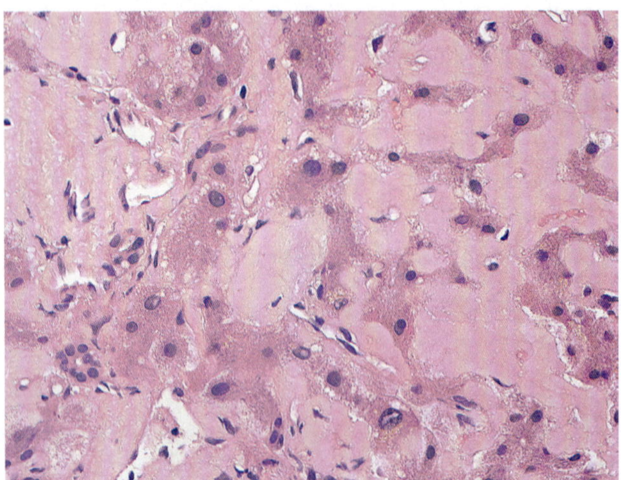

Figure 10.1. **Amyloid.** Massive amyloid deposits are seen in the sinusoids.

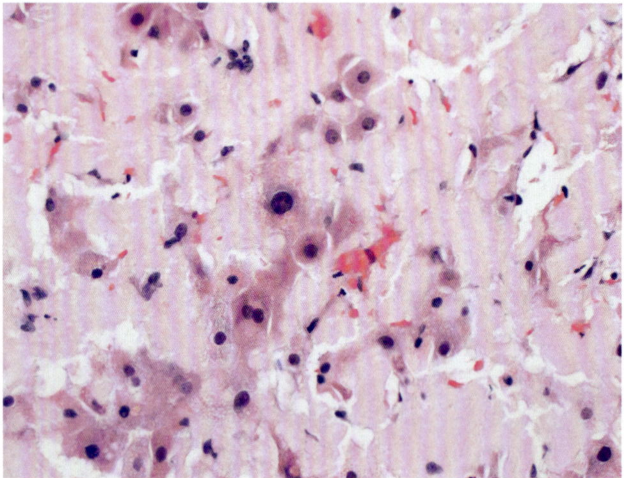

Figure 10.2. **Amyloid.** At higher power, the amyloid deposits are eosinophilic, almost acellular and often show irregular cracking.

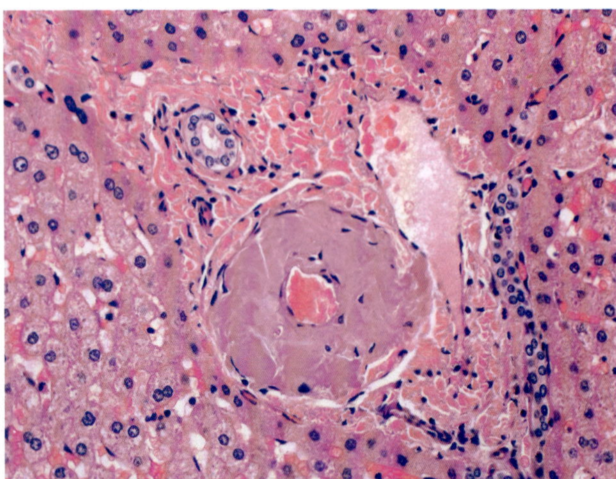

Figure 10.3. **Amyloid, Congo red.** Amyloid deposits in this case were limited to the hepatic arteries.

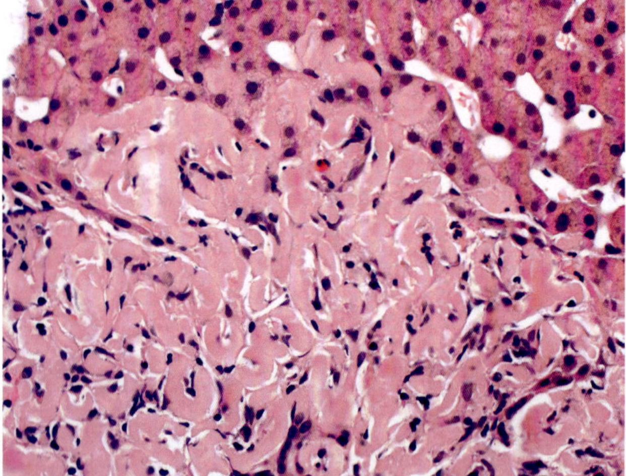

Figure 10.4. **Amyloidoma.** This case presented as an isolated mass lesion. Amlyloid deposits were limited to the nodule, at least in this biopsy specimen.

as *apple-green*, it hardly if ever really is, but instead shows a patchy, pale green color much more in line with a yellow-green lime than a green apple. In the end, the material should look like amyloid on H&E, be congophilic on Congo red stain and show apple-greenish birefringence on polarization.

PEARLS & PITFALLS

- Smooth muscle can be faintly congophilic but will not show birefringence.
- Normal collagen (for example in the portal tract) will show a silver white color on polarization (Fig. 10.8) but will not show apple-green birefringence and will not be congophilic.
- If the H&E is strongly suspicious for amyloid but the Congo red stain is negative, then (1) make sure the section was cut at 10 microns, (2) repeat the stain, and (3) turn off your office lights and turn off your filter's microscope before polarization. Still negative? Then consider Waldenström macroglobulinemia or light chain deposition disease.

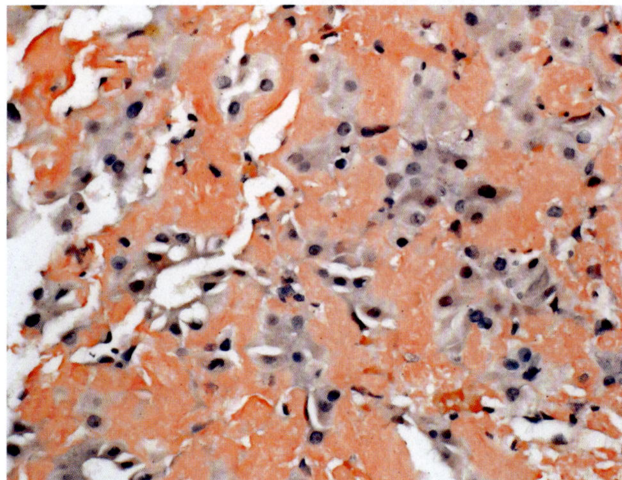

Figure 10.5. Amyloid, Congo red. The amyloid deposits have a distinctive salmon color that is called congophilia

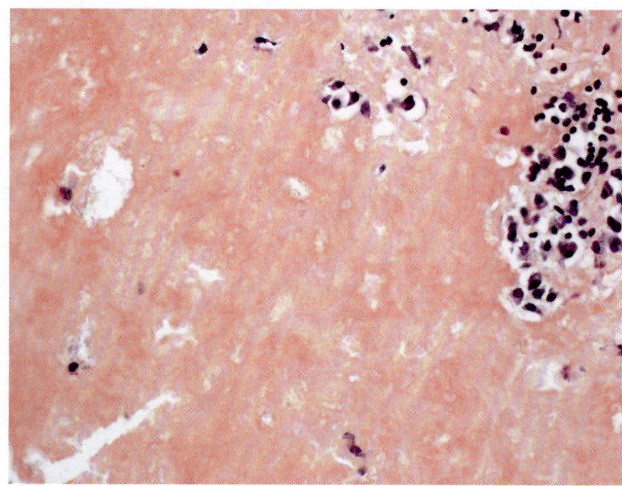

Figure 10.6. Amyloid, Congo red. A higher power view of the distinctive color that is present with amyloid deposits.

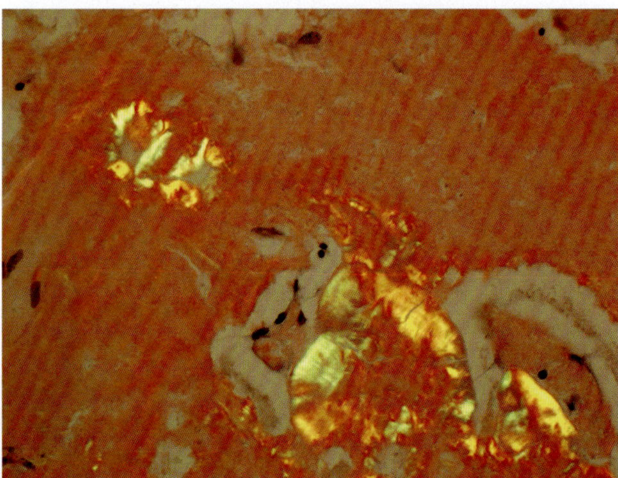

Figure 10.7. Amyloid, Congo red. When the light is polarized, a yellow green color is evident. The color is usually mottled and more yellow than green.

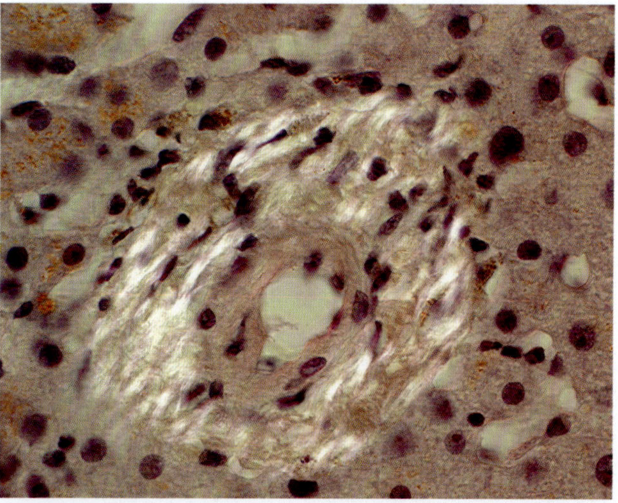

Figure 10.8. Collagen, polarized light. A silver white color is seen with polarization.

In most cases of systemic amyloidosis, the disease is diagnosed on biopsies from other organs, and the liver is not biopsied because of the risk for bleeding. However, there continues to be cases first diagnosed at liver biopsy. In this setting, the clinicians will typically want to know the amyloid subtype. Mass spectrometry is currently the best method for subtype determination[1] and is similar or cheaper in cost than a typical battery of immunostains.

LECT2 AMYLOID

LECT2 amyloid was first recognized as a morphological pattern called *globular amyloid*,[2,3] characterized by distinct round amyloid deposits in the hepatocyte cytoplasm or rarely with extracellular globular deposits in the sinusoids. The globules are round, pink to gray, and sometimes laminated (Figs. 10.9 and 10.10). They can be found anywhere but tend to have a zone 3 predilection. The globules are Congo red positive (Fig. 10.11), although they can show lighter congophilia than ordinary amyloid. An immunostain for LECT2 amyloid is available (Fig. 10.12) and is highly sensitive[4] though not completely specific, especially if staining is weak.[5] Rare cases have been reported of liver disease associated with LECT2 amyloid,[6] but typically LECT2 amyloid is an incidental finding with little or no associated liver dysfunction.

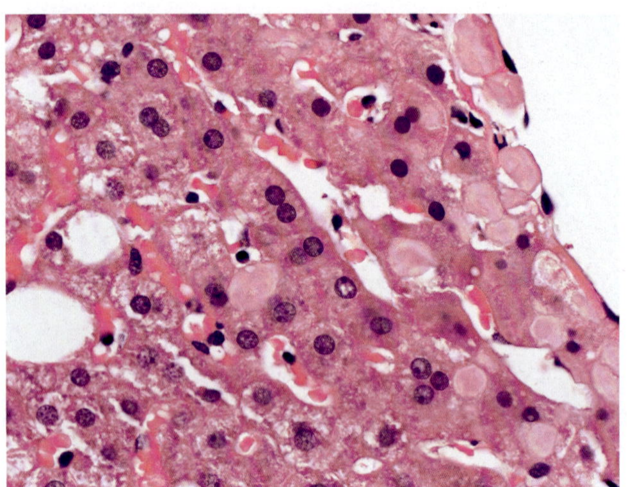

Figure 10.9. **LECT2 amyloid.** The amyloid is deposited in distinctive round pink globules in the zone 3 region of the lobules.

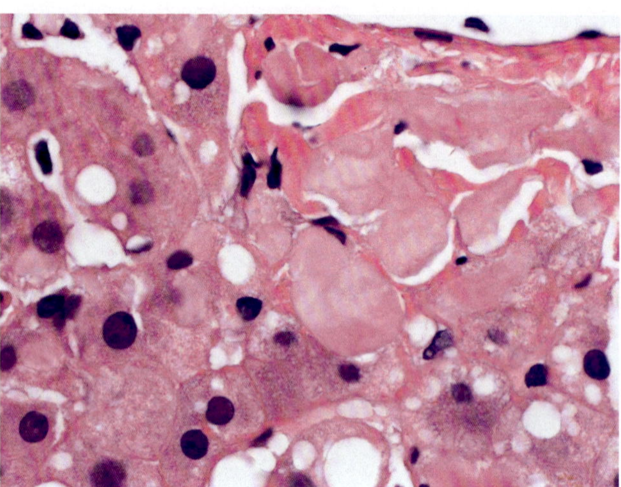

Figure 10.10. **LECT2 amyloid.** The amyloid deposits are shown here at high-power magnification.

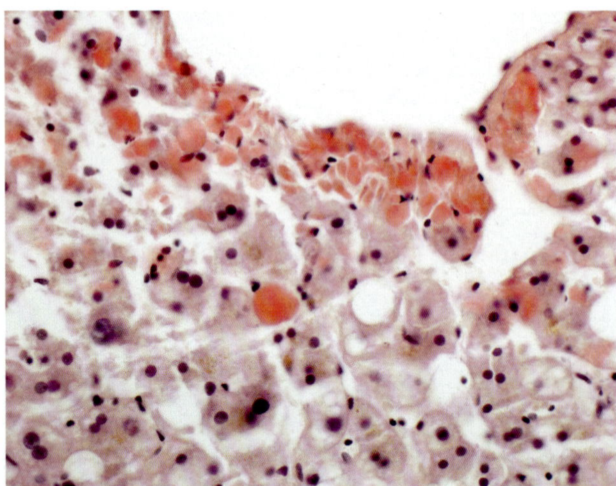

Figure 10.11. **LECT2 amyloid, Congo red.** The globules are Congo red positive.

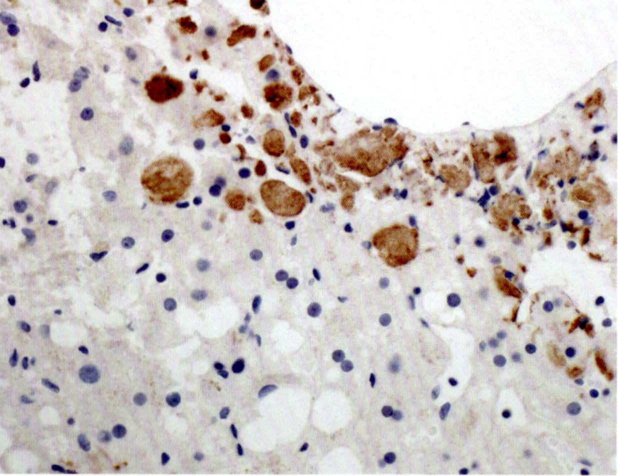

Figure 10.12. **LECT2 amyloid, LECT2 immunostain.** The deposits should be strongly positive. Weak staining can be nonspecific.

LECT2 amyloidosis has strong ethnic associations. For example, in the United States LECT is reported largely in individuals of Hispanic descent, with a frequency of 3% based on autopsy studies.[7] LECT2 amyloid also appears to be enriched in a few other populations including Egyptians.[8] LECT2 amyloidosis primarily involves the kidneys, and patients tend to first present with kidney disease. The spleen, adrenals, and lungs are also frequently involved, but not the heart.[7]

CHECKLIST: Differential for the Globular Amyloidosis Pattern. None of These Will Be Congo Red Positive

- ☐ Hepatitis B ground glass inclusions
- ☐ Glycogen psuedo-ground glass—usually a drug effect
- ☐ Type IV glycogen storage disease
- ☐ Lafora bodies

LIGHT CHAIN DEPOSITION DISEASE

Light chain deposition disease usually presents as renal disease, but liver involvement without renal disease has been reported.[9] In any case, light chain deposition disease can lead to liver dysfunction.[10] Biopsies show diffuse perisinusoidal deposits that range from subtle and easily missed to massive with marked hepatocyte atrophy (Fig. 10.13). The deposits result from an underlying plasma cell dyscrasia and are composed of Kappa light chains but are Congo red negative.[10,11]

WALDENSTRÖM MACROGLOBULINAEMIA

Waldenström macroglobulinemia is most commonly associated with lymphoplasmacytic lymphoma[12] and results from deposits of IgM heavy chains that are kappa light chain restricted. Liver involvement is uncommon[12] and is usually associated with widespread disease. The monoclonal protein deposits in Waldenström macroglobulinemia closely resemble amyloid but can be Congo red negative.[13,14]

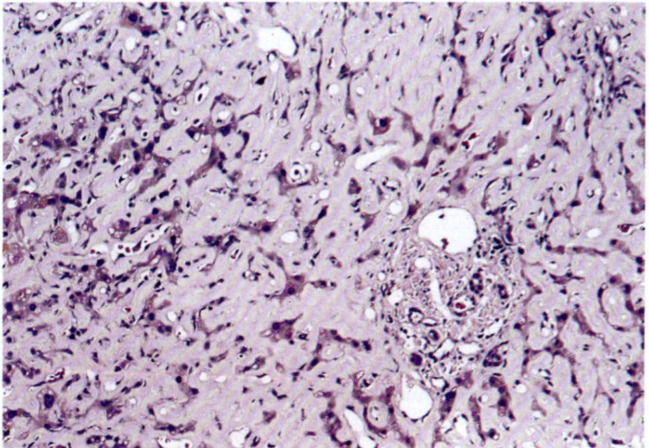

Figure 10.13. **Light chain deposition disease.** Despite the striking H&E findings, A Congo red stain showed only weak equivocal staining without birefringence.

DIABETES MELLITUS

CHECKLIST: Major Patterns of Liver Injury Associated With Diabetes Mellitus

- ☐ Fatty liver disease (type 1 or 2 diabetes mellitus)
- ☐ Glycogenic hepatopathy (type 1 diabetes mostly)
- ☐ Diabetic hepatosclerosis (type 1 or 2 diabetes mellitus)

FATTY LIVER DISEASE

Insulin resistance and/or type 2 diabetes is an important part of the metabolic syndrome, and liver biopsies in that setting show steatosis or steatohepatitis. Individuals with type 1 diabetes but no metabolic syndrome can also develop fatty liver disease. In one study that examined the cause of hepatomegaly in 99 children with type 1 diabetes, the most common cause was either moderate (22%) or marked (19%) glycogen accumulation, but mild steatosis was also present in nearly half of the cases, often accompanying the glycogenosis. In fact, the hepatomegaly in 8% of the children appeared to result primarily from fatty change.[15]

GLYCOGENIC HEPATOPATHY

CHECKLIST: There Is a Triad of Clinical Findings in Glycogenic Hepatopathy

- ☐ Poorly controlled blood sugar levels
- ☐ Elevated liver enzymes
- ☐ Hepatomegaly

Glycogenic hepatopathy (Fig. 10.14) results from poorly controlled blood sugar levels. Almost all cases result from type 1 diabetes, but rare cases can occur with type 2 diabetes (Fig. 10.15).[16] The classic history is months to years of poorly controlled blood sugars levels. At presentation, patients have elevated liver enzyme levels, predominately AST and ALT. The enzyme elevations can be very high, often greater than 10X the upper limit of normal. The enzyme levels will fluctuate over time[17] depending on the control of blood sugar levels. Many patients will get an ultrasound of the liver as part of their clinical evaluation for elevated liver enzymes. Both fatty liver disease and glycogenic hepatopathy appear echogenic on ultrasound evaluation, so the working clinical diagnosis is often fatty liver disease,[18,19] and the biopsy is performed to investigate why the enzyme levels are higher or fluctuate more than is typically seen in fatty liver disease. Once the blood sugar levels are under control, the liver enzymes will normalize and the hepatomegaly will improve or disappear.[20,21] The histological findings will also resolve.[22]

Rarely, patients will present with new onset ascites that suggests advanced liver disease, but instead the ascites results from compression of the hepatic sinusoids by the swollen hepatocytes.[23] The ascites resolves with adequate control of blood sugar.[19,23] The Mauriac syndrome is rarely encountered today because of improvements in diabetes management, but some of the first descriptions of glycogenic hepatopathy were in this setting.[23]

CHECKLIST: Mauriac Syndrome

- ☐ Growth retardation
- ☐ Delayed puberty
- ☐ Cushingoid features
- ☐ Hypercholesterolemia
- ☐ Hepatomegaly
- ☐ Abnormal liver enzymes
- ☐ Glycogenic hepatopathy on liver biopsy

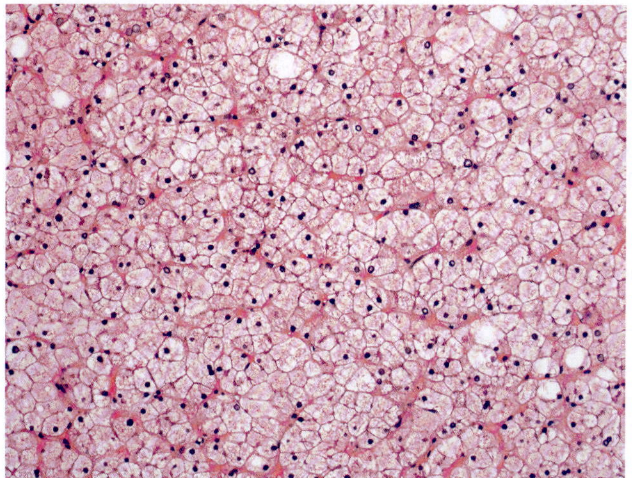

Figure 10.14. **Glycogenic hepatopathy type 1 diabetes mellitus.** The hepatocytes are enlarged and pale because of the glycogen accumulation.

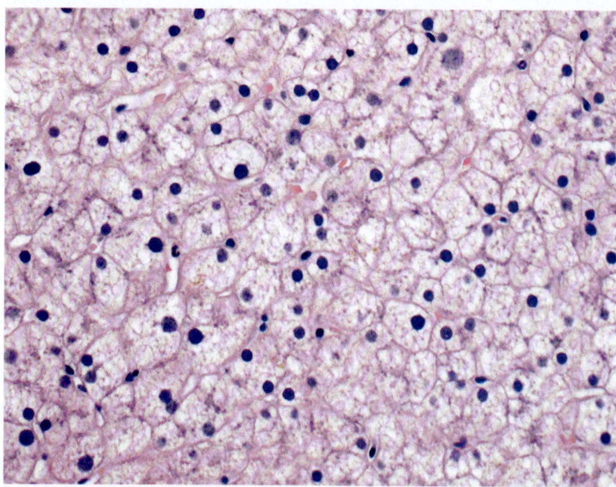

Figure 10.15. **Glycogenic hepatopathy type 2 diabetes mellitus.** This case occurred in an older adult with poorly controlled type 2 diabetes mellitus.

The histological findings of glycogenic hepatopathy are distinctive. Because of the glycogen accumulation, the hepatocytes are normal to enlarged in size and have a pale clear cytoplasm (Fig. 10.14) that tends to accentuate the cell membranes. The glycogenosis can have a zone 3 prominence. The hepatocytes can show mild macrovesicular steatosis (Fig. 10.16), but there is little or no inflammation and typically no ballooned hepatocytes. The histological diagnosis is made on the H&E. A PAS stain will highlight the glycogen, but is not necessary for the diagnosis. In addition, PAS stains can sometimes lead to diagnostic confusion, as even the normal liver will have strong PAS positivity (Fig. 10.17), so the H&E features are necessary and sufficient for the diagnosis of glycogenic hepatopathy.

When combined with the clinical findings, the histological changes are diagnostic of glycogenic hepatopathy. The histological differential for striking glycogenosis also includes glycogen storage disease and recent high-dose steroid use, but correlation with clinical findings will sort out the proper diagnosis. While hepatocyte glycogen depletion is typical in starvation,[24] a number of case reports have counterintuitively found a glycogenic hepatopathy pattern with anorexia nervosa.[25,26] Finally, adults with type 2 diabetes and fatty liver disease (or other liver diseases that lead to biopsies) can show mild subtle zone 3 hepatocyte glycogenosis (Fig. 10.18).[19] This finding most likely represents the same biological processes as seen in glycogenic hepatopathy, reflecting suboptimal control of blood sugar levels, but at this point has no clinical relevance and should not be classified as glycogenic hepatopathy.

CHECKLIST: Differential for the Glycogenosis Pattern of Injury

- ☐ Short-term high-dose steroid therapy[27,28]
- ☐ Anorexia nervosa[25,26]
- ☐ Dumping syndrome secondary to fundoplication for gastroesophageal reflux disease[29]
- ☐ Glycogen storage disease
- ☐ Urea cycle defects[30]

DIABETIC HEPATOSCLEROSIS

Hepatosclerosis is a rare complication of diabetes mellitus that results from systemic microangiopathic disease involving multiple organ systems.[31] Patients can have either type 1 or type 2 diabetes mellitus but always have long-standing histories of insulin dependence. Most patients have end-stage renal disease. Liver enzymes are mildly elevated, typically with a disproportionate elevation in alkaline phosphatase.[31] Patients can also be cholestatic[31] but do not have portal hypertension. The frequency of hepatosclerosis in diabetic patients ranges from 2% to 12% in autopsy studies,[32,33] but this frequency is much higher than is seen in routine liver biopsy specimens, as the livers in patients with end-stage diabetes are rarely biopsied. The published papers also suggest that some autopsy studies are picking up milder cases of hepatosclerosis.

The liver shows dense sinusoidal fibrosis (Fig. 10.19) that is highlighted on the trichrome stain (Fig. 10.20). The perisinusoidal fibrosis typically has a zone 3 accentuation but can extend all the way to zone 1 in severe cases. The biopsy can also show portal fibrosis or bridging fibrosis,[31] but cirrhosis with well-developed parenchymal nodularity has not been reported to date.

Cholestasis, usually mild, is common. Although there can be focal mild bile ductular proliferation, overall the biopsies do not show evidence of biliary obstruction, and the precise cause of the cholestasis is often not clear. Most cases also show diabetes-associated hyaline thickening of the small arteries. Other diabetes associated findings, such as fatty change or glycogenosis, are typically mild or absent.

FAQ: How is the fibrosis in hepatosclerosis different than ordinary pericellular fibrosis?

Answer: The fibrosis in hepatosclerosis (Fig. 10.20) is denser and more diffuse in the lobules than is true for most cases of pericellular fibrosis in the setting of steatohepatitis from the metabolic syndrome (Fig. 10.21). Nonetheless, there is some overlap between hepatosclerosis and severe pericellular fibrosis, so the diagnosis can be guided by other findings. Hepatic arteriolosclerosis is common in diabetic hepatosclerosis, while other findings of fatty liver disease are minimal or absent. The patients in diabetic hepatosclerosis have long-standing histories of diabetes mellitus with insulin dependence and microangiopathic disease in other organs.

Alcoholic liver disease with advanced fibrosis can closely mimic the dense pericellular pattern of fibrosis on trichrome stain (Fig. 10.22). Here again, the correct diagnosis becomes evident when correlated with clinical history. In addition, alcoholic liver disease is much more likely to be associated with active steatohepatitis.

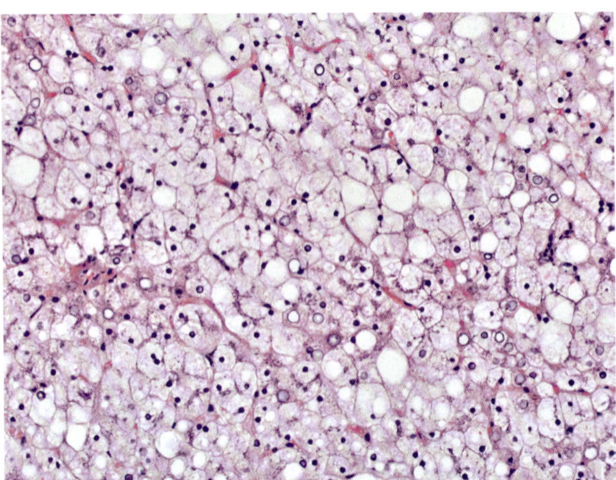

Figure 10.16. **Glycogenic hepatopathy type 1 diabetes mellitus.** Focal mild macrovesicular steatosis can sometimes be present.

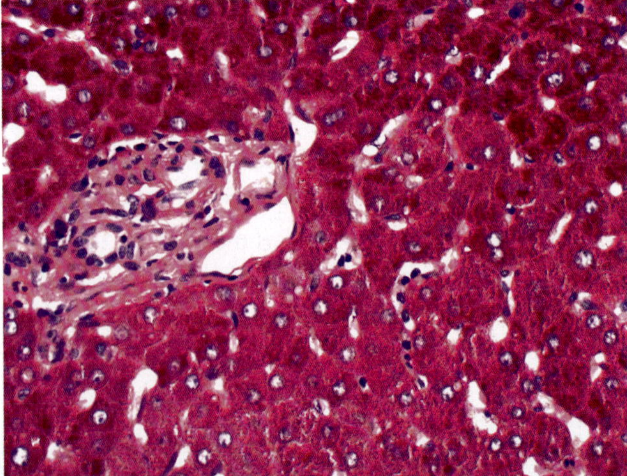

Figure 10.17. **Normal liver, PAS stain.** Normal hepatocytes have a lot of glycogen. Do not mistake this for glycogenic hepatopathy. The diagnosis of glycogenic hepatopathy should be made on the H&E.

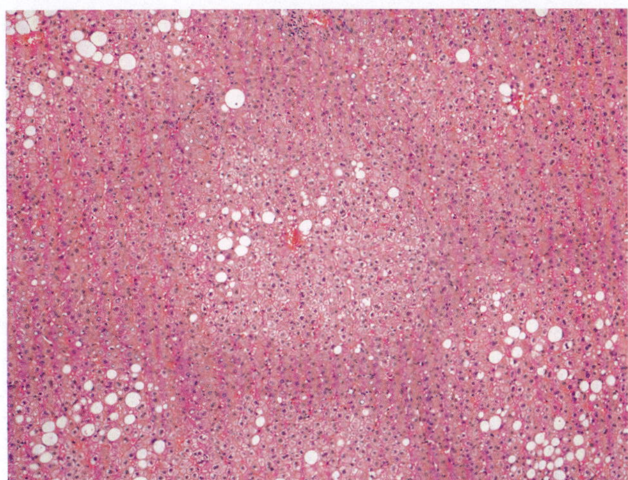

Figure 10.18. **Mild glycogen accumulation in the metabolic syndrome.** The zone 3 hepatocytes show mild glycogenosis. This pattern of subtle glycogen accumulation should not be mistaken for glycogenic hepatopathy. The patient had the metabolic syndrome, and the biopsy showed steatohepatitis as the main pattern of injury.

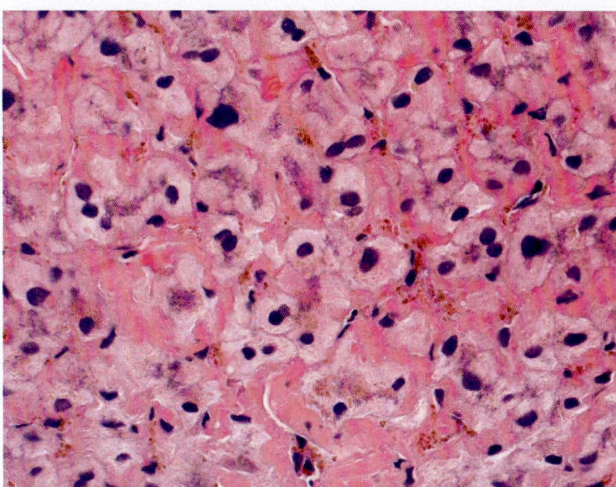

Figure 10.19. **Diabetic hepatosclerosis.** Perisinusoidal fibrosis is evident on the H&E. The biopsy otherwise showed no fat and only minimal nonspecific inflammation.

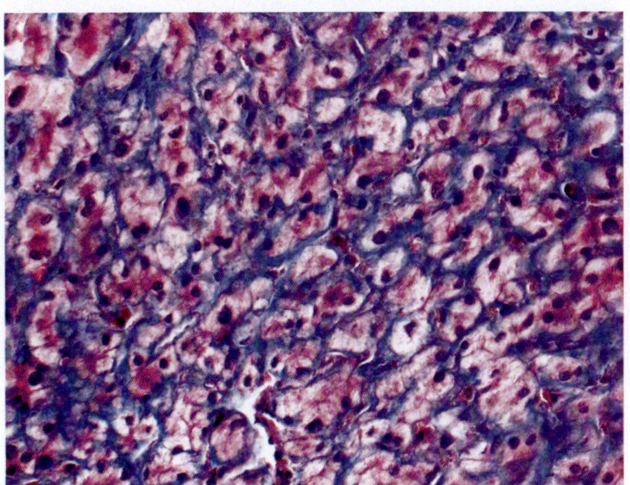

Figure 10.20. **Diabetic hepatosclerosis, trichrome stain.** The lobules show dense diffuse perisinusoidal fibrosis.

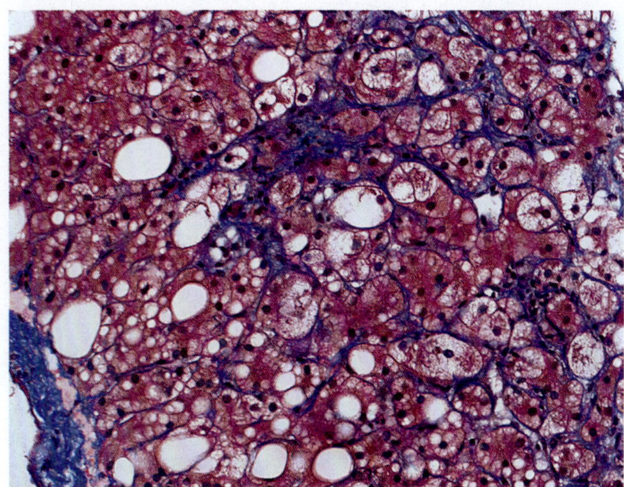

Figure 10.21. **Ordinary steatohepatitis, trichrome stain.** The pericellular fibrosis tends to be more irregular than in diabetic hepatosclerosis.

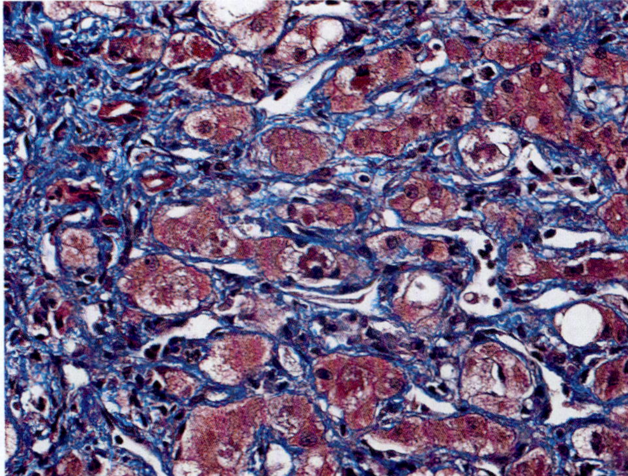

Figure 10.22. **Alcoholic liver disease, pericellular fibrosis.** In this case, the dense pericellular fibrosis does mimic that of diabetic hepatosclerosis, but correlation with the rest of the histological findings and with the clinical findings clarifies the diagnosis.

OTHER ENDOCRINE DISEASES

HYPOPITUITARY DISEASE

Hypopituitary disease affecting the liver is most commonly encountered in pediatric surgical pathology specimens. In children, the most common cause is septo-optic dysplasia, which leads to hypopituitarism as well as hypoplasia of the optic nerve and an absent septum pellucidum. Biopsies show a cholestatic pattern of injury with either a bland lobular cholestasis pattern (Fig. 10.23) or a neonatal giant cell hepatitis pattern (Fig. 10.24).[34,35] Other common findings include bile duct hypoplasia.[34,35] Fibrosis is portal based and usually mild or absent, but sometimes can be advanced. In older children, the cholestasis is minimal or absent, but there can be a wide variety of other mild changes (Fig. 10.25). Hypopituitary disease in adults is seen most commonly following trauma or pituitary surgery. In adults, fatty liver disease is the most common pattern of injury and can include either steatosis or steatohepatitis, especially when there is growth hormone deficiency.[36]

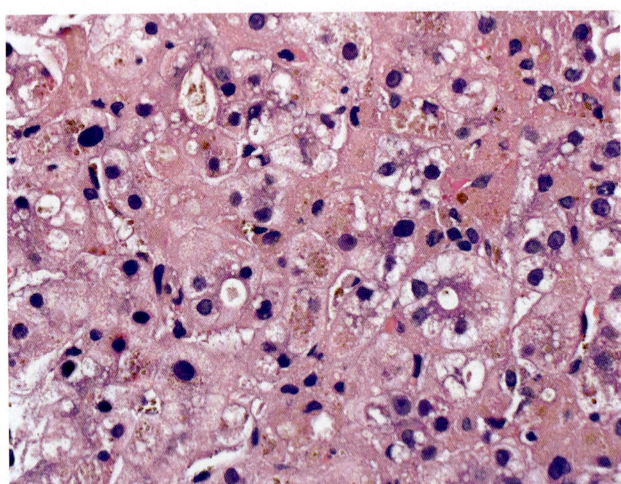

Figure 10.23. **Hypopituitary disease.** In this child with septo-optic dysplasia, the biopsy shows bland lobular cholestasis. There is no significant inflammation and no evidence for biliary obstruction.

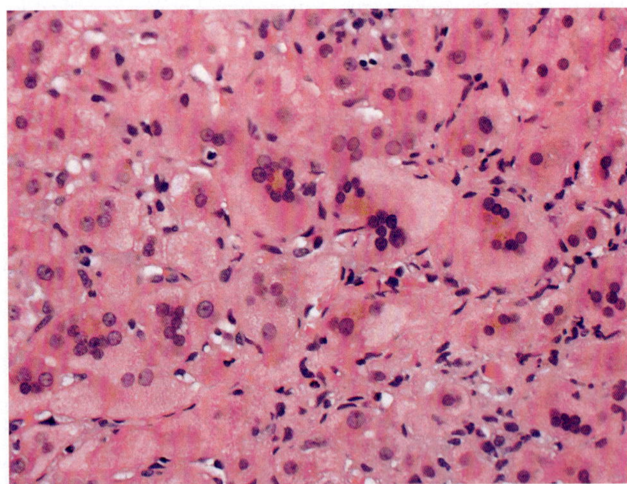

Figure 10.24. **Hypopituitary disease.** In this child with septo-optic dysplasia, the biopsy shows a neonatal giant cell hepatitis pattern of injury.

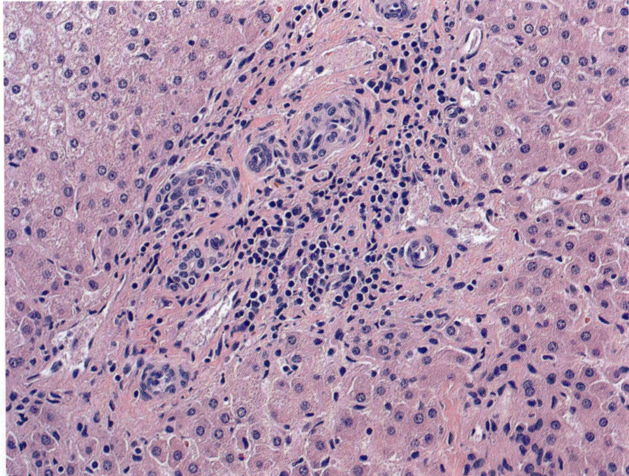

Figure 10.25. **Hypopituitary disease.** This wedge biopsy was taken in an older child and shows portal vein atrophy, mild nodular regeneration, and mild nonspecific portal inflammation, but no cholestasis.

THYROID DISEASE

Both hypothyroid disease and hyperthyroid disease can be associated with mild elevations in liver enzymes,[37,38] especially if the thyroid dysfunction is marked. The frequency of elevated liver enzymes in hyperthyroid disease is about 40%.[39] Hyperthyroid disease tends to be associated with elevated ALT and alkaline phosphatase levels, while hypothyroidism with elevated AST levels.[40] However, biopsies are rarely performed, so the histological changes are not well defined. Severe hyperthyroid disease has been associated in several studies with jaundice and a bland cholestatic pattern on biopsy, with marked cholestasis and little or no inflammation.[41–44] Treatments for thyroid disease can also lead to drug reactions, but in these cases, the enzyme elevations tend to be more significantly elevated.

INFLAMMATORY CONDITIONS

CELIAC DISEASE

Liver enzyme elevations are found in 30% of individuals with celiac disease[45] and, conversely, 4% of individuals with unexplained liver enzyme elevations will eventually be diagnosed with celiac disease. The enzyme elevations are typically mild and less than 2-3X the upper normal of limits.[46] The enzymes levels will normalize when patients have a good clinical response to a gluten-free diet, although the normalization may take several months.

The histology has been described in many papers, which have generally all found the about the same things.[47–52] The injury patterns include (1) mild nonspecific inflammation ("reactive hepatitis"), (2) a chronic hepatitis pattern, (3) fatty liver disease, (4) cryptogenic cirrhosis, (5) portal vein abnormalities and nodular regenerative hyperplasia,[53,54] (6) and finally other concomitant diseases such as primary sclerosing cholangitis, primary biliary cirrhosis, or autoimmune hepatitis. The first four patterns represent changes from a combination of malnutrition and bacterial antigens from the small bowel entering the portal circulation, both resulting from inflammation of the small bowel. In terms of concomitant diseases, meta-analysis and large epidemiological studies link celiac disease to an increased risk primarily for primary biliary cirrhosis and autoimmune hepatitis.[46]

COMMON VARIABLE IMMUNODEFICIENCY

Common variable immunodeficiency can be associated with several patterns of injury. Most cases show a mild nonspecific hepatitis pattern, especially when there is inflammatory disease of the small bowel.[55–57] Mild macrovesicular steatosis is not uncommon (Fig. 10.26). Nodular regenerative hyperplasia is also common and can lead to portal hypertension.[58–60] Granulomas are seen in about 40% of biopsies. They are typically small and epithelioid (Fig. 10.27) and can be found in both the portal tracts and the lobules.[55,61,62] Mild portal fibrosis is common but not advanced fibrosis.[55]

CROHN DISEASE

CHECKLIST: Injury Patterns in Crohn Disease

- ☐ Primary sclerosing cholangitis
- ☐ Drug effects
- ☐ Opportunistic infections
- ☐ Mild nonspecific inflammation
- ☐ Isolated granulomas
- ☐ Concurrent diseases such as fatty liver disease

Crohn disease can be associated with elevated liver enzymes for many different reasons. In cases without biochemical evidence for liver disease, biopsies show minimal nonspecific changes.[63] The most common reason to perform a biopsy is to evaluate for primary sclerosing cholangitis (Fig. 10.28). Primary sclerosing cholangitis affects 1% to 2% of individuals with Crohn disease, and the histology is essentially the same as that seen with primary sclerosing cholangitis in other settings.

A number of other injury patterns can be seen beyond biliary tract disease. Immunosuppression can lead to viral hepatitis from CMV, EBV, or other opportunistic organisms. Drug affects can cause a hepatitis or pseudo-ground glass change. Patients can have fatty liver disease resulting from medications or the metabolic syndrome. Other patterns of injury tend to be mild and nonspecific and generally do not elicit biopsies. These can include granulomas, which are usually isolated or with a background of mild nonspecific inflammation but not a true granulomatous hepatitis. A true granulomatous hepatitis pattern is not typical for Crohn disease (Fig. 10.29) and requires exclusion of infection and drug effect. Finally, a mild nonspecific hepatitis can result from inflammation of the small intestine, leading to mucosal injury and transgression of antigens from the intestinal lumen into the portal circulation.

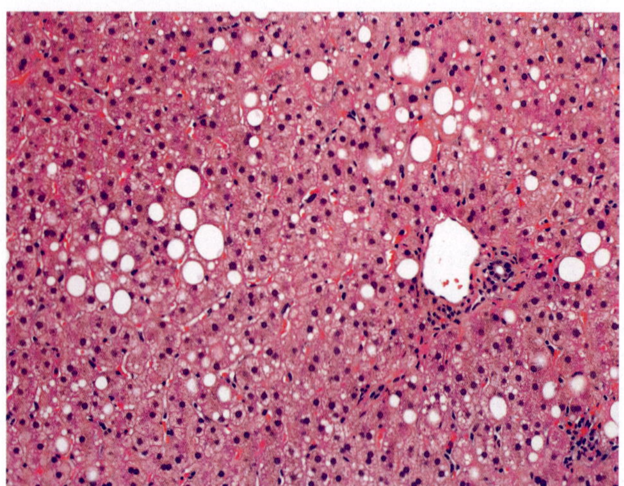

Figure 10.26. Common variable immunodeficiency. This case showed a mild nonspecific pattern of inflammation with mild patchy macrovesicular steatosis.

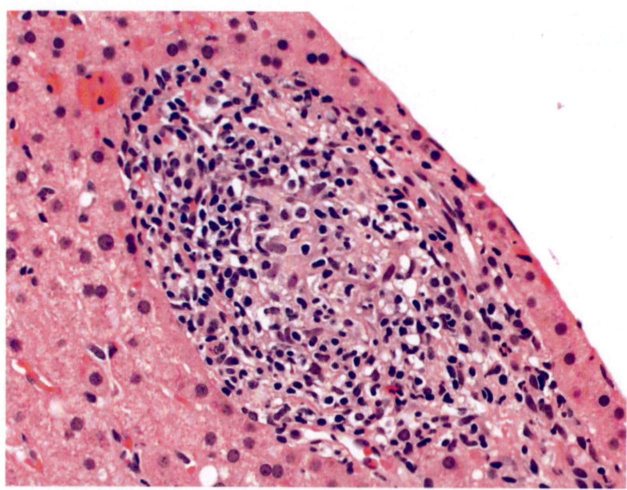

Figure 10.27. Common variable immunodeficiency. A small lobular granuloma is present. This finding is not specific for CVID of course but is a fairly common finding.

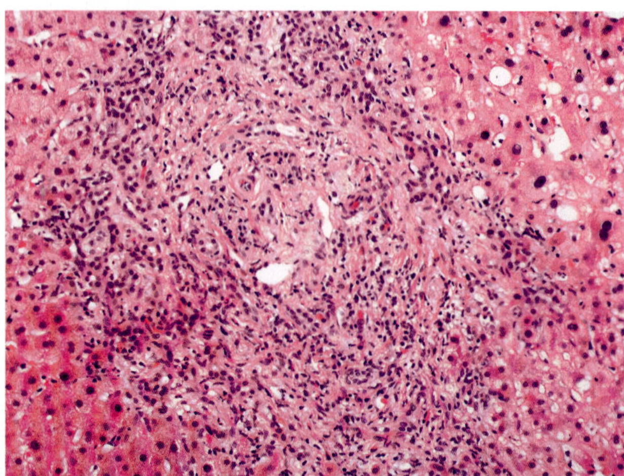

Figure 10.28. Crohn disease and primary sclerosing cholangitis. The patient had a predominant elevation in alkaline phosphatase levels and equivocal bile duct changes on imaging studies. The biopsy showed typical findings of obstructive biliary tract disease, consistent with primary sclerosing cholangitis.

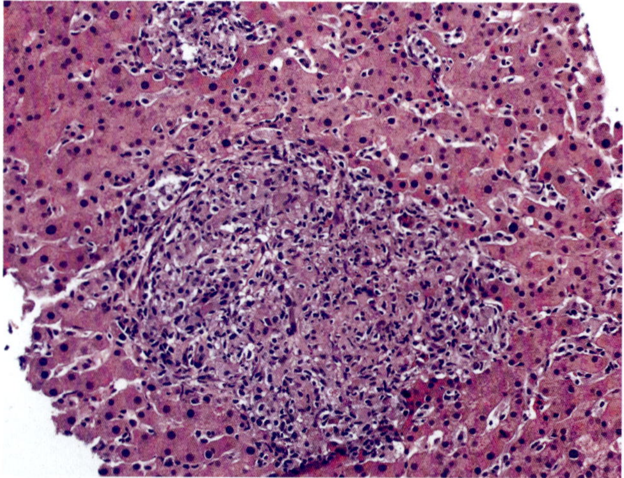

Figure 10.29. Crohn disease and granulomatous hepatitis. The patient developed marked elevations in liver enzymes, prompting a liver biopsy. This degree of inflammation and the numerous granulomas are inconsistent with Crohn disease. A GMS stain showed histoplasmosis hepatitis.

SYSTEMIC AUTOIMMUNE DISEASE

CHECKLIST: Systemic Autoimmune Conditions That Can Have Mild Nonspecific Patterns of Injury

- ☐ Common variable immunodeficiency (see also section above)
- ☐ Systemic lupus erythematosus
- ☐ Rheumatoid arthritis
- ☐ Juvenile rheumatoid arthritis
- ☐ Adult Still disease
- ☐ Various connective tissue disorders

A wide range of systemic autoimmune conditions can be associated with elevations in liver enzymes. The enzyme elevations are mild and persistent or show intermittent elevations. Serological testing for ANA can be strongly positive, reflecting the systemic autoimmune condition. Positive testing for anti-smooth muscle antibodies (do not confuse with anti-Sm antibodies, which stands for anti-Smith antibodies, and are seen in a subset of Lupus cases), while not specific, is more concerning for autoimmune hepatitis.

Liver biopsies will typically show mild changes that tend to fall into one of three basic injury patterns: mild nonspecific hepatitis, mild steatosis without steatohepatitis, or nodular regenerative hyperplasia. An individual case can sometimes show a mixed pattern, but the histological changes overall tend to be mild and nonspecific. Cases with a mild nonspecific hepatitis pattern (Fig. 10.30) should not be mistaken for autoimmune hepatitis, as they do not have either the standard clinical or histological findings, and there is no evidence that they lead to fibrosis. An older term for this pattern of mild nonspecific hepatitis is *reactive hepatitis*, but this tends to be an unsatisfying diagnosis to clinicians, so it is often better to describe what you see and write a note explaining what it means. The histological differential for the mild nonspecific hepatitis pattern can include a drug reaction. In this setting, it can be very helpful to correlate the start of the enzyme elevations with the introduction of any new medications.

Many systemic autoimmune diseases also have an increased risk for autoimmune hepatitis; in these cases, the liver enzyme elevations are more striking (>2 ULN), and the liver biopsy shows changes typical for autoimmune hepatitis. Of course, individuals with systemic autoimmune conditions can also have other diseases, such as biliary obstruction from gallstones or steatohepatitis from alcohol use or the metabolic syndrome, so the patterns of injury may reflect a superimposed injury on the background of a mild nonspecific hepatitis pattern. In these cases, there commonly is a history of recent increases in liver enzymes to levels that are significantly above baseline.

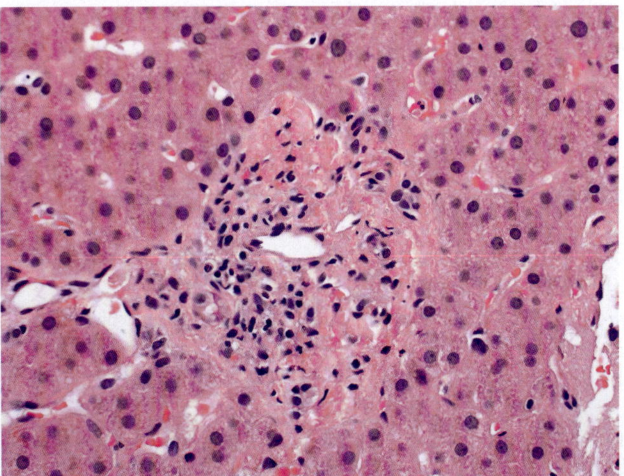

Figure 10.30. **Systemic lupus erythematosus.** A liver biopsy showed mild nonspecific portal inflammation. There was no plasma cell enrichment, and lobular inflammation was minimal. This pattern is sometimes called a *reactive hepatitis.*

LIVER DISEASE IN PREGNANCY

CHECKLIST: Liver Diseases in Pregnancy

- □ Hyperemesis gravidarum
- □ Intrahepatic cholestasis of pregnancy
- □ Preeclampsia, eclampsia, and HELLP syndrome
- □ Acute fatty liver of pregnancy
- □ Preexisting liver diseases can also be first diagnosed during pregnancy, such as autoimmune hepatitis and chronic viral hepatitis

HYPEREMESIS GRAVIDARUM

Hyperemesis gravidarum is defined as intractable nausea and vomiting that leads to dehydration, ketosis, and weight loss of at least 5%.[64] Liver enzymes are elevated in greater than 50% of individuals who require hospitalization because of the hyperemesis. ALT levels are usually higher than AST levels and range from 2 to 5 times the upper limit of normal.[64] They return to normal when the vomiting resolves.[65] If they do not return to normal, further workup is needed for other liver diseases. Liver biopsies are not part of patient management, and the histology has not been well described (Table 10.1).

INTRAHEPATIC CHOLESTASIS OF PREGNANCY

Intrahepatic cholestasis of pregnancy is the most common pregnancy-associated liver disease. The frequency of disease shows significant regional variation. For example, the frequency is about 1% in the United States but is about 15% in some parts of Chile.[66] Other risk factors include fertility treatments, multiple gestations, and a prior pregnancy with intrahepatic cholestasis of pregnancy. Patients present in the second or third trimester with pruritis, which is often worse on the palms and soles. Bilirubin levels can be normal or mildly elevated, while serum bile acid levels are invariably elevated. Liver enzyme levels can also be elevated, but risk for poor perinatal outcomes is related to bile acid levels and not liver enzyme levels. The patients' symptoms resolve within 6 weeks of delivery.

Liver biopsies are not part of patient management, so the histology has not been well described but shows a bland lobular cholestasis pattern with little or no portal or lobular inflammation.[67,68] There can be mild lobular spotty necrosis. There is no risk for fibrosis. Of note, some patients will have underlying liver diseases, with enrichment for chronic hepatitis C[64] and possibly primary biliary cirrhosis,[69] and in these cases, the liver biopsies will also show changes of their underlying disease.

About 15% of patients with a diagnosis of intrahepatic cholestasis of pregnancy have defects in bile transport proteins, mostly ABCB11 or ABCB4, but also a number of others.[64] These patients are at increased risk for gallstones and cholestatic liver disease, even after delivery.

FAQ: What is the difference between bile salts and bilirubin?

Answer: Bile acids are produced in the liver by modifying steroids. When they are conjugated, they are called bile salts. The major bile acids are the following: taurocholic acid, glycocholic acid (or cholic acid), taurochenodeoxycholic acid, and glycochenodeoxycholic acid. These bile salts are secreted into the bile and move to the small bowel where they play a critical role in digestion by emulsifying various fats and oils.

In contrast, bilirubin results from the breakdown of heme and is excreted into the bile. Bilirubin is conjugated to make it water soluble and is not reabsorbed in the terminal ileum, in contrast to most of the bile acids.

TABLE 10.1: Liver Disease in Pregnancy

Disease	Trimester	Frequency	Clinical Risk	Major Liver Findings
Hyperemesis gravidarum	First	1% to 2%	Dehydration	ALT 2-5 ULN Total bilirubin: Normal Serum bile acids: Normal Histology not described
Intrahepatic cholestasis of pregnancy	Second or more commonly third	1% to 15%, strong regional variation	Preterm labor Still birth	ALT 2-8 ULN Total bilirubin: Normal or mildly elevated Serum bile acids: Elevated Histology: bland lobular cholestasis pattern
Preeclampsia/ HELLP	Third	7%	Renal dysfunction Cerbral hemmorrage Hepatic infarct/ rupture Maternal death Fetal death	ALT 2-30 ULN Total bilirubin: Normal (preeclampsia) to 10 ULN (HELLP) Serum bile acids: Normal Histology: periportal hemorrhage with fibrin deposition
Acute fatty liver of pregnancy	Third	<1%	Maternal death Fetal death	ALT 2-20 ULN Total bilirubin: 2-10 ULN Serum bile acids: Normal Histology: microvesicular steotosis

HELLP, hemolysis, elevated liver enzymes, low platelets.

PREECLAMPSIA, ECLAMPSIA, AND HELLP SYNDROME

Preeclampsia is defined as de novo hypertension developing after the 20th week of pregnancy, with a blood pressure of 140/90 or greater, plus proteinuria. A smaller group of cases are diagnosed based on new-onset blood pressure elevations without proteinuria when other clinical findings are present, such as pulmonary edema, visual symptoms, elevated liver enzymes 2X baseline, or thrombocytopenia. The disease can occasionally present after delivery. Preeclampsia appears to result from abnormal placentation, leading the placenta to secrete factors that lead to hypertension, such as nitric oxide and prostaglandins. Recognized risk factors include a prior pregnancy with hypertension or preeclampsia, diabetes, body mass index (BMI) >35, twin pregnancy, and maternal age >40 years. About 30% of patients with preeclampsia will have elevated liver enzymes, and about half of these will have a severe form of preeclampsia called the HELLP syndrome (hemolysis, elevated liver enzymes, low platelets). Eclampsia is defined as the additional presence of seizures.

Liver biopsies are not part of routine patient management because the diagnosis is based on clinical and laboratory findings, and there is a risk for bleeding in patients with low platelet counts. However, the pathology has been reasonably well described for both preeclampasia and the HELLP syndrome.[70,71] The liver biopsy shows zone 1 hemorrhage and fibrin deposition (Fig. 10.31) with minimal or no inflammation. Lobular cholestasis is common. There is no macrovesicular steatosis, unless the patient has the metabolic syndrome or other risk factors, but in about 25% of cases, the hepatocytes can show some degree of microvesicular steatosis.[71,72] Severe cases can develop liver infarction and intrahepatic bleeding with hematoma formation, usually in a subcapsular location. The hemorrhage and necrosis can also lead to spontaneous rupture of the liver.

ACUTE FATTY LIVER OF PREGNANCY

Acute fatty liver of pregnancy is rare, with a frequency of approximately 1 per 20,000 deliveries.[64] The disease usually presents between the 30th and 38th week of pregnancy but can develop after delivery in 20% of cases. Risk factors include twins or triplets, nulliparity, and male infants. Preecclampsia is commonly present. The disease etiology is not entirely clear, but it leads to mitochondrial failure and high concentrations of beta fatty acid oxidation metabolites. Inherited defects in beta-oxidation of fatty acids increase the risk for fatty liver of pregnancy, including mutations in the alpha subunit of long-chain 3-hyroxyacly-CoA dehydrogenase (HADHA gene), carnitine paalmitoyltransferaase I, and short and medium chain acyl-CoA dehydrogenase deficiency.[66] After delivery, infants with these mutations can develop a life-threatening metabolic crisis, so genetic testing has been recommended for all babies born to a mother with acute fatty liver of pregnancy.[66]

Historically, the diagnosis of acute fatty liver of pregnancy was based on liver biopsy, but this has shifted to a clinical diagnosis based a variety of clinical findings and laboratory testing (Swansea criteria).[73] When the liver is biopsied, the main histological finding is diffuse microvesicular steatosis (Fig. 10.32),[74–76] sometimes with a zone 3 accentuation. Macrovesicular steatosis can also be present, but the predominant pattern is microvesicular steatosis. Mild to moderate lobular cholestasis is common and is usually accompanied by Kupffer cell hyperplasia. Other findings include scattered acidophil bodies and prominent megamitochondria.[75] Cases can also have zone 1 hemorrhage when there is coexisting HELLP syndrome.

The histological diagnosis of acute fatty liver of pregnancy is based on H&E findings, and an Oil red O stain is not necessary. In fact, if your laboratory does not use the Oil red O stain often, then using the stain in this setting will often lead to more confusion than clarity (Fig. 10.33). Finally, several studies have reported a lymphoplasmacytic lobular hepatitic pattern that mimicked viral hepatitis but was interpreted as acute fatty liver of pregnancy.[74,76,77] However, it is not clear if these cases only had acute fatty liver disease of pregnancy or perhaps had another concomitant disease. In any case, if you see this pattern, coexisting hepatic diseases should be carefully excluded. After delivery, the histological findings rapidly improve and largely disappear by three weeks, leaving no residual disease and no fibrosis.

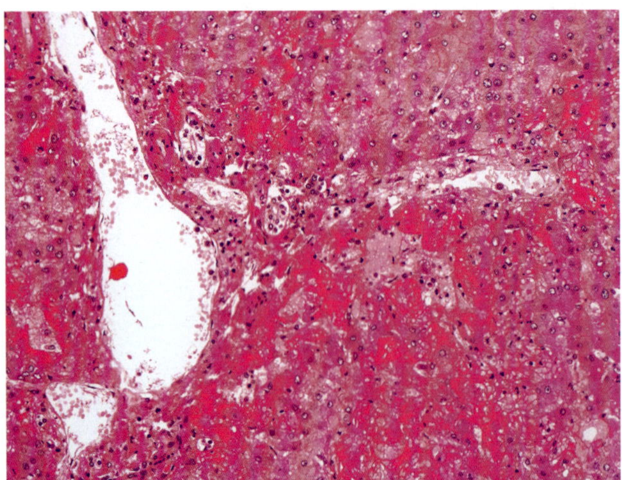

Figure 10.31. **HELLP (hemolysis, elevated liver enzymes, low platelets) syndrome.** The zone 1 region shows hemorrhage and fibrin deposition.

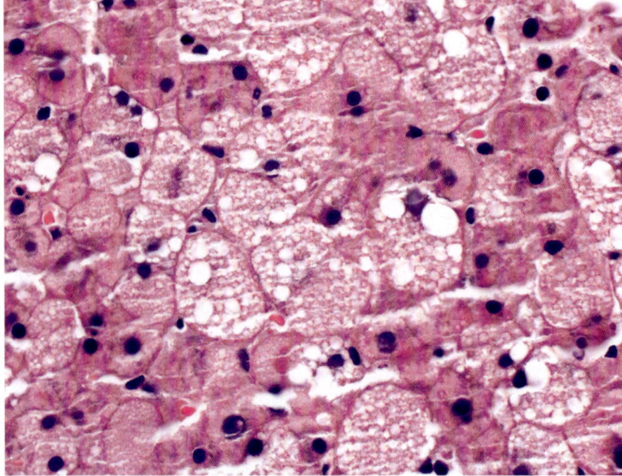

Figure 10.32. **Acute fatty liver of pregnancy.** The hepatocytes show diffuse microvesicular steatosis.

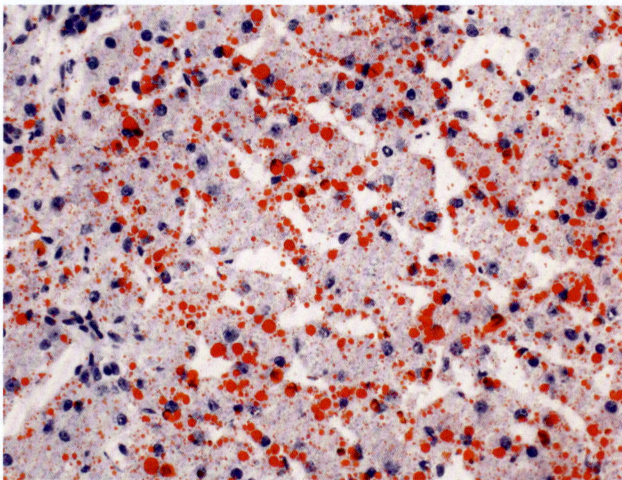

Figure 10.33. **Normal liver, Oil red O stain.** This liver wedge biopsy from a donor liver shows abundant staining but was histologically normal. Fundamentally, microvesicular steatosis is an H&E diagnosis.

HEMATOPATHOLOGY-RELATED DISEASES

LANGERHANS HISTIOCYTOSIS

Langerhans histiocytosis is a systemic disease but frequently has liver involvement, which is a negative prognostic indicator.[78] Clinically, hepatomegaly is present in many cases and blood testing shows a cholestatic pattern of liver enzyme elevations.[79,80] On biopsy, the histiocytosis tends to fall into several major patterns. In early disease, there can be a subtle infiltration of mainly the portal tracts. As the disease progresses, there is bile duct injury with changes of secondary biliary sclerosis (Fig. 10.34). In biopsy specimens, the latter pattern is more common.[78] The portal tracts often show mixed inflammation, and eosinophils are prominent in some cases (Fig. 10.35). The bile ducts can be infiltrated and injured by the Langerhans cells. The portal tracts can also show a bile ductular reaction, and the overall findings can mimic primary sclerosing cholangitis. Rarely, granulomas can be found (Fig. 10.36).[81] While hard to see on H&E (Fig. 10.37), Langerhans cells are also found in the lobules. In addition, the lobules often show cholestasis. Langerhans histiocytosis in some cases can lead to fibrosis and cirrhosis.[81]

The changes can be very subtle on H&E, and immunostains can be very helpful in making the diagnosis. The Langerhans cells are positive for Langerin (Fig. 10.38), CD1a, and S100.

ROSAI DORFMAN DISEASE

Rosai Dorfman disease results from a proliferation of histiocytes and is also called sinus histiocytosis with massive lymphadenopathy. The disease is somewhat more common in children less than 10 years of age, but can affect all ages. The cause is unknown, but patients present with infection-like symptoms including fever and elevated white blood cell counts. There is typically no history of immunosuppression, but a subset of patients will have cooccurring lymphoma.[82] Patients have enlarged lymph nodes, especially cervical lymph nodes, skin disease, and upper respiratory tract disease.[83]

When the liver is involved, it is usually part of systemic disease. Liver involvement typically manifests as hepatomegaly, but rarely there can be a mass lesion.[84] Biopsies show mixed portal inflammation with histiocytes predominating but also lymphocytes, plasma cells, and eosinophils (Fig. 10.39). Bile duct injury is common and, in some cases, can be striking. In some cases, the inflammation can appear granulomatous.[84] The portal veins can be atrophic or absent. The abnormal histiocytes can be subtle and focal, so a high degree of suspicion is often needed. The histiocytes have moderately abundant pale to

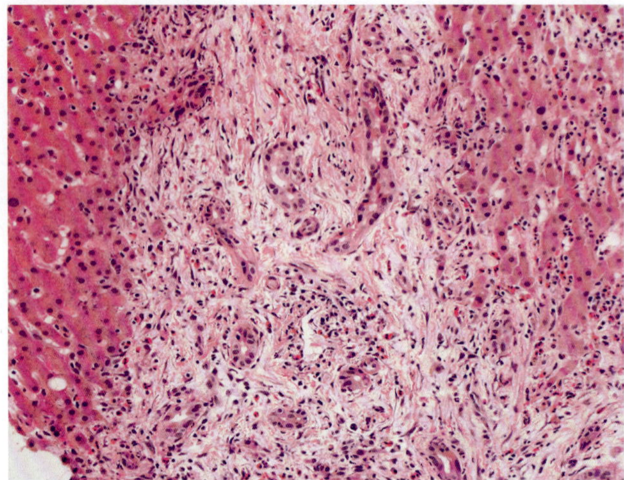

Figure 10.34. **Langerhans histiocytosis.** At low power, the portal tracts show bile ductular proliferation and fibrosis, mimicking biliary obstruction.

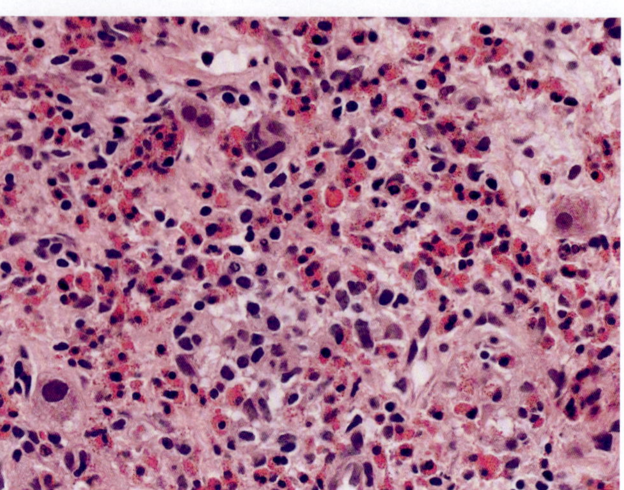

Figure 10.35. **Langerhans histiocytosis.** In this case the portal tracts had dense inflammation that was rich in eosinophils.

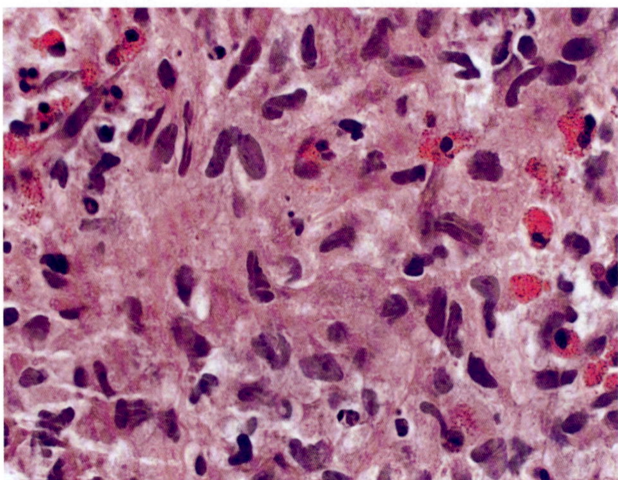

Figure 10.36. **Langerhans histiocytosis.** At higher power, the inflammation was vaguely granulomatous with clusters of Langerhan cells showing abundant eosinophilic cytoplasm and elongated nuclei.

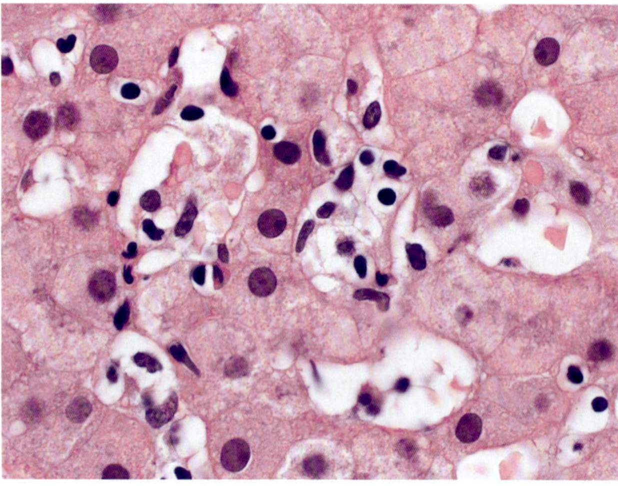

Figure 10.37. **Langerhans histiocytosis.** In this case, Langerhans cells in the sinusoids were also evident in retrospect on H&E and show clear cytoplasm.

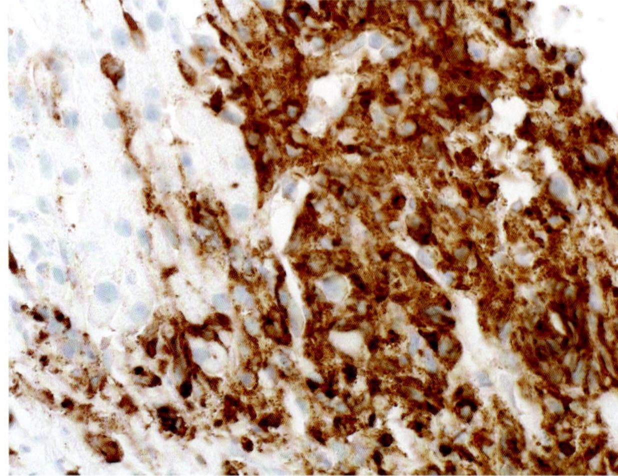

Figure 10.38. **Langerhans histiocytosis.** A Langerin stain is strongly positive.

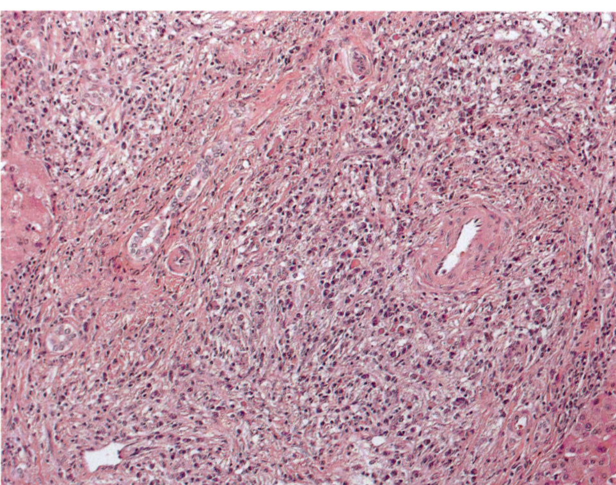

Figure 10.39. **Rosai Dorfman disease.** The portal tracts show dense mixed inflammation with histiocytes, lymphocytes, eosinophils, and a mild prominence in plasma cells.

eosinophilic cytoplasm and typically well rounded nuclei, but also commonly show some degree of nuclear irregularities. Nucleoli are often prominent. In contrast to the changes seen in lymph nodes, lymphophagocytosis is rarely seen on liver biopsy specimens.[84] The histiocytes cells are strongly S100 (Fig. 10.40) and CD68 positive but are CD1a negative.

MAST CELL DISEASE

The liver can be involved whenever there is systemic mastocytosis. Most patients will have hepatomegaly and alkaline phosphatase elevations.[85] Mast cells are found in both the portal tracts and the sinusoids. There can be bile duct injury, bile ductular proliferation, and portal fibrosis, with a pattern that resembles primary sclerosing cholangitis.[86–88] Other findings can include portal venopathy, nodular regenerative hyperplasia, and venoocclusive disease.[89] In some patients, cirrhosis can develop.[90]

In some cases, the liver biopsy is essentially normal on H&E or shows only mild nonspecific changes, with mast cells only evident on special stains. When they are visible on H&E, the mast cells tend to have moderately abundant pale to clear cytoplasm with round to oval nuclei and small nucleoli (Figs. 10.41 and 10.42). Immunostains are very helpful in confirming the diagnosis, as the mast cells are positive for CKIT (Fig. 10.43), mast cell tryptase, and CD25.

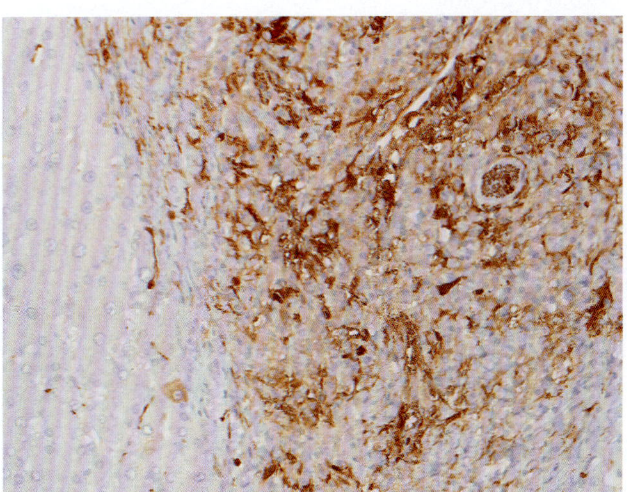

Figure 10.40. **Rosai Dorfman disease, S100.** An S100 stain is strongly positive.

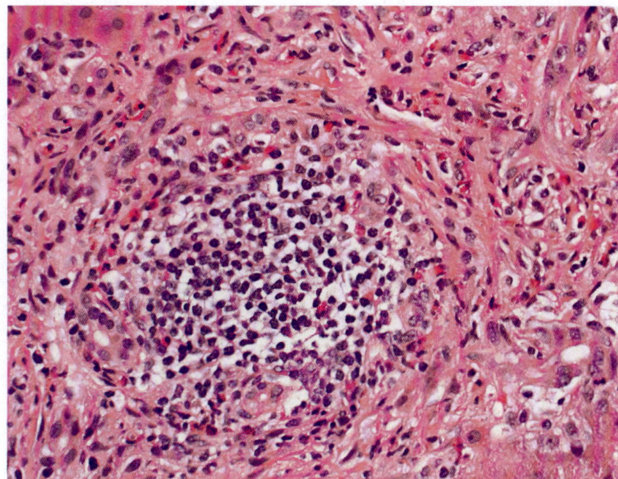

Figure 10.41. **Mast cell disease.** The portal track shows an infiltrate of round to oval cells with clear cytoplasm. A lot of eosinophils are also present.

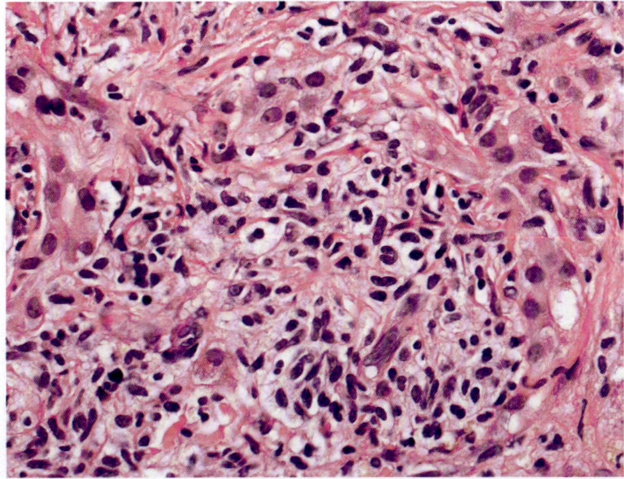

Figure 10.42. **Mast cell disease.** On higher power, the mast cells show moderately abundant clear cytoplasm with oval to round nuclei and inconspicuous nucleoli.

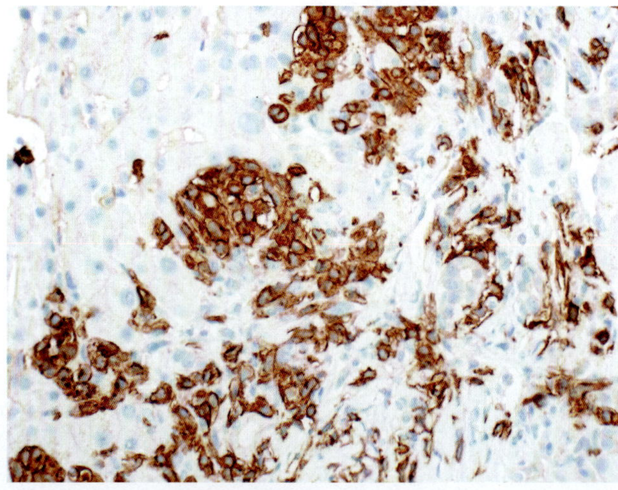

Figure 10.43. **Mast cell disease, CKIT stain.** The mast cells are strongly CKIT positive. A lot more positivity is seen on the immunostain than was expected based on the H&E, a common finding.

OTHER SYSTEMIC DIEASES

CYSTIC FIBROSIS

Cystic fibrosis results from *CFTR* mutations and leads to thick viscus secretions that "clog up the pipes," with inspissated secretions accumulating in the airways, pancreas, and biliary tree. Liver involvement leads to mildly elevated liver enzymes. Liver disease can present in infancy but tends to resolve temporarily, becoming evident again in the early teenage years.[91] Overall, approximately 40% of teenagers and young adults develop elevated liver enzymes. Elevated liver enzymes do not usually prompt a liver biopsy unless there also is hepatomegaly, splenomegaly, or esophageal varices. Even in these situations, noninvasive methods for evaluating fibrosis have largely replaced liver biopsies, which are now performed mostly to rule out other diseases or when the results of clinical and imaging findings are discordant.

Liver biopsies show a biliary obstruction pattern of injury with bile ductular proliferation, mixed portal inflammation, and portal-based fibrosis (Fig. 10.44). The biliary changes can be very patchy on biopsy. It is unusual to actually find inspissated secretions in the bile ducts in needle biopsies, being found in about 5% of cases at best (Fig. 10.45).[92] With disease progression, imaging studies can show both intrahepatic and extrahepatic bile duct dilatation and strictures.[93] Imaging also shows a microgallbladder in about one-fourth of cases. Cholelithiasis develops in 10% of patients.

In addition to biliary tract disease, macrovesicular steatosis is common, being present in 60% of cases (Fig. 10.46), and can be moderate or severe in 30% of cases.[91,92] Steatohepatitis can be seen but is less common. It is unclear how much the fatty liver contributes to fibrosis, but most of the fibrosis risk appears to be driven by the biliary tract disease. Other findings can include portal vein loss and nodular regenerative hyperplasia.[94,95]

In most cases, fibrosis starts in late childhood and early teenage years.[91] As fibrosis progresses, it can be very patchy early on with portal and bridging fibrosis in some needle cores, yet no fibrosis in other cores, a pattern sometimes called "focal biliary cirrhosis" in the cystic fibrosis literature. Fibrosis can be present even if liver enzymes are normal, but fibrosis is more common in those individuals with persistently elevated liver enzymes (about 50% of all patients). In the subgroup of patients with persistently elevated liver enzymes, about 10% develop advanced fibrosis.[91,92]

HYPERTENSION, SYSTEMIC

A liver biopsy is not part of the clinical management for systemic hypertension, but individuals with systemic hypertension can be biopsied for other reasons. While the changes of systemic hypertension are usually incidental findings, they are distinctive (Fig. 10.47). The smaller arteries sampled in liver biopsy specimens sometimes show striking hyalinosis.[96] Most affected patients also have type 2 diabetes mellitus. Sometimes the hyalinosis can resemble amyloid deposits, which can be ruled out with Congo red stains. About 1/3 of patients also show mild bile duct changes, with focal bile duct loss and/or mild patchy bile ductular proliferation. These changes may represent low-grade ischemia secondary to the arteriolosclerosis.

SEPSIS

Liver biopsies are not typically performed as part of the workup for sepsis, but the histology has been describe in cases biopsied for other reasons and at autopsy. The most common patterns of injury are a nonspecific hepatitis, fatty change (Figs. 10.48 and 10.49), or bland lobular cholestasis.[97] In fact, sepsis is a common cause of jaundice in hospitalized patients. A cholangiolar pattern of cholestasis, where the proliferating bile ductules have bile plugs, can be seen in patients with debilitating, long-standing illness, with or without sepsis (Fig. 10.50). Rarely, fibrin thrombi can be seen in the smaller branches of the portal veins in patient with sepsis (Fig. 10.51). Finally, zone 3 necrosis can be present in cases with significant hypotension.

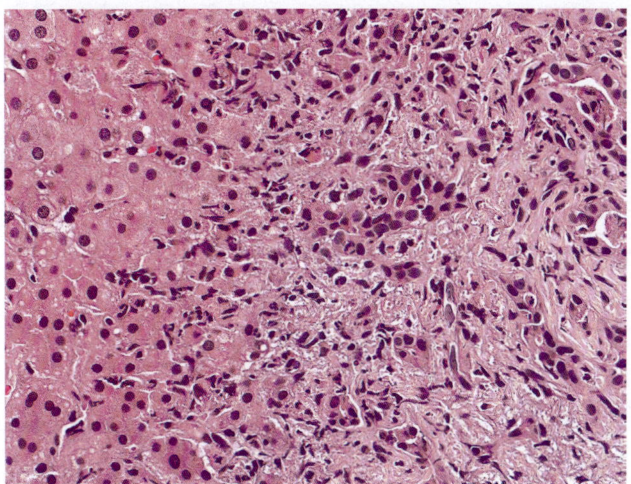

Figure 10.44. **Cystic fibrosis.** The biopsy shows a biliary obstruction pattern with bile ductular proliferation and mild mixed portal inflammation.

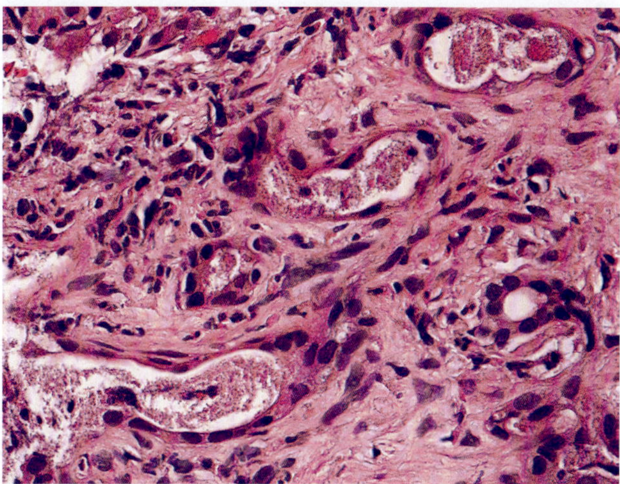

Figure 10.45. **Cystic fibrosis.** In rare portal tracts, this biopsy showed granular eosinophilic secretions, inspissated within the bile ducts and ductules.

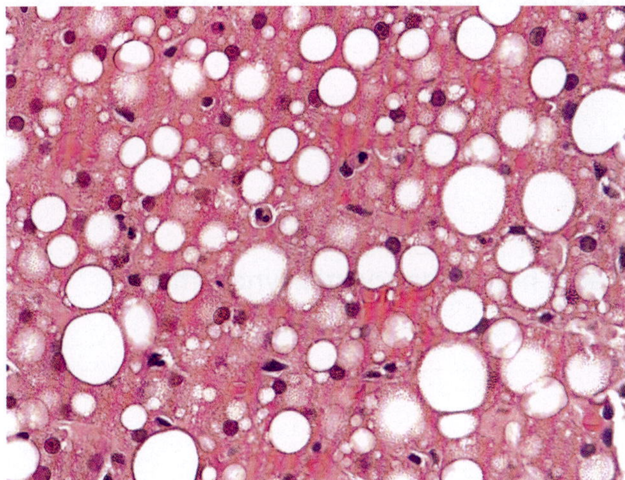

Figure 10.46. **Cystic fibrosis.** The lobules in this case show macrovesicular steatosis without steatohepatitis.

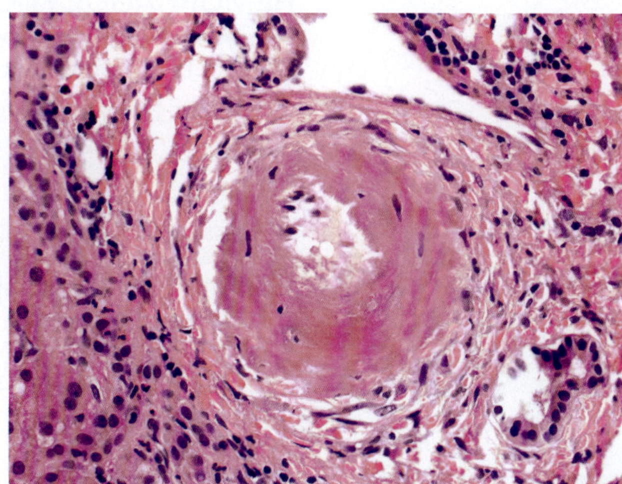

Figure 10.47. **Hypertensive changes.** The hepatic artery is thickened and hyalinized in this patient with hypertension and diabetes.

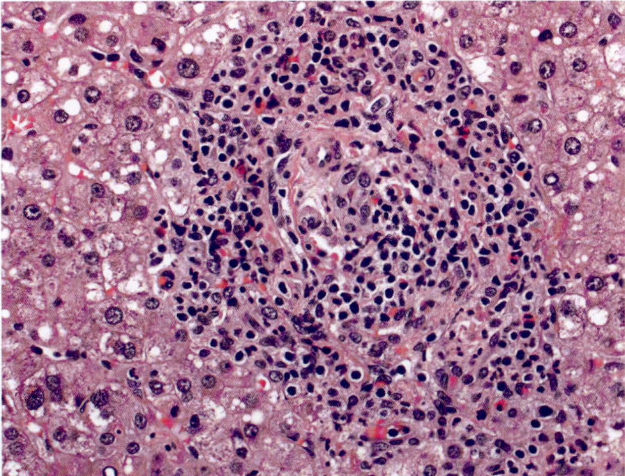

Figure 10.48. **Sepsis-related changes.** This patient presented with staphylococcus sepsis. The portal tracts showed mild to moderate lymphocytic inflammation.

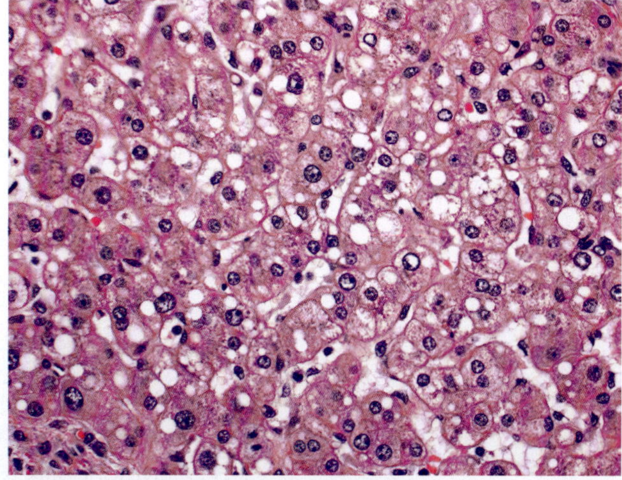

Figure 10.49. **Sepsis-related changes.** The lobules show mild fatty change (same case as Fig. 10.48).

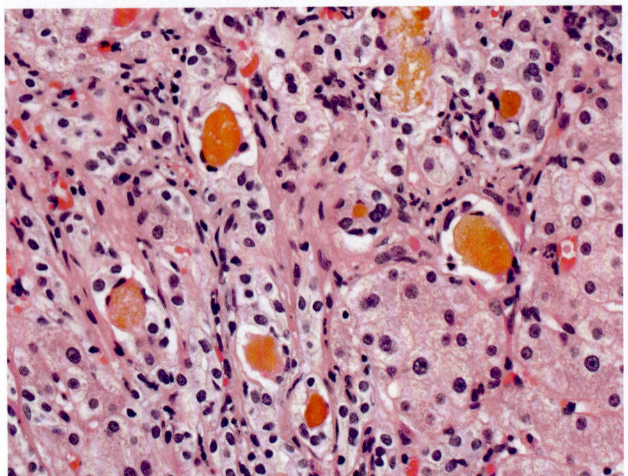

Figure 10.50. **Sepsis-related changes.** Cholangiolar cholestasis has also been described as a sepis-related change. This finding can be found with sepsis but is neither sensitive nor specific. In fact, it is very nonspecific.

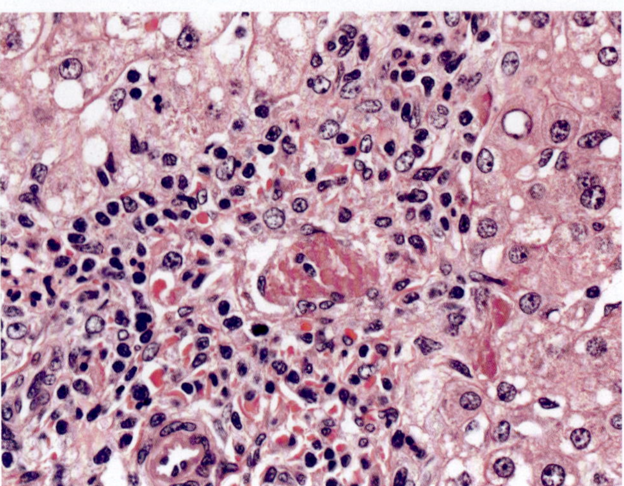

Figure 10.51. **Sepsis-related changes.** In this case, the portal tracts showed small fibrin thrombi in several of the portal veins.

HEMOPHAGOCYTIC SYNDROME

CHECKLIST: Hemophagocytic Syndrome

- ☐ Kupffer cell hyperplasia
- ☐ Hemophagocytosis
- ☐ Rare cases are familial
- ☐ Most cases are sporadic

Common causes of sporadic hemophagocytic syndrome

- ☐ Viral infections
  - CMV
  - EBV
  - HHV8
  - Varicella zoster
- ☐ Bacterial infections
  - *Mycobacteria tuberculosis*
  - *Escherichia coli*
  - *Shigella*
  - *Nocardiosis*
  - *Coxiellaburnetii* (Q fever)
- ☐ Autoimmune conditions
  - Rheumatoid arthritis
  - Ankylosing spondylitis
  - Dermatomyositis
  - Sarcoidosis
  - CVID
  - Crohn disease
- ☐ Drug effects
- ☐ Malignancies (usually hematopathology malignancies)
  - B cell lymphomas, Hodgkin disease, T cell lymphomas, and myeloproliferative disorders
  - Castleman disease

The hemophagocytic syndrome results from macrophage activation that escapes or exceeds normal downregulation controls, leading to Kupffer cell hyperplasia with prominent hemophagocytosis. Most cases are sporadic and are caused by viral infections, malignancies, autoimmune conditions, or drug effects, but rare cases of familial hemophagocytic disease have been identified. Of the many different potential causes for sporadic hemophagocytic syndrome, the most common is infection. In immunocompetent individuals, most infections are viral related, such as CMV or EBV, but in immunosuppressed individuals, infectious causes can be bacterial, parasitic, or viral. The hemophagocytic syndrome is rare in general liver biopsy specimens but is considerably higher in immunosuppressed individuals. For example, in the HIV (human immunodeficiency virus)-infected population, up to 8% of liver biopsies show the hemophagocytic syndrome.[98]

Patients tend to present with hepatosplenomegaly, prolonged fever, and cytopenias that typically involve at least two of the three cell lineages (red blood cells, white blood cells, platelets). AST and ALT levels can show mild elevations, while the alkaline phosphates levels are often very high. In addition, serum ferritin and triglyceride are typically elevated and can be very high, while fibrinogen and albumin levels tend to be low.

The histological findings show diffuse Kupffer cell hyperplasia with erythrophagocytosis (Fig. 10.52). The erythrophagocytosis can range from subtle to striking. If the erythrophagocytosis is minimal or absent, then the findings are typically classified as Kupffer cell hyperplasia, whereas cases with prominent erythrophagocytosis are classified as the hemophagocytic syndrome. Clearly there is a spectrum of findings, and there can be some tweeners, with findings that could be reasonably classified as either Kupffer cell hyperplasia or the hemophagocytic syndrome, as the erythrophagocytosis is clearly present and easily found, but not very prominent overall. As the differential for both is largely the same, such cases can be appropriately handled with a descriptive diagnosis and an explanatory note. Other findings in the hemophagocytic syndrome typically include mild sinusoidal congestion and minimal nonspecific portal and lobular inflammation. Individuals can also have other underlying liver diseases, such as fatty liver diseases, and in these cases, the changes of the underlying liver disease will also be present.

The most common mimic of the hemophagocytic syndrome is a nonspecific Kupffer cell hyperplasia, which is not surprising as one of the key findings in both disease patterns is Kupffer cell hyperplasia. The most common causes for a Kupffer cell hyperplasia pattern are systemic infections, usually viral infections such as CMV or EBV. In contrast to the hemophagocytic syndrome (which can also be viral induced), hemophagocytosis is minimal. Kupffer cell hyperplasia is also common in chronic cholestatic liver disease and with acute hepatitis from many different causes, but in these settings, the Kupffer cell changes are considered a secondary component of the main pattern of injury.

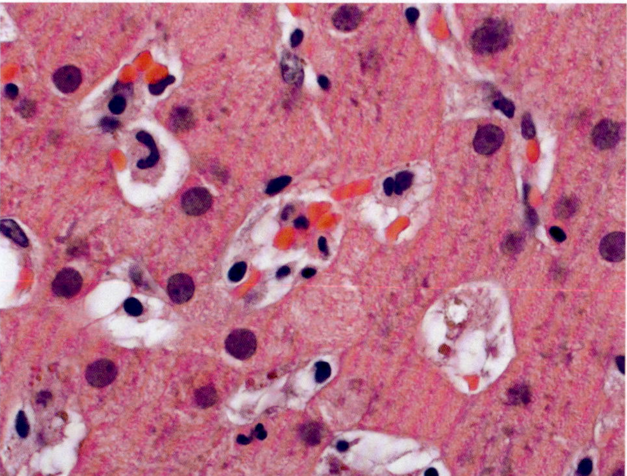

Figure 10.52. **Hemophagocytosis syndrome.** The liver biopsy shows diffuse Kupffer cell hyperplasia with prominent erythrophagocytosis. The patient's alkaline phosphatase was 600 and serum ferritin 2000. The cause was not evident at the time of the biopsy, so a differential was provided in the note.

NEAR MISSES

CASE 1. This liver biopsy was performed for mildly elevated liver enzymes in a 53-year-old woman. The patient had the metabolic syndrome, with hypertension, diabetes, and mild obesity. The biopsy showed mildly active fatty liver disease. In addition, several of the portal tracts were thickened by dense acellular eosinophilic deposits (Fig. 10.53). The case was sent in for consultation to rule out amyloid, after the outside Congo red stain was negative. A repeat Congo red stain was also negative, and a final diagnosis of arterial hyalinosis was made.

Arterial hyalinosis is usually an incidental finding, as it was in this case, but can closely mimic amyloid. Arterial hyalinosis is usually seen in patients with hypertension and diabetes mellitus. To rule out amyloid, Congo red stains should be performed on 10-micron-thick sections for optimal performance. If there is amyloid, it will show a distinctive salmon color on routine light microscopy. Polarization will show a pale green birefringence that is often referred to as "apple-green." To see the birefringence, any built in light filters within the microscope often have to be turned off. Dimming the room lights is also helpful.

CASE 2. A liver biopsy was performed in a 25-year-old man for mildly elevated AST and ALT levels. He was not taking any medications, and viral serologies were negative. Clinic notes indicated possible malabsorption type gastrointestinal (GI) symptoms. He also had a clinical diagnosis of probable obstructive lung disease, with several pulmonary infections in teenage years. His BMI was normal.

The biopsy showed mild patchy macrovesicular steatosis along with mild nonspecific lobular inflammation (Fig. 10.54). There was mild patchy lymphocytic portal inflammation, but the portal tracts were otherwise normal. Given the normal BMI, the lack of medications, and negative viral serologies, the cause of the steatosis and mild inflammation was not clear. However, after the case was signed out, follow-up information was received that the patient had been diagnosed with common variable immunodeficiency based on concurrent clinical workup.

Many systemic diseases that involve the GI tract can lead to mild nonspecific changes on liver biopsy, including mild steatosis and mild nonspecific inflammation. Examples include celiac disease, small bowel bacterial overgrowth, Crohn disease of the small bowel, and common variable immunodeficiency. Cases of common variable immunodeficiency also frequently have noncaseating granulomas, although none were evident on this biopsy. In all of these cases, as well as with other causes that lead to small bowel inflammation, it

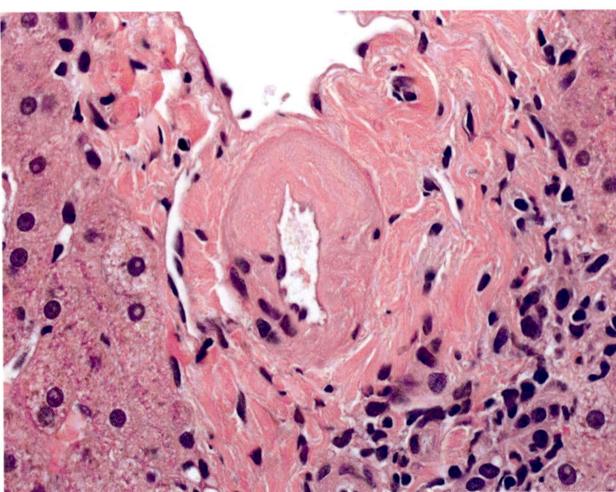

Figure 10.53. **Near miss case 1, arterial hyalinosis.** Arterial hyalinosis can mimic amyloid disease but is associated with diabetes mellitus and hypertension.

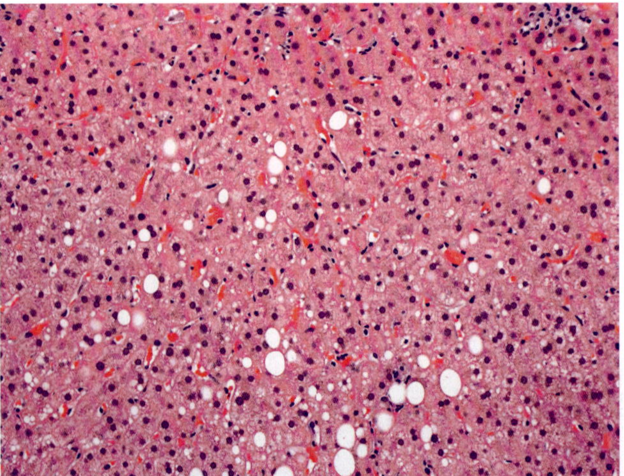

Figure 10.54. **Near miss case 2, common variable immunodeficiency.** The biopsy shows very mild macrovesicular steatosis, a disease pattern that is not specific but can result from a number of different causes of inflammation of the small bowel.

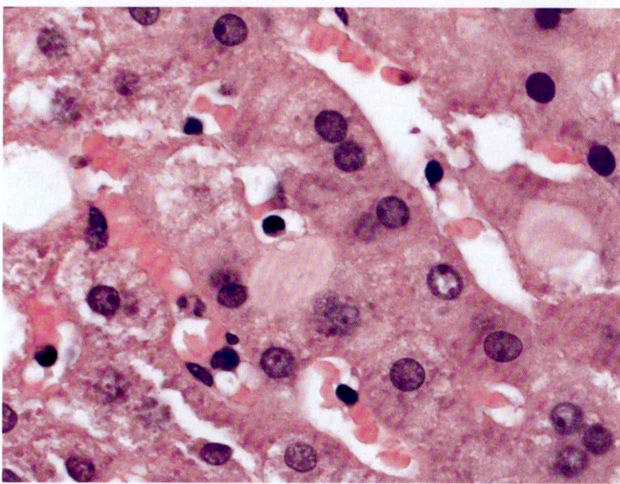

Figure 10.55. Near miss case 3, LECT amyloidosis. The hepatocytes have distinctive inclusions.

is thought that the inflammation in the small bowel leads to bacterial and other antigens breaching the mucosal barrier and causing mild inflammatory changes when they reach the liver. The fatty change is presumed to represent a component of malabsorption resulting from small bowel inflammation.

The differential is broad for a liver specimen that shows a pattern of mild inflammatory changes with or without mild fatty liver. In addition to inflammatory diseases involving the small bowel, the differential includes the metabolic syndrome, medication effect, and viral hepatitis C. In most of these cases, a final diagnosis is only established by correlation of clinical, imaging, and histology findings.

CASE 3. A 47-year-old man died from traumatic injury. In addition to documenting the traumatic injury, the autopsy found mild atherosclerotic heart disease, diverticular disease of the colon, and occasional pale amphophilic inclusions in hepatocytes (Fig. 10.55). Based on the liver biopsy findings, a presumptive diagnosis of LECT2 amyloidosis was made. A Congo red stain confirmed amyloid deposits, and mass spectrometry analysis confirmed LECT2 amyloid. A subsequent Congo red stain on the kidney showed mild patchy interstitial and mesangial amyloid deposits.

LECT2 amyloid deposits in the liver can be very subtle, as seen in this specimen. This case also illustrates the point that LECT amyloid in the liver is often an incidental finding. If clinical disease develops, patients usually present with renal disease. There are strong ethnic associations with LECT2 amyloidosis, in particular with Mexican heritage. The liver findings consist of distinctive round globules of amyloid deposited in the lobules. The amyloid appears to be within either the hepatocytes or the sinusoids. The H&E differential includes hepatitis B-related ground glass changes and medication-related pseudo-ground glass changes, but clinical history and immunohistochemical stains readily sort out the proper diagnosis. If needed, the amyloid can be subtyped and confirmed to be LECT2 by either immunostains (when available) or mass spectrometry.

References

1. Gilbertson JA, Theis JD, Vrana JA, et al. A comparison of immunohistochemistry and mass spectrometry for determining the amyloid fibril protein from formalin-fixed biopsy tissue. *J Clin Pathol*. 2015;68:314-317.
2. French SW, Schloss GT, Stillman AE. Unusual amyloid bodies in human liver. *Am J Clin Pathol*. 1981;75:400-402.
3. Makhlouf HR, Goodman ZD. Globular hepatic amyloid: an early stage in the pathway of amyloid formation: a study of 20 new cases. *Am J Surg Pathol*. 2007;31:1615-1621.
4. Chandan VS, Shah SS, Lam-Himlin DM, et al. Globular hepatic amyloid is highly sensitive and specific for LECT2 amyloidosis. *Am J Surg Pathol*. 2015;39(4):558-564.

5. Paueksakon P, Fogo AB, Sethi S. Leukocyte chemotactic factor 2 amyloidosis cannot be reliably diagnosed by immunohistochemical staining. *Hum Pathol*. 2014;45:1445-1450.

6. Damlaj M, Amre R, Wong P, How J. Hepatic ALECT-2 amyloidosis causing portal hypertension and recurrent variceal bleeding: a case report and review of the literature. *Am J Clin Pathol*. 2014;141:288-291.

7. Larsen CP, Beggs ML, Wilson JD, Lathrop SL. Prevalence and organ distribution of leukocyte chemotactic factor 2 amyloidosis (ALECT2) among decedents in New Mexico. *Amyloid*. 2016;23:119-123.

8. Larsen CP, Ismail W, Kurtin PJ, Vrana JA, Dasari S, Nasr SH. Leukocyte chemotactic factor 2 amyloidosis (ALECT2) is a common form of renal amyloidosis among Egyptians. *Mod Pathol*. 2016;29:416-420.

9. Girelli CM, Lodi G, Rocca F. Kappa light chain deposition disease of the liver. *Eur J Gastroenterol Hepatol*. 1998;10:429-430.

10. Mena-Duran A, Munoz Vicente E, Pareja Llorens G, Sanchis Cervera J. Liver failure caused by light chain deposition disease associated with multiple myeloma. *Intern Med*. 2012;51:773-776.

11. Talukdar A, Mukherjee K, Khanra D, Saha M. Portal hypertension related to light chain deposition disease of liver: an enlightening experience. *BMJ Case Rep*. 2013;2013.

12. Lin P, Bueso-Ramos C, Wilson CS, Mansoor A, Medeiros LJ. Waldenstrom macroglobulinemia involving extramedullary sites: morphologic and immunophenotypic findings in 44 patients. *Am J Surg Pathol*. 2003;27:1104-1113.

13. Yowell RL, Hammond EH. Cardiac paraprotein associated with Waldenstrom's macroglobulinemia: a case report. *Ultrastruct Pathol*. 1994;18:229-232.

14. Figueroa JJ, Bosch EP, Dyck PJ, et al. Amyloid-like IgM deposition neuropathy: a distinct clinico-pathologic and proteomic profiled disorder. *J Peripher Nerv Syst*. 2012;17:182-190.

15. Lorenz G, Barenwald G. Histologic and electron-microscopic liver changes in diabetic children. *Acta Hepatogastroenterol (Stuttg)*. 1979;26:435-438.

16. Umpaichitra V. Unusual glycogenic hepatopathy causing abnormal liver enzymes in a morbidly obese adolescent with well-controlled type 2 diabetes: resolved after A1c was normalized by metformin. *Clin Obes*. 2016;6:281-284.

17. van den Brand M, Elving LD, Drenth JP, van Krieken JH. Glycogenic hepatopathy: a rare cause of elevated serum transaminases in diabetes mellitus. *Neth J Med*. 2009;67:394-396.

18. Carcione L, Lombardo F, Messina MF, Rosano M, De Luca F. Liver glycogenosis as early manifestation in type 1 diabetes mellitus. *Diabetes Nutr Metab*. 2003;16:182-184.

19. Chatila R, West AB. Hepatomegaly and abnormal liver tests due to glycogenosis in adults with diabetes. *Medicine (Baltimore)*. 1996;75:327-333.

20. Tomihira M, Kawasaki E, Nakajima H, et al. Intermittent and recurrent hepatomegaly due to glycogen storage in a patient with type 1 diabetes: genetic analysis of the liver glycogen phosphorylase gene (PYGL). *Diabetes Res Clin Pract*. 2004;65:175-182.

21. Olsson R, Wesslau C, William-Olsson T, Zettergren L. Elevated aminotransferases and alkaline phosphatases in unstable diabetes mellitus without ketoacidosis or hypoglycemia. *J Clin Gastroenterol*. 1989;11:541-545.

22. Fridell JA, Saxena R, Chalasani NP, Goggins WC, Powelson JA, Cummings OW. Complete reversal of glycogen hepatopathy with pancreas transplantation: two cases. *Transplantation*. 2007;83:84-86.

23. Torbenson M, Chen YY, Brunt E, et al. Glycogenic hepatopathy: an underrecognized hepatic complication of diabetes mellitus. *Am J Surg Pathol*. 2006;30:508-513.

24. Rautou PE, Cazals-Hatem D, Moreau R, et al. Acute liver cell damage in patients with anorexia nervosa: a possible role of starvation-induced hepatocyte autophagy. *Gastroenterology*. 2008;135:840-848, 888.e1-3.

25. Kransdorf LN, Millstine D, Smith ML, Aqel BA. Hepatic glycogen deposition in a patient with anorexia nervosa and persistently abnormal transaminase levels. *Clin Res Hepatol Gastroenterol*. 2016;40:e15-e18.

26. Komuta M, Harada M, Ueno T, et al. Unusual accumulation of glycogen in liver parenchymal cells in a patient with anorexia nervosa. *Intern Med*. 1998;37:678-682.

27. Torous VF, Farahmand A, Tatishchev S, Wang HL. Glucocorticoid-induced rapid development of glycogenic hepatopathy in a liver transplant patient with no prior history of diabetes mellitus: a case report. *Am J Digest Dis*. 2016;3:24-28.

28. Iancu TC, Shiloh H, Dembo L. Hepatomegaly following short-term high-dose steroid therapy. *J Pediatr Gastroenterol Nutr*. 1986;5:41-46.

29. Resnick JM, Zador I, Fish DL. Dumping syndrome, a cause of acquired glycogenic hepatopathy. *Pediatr Dev Pathol*. 2011;14:318-321.

30. Miles L, Heubi JE, Bove KE. Hepatocyte glycogen accumulation in patients undergoing dietary management of urea cycle defects mimics storage disease. *J Pediatr Gastroenterol Nutr*. 2005;40:471-476.

31. Harrison SA, Brunt EM, Goodman ZD, Di Bisceglie AM. Diabetic hepatosclerosis: diabetic microangiopathy of the liver. *Arch Pathol Lab Med*. 2006;130:27-32.

32. Hudacko RM, Sciancalepore JP, Fyfe BS. Diabetic microangiopathy in the liver: an autopsy study of incidence and association with other diabetic complications. *Am J Clin Pathol*. 2009;132:494-499.

33. Chen G, Brunt EM. Diabetic hepatosclerosis: a 10-year autopsy series. *Liver Int*. 2009;29:1044-1050.

34. Torbenson M, Hart J, Westerhoff M, et al. Neonatal giant cell hepatitis: histological and etiological findings. *Am J Surg Pathol*. 2010;34:1498-1503.

35. Wada K, Kobayashi H, Moriyama A, et al. A case of an infant with congenital combined pituitary hormone deficiency and normalized liver histology of infantile cholestasis after hormone replacement therapy. *Clin Pediatr Endocrinol*. 2017;26:251-257.

36. Nishizawa H, Iguchi G, Murawaki A, et al. Nonalcoholic fatty liver disease in adult hypopituitary patients with GH deficiency and the impact of GH replacement therapy. *Eur J Endocrinol*. 2012;167:67-74.

37. Bayraktar M, Van Thiel DH. Abnormalities in measures of liver function and injury in thyroid disorders. *Hepatogastroenterology*. 1997;44:1614-1618.

38. Soylu A, Taskale MG, Ciltas A, Kalayci M, Kumbasar AB. Intrahepatic cholestasis in subclinical and overt hyperthyroidism: two case reports. *J Med Case Rep*. 2008;2:116.

39. Lin TY, Shekar AO, Li N, et al. Incidence of abnormal liver biochemical tests in hyperthyroidism. *Clin Endocrinol (Oxf)*. 2017;86:755-759.

40. Huang MJ, Liaw YF. Clinical associations between thyroid and liver diseases. *J Gastroenterol Hepatol*. 1995;10:344-350.

41. Soleimanpour SA. Fulminant liver failure associated with delayed identification of thyroid storm due to heterophile antibodies. *Clin Diabetes Endocrinol*. 2015;1.

42. Hull K, Horenstein R, Naglieri R, Munir K, Ghany M, Celi FS. Two cases of thyroid storm-associated cholestatic jaundice. *Endocr Pract*. 2007;13:476-480.

43. Hasan MK, Tierney WM, Baker MZ. Severe cholestatic jaundice in hyperthyroidism after treatment with 131-iodine. *Am J Med Sci*. 2004;328:348-350.

44. Majeed M, Babu A. Cholestasis secondary to hyperthyroidism made worse by methimazole. *Am J Med Sci*. 2006;332:51-53.

45. Sainsbury A, Sanders DS, Ford AC. Meta-analysis: coeliac disease and hypertransaminasaemia. *Aliment Pharmacol Ther*. 2011;34:33-40.

46. Duggan JM, Duggan AE. Systematic review: the liver in coeliac disease. *Aliment Pharmacol Ther*. 2005;21:515-518.

47. Majumdar K, Sakhuja P, Puri AS, Gaur K, Haider A, Gondal R. Coeliac disease and the liver: spectrum of liver histology, serology and treatment response at a tertiary referral centre. *J Clin Pathol*. 2017.

48. Ivanova II, Dukova DY, Boikova PG, Grudeva LS, Shalev IB, Kotzev IA. Chronic hepatitis due to gluten enteropathy–a case report. *Folia Med (Plovdiv)*. 2017;59:228-231.

49. Gaur K, Sakhuja P, Puri AS, Majumdar K. Gluten-Free hepatomiracle in "celiac hepatitis": a case highlighting the rare occurrence of nutrition-induced near total reversal of advanced steatohepatitis and cirrhosis. *Saudi J Gastroenterol*. 2016;22:461-464.

50. Mounajjed T, Oxentenko A, Shmidt E, Smyrk T. The liver in celiac disease: clinical manifestations, histologic features, and response to gluten-free diet in 30 patients. *Am J Clin Pathol*. 2011;136:128-137.

51. Sedlack RE, Smyrk TC, Czaja AJ, Talwalkar JA. Celiac disease-associated autoimmune cholangitis. *Am J Gastroenterol*. 2002;97:3196-3198.

52. Hagander B, Berg NO, Brandt L, Norden A, Sjolund K, Stenstam M. Hepatic injury in adult coeliac disease. *Lancet*. 1977;2:270-272.

53. Riestra S, Dominguez F, Rodrigo L. Nodular regenerative hyperplasia of the liver in a patient with celiac disease. *J Clin Gastroenterol*. 2001;33:323-326.

54. Biecker E, Trebicka J, Fischer HP, Sauerbruch T, Lammert F. Portal hypertension and nodular regenerative hyperplasia in a patient with celiac disease. *Z Gastroenterol*. 2006;44:395-398.

55. Daniels JA, Torbenson M, Vivekanandan P, Anders RA, Boitnott JK. Hepatitis in common variable immunodeficiency. *Hum Pathol*. 2009;40:484-488.

56. Ebrahimi Daryani N, Aghamohammadi A, Mousavi Mirkala MR, et al. Gastrointestinal complications in two patients with common variable immunodeficiency. *Iran J Allergy Asthma Immunol*. 2004;3:149-152.

57. Bjoro K, Haaland T, Skaug K, Froland SS. The spectrum of hepatobiliary disease in primary hypogammaglobulinaemia. *J Intern Med*. 1999;245:517-524.

58. Fuss IJ, Friend J, Yang Z, et al. Nodular regenerative hyperplasia in common variable immunodeficiency. *J Clin Immunol*. 2013;33:748-758.

59. Ward C, Lucas M, Piris J, Collier J, Chapel H. Abnormal liver function in common variable immunodeficiency disorders due to nodular regenerative hyperplasia. *Clin Exp Immunol*. 2008;153:331-337.

60. Malamut G, Ziol M, Suarez F, et al. Nodular regenerative hyperplasia: the main liver disease in patients with primary hypogammaglobulinemia and hepatic abnormalities. *J Hepatol*. 2008;48:74-82.

61. Ardeniz O, Cunningham-Rundles C. Granulomatous disease in common variable immunodeficiency. *Clin Immunol*. 2009;133:198-207.

62. Baron-Ruiz I, Martin-Mateos MA, Plaza-Martin AM, Giner-Munoz MT, Piquer M. Lymphoma as presentation of common variable immunodeficiency. *Allergol Immunopathol (Madr)*. 2009;37:51-53.

63. Ribaldone DG, Garavagno M, Pellicano R, et al. Prevalence and prognostic value of hepatic histological alterations in patients with Crohn's disease. *Scand J Gastroenterol*. 2015;50:1463-1468.

64. Westbrook RH, Dusheiko G, Williamson C. Pregnancy and liver disease. *J Hepatol*. 2016;64:933-945.

65. Conchillo JM, Pijnenborg JM, Peeters P, Stockbrugger RW, Fevery J, Koek GH. Liver enzyme elevation induced by hyperemesis gravidarum: aetiology, diagnosis and treatment. *Neth J Med*. 2002;60:374-378.

66. Bacq Y. Liver diseases unique to pregnancy: a 2010 update. *Clin Res Hepatol Gastroenterol*. 2011;35:182-193.

67. Bacq Y, Sapey T, Brechot MC, Pierre F, Fignon A, Dubois F. Intrahepatic cholestasis of pregnancy: a French prospective study. *Hepatology*. 1997;26:358-364.

68. Keitel V, Vogt C, Haussinger D, Kubitz R. Combined mutations of canalicular transporter proteins cause severe intrahepatic cholestasis of pregnancy. *Gastroenterology*. 2006;131:624-629.

69. Ropponen A, Sund R, Riikonen S, Ylikorkala O, Aittomaki K. Intrahepatic cholestasis of pregnancy as an indicator of liver and biliary diseases: a population-based study. *Hepatology*. 2006;43:723-728.

70. Tsokos M, Longauer F, Kardosova V, Gavel A, Anders S, Schulz F. Maternal death in pregnancy from HELLP syndrome. A report of three medico-legal autopsy cases with special reference to distinctive histopathological alterations. *Int J Legal Med*. 2002;116:50-53.

71. Barton JR, Riely CA, Adamec TA, Shanklin DR, Khoury AD, Sibai BM. Hepatic histopathologic condition does not correlate with laboratory abnormalities in HELLP syndrome (hemolysis, elevated liver enzymes, and low platelet count). *Am J Obstet Gynecol*. 1992;167:1538-1543.

72. Minakami H, Oka N, Sato T, Tamada T, Yasuda Y, Hirota N. Preeclampsia: a microvesicular fat disease of the liver? *Am J Obstet Gynecol*. 1988;159:1043-1087.

73. Ch'ng CL, Morgan M, Hainsworth I, Kingham JG. Prospective study of liver dysfunction in pregnancy in Southwest Wales. *Gut*. 2002;51:876-880.

74. Burroughs AK, Seong NH, Dojcinov DM, Scheuer PJ, Sherlock SV. Idiopathic acute fatty liver of pregnancy in 12 patients. *Q J Med*. 1982;51:481-497.

75. Reyes H, Sandoval L, Wainstein A, et al. Acute fatty liver of pregnancy: a clinical study of 12 episodes in 11 patients. *Gut*. 1994;35:101-106.

76. Rolfes DB, Ishak KG. Acute fatty liver of pregnancy: a clinicopathologic study of 35 cases. *Hepatology*. 1985;5:1149-1158.

77. Riely CA, Latham PS, Romero R, Duffy TP. Acute fatty liver of pregnancy. A reassessment based on observations in nine patients. *Ann Intern Med.* 1987;106:703-706.

78. Abdallah M, Genereau T, Donadieu J, . Langerhans' cell histiocytosis of the liver in adults. *Clin Res Hepatol Gastroenterol.* 2011;35:475-481.

79. Braier J, Ciocca M, Latella A, de Davila MG, Drajer M, Imventarza O. Cholestasis, sclerosing cholangitis, and liver transplantation in Langerhans cell Histiocytosis. *Med Pediatr Oncol.* 2002;38:178-182.

80. Yi X, Han T, Zai H, Long X, Wang X, Li W. Liver involvement of Langerhans' cell histiocytosis in children. *Int J Clin Exp Med.* 2015;8:7098-7106.

81. Heyn RM, Hamoudi A, Newton WA. Pretreatment liver biopsy in 20 children with histiocytosis X: a clinicopathologic correlation. *Med Pediatr Oncol.* 1990;18:110-118.

82. Di Tommaso L, Rahal D, Bossi P, Roncalli M. Hepatic Rosai-Dorfman disease with coincidental lymphoma: report of a case. *Int J Surg Pathol.* 2010;18:540-543.

83. Foucar E, Rosai J, Dorfman R. Sinus histiocytosis with massive lymphadenopathy (Rosai-Dorfman disease): review of the entity. *Semin Diagn Pathol.* 1990;7:19-73.

84. Lauwers GY, Perez-Atayde A, Dorfman RF, Rosai J. The digestive system manifestations of Rosai-Dorfman disease (sinus histiocytosis with massive lymphadenopathy): review of 11 cases. *Hum Pathol.* 2000;31:380-385.

85. Yam LT, Chan CH, Li CY. Hepatic involvement in systemic mast cell disease. *Am J Med.* 1986;80:819-826.

86. Marbello L, Anghilieri M, Nosari A, et al. Aggressive systemic mastocytosis mimicking sclerosing cholangitis. *Haematologica.* 2004;89:ECR35.

87. Kyriakou D, Kouroumalis E, Konsolas J, et al. Systemic mastocytosis: a rare cause of noncirrhotic portal hypertension simulating autoimmune cholangitis–report of four cases. *Am J Gastroenterol.* 1998;93:106-108.

88. Safyan EL, Veerabagu MP, Swerdlow SH, Lee RG, Rakela J. Intrahepatic cholestasis due to systemic mastocytosis: a case report and review of literature. *Am J Gastroenterol.* 1997;92:1197-1200.

89. Mican JM, Di Bisceglie AM, Fong TL. Hepatic involvement in mastocytosis: clinicopathologic correlations in 41 cases. *Hepatology.* 1995;22:1163-1170.

90. Horny HP, Kaiserling E, Campbell M, Parwaresch MR, Lennert K. Liver findings in generalized mastocytosis. A clinicopathologic study. *Cancer.* 1989;63:532-538.

91. Lindblad A, Glaumann H, Strandvik B. Natural history of liver disease in cystic fibrosis. *Hepatology.* 1999;30:1151-1158.

92. Potter CJ, Fishbein M, Hammond S, McCoy K, Qualman S. Can the histologic changes of cystic fibrosis-associated hepatobiliary disease be predicted by clinical criteria? *J Pediatr Gastroenterol Nutr.* 1997;25:32-36.

93. Moyer K, Balistreri W. Hepatobiliary disease in patients with cystic fibrosis. *Curr Opin Gastroenterol.* 2009;25:272-278.

94. Schwarzenberg SJ, Wielinski CL, Shamieh I, et al. Cystic fibrosis-associated colitis and fibrosing colonopathy. *J Pediatr.* 1995;127:565-570.

95. Witters P, Libbrecht L, Roskams T, et al. Noncirrhotic presinusoidal portal hypertension is common in cystic fibrosis-associated liver disease. *Hepatology.* 2011;53:1064-1065.

96. Balakrishnan M, Garcia-Tsao G, Deng Y, Ciarleglio M, Jain D. Hepatic arteriolosclerosis: a small-vessel complication of diabetes and hypertension. *Am J Surg Pathol.* 2015;39:1000-1009.

97. Koskinas J, Gomatos IP, Tiniakos DG, et al. Liver histology in ICU patients dying from sepsis: a clinico-pathological study. *World J Gastroenterol.* 2008;14:1389-1393.

98. Prendki V, Stirnemann J, Lemoine M, et al. Prevalence and clinical significance of Kupffer cell hyperplasia with hemophagocytosis in liver biopsies. *Am J Surg Pathol.* 2011;35:337-345.

TRANSPLANT PATHOLOGY 11

CHAPTER OUTLINE

DONOR LIVER EVALUATION

CHECKLIST: Donor Liver Evaluation

- ☐ Macrovesicular steatosis, estimated to the nearest 10%
- ☐ Inflammation, portal and lobular. Grade as minimal, mild, moderate, or marked
- ☐ Necrosis—estimated to nearest 10% and indicates zonation and distribution (e.g., focal, diffuse, etc.)
- ☐ Fibrosis
- ☐ Other findings
  - ○ Examples include granulomas, excess pigment that suggests iron, cholestasis

The use of biopsies to evaluate livers of deceased donors for transplantation varies widely between different medical centers. In part, this depends on whether the center regularly considers using clinically marginal livers in their transplant program. In this setting in particular, the liver biopsy can provide useful information. The purpose is straightforward: provide additional data on the suitability of the donor liver for transplantation. Of note, the clinical team considers a variety of factors before making their final decision on whether to use the liver, and the histology findings are often not the only factor. Other factors include age of the deceased donor, the cause of death, the amount of warm ischemia time, the gross appearance of the liver, and the status of the recipient.

Your job is to determine the amount of fat, inflammation, necrosis, and fibrosis in every biopsy, as well as to comment on any other unusual findings. Only the macrovesicular steatosis is scored, as smaller droplet fat has minimal or no effect on clinical outcomes (Fig. 11.1). There is a persistent sprinkling of papers over the year saying otherwise, but the center mass of the data is pretty clear: it is only the macrovesicular component that matters. For instance, one study examined nearly 12,000 allografts and found that donor livers with microvesicular steatosis perform essentially the same as those without any fat.[1] Macrovesicular fat should be estimated to the nearest 10%. A common clinical cutoff for donor suitability is less than 30%, but other factors also come into play, so livers with more fat can also be suitable organs for transplantation in some situations. Some centers use the Oil red O or similar stains for fat assessment. This stain can work well for those centers that use it a lot, but the Oil red O is a dirty stain and can lead to significant fat overcalls (and thus potential organ wastage), so it is hard to recommend its usage by most centers. Besides, the H&E works just as well.

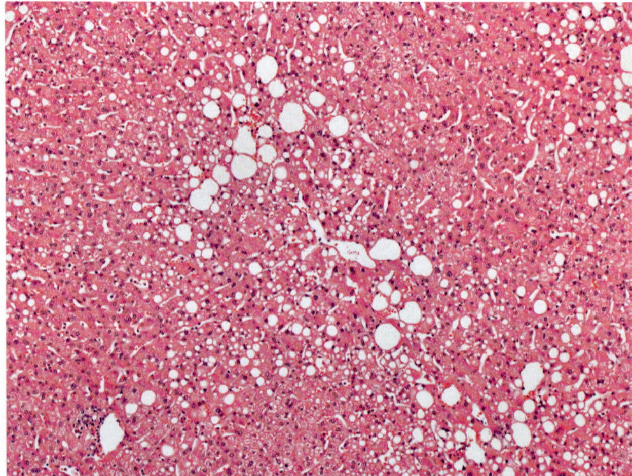

Figure 11.1. **Steatosis in donor liver biopsies.** Only the macrovesicular component is relevant for predicting graft and patient outcomes. This case was estimated to have between 5% and 10% macrovesicular steatosis.

The inflammation can be scored as minimal to marked, with the portal and lobular inflammation evaluated separately. A formal grading system for inflammation (e.g., Ishak score) is fine to use but is not necessary. Donor livers commonly show minimal to mild nonspecific inflammation, but moderate or greater inflammation suggests an underlying liver disease. When present, necrosis is usually focal and mild and located in zone 3 or is immediately beneath the liver capsule. Necrosis should be estimated to the nearest 10% and the location provided. Fibrosis is staged in the usual fashion (pericellular, portal, bridging, cirrhosis).

PRESERVATION CHANGES

CHECKLIST: Preservation Changes

- ☐ Lobular changes are often accentuated in zone 3
    - ○ Minimal to mild inflammation
    - ○ Mild Kupffer cell hyperplasia
    - ○ Occasional apoptotic hepatocytes
    - ○ Mild lobular cholestasis
- ☐ Minimal to mild nonspecific portal inflammation

Preservation changes are usually seen within the first 7 or so days after transplantation. They are usually an incidental finding when some other factor leads to a liver biopsy, such as concern for graft nonfunction or rejection. Centers that do protocol day 7 biopsies also commonly see preservation changes. The changes are usually mild and consist of mild lobular cholestasis, inflammation, and Kupffer cell hyperplasia, along with occasional apoptotic hepatocytes (Fig. 11.2).[2] Severe preservation changes can lead to hepatocyte dropout. However, significant loss of zone 3 hepatocytes plus central venulitis should be interpreted as rejection and not preservation changes.[2]

These early biopsies can also have fat, with the amount of fat dependent to some degree on the amount of fat in the donor liver. In routine liver transplants, the fat can be quickly cleared (usually less than a week), so there may be little or no fat, even if there was a fair amount of fat at baseline. Donor livers that have a lot of fat plus other injuries that prevent adequate graft function can have higher degrees of zone 3 necrosis. The dying hepatocytes can release the fat, and rarely this can lead to sinusoidal obstruction[3] or pulmonary fat emboli.[4] The term "pseudopeliotic steatosis" (Fig. 11.3) has been used to describe the dilated, obstructed sinusoids.[4]

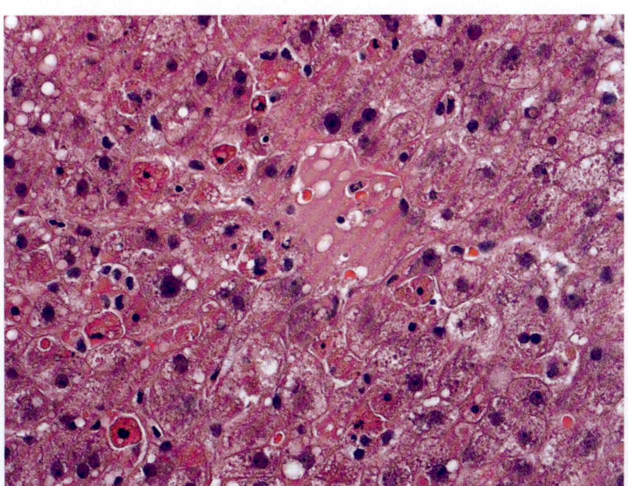

Figure 11.2. Preservation changes. The biopsy shows zone 3 cholestasis and apoptosis.

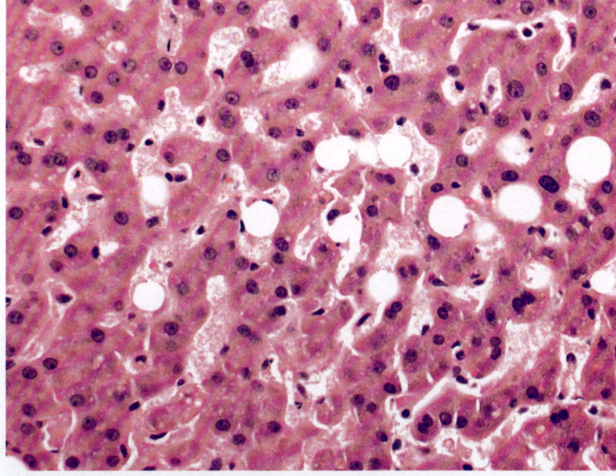

Figure 11.3. Pseudopeliotic changes. This finding is very rare, but the sinusoids are distended by fat droplets.

ACUTE CELLULAR REJECTION

CHECKLIST: Acute Cellular Rejection

- ☐ Clinical triggers
  - ○ Reduced immunosuppression
  - ○ Anything that upregulates the immune system
  - ○ In many cases, no trigger is found
- ☐ Definite diagnosis is made only on biopsy
  - ○ Some centers will treat presumed rejections without biopsy if the clinical and biochemistry findings are typical
- ☐ Rejection can occur any time but rejection is most common in the first 3 months following transplantation
- ☐ Biochemical findings: Alkaline phosphatase–predominant elevations in liver enzymes
- ☐ Histological findings in typical acute cellular rejection include these:
  - ○ Portal inflammation
  - ○ Bile duct lymphocytosis and injury
  - ○ Endothelialitis
- ☐ Atypical forms of acute cellular rejection
  - ○ Lobular variant
  - ○ Central perivenulitis variant
  - ○ Plasma cell–rich variant

The Banff Group has recently recommended that the term *T cell–mediated rejection* replace the term *acute cellular rejection*.[5] However, since the term acute cellular rejection is so widely used in the pathology and clinical community, that term will be used in this chapter.

The single most common indication for an allograft liver biopsy is to evaluate for acute cellular rejection. For that reason, most liver transplant biopsies will be comfortably handled if you take the time to master the patterns of acute cellular rejection. Of note, transplant pathology seems to be unusually enriched for center-specific, idiosyncratic, and often times inscrutable beliefs on the histology of acute cellular rejection. This is particularly unfortunate because the Banff Society has done an outstanding job in providing guidelines, position statements, and timely reviews on important aspects of transplant pathology.

PEARLS & PITFALLS

There are a lot of idiosyncratic beliefs when it comes to liver transplant pathology, many of them closely held by pathologists and sometimes clinical colleagues. Here are some of the more common ones. While none of them are true, they all have just enough charm that pathologist can be quite committed to them.

- If there are eosinophils in the portal tracts, even just a few, the diagnosis should be acute cellular rejection.
- If there are neutrophils in the portal tracts, even just a few, the diagnosis should be acute cellular rejection (Fig. 11.4).
- Portal inflammation in the first year after transplant has to be rejection.
  - Once, this point of view intrigued me enough to ask a pathologist why he felt that way. Answer: "There is no other reason for the inflammation to be there besides rejection" (Fig. 11.5). But of course there are other reasons, in fact many.
- If the portal inflammation looks "activated," then the diagnosis is rejection, even if there is no duct injury or endothelialitis.
- The number of "portal tracts with rejection" should be part of the pathology report. For example, "3 out of 10 portal tracts show rejection."

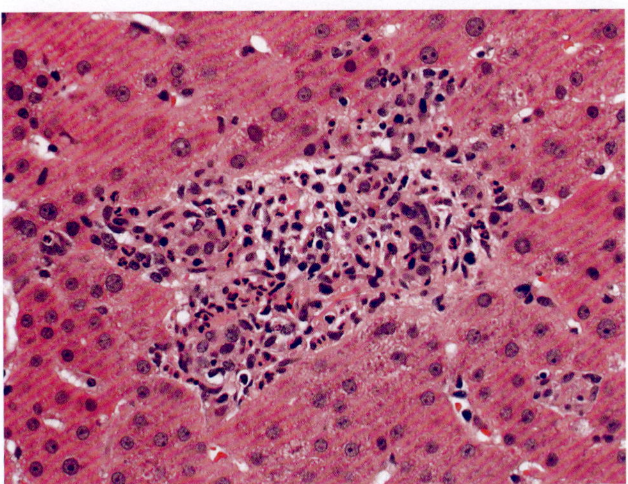

Figure 11.4. Mixed portal inflammation mimicking acute cellular rejection. This case was misdiagnosed as acute cellular rejection because there was mild patchy neutrophilic inflammation. The diagnosis turned out to be biliary obstruction. Enzymes normalized not with steroids but with stenting.

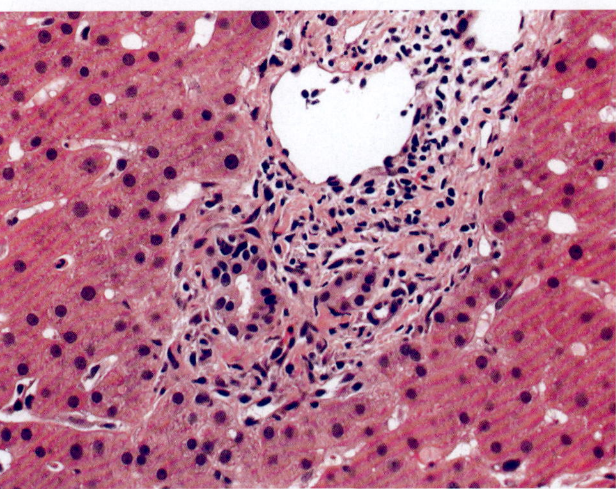

Figure 11.5. Mild portal chronic inflammation mimicking acute cellular rejection. This case was misdiagnosed as acute cellular rejection because there was mild patchy portal chronic inflammation. Once again, the diagnosis turned out to be biliary obstruction, and liver enzymes normalized not with steroids but with stenting.

Typical acute cellular rejection is a portal-based inflammatory disease (Fig. 11.6) with active bile duct injury and sometimes endothelialitis. The portal inflammation is predominately lymphocytic, but a few eosinophils or neutrophils or plasma cells are not uncommon. They are also not that relevant, unless they are prominent, as they have no specific diagnostic value when few in number.

In the Banff classification, a diagnosis of acute cellular rejections requires at least 2 of 3 key findings to be present: portal inflammation, bile duct injury, and endothelialitis.[6] At a practical level, essentially all cases show one of these patterns (1) portal inflammation plus bile duct injury (most common); (2) portal inflammation plus duct injury plus endothelialitis (second most common); or (3) portal inflammation plus endothelialitis, but no duct injury (least common).

The portal inflammation is composed mostly of lymphocytes, but occasional eosinophils or neutrophils are seen (Fig. 11.7). The lymphocytes can appear activated (Fig. 11.8) in that they appear larger and have more prominent nuclei and vesiculated chromatin. This histological finding is easiest to see in cases of early and severe rejection.

Bile duct injury is identified by looking for bile duct lymphocytosis and/or injury (Figs. 11.9–11.11). The portal inflammation can be accentuated around the bile duct. The affected bile ducts will typically have a few intraepithelial lymphocytes, mild reactive changes, and rare apoptotic bodies. You do not have to wait for the duct to be severely injured or destroyed before identifying bile duct injury. On the other hand, you will overcall rejection if you insist that any duct that is not picture perfect is injured, as mild bile duct reactive changes are common and nonspecific (Fig. 11.12).

It is well recognized that bile duct lymphocytosis and injury are also present in some cases of viral hepatitis and drug effect. However, in these cases the duct lymphocytosis and injury is unusually mild and focal and present mostly in portal tracts that show moderate or greater inflammation. In contrast, the duct injury in acute cellular rejection is more widespread and present in portal tracts that have only mild inflammation. Other histological changes, such as lobular hepatitis in viral infections, will also help clarify the diagnosis.

Endothelialitis can be present in either portal veins or central veins. The affected veins show injured or reactive appearing endothelial cells associated with lymphocytes, which can be adjacent and underneath the endothelial cells, sometimes appearing to lift them off their basement membrane, or the lymphocytes can be within the lumen, adherent to the endothelial cells (Figs. 11.13 and 11.14). To be diagnostically useful, the endothelialitis should be definite. If a focus in question shows equivocal endothelialitis, then do not score that one and move on to other parts of the biopsy. In most cases with adequate biopsies, endothelialitis is not limited to single vein. If the diagnosis of endothelialitis is still equivocal, then it is best to base your diagnosis on other findings. There is a very strong tendency

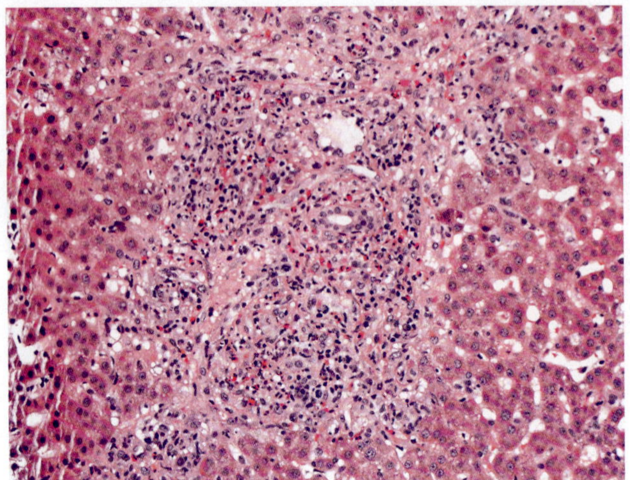

Figure 11.6. **Acute cellular rejection, low-power view.** Acute cellular rejection in most cases is a portal-based disease process.

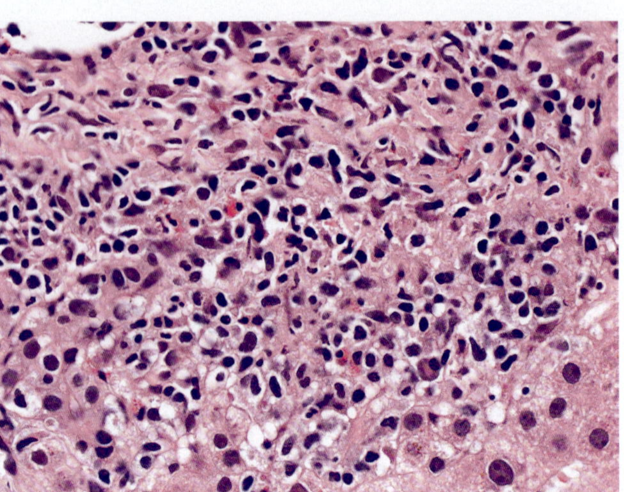

Figure 11.7. **Acute cellular rejection, portal inflammation.** The inflammation in acute cellular rejection is predominately lymphocytic, but occasional neutrophils, eosinophils, and plasma cells are common. Eosinophils are more likely to be seen in rejection occurring soon after transplant.

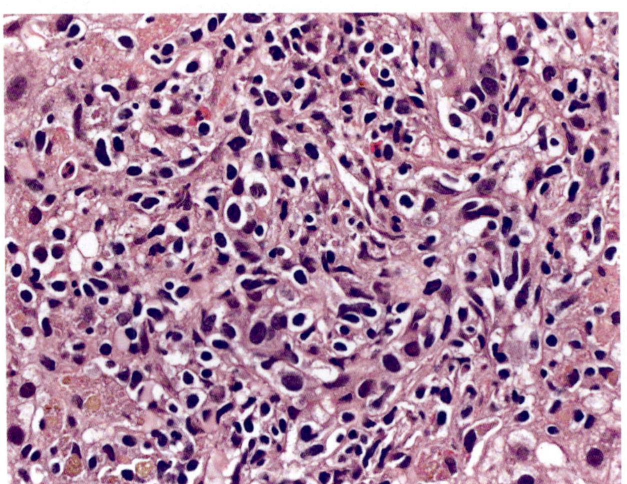

Figure 11.8. **Acute cellular rejection, lymphocytes.** The lymphocytes are large and activated.

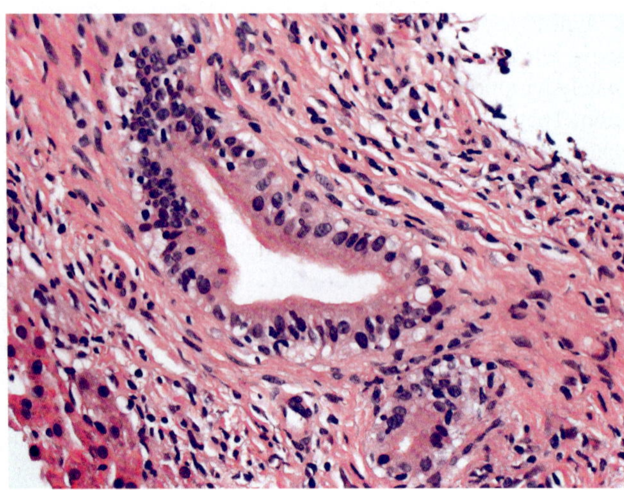

Figure 11.9. **Acute cellular rejection, bile duct injury.** The bile duct shows lymphocytosis and injury.

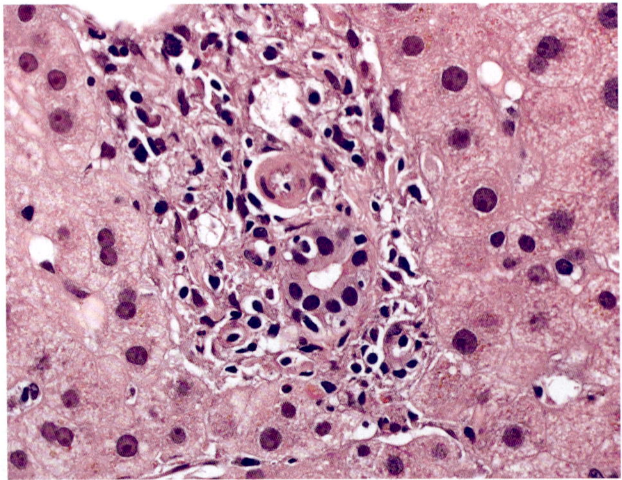

Figure 11.10. **Acute cellular rejection, bile duct injury.** Another example of mild bile duct inflammation and injury.

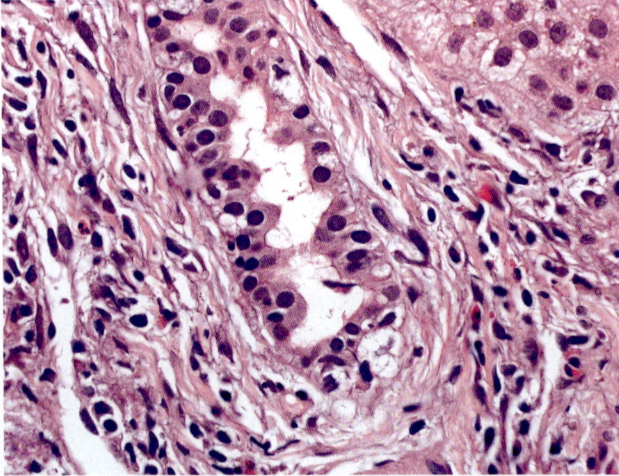

Figure 11.11. **Acute cellular rejection, bile duct injury.** In this case, the epithelium also shows vacuolization, as well as mild lymphocytosis and rare apoptotic bodies.

to overdiagnose endothelialitis. However, inflammatory cells in portal tracts are frequently near the vessels, even if there is no rejection, so a diagnostic focus should show definite endothelial injury/reactive changes. Rarely,[7] endothelialitis can involve a hepatic artery (Fig. 11.15), often in the setting of other features of acute cellular rejection.[8] In cases with severe arteritis, the liver can also show ischemic patterns of injury.[9]

The differential for acute cellular rejection can include recurrent disease, such as hepatitis B, hepatis C, autoimmune hepatitis, or a drug effect. While specific findings can have areas of overlap between acute cellular rejection and other etiologies, such as duct injury, the overall histological patterns of injury are sufficiently different that a definite diagnosis can be rendered in most cases. For example, a predominately lobular-based injury pattern would be unusual for typical acute cellular rejection, and other diseases, such as viral hepatitis, need to be clinically excluded. As another example, a biopsy with disproportionately heavy bile duct injury and mixed neutrophilic and lymphocytic inflammation of the bile duct would be unusual for acute cellular rejection and suggest a drug reaction.

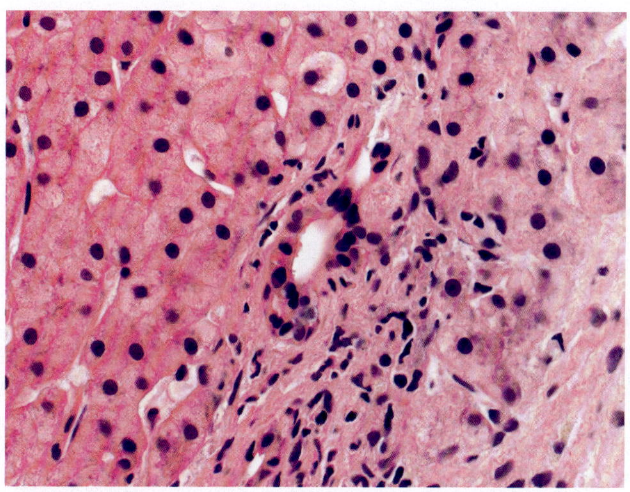

Figure 11.12. **Minimal nonspecific bile duct changes.** The bile duct in this case is not pristine, but there is no active duct injury.

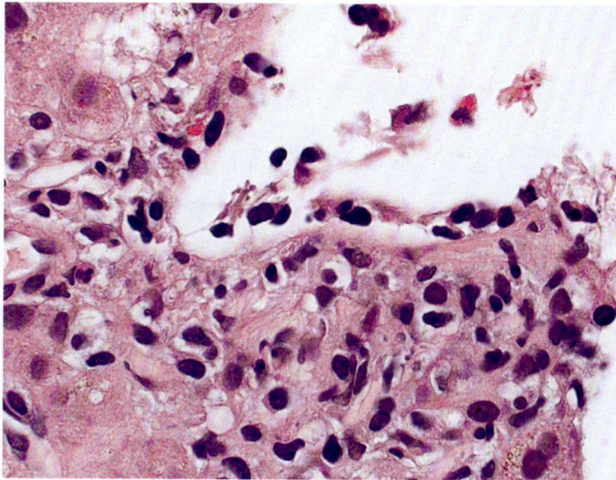

Figure 11.13. **Acute cellular rejection, endothelialitis.** On high power, endothelialitis has led to marked endothelial injury.

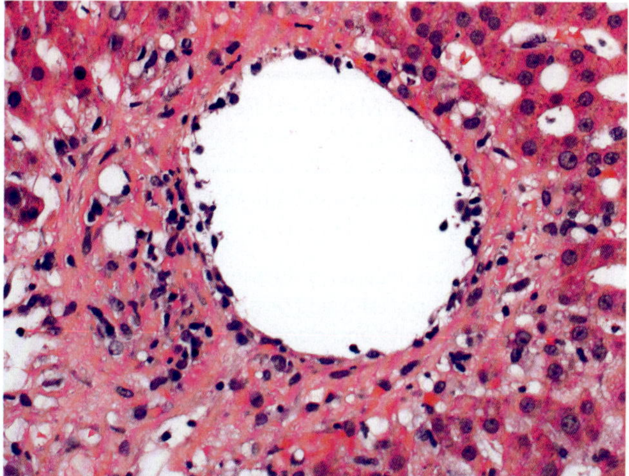

Figure 11.14. **Acute cellular rejection, endothelialitis.** A central vein shows endothelialitis, with lymphocytes attached to luminal surface of the endothelial cells.

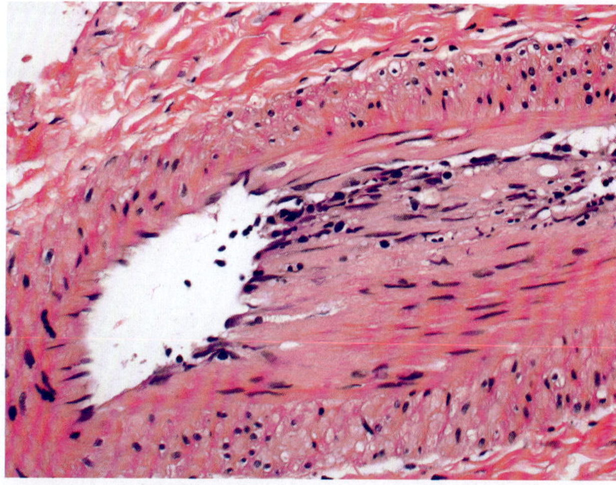

Figure 11.15. **Acute cellular rejection, arteritis.** In this case, an artery shows endothelialitis.

GRADING ACUTE CELLULAR REJECTION

After making a diagnosis of acute cellular rejection, the amount of inflammation and injury is graded as mild, moderate, or severe (Table 11.1). The grade of rejection does not necessarily guide therapy, as rejections at many centers are initially all treated in fundamentally the same way regardless of the grade. However, the grade of rejection does provide useful information about the severity of allograft injury.

Some centers also report out the rejection activity index (RAI) (Table 11.2) in the surgical pathology report. Reporting the RAI is not necessary for clinical care but is an important research tool. The RAI score is not used to make a diagnosis of rejection but can be applied after a diagnosis is made using the overall pattern of injury. To calculate the RAI, each feature of acute cellular rejection is summed on a scale of 0 to 3, with a maximum score of 9.

ATYPICAL PATTERNS OF ACUTE CELLULAR REJECTION

CHECKLIST: Atypical Patterns of Acute Cellular Rejection

- ☐ Lobular variant, a pattern that is most common in these settings:
  - ○ Children
  - ○ Adults who have stopped their antirejection medicines
- ☐ Central perivenulitis variant
- ☐ Plasma cell–rich variant

There are several uncommon patterns of acute cellular rejection. Because these patterns are rare and because they tend to show less specific features, other disease processes have to be excluded. In typical acute cellular rejection, the lobules often show minimal inflammation or sometimes very mild patchy inflammation. However, with the lobular variant of acute cellar rejection, the lobular hepatitis tends to dominate the histological findings (Fig. 11.16). The portal inflammation can range from mild and nonspecific to showing more typical findings of duct injury and/or endothelialitis. This rare pattern is seen sometimes in children, where biopsies also tend to show portal-based rejection. The second setting is adults who stop taking their medications suddenly, going from full immunosuppression to no immunosuppression. In this setting, the rejection can be largely limited to the lobules. Outside of these two settings, a lobular hepatitis is not typical for acute cellular rejection and suggests a different cause of liver injury. Even within these two known settings, drug effects and viral hepatitis should still be carefully excluded.

TABLE 11.1: Acute Cellular Rejection (T Cell–Mediated Rejection)

Grade	Comment
Indeterminate	Portal and/or perivenular inflammation with no other likely etiology, but without enough tissue damage to qualify for rejection.
Mild	Rejection-type inflammation (including duct injury, endothelialitis) in less than half of portal tracts or perivenular areas. Inflammation is generally mild and does not lead to expansion of the portal tracts. There is no necrosis in cases with a perivenular pattern of rejection.
Moderate	Rejection-type inflammation (including duct injury, endothelialitis) in 50% or more of the portal tracts or perivenular areas. The inflammation often expands the portal regions. In cases of perivenular pattern of rejection, there can be perivenular necrosis in a minority of zone 3 regions.
Severe	Similar to moderate rejection, but now with spillover of the portal inflammation into the periportal regions or pervenular necrosis involving more than 50% of zone 3 regions.

TABLE 11.2: Rejection Activity Index (RAI) for Typical Acute Cellular Rejection

Score	Comment
Portal Inflammation	
1	Inflammation is mostly lymphocytic. Inflammation is present in less than 50% of portal tracts and does not lead to portal tract expansion.
2	Inflammation is mostly lymphocytic but now contains occasional lymphoblasts, neutrophils, and eosinophils. Note: Also consider antibody-mediated rejection if eosinophils are prominent or if there is prominent portal tract edema or endothelial cell hypertrophy in the capillaries.
3	Inflammation is as in grade 2 but involves most of the portal tracts.
Bile Duct Injury	
1	Less than 50% of bile ducts are either cuffed or infiltrated by lymphocytes. The bile ducts show mild focal injury and mild reactive changes.
2	More than 50% of the bile ducts are either cuffed or infiltrated by lymphocytes. The ducts also show more than rare damage, but damage is present in less than 50% of ducts. Duct damage includes apoptotic cells, nuclear pleomorphism, and cytoplasmic vacuolization.
3	As in grade 2, but greater than 50% of ducts show damage.
Venous Endothelialitis	
1	Endothelialitis is present in some portal tracts or central veins but less than 50%. Endothelialitis can be subendothelial inflammation or endothelial cells attached to the luminal surface of the endothelial cells.
2	As for 1, but greater than 50% of portal/central veins show damage endothelialitis. There may be focal zone 3 confluent necrosis in less than 50% of perivenular areas.
3	As for 2, but there is zone 3 confluent necrosis in 50% or more of the perivenular areas.

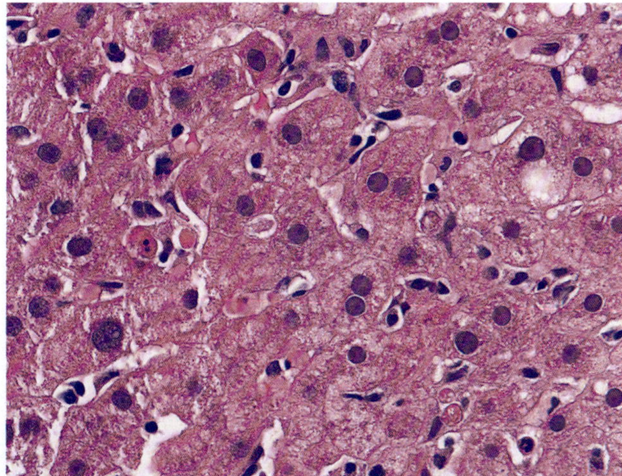

Figure 11.16. **Acute cellular rejection, lobular pattern.** The portal tracts showed mild nonspecific lymphocytic inflammation without duct injury or endothelialitis, but the lobules show diffuse mild to moderate hepatitis. The hepatitis responded to antirejection therapy (immunosuppressive drugs had been stopped while on vacation).

The central perivenulitis pattern of acute cellular rejection shows zone 3 hepatocyte drop out, with inflammation in the loose edematous fibrous tissue where the hepatocytes should be located (Fig. 11.17). A true endothelialitis is uncommon. The central perivenulitis pattern of injury can be an isolated finding, or it can be associated with typical acute cellular rejection in the portal tracts. Overall, isolated central perivenulitis tends to be more common in allograft biopsies taken a year or more after transplantation. If there are subsequent rejections in the same allograft, they also tend to have a central perivenulitis pattern. This pattern of rejection responds to conventional antirejection therapy.[10] If untreated or undertreated, the central perivenulitis pattern of rejection pattern can lead to central vein fibrosis.[11] This pattern is also associated with an increased risk for ductopenia.[11]

Plasma cell–rich rejection looks like typical acute cellular rejection except that plasma cells are prominent (Fig. 11.18). A few plasma cells are common in ordinary rejection, where the number of plasma cells roughly correlates with the amount of portal inflammation and the severity of the rejection.[12] However, the plasma cells are never particularly striking in typical rejection, in contrast to the plasma cell–rich variant of rejection.

This pattern of rejection has several known associations. First, some individuals appear predisposed to a plasma cell-rich autoimmune response to antigens. For example, individuals with increased numbers of plasma cells in their native livers have an increased risk for the plasma cell–rich pattern of rejection, particularly if the native liver had portal tracts showing greater than 30% plasma cells.[13] Although not relevant anymore because of new antiviral medications, historically, interferon-based therapy for the treatment of recurrent hepatitis C could trigger a plasma cell–rich variant of rejection,[14–16] in particular when immunosuppression levels were reduced before interferon treatment. Finally, there are some cases of steroid-resistant, difficult-to-manage rejections that are frequently recurrent and tend to develop a plasma cell–rich pattern over time. In these cases, the duct injury and endothelialitis tends to diminish as the plasma cells increase. Some of these cases can also have a central perivenulitis pattern of injury.[17] Because these cases can be difficult to manage, graft failure can develop.[13,17]

The histological differential includes recurrent autoimmune hepatitis as well as de novo autoimmune hepatitis. The therapies used to treat rejection are broadly similar but not identical to those used for recurrent autoimmune hepatitis or de novo autoimmune hepatitis, so the distinction does have clinical relevance. Although there is some histological overlap, cases of recurrent and de novo autoimmune hepatitis lack the degree of duct injury and/or endothelialitis that is present in the plasma cell–rich variant of rejection. Likewise, recurrent autoimmune hepatitis or de novo autoimmune hepatitis has more lobular hepatitis than rejection and often has more portal inflammation, with little or no duct injury or endothelialitis. The clinical course is also relevant, as most cases of plasma cell–rich rejection are associated with low levels of immunosuppression and occur within the first two

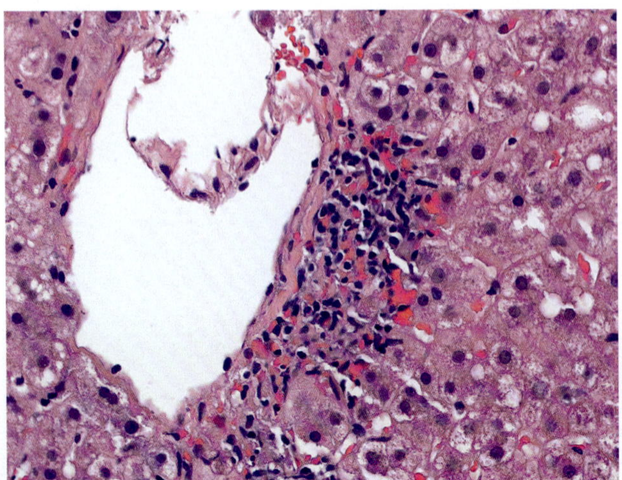

Figure 11.17. Acute cellular rejection, perivenulitis pattern. The central vein endothelial cells looked normal throughout the biopsy, but perivenulitis was present in most central vein areas.

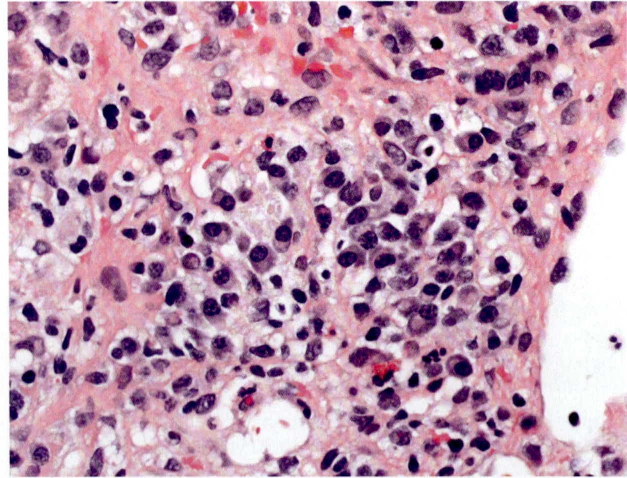

Figure 11.18. Acute cellular rejection, plasma cell–rich pattern. Plasma cells were prominent in this case.

years of transplantation, while recurrent autoimmune hepatitis is not specifically associated with immunosuppression levels and typically occurs 3 years or more after transplantation.[17] Serological findings can also be factored in, as autoantibody titers are commonly high titer in true autoimmune hepatitis, while negative or low titer in plasma cell–rich rejection.

IDIOPATHIC POSTTRANSPLANT HEPATITIS

Late allografts can develop a chronic hepatitis pattern of injury called *idiopathic posttransplant hepatitis*. This pattern shows nonspecific portal chronic inflammation with no endothelialitis and no or minimal bile duct injury (Fig. 11.19). The portal chronic inflammation is typically mild to moderate and predominately lymphocytic, though plasma cells can be mildly prominent. Mild interface activity is common when there is moderate portal chronic inflammation. The lobular inflammation is absent or mild. The idiopathic posttransplant hepatitis pattern appears to be a mixture of different disease processes, but a subset can develop fibrosis progression.[18,19] In all cases, chronic viral hepatitis, including hepatitis E, has to be clinically excluded, as should drug effects. If there is a component of central perivenulitis, then immunosuppression should be optimized to see if there is improvement in live enzymes.

ANTIBODY-MEDIATED REJECTION

Antibody-mediated rejection results from circulating antibodies that recognize donor antigens in the transplanted liver, leading to graft injury. Of note, the detection of donor-specific antibodies alone does not equal a diagnosis of antibody-mediated rejection. A diagnosis is made when the following criteria are met: (1) the patient has donor-specific antibodies; (2) there is laboratory evidence of graft dysfunction; (3) the liver biopsy shows changes that are consistent with antibody-mediated rejection and provide no other explanation for the graft dysfunction; and (4) a C4d stain shows a compatible pattern of C4d deposition in the liver.

Most cases of antibody-mediated rejection result from de novo antibodies that develop after transplantation. Antibody-mediated rejection can be associated with other clinical and histological findings of acute cellular rejection or chronic rejection.[20] In rare cases, the specific antigen has been identified that led to the formation of donor-specific antibodies. The best characterized setting is when the donor liver expresses a normal liver protein that was not expressed in the patient's native liver, owing to either polymorphism, such as with glutathione-S-transferase T1 (GSTT1),[21,22] or genetic diseases that lead to lack of protein expression, such as bile salt export proteins.[23] These cases are can also have de novo autoimmune hepatitis pattern of injury.

The histological findings in cases of antibody-mediated rejection will vary and can be divided into early and late changes. Early findings are characterized by endothelial injury.[24] In severe cases, the endothelial injury can lead to hemorrhagic necrosis, but most cases show milder changes with neutrophil-rich inflammation in the portal tracts, rare microvascular thrombi, and sometimes mild sinusoidal dilatation and congestion. The zone 3 hepatocytes can show changes that resemble preservation injury, with mild hepatocyte ballooning, mild cholestasis, and scattered acidophil bodies.[20,25]

Later on, the pattern of injury resembles that of biliary obstruction (Fig. 11.20). The portal tract shows mixed inflammation with a neutrophilic component, edema, and ductular proliferation.[20,26,27] The lobules can show cholestasis and mild sinusoidal dilatation. If the diagnosis is not made or the patient is resistant to therapy, antibody-mediated rejection can lead to thrombosis of the portal vein and/or hepatic artery. This in turn can lead to ischemic strictures or necrosis of the bile ducts.

C4d staining can be challenging to interpret because many diseases that are not antibody-mediated rejection can also show C4d staining, so both the presence of staining and the pattern of staining need to be evaluated. The C4d should have a strong and diffuse

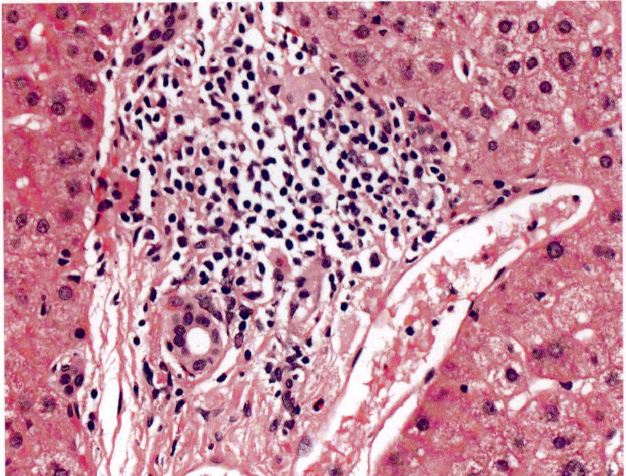

Figure 11.19. **Idiopathic posttransplant hepatitis pattern.** A chronic hepatitis developed 5 years after liver transplantation for autosomal dominant polycystic liver disease. There was mild but persistent portal chronic inflammation.

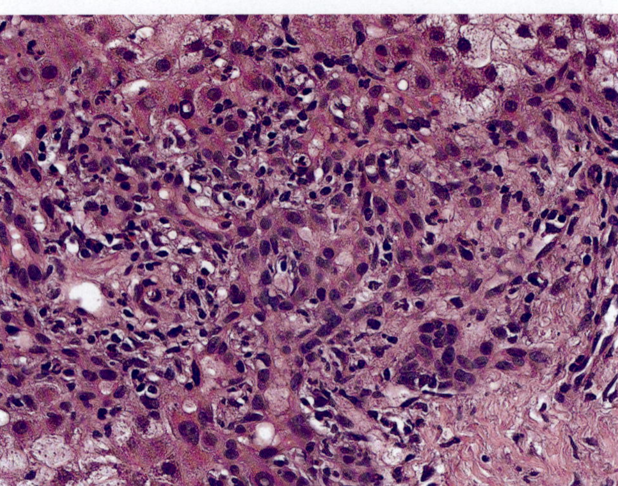

Figure 11.20. **Antibody-mediated rejection mimicking biliary obstruction.** The first impression on this biopsy was that of biliary obstruction, but there was no obstruction on imaging, and further testing showed antibody-mediated rejection.

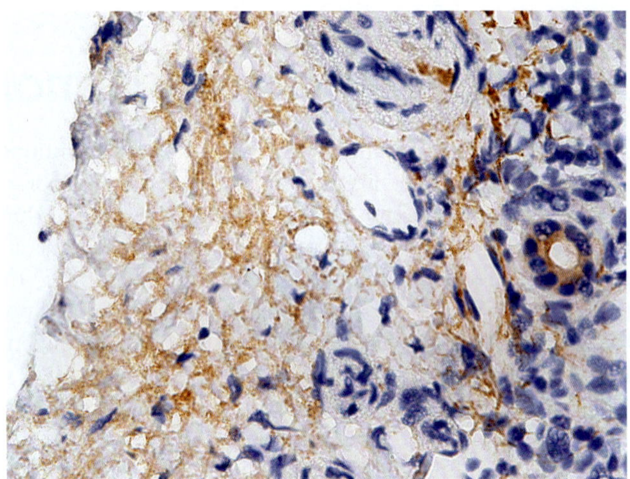

Figure 11.21. **Antibody-mediated rejection mimicking biliary obstruction, C4d stain.** An immunostain for C4d was positive in most of the portal tracts.

pattern of staining to support a diagnosis of antibody-mediated rejection. Using this approach, most cases of antibody-mediated rejection can be distinguished from nonspecific staining.[28] Diffuse staining is defined as greater than 50% of portal tracts showing positive staining.[20] C4d positivity can be seen in the portal veins and the capillaries/stroma of the portal tracts (Fig. 11.21). Sinusoidal staining or central vein staining is less common but, if strong and diffuse, can also be clinically significant.[28]

CHRONIC REJECTION

With chronic rejection, the serum alkaline phosphatase levels are chronically elevated and imaging can show pruning of the intrahepatic biliary tree, which is defined as less than normal numbers of the smaller branches of the biliary tree. In all cases, biliary strictures need to be excluded before a final diagnosis of chronic rejection is achieved.

On peripheral needle biopsy, the chronic rejection pattern of injury is essentially that of bile duct atrophy (Fig. 11.22), bile duct loss, and lobular cholestasis. Inflammation in the

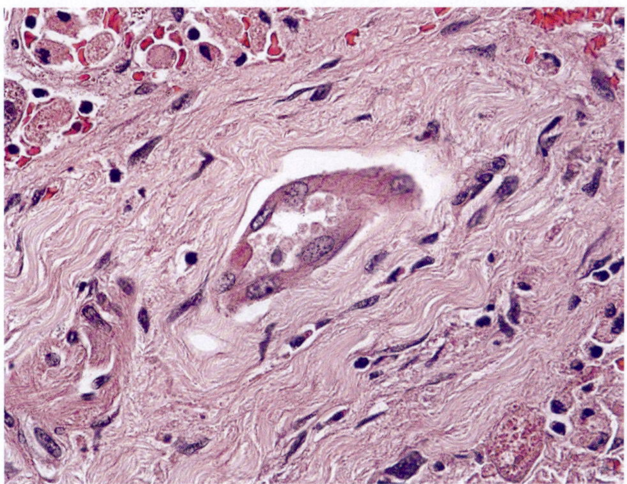

Figure 11.22. **Chronic rejection, bile duct atrophy.** The bile duct is still there but looks abnormal, with atrophic and reactive changes.

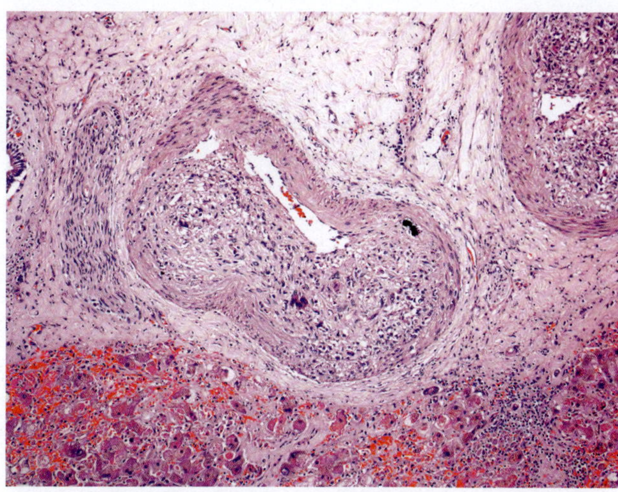

Figure 11.23. **Chronic rejection, foam cell arteriopathy.** The arteries are markedly thickened by a histocytic/fibrotic reaction.

portal tracts is usually absent or mild and patchy. The diagnosis of chronic rejection can be made using any of the following patterns:[29] (1) bile duct atrophy in >50% of bile ducts, with or without bile duct loss, where the first changes of senescence/atrophy are found in the smallest branches of the biliary tree; (2) bile duct loss in >50% of bile ducts; or (3) foam cell obliterative arteriopathy. Foam cell arteriopathy is usually seen only on resection specimens (Fig. 11.23), as it is the larger branches of the hepatic artery that are affected. The lobules can show cholestasis, especially in later stages of the disease. The lobules can also show a central perivenulitis pattern of injury, and the central vein injury can eventually lead to zone 3 fibrosis.

VASCULAR PROBLEMS

HEPATIC ARTERY INSUFFICIENCY

There can be a number of different hepatic artery problems following transplantation, the most common being hepatic artery thrombosis (HAT). Most cases of HAT occur within the first three weeks of transplantation, with a median of about 7 days.[30] However, there is a smaller group of cases that present with delayed or late HAT, commonly defined as occurring greater than 4 weeks after transplantation.[31] The frequency of early HAT is 8% in children and 3% in adults,[30] but is variable from center to center depending on the experience of the surgical team[32] and the patient population receiving transplants. Most cases are diagnosed by imaging findings alone, and biopsies do not play a major role. Many cases lead to fulminant hepatic failure and retransplantation.[32] In those cases with less severe allograft ischemia, the histological findings fall into two broad categories of early and late changes. In early hepatic arterial thrombosis, the biopsy shows increased lobular hepatocyte spotty necrosis without significant inflammation, but with the additional finding of increased cell cycling (Fig. 11.24) with increased mitotic figures.[8,33,34] Rarely, arteritis from acute cellular rejection can lead to similar findings.[8] If the arterial blood flow is not adequately restored, then over time (weeks, months) the liver can show zone 3 hepatocyte necrosis and/or dropout along with ischemic strictures that lead to biliary obstructive type changes on biopsy.[35,36] Individuals who develop delayed or late HAT (>4 weeks after transplantation) tend to present with cholestasis or biliary strictures,[31] although many patients can be clinically asymptomatic and identified only after evaluation for biochemical abnormalities.

SMALL-FOR-SIZE GRAFT

This pattern of injury results from too much blood flow coming through the portal vein and happens when a small liver allograft is used, usually one that is less than 30% of the

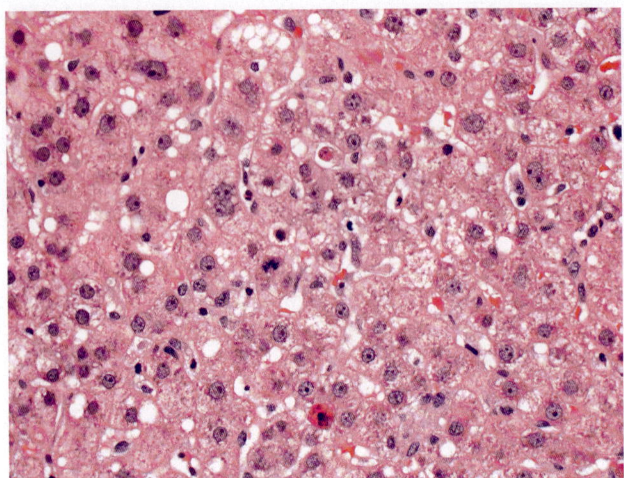

Figure 11.24. **Hepatic artery thrombosis.** After a recent hepatic artery thrombosis, the lobules show both numerous apoptotic bodies and mitotic figures.

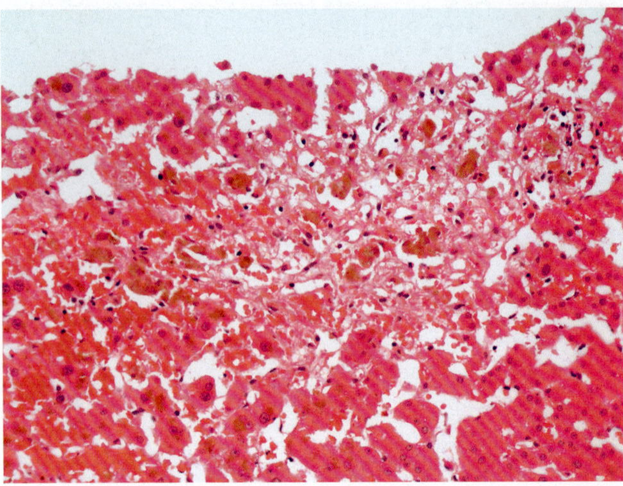

Figure 11.25. **Piggyback graft, outflow changes.** The biopsy shows zone 3 hepatocyte dropout, numerous pigmented macrophages, and sinusoidal congestion.

native liver volume or 0.8% of the recipient's body weight.[37] Other risk factors include prolonged ischemia time and greater than 30% steatosis in the donor liver.[38] The clinical findings are that of ascites and graft dysfunction (defined as having at least two of these: elevated bilirubin levels, coagulopathy, encephalopathy) within the first week or so after transplant, with a small-for-size graft and all other causes excluded.[39] Clinically, this is called the *small-for-size syndrome*.

The histological changes are also subtle, especially in cases with mild disease. The histological changes include portal vein dilatation, zone 1 sinusoidal dilatation, and hemorrhage into the portal tract connective tissue. Of note, these finding are seen primarily in the larger portal tracts, which are usually not well sampled in peripheral liver biopsies. The findings in the liver periphery are mild and nonspecific but can include mild bile ductular proliferation and nodular regenerative hyperplasia. A component of mild acute cellular rejection is also commonly seen.[37] In cases with severe hyperperfusion, there can be thrombosis or vasospasm of the hepatic artery, leading to ischemic necrosis of the larger sized bile ducts, along with bile leaks and peribiliary abscesses.

PIGGYBACK GRAFTS AND CONGESTIVE HEPATOPATHY

The transplant surgery can preserve the recipient's vena cava using the "piggyback" technique, where the recipient's vena cava is directly sewn to the donor's inferior vena cava, an approach that improves operating time, blood loss, and time in hospital. In early studies, 8% of patients transplanted with the piggyback method developed refractory ascites,[29] due either to Budd–Chiari or to insufficient blood outflow at the vascular reconstruction, even if no anastomotic stricture was detected by imaging studies.[40,41] Histologically, the liver biopsies show a vascular outflow pattern of injury with zone 3 sinusoidal dilatation, congestion, and hepatocyte dropout (Fig. 11.25). The degree of these changes will reflect the severity of vascular outflow disease and can range from mild and patchy to striking. As it is true for vascular outflow disease in general, the portal tracts can also show a mild reactive bile ductular proliferation.

OTHER FINDINGS

OPPORTUNISTIC VIRAL INFECTIONS

Immunosuppression leads to an increased risk for certain viral infections within the allograft, in particular cytomegalovirus (CMV) and EBV. CMV infection is the most common, and the histological findings can range from mild nonspecific hepatitis to numerous neutrophilic microabscesses in the liver to a marked hepatitis. CMV can infect hepatocytes, endothelial cells, and bile ducts, but viral cytopathic effect is not always present, so immunostains should be performed whenever there is clinical or histological concern for infection. The neutrophilic microabscesses pattern of injury (Fig. 11.26) is not a sensitive or specific finding for CMV infection and is idiopathic in most cases anyway.[42] In contrast, numerous microabscesses (>10) is more suggestive of CMV infection.

EBV hepatitis can be subtle, with mild nonspecific portal inflammation and patchy mild lobular inflammation. In a subset of cases, there will be patchy but dense sinusoidal infiltrates with relatively little hepatocyte damage. Lobular granulomas can occasionally be seen. Because the histological findings are often nonspecific, in situ hybridization for EBV or immunostains are important tests in any case of unexplained hepatitis, even if mild.

Other opportunistic viral infections include herpes simplex virus and adenovirus. These viruses show extensive azonal areas of necrosis. The hepatocytes at the edges of the necrotic areas are the best place to hunt for viral inclusions on H&E, but viral inclusions are often hard to see, so immunostains should be used to confirm the diagnosis. Finally, human herpesvirus 6 (HHV6) has rarely been reported after transplantation and at least sometimes can lead to a giant cell hepatitis pattern of injury.[43]

Hepatitis E virus (HEV) infection can lead to chronic hepatitis in immunosuppressed patients, including those with liver transplants. The frequency has not been well defined but overall appears to be rare, probably less than 1% in most centers. The histological findings are variable but usually consist of mild nonspecific portal and lobular hepatitis, sometimes with mild unexplained lobular cholestasis.[44–46] Rapid fibrosis progression has been reported[44] but does not seem to be typical, as most cases tend to have mild persistent unexplained hepatitis with slow or no fibrosis progression. An exposure history or other risk factors are not evident in most cases, so a high index of suspicion is the best way to pick up HEV infections, in particular if there is an unexplained chronic hepatitis or unexplained fibrosis progression. The most common method to establish the diagnosis is serological testing, but some centers also have available in situ hybridization or immunostains.

RECURRENT DISEASE

CHECKLIST: Recurrent Disease in the Liver Allograft

- ☐ Viral hepatitis
  - ○ HCV; historically, recurrence around 4 to 12 weeks in most cases, some later out to 6 months; recurrent HCV is now rare with current antivirals
  - ○ HBV: Historically there was a high rate or recurrence and graft failure, but not now. With current antivirals less than 5% of cases recur[47]
  - ○ HAV: very rare, in individuals transplanted for fulminant HAV
- ☐ Autoimmune hepatitis
  - ○ About 30% of cases recur[48]
  - ○ Average time of recurrence is ~5 years, range ~3 to 10 years
- ☐ Primary sclerosing cholangitis
  - ○ About 40% of cases recur
  - ○ Average time of recurrence is ~5 years, ~range 0.5 to 10 years[49,50]
- ☐ Primary biliary cirrhosis
  - ○ About 30% of cases recur[48]
  - ○ Average time of recurrence is ~5 years, range ~3 to 10 years
- ☐ Fatty liver disease
  - ○ Nonalcoholic (nearly 100% if followed long enough and the metabolic syndrome is not adequately controlled)[51,52]
  - ○ Alcoholic (about 30% to 45%)[53,54]

Recurrent diseases can include chronic viral hepatitis B or C (less so now with effective antiviral therapy), autoimmune hepatitis, primary biliary cirrhosis, primary sclerosing cholangitis, and fatty liver disease. In each of these diseases, the histological patterns in the allograft are essentially the same as they are in the native liver, and the diagnostic approach is also essentially the same.

Recurrent hepatitis C and B are now very rare because of effective antiviral thereapies. Before the advent of the highly effective antiretrovirals, recurrent viral hepatitis would present with a spike in liver enzymes above baseline, with AST and ALT levels greater than alkaline phosphatase levels. Most cases recurred biochemically and histologically between 3 and 6 months after transplantation. The early changes showed increased lobular apoptosis (Fig. 11.27), often with a mild lobular hepatitis pattern, while later changes show a typical chronic hepatitis pattern.

A fibrosing cholestatic pattern of chronic viral hepatitis (can be either B or C) can develop when there are very high levels of viral replication. This pattern of injury is now very rare because of effective antiviral drugs. Nonetheless, the earliest changes in the fibrosing cholestatic pattern are lobular cholestasis and early lobular fibrosis.[55] In later cases, the biopsy often mimics biliary obstruction (Fig. 11.28), with bile ductular proliferation, minimal to mild portal inflammation, minimal lobular inflammation, moderate lobular cholestasis, and often prominent ballooned hepatocytes. A trichrome can show portal fibrosis and pericellular fibrosis (Fig. 11.29), often a with zone 1 pattern, but sometimes with more diffuse lobular fibrosis, or a zone 3 pattern.

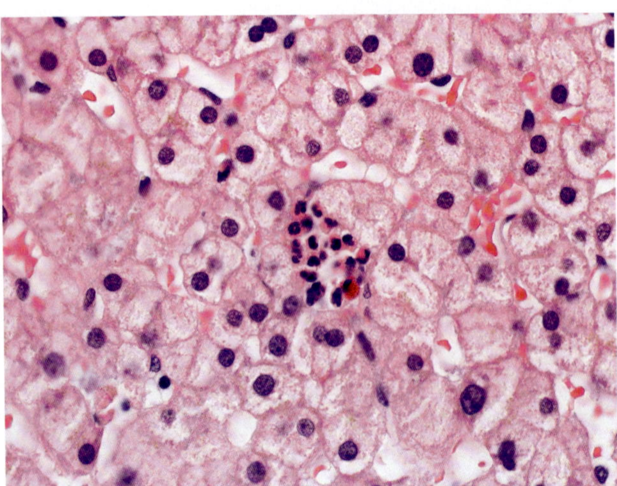

Figure 11.26. **Microabscess pattern of injury.** The lobules show scattered small cluster of neutrophils. This pattern is not specific for cytomegalovirus (CMV), but prominent microabscesses have been associated with CMV infection.

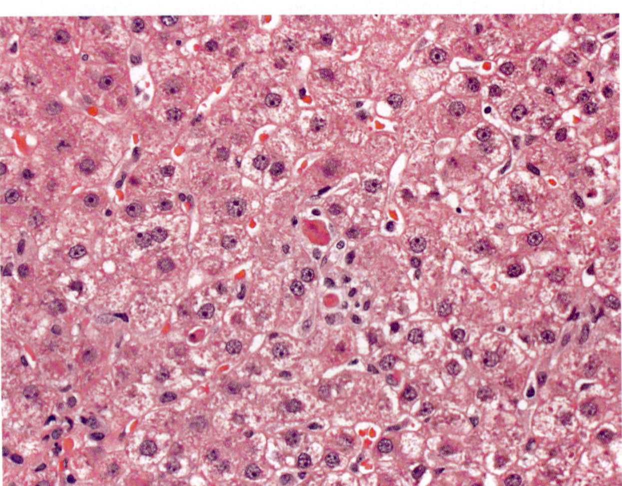

Figure 11.27. **Recurrent hepatitis C.** This biopsy was obtained at 4 months after transplant and shows increased hepatocyte apotosis with mild Kupffer cell hyperplasia and mild lobular inflammation.

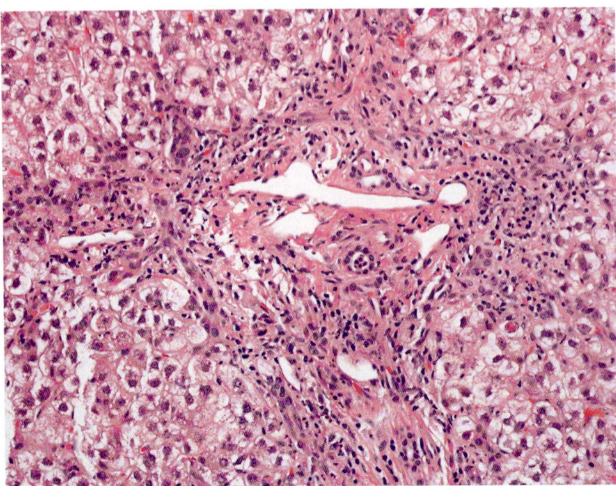

Figure 11.28. **Fibrosing cholestatic hepatis C.** The biopsy shows bile ductular proliferation and cholestasis, with relatively little portal or lobular inflammation.

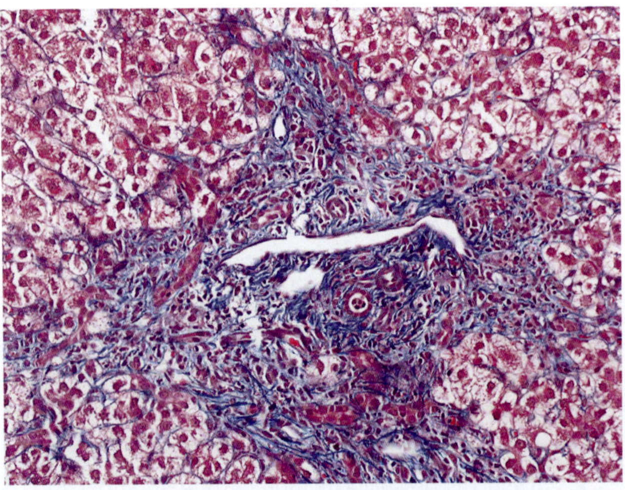

Figure 11.29. **Fibrosing cholestatic hepatis C, trichrome stain.** The portal tracts showed portal and zone 1 fibrosis (same case as above)

Fatty liver disease occurs in about 1/3 of individuals transplanted for alcohol cirrhosis due to recidivism. With nonalcoholic fatty liver disease, almost all individuals who continue to have the metabolic syndrome will develop recurrent fatty liver disease steatosis. Fatty liver disease typically reoccurs histologically within 5 years after liver transplantation,[56] even if enzyme levels are normal or near normal.[51] Steroid use for antirejection therapy is also a risk factor.[56] Steatosis or steatohepatitis can be seen, and the diagnosis is made in the usual fashion.

Although not recurrent disease per se, de novo steatosis or steatohepatitis can develop in individuals transplanted for FIC1 deficiency.[57] Often times the steatohepatitis is severe. Portal vein thrombosis and steroid use can also contribute to fatty liver disease in individuals with the metabolic syndrome.

For recurrent autoimmune hepatitis, primary sclerosing cholangitis and primary biliary cirrhosis, the histological changes are fundamentally the same as those seen in nontransplanted patients, and the diagnosis is made using usual criteria.[29] In cases of recurrent chronic biliary tract disease, biliary anastomotic obstruction has to be excluded by imaging findings. Imaging findings can also help support a diagnosis of recurrent primary sclerosing cholangitis by demonstrating nonanastomotic biliary strictures. In general, most surgical-related strictures present clinically within the first 90 days following transplantation.

In cases where the main pattern of injury is ductopenia, the differential includes recurrent biliary tract disease and chronic rejection. Chronic rejection is usually associated with a history of multiple episodes of acute cellar rejection or a long history of suboptimal immunosuppression. Histologically, findings that would favor recurrent biliary tract disease over chronic rejection include ductular proliferation (PSC), mild to moderate portal inflammation (PBC), florid duct lesions (PBC) granulomas (PBC), and fibrosis (either PSC or PBC). On the other hand, chronic rejection is more likely to have a component of central perivenulitis and/or central perivenular fibrosis. Periductal fibrosis or fibro-obliterative duct lesions are not part of the pathology of chronic rejection and suggest either PSC or chronic anastomotic strictures.

The differential for recurrent autoimmune hepatitis includes plasma cell–rich rejection. Recurrent autoimmune hepatitis looks like autoimmune hepatitis, with plasma cell–rich portal inflammation and a brisk lobular hepatitis. In contrast, plasma cell–rich rejection has little or no lobular hepatitis (other than some cases having perivenulitis), and the portal tracts often show other findings typical for acute cellar rejection, including prominent duct injury and/or endothelialitis. Elevated serum autoantibodies (ANA, ASMA, etc.) and serum IgG levels are essentially always present with recurrent autoimmune hepatitis, so negative serologies make autoimmune hepatitis unlikely. However, serologies can also be persistently elevated in patients who were transplanted for autoimmune hepatitis, but who have rejection and not recurrent autoimmune hepatitis, although in this setting the autoantibodies are generally low titer.[17]

GLYCOGENIC HEPATOPATHY

Glycogenic hepatopathy after steroid therapy for rejection can cause transient histological changes and mild AST and ALT elevations. The histological changes are similar to that of diabetic glycogenic hepatopathy with enlarged pale hepatocytes but are usually less pronounced. The histological findings rapidly resolve with stopping of steroids, and there are no lasting clinical or histological sequelae. Anecdotally, patients with diabetes and poor glycemic control are predisposed to this finding. In many cases, the finding is subclinical and seen mostly on follow-up biopsies to evaluate the effectiveness of antirejection steroid therapy.

DRUG REACTION

Drug reactions can be very challenging to diagnose after liver transplantation, as they can closely mimic acute cellular rejection and recurrent diseases. Data on this topic are sparse, but one study found a drug-induced liver injury (DILI) frequency of 1.7% after liver transplantation.[58] In this study, patients presented with nonspecific findings of nausea or diarrhea (31%), jaundice (24%), and pruritus (10%). The most common class of drug was antibiotics (48%), followed by immunosuppressive agents (14%), and antihyperlipidemic drugs (7%). Of the antibiotics, trimethoprim–sulfamethoxazole was the most common cause of DILI. The median time for liver enzymes to return to baseline after stopping the drug was 34 days.[58] Another study identified antifungal agents as a common cause of DILI.[59]

Histologically, the possibility of DILI is usually suggested when biopsy findings do not fit for any other of the common patterns of injury, such as rejection or recurrent disease. The two most common DILI patterns seem to be bland lobular cholestasis or a cholangitic pattern of injury, with mixed portal inflammation (neutrophils and lymphocytes) and injury of the bile duct. In other cases, failure to respond to antirejection therapy can prompt reevaluation of the biopsy to look for a possible drug reaction.

POSTTRANSPLANT LYMHOPROLIFERATIVE DISORDER

Posttransplant lymphoproliferative disorders (PTLDs) are usually EBV-driven proliferations of B cells. However, some cases of PTLD are EBV negative (10%),[60] and rare cases are of T cell or NK cell origin.[60] The histological findings can vary from hepatitic-like patterns to mass-forming lesions (Figs. 11.30 and 11.31). The hepatitic pattern is the most challenging to identify because it can mimic other causes of hepatitis. In general, the biopsy shows moderate or greater portal and lobular inflammation. Some cases can have plasma cell–rich portal infiltrates.[61] Rarely the lymphocytes will be cytologically atypical, with large nuclei and irregular nuclear contours, but in most cases with a hepatitic pattern, the cytological atypia is mild and not clearly beyond that of reactive changes. For that reason, the best way to identify PTLD is to have a high index of suspicion and a low threshold for doing EBV stains (Fig. 11.32). In particular, PTLD should be ruled out in cases of unexplained hepatitis. PTLD is further subclassified as per the current WHO system. Finally, patients can rarely develop PTLD in a lymph node or other organ without involvement of the allograft liver. Liver biopsies in this setting can show a range of findings from acute cellular rejection, to recurrent disease, to mild nonspecific inflammatory changes.[62]

GRAFT VERSUS HOST DISEASE

Graft versus host disease (GVHD) affects allogenic bone marrow transplant recipients when engrafted donor immune cells attack the recipient's liver. GVHD most commonly involves the skin, gastrointestinal (GI) tract, and liver. When there is liver disease, the skin and/or the GI tract are almost always affected, although rare cases of isolated liver GVHD have been reported.[63] Isolated GVHD is always a diagnosis of exclusion and should be made with caution.

Clinically, liver involvement by GVHD manifests with elevations in alkaline phosphatase and bilirubin. The histological findings are bile duct–centered injury (Fig. 11.33).

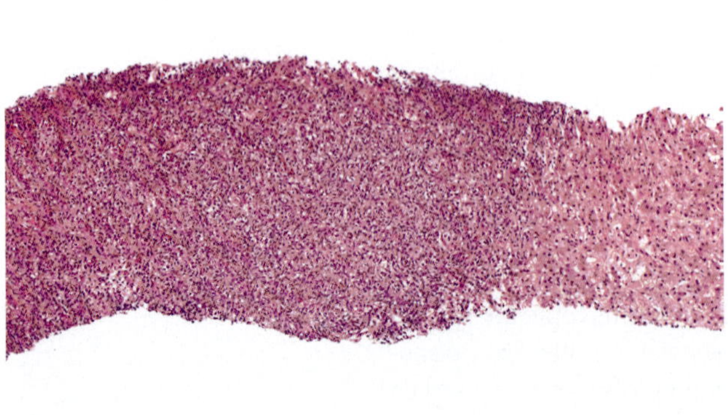

Figure 11.30. Posttransplant lymphoproliferative disorder. A liver mass was targeted in this biopsy.

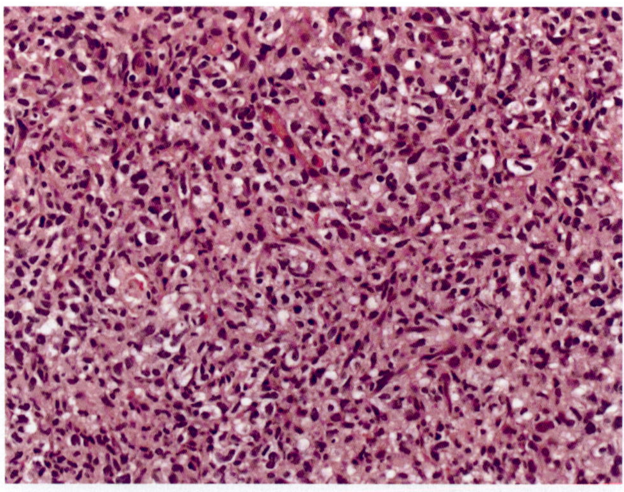

Figure 11.31. Posttransplant lymphoproliferative disorder. The liver mass is composed of atypical lymphocytes.

While portal inflammation and bile duct lymphocytosis are generally minimal, there is bile duct apoptosis, reactive epithelial changes, and bile duct atrophy. The lobules often show cholestasis.

A hepatitic variant of GVHD can be seen after donor lymphocyte infusion, where the main pattern of injury is lobular hepatitis.[64] The portal tracts can show either mild nonspecific changes or the typical changes of GVHD. In chronic GVHD, the pattern of injury is predominately duct atrophy and ductopenia.

ENGRAFTMENT SYNDROME

The engraftment syndrome is a clinical finding that occurs 4 to 10 days after bone marrow engraftment. The syndrome is well recognized clinically, and the liver is usually not biopsied. The engraftment syndrome results from a big burst of cytokines released by the engrafted marrow cells, and these lead to fever, an erythematous rash that covers >25% of the body, and pulmonary edema. Additional findings include elevated liver enzyme (bilirubin >2 mg/dl or AST or ALT >2 ULN), renal insufficiency, and rapid weight gain. On biopsy, the liver findings can mimic veno-occlusive disease, with marked sinusoidal congestion and congestion (Fig. 11.34).

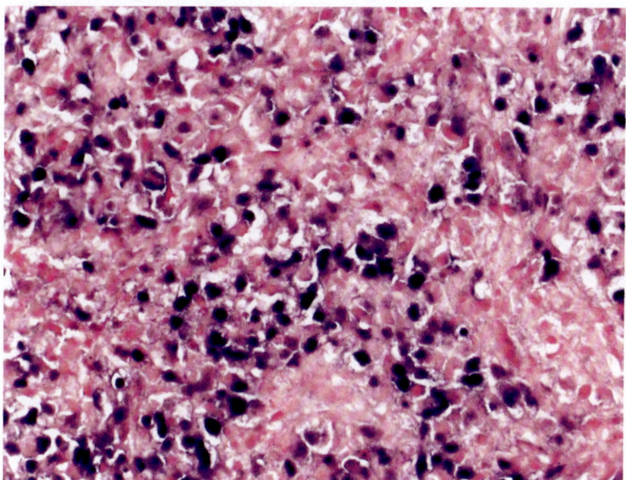

Figure 11.32. **Posttransplant lymphoproliferative disorder (PTLD), EBV in situ hybridization.** The PTLD is strongly positive.

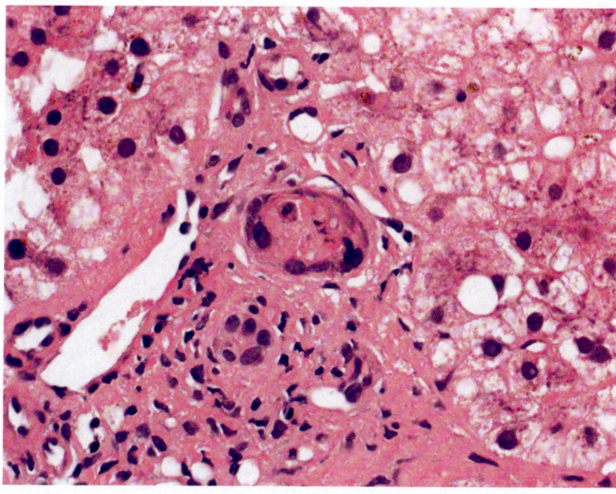

Figure 11.33. **Graft versus host disease.** There is almost no inflammation, but the bile ducts are atrophic and one of them has several apoptotic bodies.

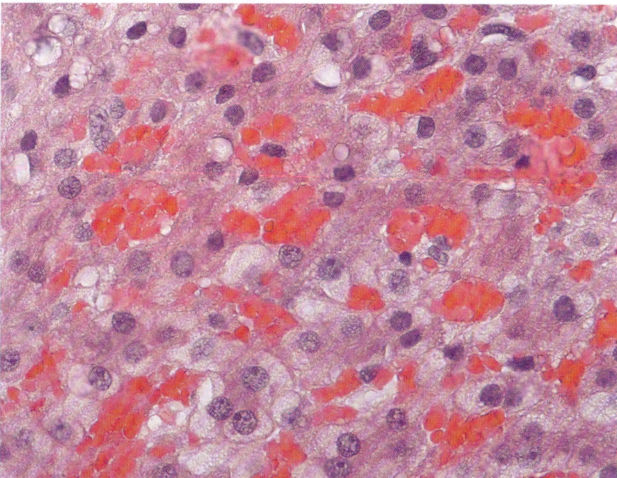

Figure 11.34. **Engraftment syndrome.** The sinusoids show congestion, mostly in zone 3 regions.

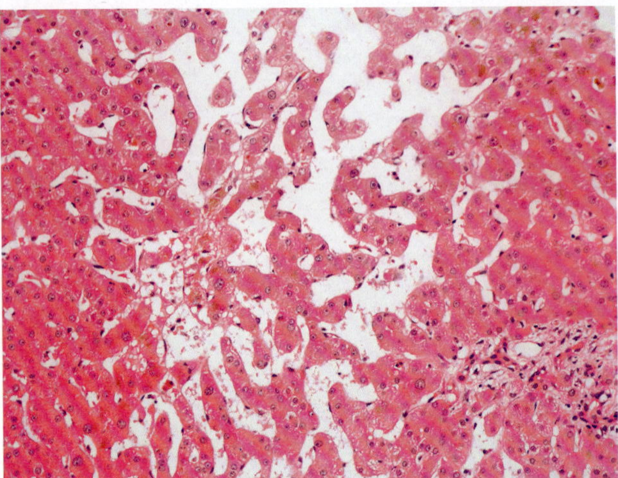

Figure 11.35. **Near miss case 1, vascular outflow disease.** The biopsy showed changes that strongly indicated vascular outflow disease. Even though imaging findings could not confirm vascular outflow disease, the pathology findings led to the correct management.

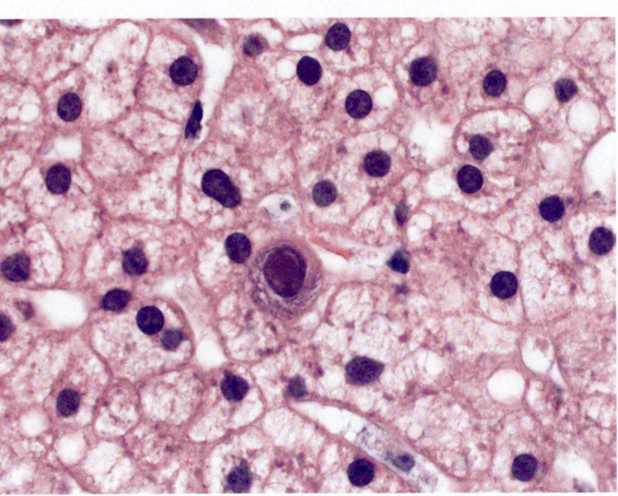

Figure 11.36. **Near miss case 2, cytomegalovirus (CMV) hepatitis.** The biopsy showed only a single convincing hepatocyte with viral cytopathic effect.

NEAR MISSES

CASE 1. A 47-year-old woman underwent liver transplantation for cirrhosis from chronic hepatitis C. The clinical course was smooth after transplantation, other than for mild intermittent ascites that seemed to resolve on its own for the most part. Several biopsies were obtained during this clinical course and were essentially normal. Likewise, imaging of the vasculature was essentially normal. In time, the ascites worsened and became persistent. A transjuglar biopsy was performed. Although the biopsy was small and fragmented, there was marked zone 3 dilatation in several of the fragments (Fig. 11.35) leading to a diagnosis of impaired vascular outflow. Venography was, however, normal and the pressure gradients across the anastomosis were only minimally elevated. Nonetheless, given the overall findings, in particular the biopsy findings, the anastomosis was stented, which led to resolution of the ascites.

This case illustrates the challenges of identifying vascular flow changes in the liver allograft. Imaging and pressure gradients are important parts of the evaluation, but the histological findings can often help clarify difficult cases. On the other hand, the histological changes of vascular outflow disease can be absent or mild in early disease, as seen in this case, and sometimes the final diagnosis is only clear after some time.

CASE 2. A 5-year-old child was transplanted for biliary atresia. The transplant went well, but there was a mild bump in liver enzymes at day 14, leading to a liver biopsy. The biopsy findings were very mild, with minimal nonspecific inflammation in the portal tracts and lobules, providing no evidence for acute cellular rejection. However, a sharp-eyed fellow noted a single hepatocyte with viral cytopathic effect (Fig. 11.36). A CMV immunostain showed two cells that seemed to be positive, but the biopsy also had some nonspecific staining. A repeat stain was negative. However, based on the cytology, a diagnosis of early CMV infection was made and was subsequently confirmed on serum PCR. Follow-up information indicated the patient and donor were CMV seronegative, indicating a new infectious exposure.

As shown in this case, early CMV infection can be very subtle with little or no inflammatory response. In later infection, there can definite lobular hepatitis, including clusters of neutrophils, as well as more evident viral cytopathic effect. On the other hand, viral cytopathic effect is not always evident, and a reasonable approach is to obtain a CMV immunostain whenever there is clinical concern for CMV or an unexplained acute onset hepatitis. The seronegative status of the patient and donor increased the risk of CMV infection.

References

1. Dutkowski P, Schlegel A, Slankamenac K, et al. The use of fatty liver grafts in modern allocation systems: risk assessment by the balance of risk (BAR) score. *Ann Surg*. 2012;256:861-868; discussion 8-9.
2. Neil DA, Hubscher SG. Are parenchymal changes in early post-transplant biopsies related to preservation-reperfusion injury or rejection? *Transplantation*. 2001;71:1566-1572.
3. Cha I, Bass N, Ferrell LD. Lipopeliosis. An immunohistochemical and clinicopathologic study of five cases. *Am J Surg Pathol*. 1994;18:789-795.
4. Bioulac-Sage P, Balabaud C, Ferrell L. Lipopeliosis revisited: should we keep the term? *Am J Surg Pathol*. 2002;26:134-135.
5. Demetris AJ, Bellamy C, Hubscher SG, et al. 2016 comprehensive update of the Banff Working Group on liver allograft pathology: introduction of antibody-mediated rejection. *Am J Transpl*. 2016;16:2816-2835.
6. Group BW. Banff schema for grading liver allograft rejection: an international consensus document. *Hepatology*. 1997;25:658-663.
7. Demetris AJ, Belle SH, Hart J, et al. Intraobserver and interobserver variation in the histopathological assessment of liver allograft rejection. The Liver Transplantation Database (LTD) investigators. *Hepatology*. 1991;14:751-755.
8. Liu TC, Nguyen TT, Torbenson MS. Concurrent increase in mitosis and apoptosis: a histological pattern of hepatic arterial flow abnormalities in post-transplant liver biopsies. *Mod Pathol*. 2012;25:1594-1598.
9. Morse SS, Reuben A, Strauss EB, et al. Liver transplant rejection arteritis: serial hepatic arteriography. *Cardiovasc Intervent Radiol*. 1986;9:191-194.
10. Sundaram SS, Melin-Aldana H, Neighbors K, Alonso EM. Histologic characteristics of late cellular rejection, significance of centrilobular injury, and long-term outcome in pediatric liver transplant recipients. *Liver Transpl*. 2006;12:58-64.
11. Krasinskas AM, Demetris AJ, Poterucha JJ, Abraham SC. The prevalence and natural history of untreated isolated central perivenulitis in adult allograft livers. *Liver Transpl*. 2008;14:625-632.
12. Alexander J, Chu W, Swanson PE, Yeh MM. The significance of plasma cell infiltrate in acute cellular rejection of liver allografts. *Hum Pathol*. 2012;43:1645-1650.
13. Ward SC, Schiano TD, Thung SN, Fiel MI. Plasma cell hepatitis in hepatitis C virus patients post-liver transplantation: case-control study showing poor outcome and predictive features in the liver explant. *Liver Transpl*. 2009;15:1826-1833.
14. Cholongitas E, Samonakis D, Patch D, et al. Induction of autoimmune hepatitis by pegylated interferon in a liver transplant patient with recurrent hepatitis C virus. *Transplantation*. 2006;81:488-490.
15. Kontorinis N, Agarwal K, Elhajj N, Fiel MI, Schiano TD. Pegylated interferon-induced immune-mediated hepatitis post-liver transplantation. *Liver Transpl*. 2006;12:827-830.
16. Berardi S, Lodato F, Gramenzi A, et al. High incidence of allograft dysfunction in liver transplanted patients treated with pegylated-interferon alpha-2b and ribavirin for hepatitis C recurrence: possible de novo autoimmune hepatitis? *Gut*. 2007;56:237-242.
17. Fiel MI, Agarwal K, Stanca C, et al. Posttransplant plasma cell hepatitis (de novo autoimmune hepatitis) is a variant of rejection and may lead to a negative outcome in patients with hepatitis C virus. *Liver Transpl*. 2008;14:861-871.
18. Syn WK, Nightingale P, Gunson B, Hubscher SG, Neuberger JM. Natural history of unexplained chronic hepatitis after liver transplantation. *Liver Transpl*. 2007;13:984-989.
19. Seyam M, Neuberger JM, Gunson BK, Hubscher SG. Cirrhosis after orthotopic liver transplantation in the absence of primary disease recurrence. *Liver Transpl*. 2007;13:966-974.
20. Hubscher SG. Antibody-mediated rejection in the liver allograft. *Curr Opin Organ Transpl*. 2012;17:280-286.
21. Aguilera I, Sousa JM, Gavilan F, Bernardos A, Wichmann I, Nunez-Roldan A. Glutathione S-transferase T1 genetic mismatch is a risk factor for de novo immune hepatitis in liver transplantation. *Transpl Proc*. 2005;37:3968-3969.
22. Aguilera I, Wichmann I, Sousa JM, et al. Antibodies against glutathione S-transferase T1 (GSTT1) in patients with de novo immune hepatitis following liver transplantation. *Clin Exp Immunol*. 2001;126:535-539.

23. Keitel V, Burdelski M, Vojnisek Z, Schmitt L, Haussinger D, Kubitz R. De novo bile salt transporter antibodies as a possible cause of recurrent graft failure after liver transplantation: a novel mechanism of cholestasis. *Hepatology*. 2009;50:510-517.

24. Demetris AJ, Zeevi A, O'Leary JG. ABO-compatible liver allograft antibody-mediated rejection: an update. *Curr Opin Organ Transpl*. 2015;20:314-324.

25. Kozlowski T, Andreoni K, Schmitz J, Hayashi PH, Nickeleit V. Sinusoidal C4d deposits in liver allografts indicate an antibody-mediated response: diagnostic considerations in the evaluation of liver allografts. *Liver Transpl*. 2012;18:641-658.

26. Demetris AJ, Nakamura K, Yagihashi A, et al. A clinicopathological study of human liver allograft recipients harboring preformed IgG lymphocytotoxic antibodies. *Hepatology*. 1992;16:671-681.

27. Hubscher SG. Transplantation pathology. *Semin Liver Dis*. 2009;29:74-90.

28. Dah N, Co B, Smith M, et al. Global quality assessment of liver allograft C4d staining during acute antibody mediated rejection in formalin-fixed paraffin-embedded tissue. *Hum Pathol*. 2017.

29. Demetris AJ, Adeyi O, Bellamy CO, et al. Liver biopsy interpretation for causes of late liver allograft dysfunction. *Hepatology*. 2006;44:489-501.

30. Bekker J, Ploem S, de Jong KP. Early hepatic artery thrombosis after liver transplantation: a systematic review of the incidence, outcome and risk factors. *Am J Transpl*. 2009;9:746-757.

31. Bhattacharjya S, Gunson BK, Mirza DF, et al. Delayed hepatic artery thrombosis in adult orthotopic liver transplantation-a 12-year experience. *Transplantation*. 2001;71:1592-1596.

32. Pareja E, Cortes M, Navarro R, Sanjuan F, Lopez R, Mir J. Vascular complications after orthotopic liver transplantation: hepatic artery thrombosis. *Transpl Proc*. 2010;42:2970-2972.

33. Sedivy R, Gollackner B, Casati B, et al. Apoptotic hepatocytes in rejection and vascular occlusion in liver allograft specimens. *Histopathology*. 1998;32:503-507.

34. Gollackner B, Sedivy R, Rockenschaub S, et al. Increased apoptosis of hepatocytes in vascular occlusion after orthotopic liver transplantation. *Transpl Int*. 2000;13:49-53.

35. Valente JF, Alonso MH, Weber FL, Hanto DW. Late hepatic artery thrombosis in liver allograft recipients is associated with intrahepatic biliary necrosis. *Transplantation*. 1996;61:61-65.

36. Adeyi O, Fischer SE, Guindi M. Liver allograft pathology: approach to interpretation of needle biopsies with clinicopathological correlation. *J Clin Pathol*. 2010;63:47-74.

37. Demetris AJ, Kelly DM, Eghtesad B, et al. Pathophysiologic observations and histopathologic recognition of the portal hyperperfusion or small-for-size syndrome. *Am J Surg Pathol*. 2006;30:986-993.

38. Gonzalez HD, Liu ZW, Cashman S, Fusai GK. Small for size syndrome following living donor and split liver transplantation. *World J Gastrointest Surg*. 2010;2:389-394.

39. Dahm F, Georgiev P, Clavien PA. Small-for-size syndrome after partial liver transplantation: definition, mechanisms of disease and clinical implications. *Am J Transpl*. 2005;5:2605-2610.

40. Cescon M, Grazi GL, Varotti G, et al. Venous outflow reconstructions with the piggyback technique in liver transplantation: a single-center experience of 431 cases. *Transpl Int*. 2005;18:318-325.

41. Audet M, Piardi T, Panaro F, et al. Four hundred and twenty-three consecutive adults piggy-back liver transplantations with the three suprahepatic veins: was the portal systemic shunt required? *J Gastroenterol Hepatol*. 2010;25:591-596.

42. MacDonald GA, Greenson JK, DelBuono EA, et al. Mini-microabscess syndrome in liver transplant recipients. *Hepatology*. 1997;26:192-197.

43. Potenza L, Luppi M, Barozzi P, et al. HHV-6A in syncytial giant-cell hepatitis. *N Engl J Med*. 2008;359:593-602.

44. Schlosser B, Stein A, Neuhaus R, et al. Liver transplant from a donor with occult HEV infection induced chronic hepatitis and cirrhosis in the recipient. *J Hepatol*. 2012;56:500-502.

45. Pischke S, Suneetha PV, Baechlein C, et al. Hepatitis E virus infection as a cause of graft hepatitis in liver transplant recipients. *Liver Transpl*. 2010;16:74-82.

46. Kamar N, Selves J, Mansuy JM, et al. Hepatitis E virus and chronic hepatitis in organ-transplant recipients. *N Engl J Med*. 2008;358:811-817.

47. Zhou K, Terrault N. Management of hepatitis B in special populations. *Best Pract Res Clin Gastroenterol*. 2017;31:311-320.

48. Silveira MG, Talwalkar JA, Lindor KD, Wiesner RH. Recurrent primary biliary cirrhosis after liver transplantation. *Am J Transpl*. 2010;10:720-726.

49. Alexander J, Lord JD, Yeh MM, Cuevas C, Bakthavatsalam R, Kowdley KV. Risk factors for recurrence of primary sclerosing cholangitis after liver transplantation. *Liver Transpl*. 2008;14:245-251.

50. Alabraba E, Nightingale P, Gunson B, et al. A re-evaluation of the risk factors for the recurrence of primary sclerosing cholangitis in liver allografts. *Liver Transpl*. 2009;15:330-340.

51. Malik SM, Devera ME, Fontes P, Shaikh O, Sasatomi E, Ahmad J. Recurrent disease following liver transplantation for nonalcoholic steatohepatitis cirrhosis. *Liver Transpl*. 2009;15:1843-1851.

52. Contos MJ, Cales W, Sterling RK, et al. Development of nonalcoholic fatty liver disease after orthotopic liver transplantation for cryptogenic cirrhosis. *Liver Transpl*. 2001;7:363-373.

53. Bjornsson E, Olsson J, Rydell A, et al. Long-term follow-up of patients with alcoholic liver disease after liver transplantation in Sweden: impact of structured management on recidivism. *Scand J Gastroenterol*. 2005;40:206-216.

54. Faure S, Herrero A, Jung B, et al. Excessive alcohol consumption after liver transplantation impacts on long-term survival, whatever the primary indication. *J Hepatol*. 2012;57:306-312.

55. Dixon LR, Crawford JM. Early histologic changes in fibrosing cholestatic hepatitis C. *Liver Transpl*. 2007;13:219-226.

56. Dureja P, Mellinger J, Agni R, et al. NAFLD recurrence in liver transplant recipients. *Transplantation*. 2011;91:684-689.

57. Miyagawa-Hayashino A, Egawa H, Yorifuji T, et al. Allograft steatohepatitis in progressive familial intrahepatic cholestasis type 1 after living donor liver transplantation. *Liver Transpl*. 2009;15:610-618.

58. Sembera S, Lammert C, Talwalkar JA, et al. Frequency, clinical presentation, and outcomes of drug-induced liver injury after liver transplantation. *Liver Transpl*. 2012;18:803-810.

59. Zhenglu W, Hui L, Shuying Z, Wenjuan C, Zhongyang S. A clinical-pathological analysis of drug-induced hepatic injury after liver transplantation. *Transpl Proc*. 2007;39:3287-3291.

60. Nalesnik MA. The diverse pathology of post-transplant lymphoproliferative disorders: the importance of a standardized approach. *Transpl Infect Dis*. 2001;3:88-96.

61. Vishnu P, Jiang L, Cortese C, Menke DM, Tun HW. Plasmacytoma-like posttransplant lymphoproliferative disorder following orthotopic liver transplantation: a case report. *Transpl Proc*. 2011;43:2806-2809.

62. Randhawa P, Blakolmer K, Kashyap R, et al. Allograft liver biopsy in patients with Epstein-Barr virus-associated posttransplant lymphoproliferative disease. *Am J Surg Pathol*. 2001;25:324-330.

63. Yeh KH, Hsieh HC, Tang JL, Lin MT, Yang CH, Chen YC. Severe isolated acute hepatic graft-versus-host disease with vanishing bile duct syndrome. *Bone Marrow Transpl*. 1994;14:319-321.

64. Akpek G, Boitnott JK, Lee LA, et al. Hepatitic variant of graft-versus-host disease after donor lymphocyte infusion. *Blood*. 2002;100:3903-3907.

12 GENETIC DISEASES

CHAPTER OUTLINE

GENETIC DISEASES OF THE LIVER, OVERVIEW

Many of the genetic diseases of the liver are covered in other chapters, such as bile salt deficiencies that are covered in the chapter on biliary tract disease. This chapter focuses on those genetic diseases of the liver that lead to abnormal accumulation of material in the liver, including hepatocytes and/or Kupffer cells. The emphasis is on the histological pattern of injury and the key clinical, genetic, and histological findings, as well as the major diseases in the differential, but a comprehensive review of each disease is beyond the scope of any single chapter. In fact, many of these diseases have entire books written solely about that disease, underscoring the complexity and breadth of genetic diseases of the liver. Nonetheless, the fundamental pathology diagnosis can be made in most cases based on the pattern of injury combined with a few key clinical or laboratory findings.

ALPHA-1-ANTITRYPSIN DEFICIENCY

CHECKLIST: Alpha-1-Antitrypsin Deficiency

- □ Mutations in *SERPINA1* gene lead to accumulation of misfolded alpha-1-antitrypsin protein in hepatocytes
- □ Autosomal recessive inheritance
- □ Clinically, lung and/or liver disease can be prominent
- □ Testing:
  - ○ Pi typing
  - ○ Sequencing
  - ○ PASD (periodic acid–Schiff with diastase)–positive zone 1 hepatocyte globules
- □ Liver disease patterns
  - ○ Neonatal cholestatic liver disease
  - ○ Almost-normal liver
  - ○ Cryptogenic cirrhosis
  - ○ Additional finding in a liver specimen with another main injury pattern

In many pathology training programs, the alpha-1-antitrypsin deficiency pattern of injury is one of the first that is learned about genetic diseases because it is a subtle, but still easily recognized pattern: the hepatocytes show eosinophilic cytoplasmic globules, in particular the zone 1 hepatocytes (Figs. 12.1 and 12.2), that are highlighted on PASD stains (Fig. 12.3). The globules are located in the cytoplasm, are round to oval, and can range from several larger globules to many smaller globules. The globules can be patchy, especially in early disease and/or in cases with heterozygous mutations, so the zone 1 hepatocytes around multiple portal tracts should be examined. In some cases, the globules will be more widely spread throughout the cytoplasm, which is particularly true with homozygous disease. Immunostains are also available and work well (Fig. 12.4), but PASD is sufficient in most cases.

Alpha-1-antitrypsin deficiency is an autosomal recessive disease, where each gene contributes to 50% of the total protein in the blood. The M allele is the normal allele, while the S and Z alleles are the most common alleles to cause disease. Heterozygosity with a normal and an abnormal allele (MZ or MS) leads to reduced serum alpha-1-antitrypsin levels, and globules can be seen in the liver, but clinical lung or liver disease are not seen. Globules in the setting of MS disease are most likely to be seen when other concomitant liver diseases are present.[1–3] Rare alleles called Mmalton and Mduarate can also cause intrahepatocellular inclusions.[4,5] They can also be associated with liver disease and lung disease.[5] In contrast, the rare null phenotype does not lead to liver inclusions or liver disease but can cause lung disease.

Surgical pathology specimens with alpha-1-antitrypsin deficiency are seen in essentially four situations. The first situation is biopsies performed to evaluate cholestatic liver disease

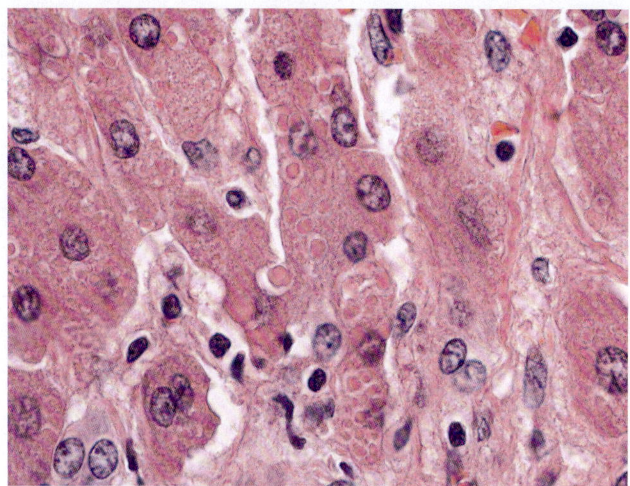

Figure 12.1. **Alpha-1-antitrypsin deficiency.** Distinct, round globules are seen in the hepatocytes adjacent to the portal tract.

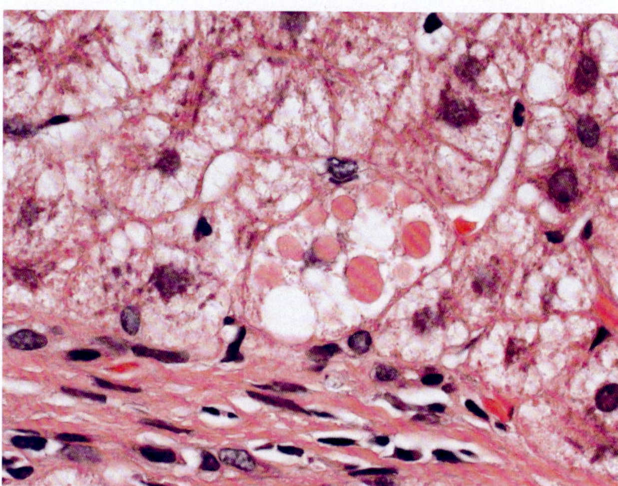

Figure 12.2. **Alpha-1-antitrypsin deficiency.** Another example at higher power shows the round hepatocyte globules.

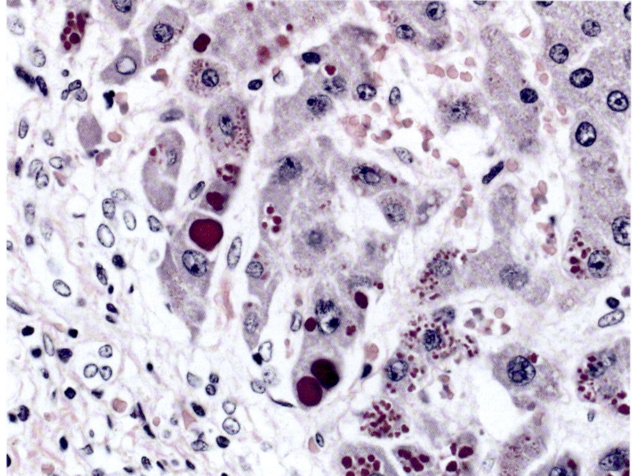

Figure 12.3. **Alpha-1-antitrypsin deficiency, periodic acid–Schiff with diastase (PASD).** The globules are bright magenta on PASD stain. Many smaller globules that were not evident on H&E are also seen.

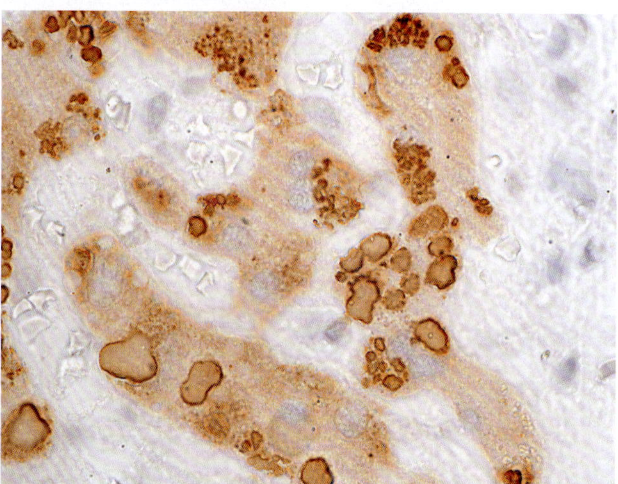

Figure 12.4. **Alpha-1-antitrypsin deficiency, immunostain.** The larger globules often stain at the edges, with less staining in the middle.

in neonates or infants.[6] About 10% of individuals with homozygous alpha-1-antitrypsin deficiency will present with neonatal cholestasis. The biopsies show various cholestatic patterns of liver injury, including cases with findings that overlap with the early changes of biliary atresia or show a neonatal giant cell hepatitis pattern of injury. Intrahepatic globules are absent to sparse in the first 3 to 4 months of life, so the diagnosis is made mostly by serum testing and ruling out other disease patterns on liver biopsy.

A second situation is when there is known disease in adults and biopsies are obtained to stage known disease or to assess for other concomitant disease processes. This situation is now relatively uncommon because of improvements in noninvasive measures of liver fibrosis.

The third setting is when globules are found in biopsies in the setting of other liver diseases that are the main pattern of liver injury, such as autoimmune hepatitis. This setting is the most common, and most cases represent heterozygous disease, where the alpha-1-antitrypsin deficiency is possibly a cofactor in fibrosis progression but not the main driver.

The final setting is when globules are identified in liver biopsies performed to assess for potential causes in cases of clinically cryptogenic cirrhosis. The clinical significance is variable: most cases represent heterozygous disease, but some can be homozygous disease. In the latter situation, the alpha-1-antitrypsin deficiency can explain the cirrhosis, but in the setting of heterozygous disease, other causes of liver disease must also have been present and were likely the main driver of liver disease, even if no longer evident on histology. Although globules tend to be more abundant and diffuse with homozygous disease, the histological findings do not reliably distinguish homozygous from heterozygous alpha-1-antitrypsin deficiency, so serological or genetic testing is needed.

Sometimes, megamitochondria can mimic the globules of alpha-1-antitrypsin deficiency. Overall, megamitochondria tend to be smaller and lack a strong zone 1 predominance. If needed, PASD or immunostains for alpha-1-antitrypsin proteins can be used to separate these two. In some cases of congestive hepatopathy, globules can also develop in the zone 3 hepatocytes. This finding has been reported in several studies, but not thoroughly examined, so the precise mechanism is unclear, but it does not appear to represent a variant of alpha-1-antitrypsin deficiency. Other extremely rare causes of hepatocyte inclusions, similar to those in alpha-1-antitrypsin deficiency, include antithrombin III deficiency and α1-antichymotrypsin deficiency, although in the latter case the inclusions are small, not visible or only barely visible on H&E, and only weakly PASD positive.[7]

AFIBRINOGENEMIA/HYPOFIBRINOGENEMIA

Afibrinogenemia and hypofibrinogenemia are both very rare diseases that can be either autosomal dominant or autosomal recessive. Mutations lead to absent plasma fibrinogen, low levels of plasma fibrinogen, or fibrinogen that is functionally impaired. There are several related fibrinogen genes: α (FGA); β (FGB), or γ (FGG), but mutations in the *FGA* gene are the most common. In most cases of afibrinogenemia, patients present with bleeding, often sporadic or following mild trauma. In contrast, in hypofibrinogenemia, fibrinogen levels are low but can provide enough function that the patients may be asymptomatic.

On the other hand, and somewhat counterintuitively, a subset of individuals with hypofibrinogenaemia can present with a history of multiple thromboses. This occurs when the fibrinogen mutations lead to fibrinogen that is fibrinolysis resistant.[8] In others cases that present with thrombotic disease, patients can have prothrombotic mutations in unrelated genes, such as factor V Leiden mutations.[9]

These fibrinogen diseases can lead to hepatocyte inclusions, which are the main finding on biopsy. The disease is so rare that genotype–phenotype studies have not been performed, but the inclusions vary in their size, shape, and color,[10–12] which appears likely to correlate with underlying mutations. The inclusions can be eosinophilic or amphophilic (Figs. 12.5 and 12.6) and small or large. They sometimes resemble the hepatocyte ground glass changes seen in hepatitis B or drug effects. However, in contrast to the ground glass changes in hepatitis B and drug effects, the inclusions in hypofibrinogenaemia are PASD negative (Fig. 12.7), or weakly positive, and are also positive on phosphotungstic acid–haematoxylin stains.

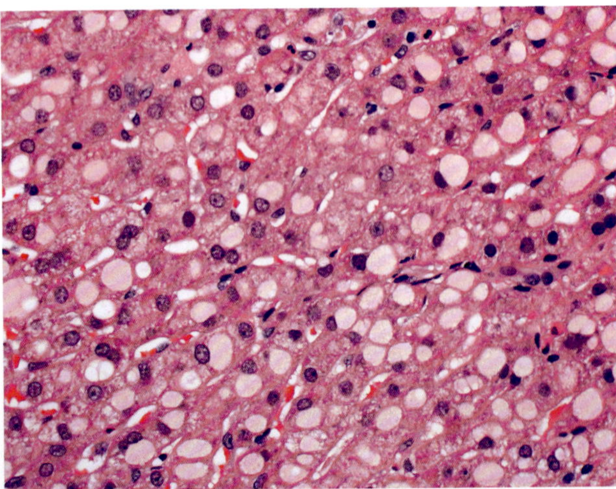

Figure 12.5. **Dysfibrinogenemia.** At low power, the hepatocytes show large cytoplasmic vacuoles.

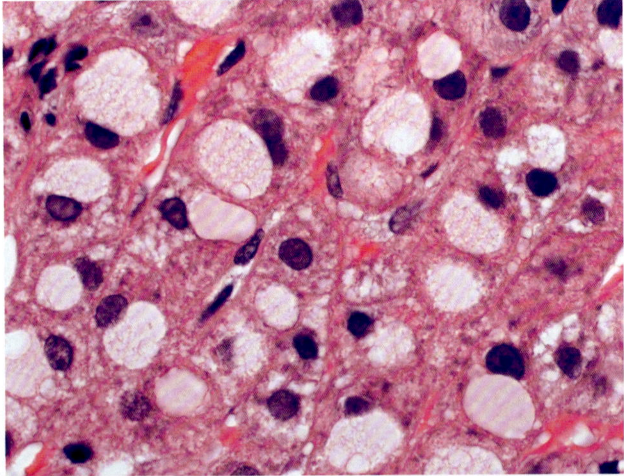

Figure 12.6. **Dysfibrinogenemia.** At high power, the vacuoles are round and resemble ground glass inclusions (hepatitis B related) or pseudo–ground glass inclusions (drug related in most cases).

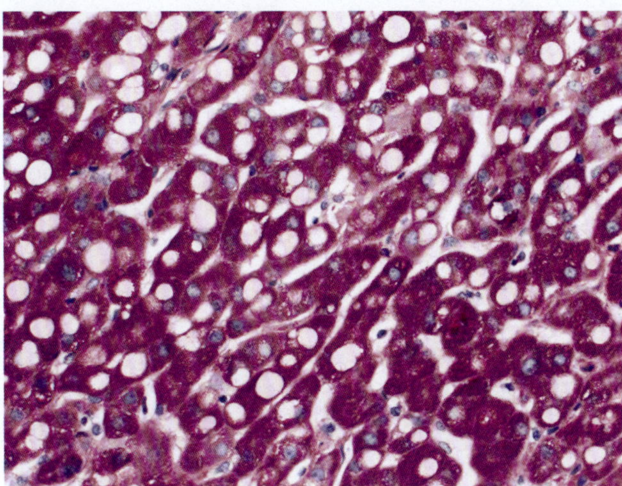

Figure 12.7. **Dysfibrinogenemia, PAS.** Same case as above. The inclusions are PAS negative, in contrast to ground glass inclusions and pseudo–ground glass inclusions, which are PAS positive.

WILSON DISEASE

CHECKLIST: Wilson Disease

- ☐ Mutations in *ATPB7* gene lead to abnormal copper accumulation
- ☐ Autosomal recessive inheritance
- ☐ Clinically, disease tends to have liver-predominant or neural-predominant signs and symptoms
- ☐ Testing:
  - ○ Low serum ceruloplasmin (<10 mg/dL is strongly suggestive; 10 to 20 mg/dL can be consistent)
  - ○ Elevated 24 urine copper (>200 μg/24 hours strongly suggestive; 100 to 200 μg/24 hours can be consistent)
  - ○ Positive tissue copper stain (can be patchy; make sure to cut at 10 microns; sections cut at 3 or 5 microns have very low sensitivity)
  - ○ Quantitative copper on liver tissue, in noncholestatic liver specimens (>209 μg/g dry wt is strongly suggestive; >100 μg/g dry wt is consistent)

Individuals with Wilson disease present clinically most often between the ages of 5 and 35 years, but presentation can be as young as 3 years of age or as late as 80 years of age.[13] Wilson disease results from abnormal copper metabolism, leading to copper deposits in various organs. Copper accumulates primarily in the liver and the basal ganglia, but other organs are affected including the eyes, kidneys, and heart. With eye disease, copper is deposited in the cornea, leading to a finding on eye examination called *Kayser–Fleischer rings*. About 2/3 of individuals with Wilson disease will have Kayser–Fleischer rings at clinical presentation. The overall frequency is >90% for individuals who present with neurological or psychiatric symptoms. In contrast, Kayser–Fleischer rings are present in about 50% of individuals who present with liver-predominant disease. Kayser–Fleischer rings are considered pathognomonic for Wilson disease, but there are several mimics that can lead to a false-positive eye examination.[14] Important laboratory testing to support a diagnosis of Wilson disease includes a low serum ceruloplasmin levels and elevated 24 urine copper levels. Of note, ceruloplasmin is an acute phase reactant, so levels can be normal in Wilson disease if there is significant active hepatitis or in the setting of increased estrogen (for example, from pregnancy or oral contraceptive pills).

FAQ: How is a diagnosis of Wilson disease made?

Answer: In general, the key components of the diagnosis are elevated urinary copper levels, elevated hepatic copper levels, low ceruloplasmin levels, and Kayser–Fleischer rings, but other findings can also be helpful. Of note, mutation analysis can be definitive if known disease causing mutations are identified on both chromosomes. However, not all mutations cause disease, and some well-defined clinical cases do not have two mutations identified by sequencing. Thus, a combined clinical, laboratory, and genetic approach is commonly used in making a diagnosis of Wilson disease.

One approach is to diagnose Wilson disease using a scoring method.[15,16] In this method, a score of >4 is considered highly likely to be Wilson disease, a score of 2 or 3 is probably Wilson disease, and score of 0 or 1 is unlikely to be Wilson disease.

- Kayser–Fleischer rings:
  - Absent: 0 points
  - Present: 2 points
- Typical brain magnetic resonance imaging (MRI) or typical clinical neuropsychiatric symptoms:
  - Absent: 0 points
  - Present: 2 points
- Serum ceruloplasmin (mg/dL):
  - >21: 0 points
  - 10 to 20: 1 point
  - >20: 2 points
- Coombs negative hemolytic anemia plus high serum copper:
  - Absent: 0 points
  - Present: 1 point
- 24 urine copper excretion (μg/24 hours) OR after penicillamine treatment (μg/24 hours):
  - <100: 0 points or <1500: 0 points
  - 100 to 200: 1 point or 1500 to 2500: 1 point
  - >200: 2 points or >2500: 2 points
- Quantitative copper on liver tissue (μg/g dry):
  - < 50: –1 points
  - 50 to 100: 0 points
  - 100 to 250: 1 point
  - > 250: 2 points
- Rhodanine copper stain (only if quant copper not available):
  - Absent: 0 points
  - Present: 1 point
- ATP7B mutations known to be disease causing:
  - No mutations: 0 points
  - 1 mutation: 1 point
  - 1 mutation on each chromosome: 4 points

In terms of liver disease, Wilson disease leads to increased deposits of copper in the hepatocytes. In early disease, the increased copper may not be evident on rhodanine or other copper stains, as the copper is finely distributed in the cytoplasm at first and only later accumulates in larger granules within the lysosomes of hepatocytes. Only the lysosomal form is identified on rhodanine stain. Thus, if there is strong clinical concern for Wilson disease, a negative rhodanine stain does not rule out Wilson disease and quantitative copper testing is important.

Wilson disease results from mutations in the *ATP7B* gene.[17] *ATP7B* encodes an ATPase that transports copper from the hepatocytes into the bile, where it is excreted, and also helps incorporate copper into ceruloplasmin in the blood. Ceruloplasmin is a key serum copper transporter. When the protein is mutated, then copper is not efficiently excreted into the bile and is not efficiently bound to ceruloplasmin in the blood. Copper subsequently accumulates in hepatocytes and other organs. Because copper is normally excreted in bile, any disease that causes chronic cholestasis can also lead to copper deposition in the liver, and in this regard can mimic Wilson disease.

Wilson disease is inherited in an autosomal recessive pattern. Disease-causing mutations can be either homozygous or compound heterozygous mutations. Clinically, disease tends to have liver-predominant or neural-predominant signs and symptoms, which correlates broadly with mutation patterns, at least in many studies.[18,19] There are over 500 mutations reported in the *ATP7B* gene, with most but not all causing disease. Carriers (those with heterozygous mutations) tend to have mild liver enzyme elevations but generally do not develop liver disease. The histological findings in livers with heterozygous mutations have not been well described in the literature but anecdotally show mild nonspecific changes, sometimes with mild patchy copper deposition. It is possible that heterozygous mutations may contribute to liver disease when another liver disease is present, but this has not been well studied to date.

CHECKLIST: Histological Patterns in Wilson Disease

- ☐ Almost-normal liver
- ☐ Mild nonspecific changes
- ☐ Fulminant liver failure
  - The liver can be noncirrhotic or cirrhotic
- ☐ Acute hepatitis or acute on chronic hepatitis
  - Sometimes with autoimmune hepatitis features
- ☐ Steatosis or steatohepatitis (most common histological pattern)
- ☐ Cryptogenic cirrhosis

Wilson disease can show several histological patterns, all of which mimic other diseases, so the histological diagnosis can be very challenging to make without clinical and laboratory findings. A good approach is to have a high index of suspicion when the histological pattern in a liver specimen from a young individual is not well explained by clinical findings, such as fatty liver disease in a young person without the metabolic syndrome, a compatible drug history, or alcohol use.

In very early disease, the histological findings in Wilson disease can be minimal and nonspecific (Fig. 12.8). These cases are usually seen in kindred with known Wilson disease when biopsies are obtained in asymptomatic individuals for quantitative copper analysis. Overall, the most common histological pattern in symptomatic individuals is that of fatty liver disease (Fig. 12.9), which can show steatosis or steatohepatitis.[20] Interestingly, the amount of steatosis correlates roughly with amount of copper in the liver.[21] A less common pattern is that of acute hepatitis, acute-on-chronic hepatitis, or chronic hepatitis. In some of these cases, the inflammation can be plasma cell rich, mimicking autoimmune hepatitis (Figs. 12.10 and 12.11). Acute hepatitis, when severe, can lead to fulminant liver failure, a finding more common in children and more common in girls than boys.[22] Finally, liver biopsies can show a cryptogenic cirrhosis pattern, sometimes with little or no inflammation and no fat (Fig. 12.12). However, in most cirrhotic livers, there is at least mild steatosis, glycogenated nuclei, mild but distinctive nuclear pleomorphism, and mild lobular cholestasis.[23] In some cases, the hepatocytes can appear slightly enlarged and oncocytic (Fig. 12.13).

Glycogenated nuclei and nuclear pleomorphism are commonly included in histological descriptions of Wilson disease in books and review articles, which is true enough, but these findings are also common in other diseases, so they lack specificity and are mostly secondary changes. They also lack sensitivity, being minimal or underwhelming in many cases. In fact, it is fair to say that it would be very unusual to have a case where the diagnosis of Wilson disease was first considered because of either of these findings.

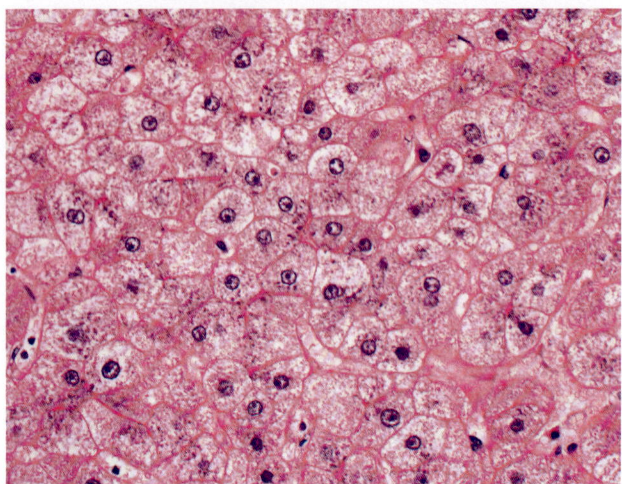

Figure 12.8. **Wilson disease.** The H&E findings in this case are mild and nonspecific.

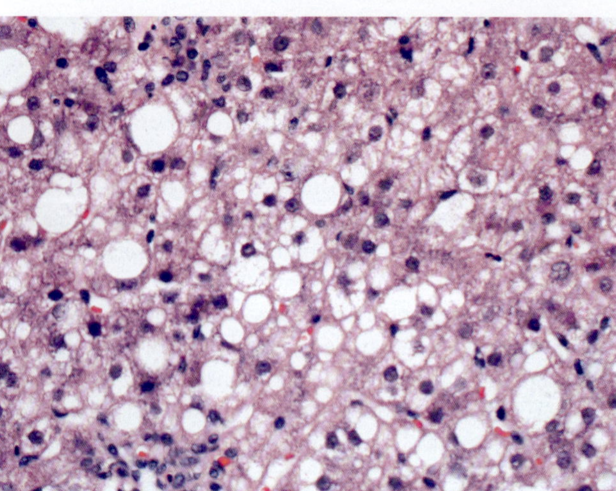

Figure 12.9. **Wilson disease.** This case shows moderate macrovesicular steatosis. An important clue was that the patient had none of the usual risk factors, such as the metabolic syndrome, alcohol use, etc.

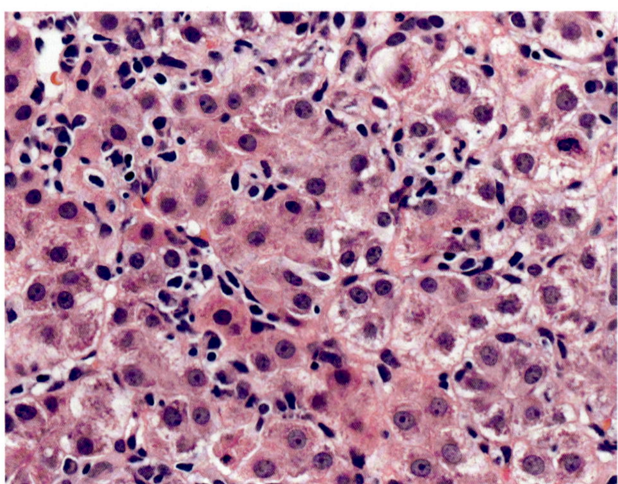

Figure 12.10. **Wilson disease.** This case presented with an acute hepatitis that is plasma cell rich and resembles autoimmune hepatitis.

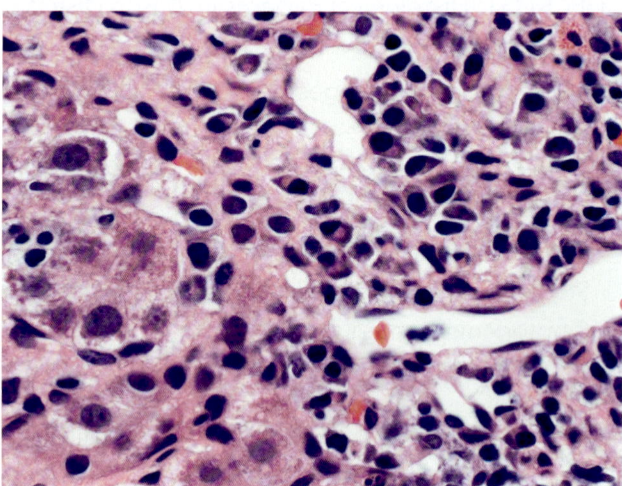

Figure 12.11. **Wilson disease.** The portal tracts have plasma cell–rich inflammation (same case as Fig. 12.10).

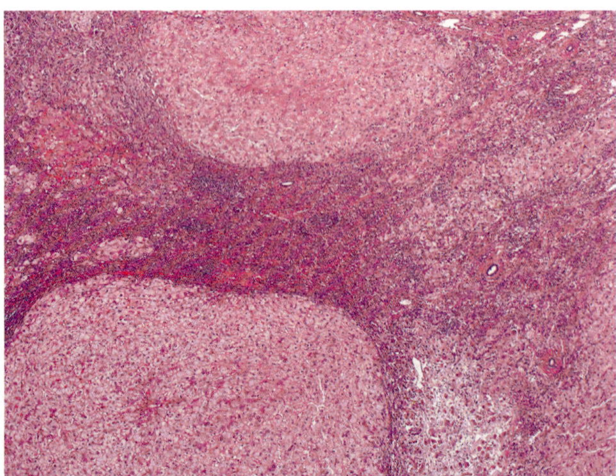

Figure 12.12. **Wilson disease.** This case presented as cryptogenic cirrhosis in a young man.

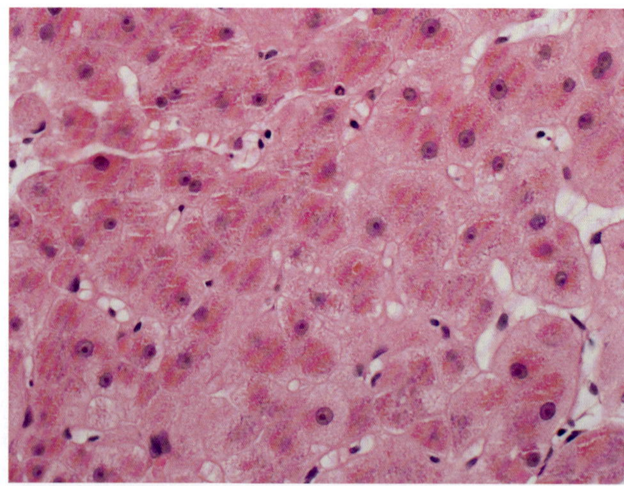

Figure 12.13. **Wilson disease.** Another case that presented as cryptogenic cirrhosis. In this case, one of the clues is that the hepatocytes have a distinctly oncocytic appearance.

COPPER STAINS

PEARLS & PITFALLS: Using a Copper Stain

There are several useful guidelines that can help interpret copper stains. Of course, these are only guidelines, so use them in context of the entire case, including the clinical and histological findings, and your common sense.

1. The pattern that most strongly supports Wilson disease is copper accumulation in the zone 1 hepatocytes (or even more widespread lobular staining) in a liver biopsy that is noncirrhotic and shows one of the typical patterns of Wilson disease (see checklist of histological patterns in Wilson disease).
2. The rhodanine copper stain, or other copper stains, can be negative in early Wilson disease, so a negative stain does not exclude Wilson disease.
3. On the other hand, a negative copper stain in the setting of an adequate biopsy and cirrhosis makes Wilson disease unlikely.
4. Copper accumulation can also be found in noncirrhotic livers in the setting of biliary obstruction, ductopenia, or chronic cholestatic liver disease, but none of these patterns are present in Wilson disease, so the H&E findings should be incorporated into your interpretation of the copper stain.
5. There can be copper accumulation in cirrhotic livers from many different underlying liver diseases[24] if the liver decompensates and becomes cholestatic.

The most commonly used copper stain is the rhodanine stain, which leads to a red–brown granular staining pattern when copper is present (Fig. 12.14). The rhodanine stain only detects copper deposits in the hepatocyte lysosomes and not the fine cytosolic copper present in early Wilson disease. The copper deposits are seen primarily in zone 1 hepatocytes but can be more widespread. In cirrhotic livers, the copper distribution is often patchy, with some nodules completely devoid of visible copper (Fig. 12.15). The rhodanine stain should be performed on sections cut at 10 microns for optimal sensitivity.

The Timm silver sulfide stain is a bit more sensitive than the rhodanine,[25] but is technically more challenging to perform. Orcein and Victoria blue stains are not as sensitive for Wilson disease and detect copper binding protein, not copper itself.

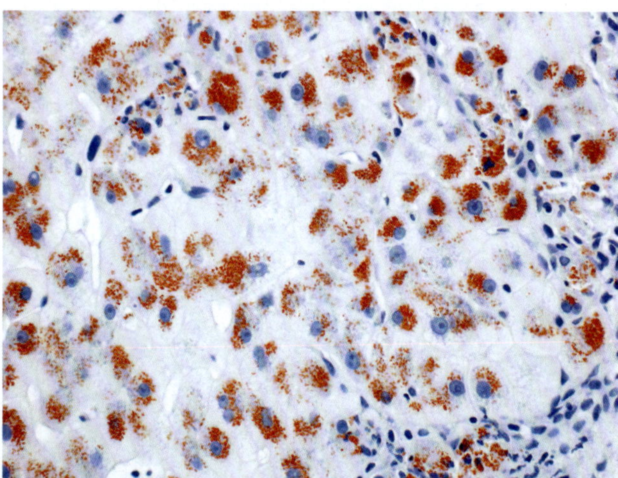

Figure 12.14. Wilson disease, rhodanine copper stain. The hepatocytes show distinctive red brown granules.

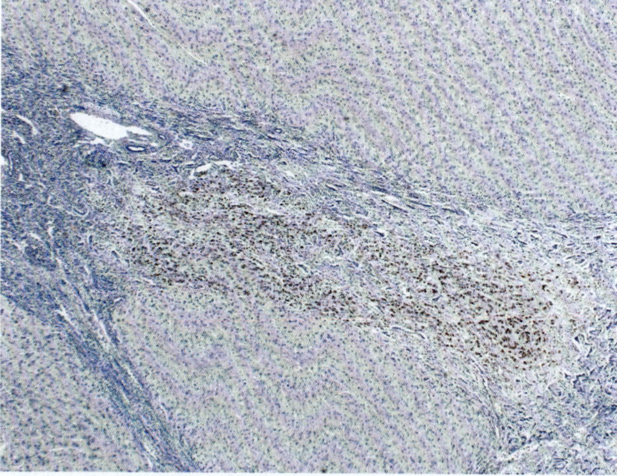

Figure 12.15. Wilson disease, rhodanine copper stain. In this case of Wilson cirrhosis, the copper deposits were not uniformly present in all nodules. In this field, the center nodule is positive, while two adjacent ones are negative.

FAQ: What is the best stain for copper?

Answer: Rhodanine is an excellent and reliable stain that is easy to interpret. The Timm silver sulfide stain shows very similar sensitivity and specificity, while the orcein stain is considerably less sensitive.[23] Some[25] but not all studies[23] have suggested the Timm stain is more sensitive than the rhodanine stain, at least in noncirrhotic livers.

Methodological considerations are important too. For example, the rhodanine stain should be performed on 10-micron-thick sections for optimal sensitivity. Studies that use 3 or 5 micron sections consistently show a high percent of negative stains in patients with known Wilson disease. This unfortunately has led to frequent disparaging of the rhodanine stain in the literature, but the stain works well and is helpful when properly performed, and not surprisingly, less helpful when not.

The Timm method benefits from increased deparaffination time.[26]

QUANTITATIVE COPPER

Quantitative copper analysis can be performed on fresh liver tissue or paraffin-embedded tissue. The results are the same, so paraffin-embedded tissue is preferred. Reference laboratory results sometimes provide slightly different information in their autogenerated notes regarding how to interpret levels. Historically, levels greater than 250 µg/g dry weight were considered highly specific for Wilson disease, but that cutoff was based on a very small number of cases (less than 10), and several subsequent studies have shown that cutoff is too high.[15,27] In the end, no cut off should be used in isolation and the current approach to diagnosis is outlined in the prior section "FAQ: How is a diagnosis of Wilson disease made?"

OTHER RARE COPPER OVERLOAD DISEASES

In addition to Wilson disease, there are several other copper overload diseases that affect children.[28,29] These include Indian childhood cirrhosis, Tyrolean infantile cirrhosis, and idiopathic copper toxiocosis. These diseases are thought to have both genetic and environmental risk factors, but the precise etiology is unclear. The overall frequency of these diseases appears to have dropped rapidly over the past several decades, at least for Indian childhood cirrhosis,[30] suggesting strong environmental risk factors, although dietary copper intake does not appear to play a strong role.[30] In all of these diseases, there is rapid fibrosis progression and most children will have advanced fibrosis or cirrhosis at first clinical presentation, which is usually at less than 2 years of age, although rare cases can present as late as 10 years of age.[29] In all cases, there are no mutations in the *ATPB7* gene and ceruloplasmin levels are normal.

Histologically, biopsies show cirrhosis with mild nonspecific inflammation and little or no fat, but abundant copper deposition. The livers can be deeply cholestatic. The cirrhosis is micronodular, with very tiny nodules, and pericellular fibrosis can be diffuse and striking. Quantitative copper analysis shows more copper than is commonly seen in Wilson disease.[30]

HEMOCHROMATOSIS

CHECKLIST: HFE Hemochromatosis

- ☐ Mutations in the HFE gene lead to accumulation of iron in the liver and other organs
- ☐ Autosomal recessive inheritance
- ☐ Clinically, liver disease is often the main manifestation, but patients can also have diabetes, heart disease, and/or arthritis

- Testing:
  - Elevated serum ferritin
  - Elevated serum transferrin
  - Sequencing of *HFE* gene
  - Quantitative tissue iron analysis
  - Tissue iron stain
- Liver disease patterns
  - Excess iron accumulation, zone 1–predominant pattern
  - Fibrosis ranges from none to cirrhosis

Hepcidin is the master regulator of iron metabolism. Hepcidin is produced in the liver, and it controls the amount of iron absorption from the intestine and the amount of iron released from body stores in the hepatocytes and Kupffer cells. Iron is stored in the body as ferritin, which can be rapidly mobilized when needed. When the body is iron replete, then hepcidin levels are high, and iron is not absorbed from the gastrointestinal (GI) tract and not released from body stores, but when the body needs more iron, then hepcidin levels decrease and more iron is absorbed from the GI tract and released from body stores.

All of the known forms of genetic hemochromatosis act at least in large part by impairing hepcidin production or function.[31,32] The low levels of hepcidin or the impaired function of hepcidin then gradually lead to excess iron absorption from the GI tract and iron deposition in the liver and other organs. On the other hand, there have been rare mutations identified that increase hepcidin function, and these lead to refractory congenital anemia due to impaired iron absorption.[33] Interestingly, hepcidin appears to be either overexpressed or its function otherwise enhanced in a subset of hepatic adenomas that are associated with anemia at clinical presentation,[34,35] as resection of the adenoma leads to resolution of clinical anemia.

Hemochromatosis can lead to liver cirrhosis and to hepatocellular carcinoma.[36–39] Other clinical manifestations include heart failure and diabetes, which results from iron deposits in the heart and the islet cells, respectively. Patients with clinical hemochromatosis also can develop an arthropathy that results from iron deposits in the cartilage and synovial cells, with a strong predilection for the 2nd and 3rd metacarpophalangeal joints and the interphalangeal joints.

The vast majority of clinical cases of genetic hemochromatosis are caused by *HFE* mutations. Mutations in the *HFE* gene lead to abnormal HFE proteins that lack normal binding to b2-microglobulin, which in turn makes the protein unstable. There are close to 40 known mutations in the HFE gene,[40] but the most important disease-causing mutations are C282Y, H63D, and possibly S65C. The C282Y mutation has a strong association with northern European genetic ancestry,[40] while the H63D mutation has a much wider geographic distribution.[41] S65C mutations are more common in populations from Brittany, France.[42]

In clinical practice, 80% of hemochromatosis cases that are caused by genetic mutations have homozygous C282Y mutations, while another 5% of cases result from compound C282Y and H63D mutations.[42] Of note, most individuals with C282Y mutations do not develop clinical hemochromatosis, underscoring the important role of other genetic and/or environmental factors. For example, one meta-analysis found a clinical disease penetrance for C282Y homozygosity of only 13.5%.[42]

In contrast to C282Y mutations, homozygous H63D mutations are usually insufficient on their own to cause hemochromatosis but can lead to iron overload when other chronic liver diseases are present. Of the many other *HFE* mutations, S65C mutations have also been associated with iron accumulation,[43,44] but its role in causing clinical disease remains controversial.[45] The center mass of the data suggests that S65C mutations by themselves do not lead to clinical hemochromatosis, but they can contribute to excess iron deposits when other liver diseases are present or when there are additional mutations in iron metabolism genes.

HISTOLOGICAL FINDINGS

On H&E, iron is seen as granular, brown, and somewhat refractile cytoplasmic deposits (Fig. 12.16). Special stains are used to both identify low levels of iron that are not readily visible on H&E and to distinguish iron from lipofuschin. Iron is visualized in most centers using the Perls iron stain. The iron deposits in genetic hemochromatosis are predominantly hepatocellular, at least in the beginning, and begin in the zone 1 hepatocytes (Fig. 12.17). In addition, the iron deposits are often accentuated around the bile canaliculi (Fig. 12.18). The classic zone 1 to zone 3 gradient can be less evident with marked iron accumulation but is often still discernable. Cirrhotic nodules can retain a similar gradation of iron, with heavy deposits at the edges that taper toward the center of the nodule.

The Perls iron stain can sometimes show a light, diffuse, blue blush in hepatocytes or Kupffer cells. This finding is generally considered to represent ferritin (Fig. 12.19). In contrast to hemosiderin, with ferritin there are no findings visible on H&E, and the deposits are more diffuse in the cytoplasm, are nongranular, and have no clinical relevance, other than as a potential diagnostic pitfall.

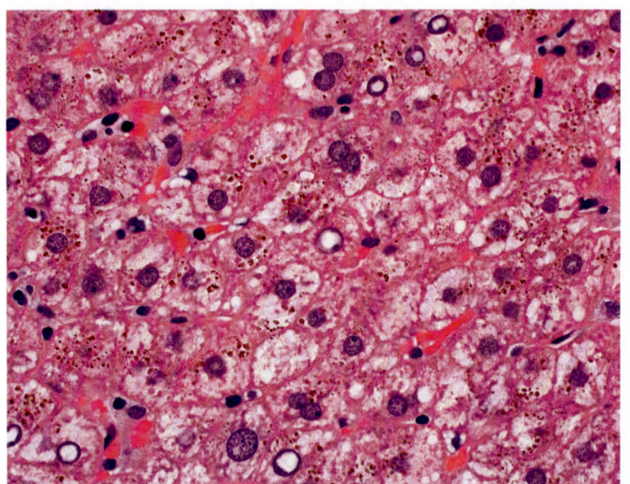

Figure 12.16. **Iron in hepatocytes.** The hepatocytes have granular brown deposits. From a case with C282Y homozygous disease.

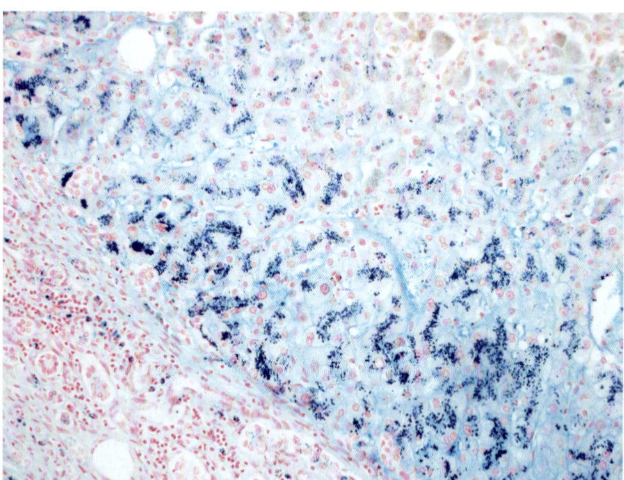

Figure 12.17. **Hemochromatosis, Perls iron stain.** The hepatocytes show a gradient of iron deposition, with heavier iron in zone 1 and diminishing iron toward zone 3 (upper right corner of image).

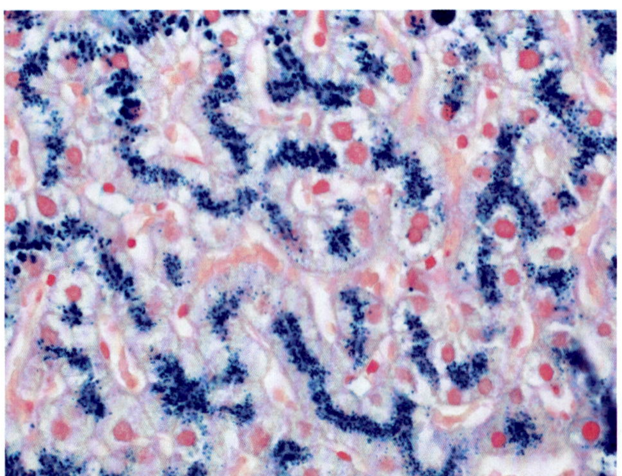

Figure 12.18. **Hemochromatosis, Perls iron stain.** The iron is accentuated around the bile canaliculi.

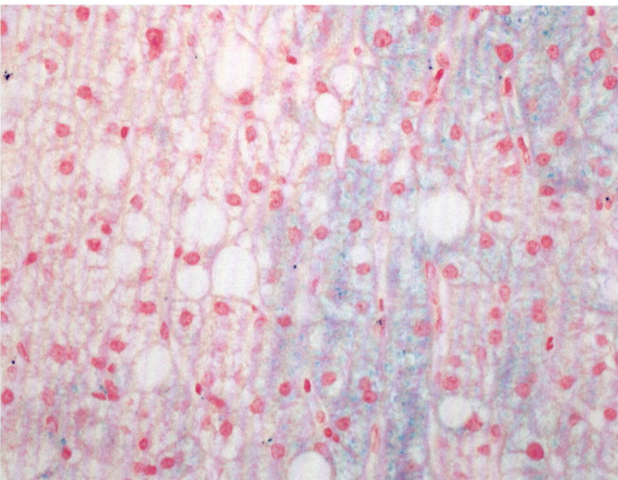

Figure 12.19. **Ferritin, Perls iron stain.** The hepatocytes show a faint blue blush. The hepatocytes do not show the typical granular deposits of hemosiderin.

Iron in Nonhepatocytes

Iron can also be seen in the epithelium of the bile duct proper, usually in cases with moderate or marked iron accumulation (Figs. 12.20 and 12.21). Most but not all of these cases will be a result of HFE hemochromatosis (Fig. 12.22). In contrast, when there is a significant hepatitis, especially with parenchymal collapse, iron is commonly observed in the reactive, proliferating bile ductules (do not confuse with the bile duct proper). However, this finding is nonspecific and does not indicate genetic hemochromatosis or other causes of iron overload are present.

When there is severe iron overload from any cause, iron can be deposited in many cell types including the endothelial cells, smooth muscle of vessel walls (Fig. 12.23), Kupffer cells, cholangiocytes, and hepatocytes. In particular, Kupffer cell iron is common in all forms of iron overload. In cases of secondary iron overload, Kupffer cell iron is often more abundant than hepatocellular iron. Likewise, in ferroportin disease, the iron deposits are predominately found in Kupffer cells. Finally, in some specimens, iron is present exclusively in portal endothelial cells (Fig. 12.24). To date, this finding does not have any specific linkage to an environmental etiology or to a genetic mutation.

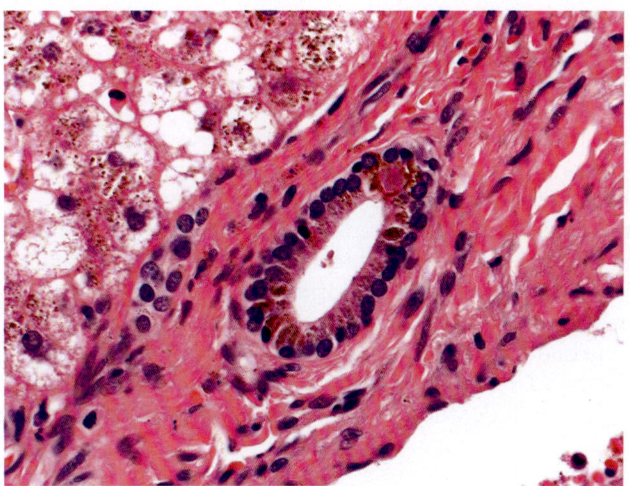

Figure 12.20. **Iron in bile ducts.** The bile ducts have granular brown iron deposits, from a case with C282Y homozygous disease and marked hepatocellular iron deposits.

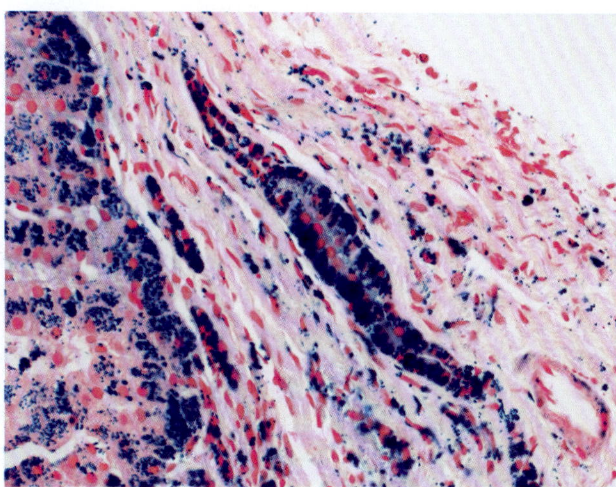

Figure 12.21. **Iron in bile ducts, Perls iron stain.** The bile ducts and hepatocytes are strongly positive in case with C282Y homozygous disease.

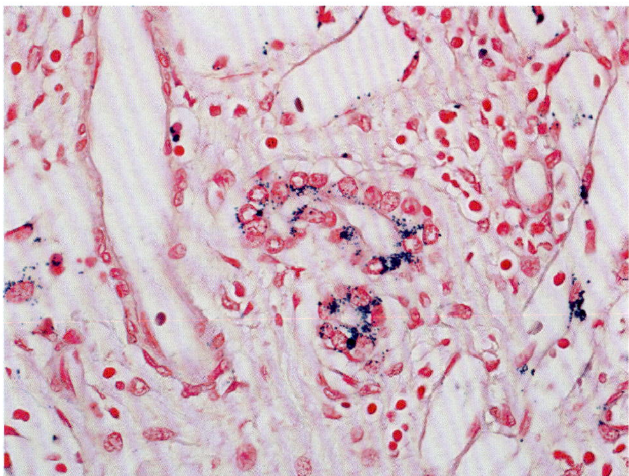

Figure 12.22. **Iron in bile ducts, Perls iron stain.** The bile ducts showed patchy iron accumulation in this liver with marked secondary iron overload. Testing was negative for HFE mutations.

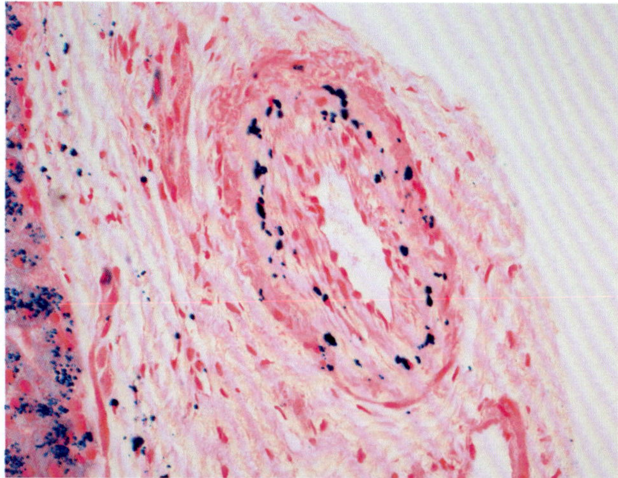

Figure 12.23. **Iron in endothelial cells, Perls iron stain.** There is iron present in an artery wall in this case of marked iron overload resulting from C282Y homozygous disease.

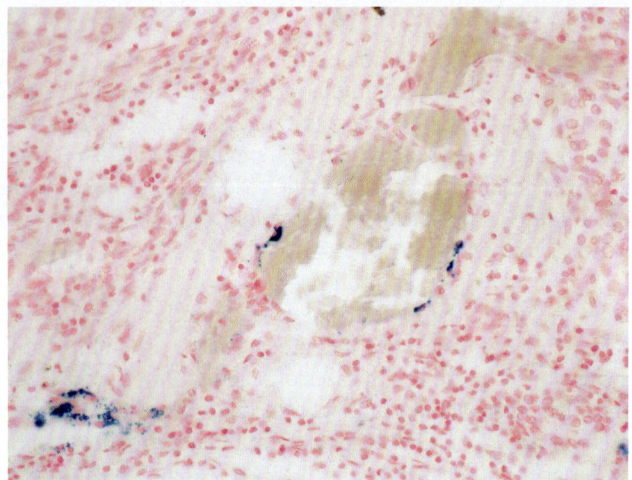

Figure 12.24. **Iron in endothelial cells, Perls iron stain.** In this biopsy, iron was present only in the endothelial cells of portal veins.

PEARLS & PITFALLS: the Perls Iron Stain

The classic pattern of iron deposition in genetic hemochromatosis includes these elements (not all need to be present): (1) predominately hepatic iron deposits; (2) a zone 1–predominant pattern; (3) iron deposits accentuated around the bile canaliculi; and (4) iron deposits in the bile duct epithelium.

While the above pattern is most commonly seen in the setting of HFE hemochromatosis, none of these findings are entirely specific, and nor is the overall pattern. For example, the zone 1–predominant deposition of iron is seen whenever the iron accumulation is driven by abnormal hepcidin levels. Likewise, iron deposits clustering around the bile canaliculi are found in a variety of genetic and nongenetic causes of iron overload. Finally, iron deposits in the bile duct epithelium correlate better with the overall duration and degree of iron accumulation than with HFE mutations.

Nonetheless, these pitfalls should not lead to a nihilistic approach to evaluating patterns of iron deposition, as patterns of iron deposition can still help guide subsequent clinical testing.

FAQ: Is an iron stain necessary as an up-front stain on all medical liver biopsies?

Answer: There are no validated data to answer this question, but there are several settings where an iron stain is not necessary as an up-front stain. The most common are biopsies in the liver transplant setting that were obtained to evaluate for rejection.

In the nontransplant setting, iron stains are very helpful for detecting mild iron, but cases with moderate or greater iron will have H&E findings to trigger an iron stain. If mild or less iron is not going to be clinically important, for example, in the setting of cirrhosis, then an iron stain may not be needed. Other clinical findings that should trigger an iron stain include unexplained heart disease, gonadal dysfunction, or significantly elevated serum ferritin (>1000) or transferrin saturation levels (>45%).

GENETIC VERSUS SECONDARY CAUSES OF IRON OVERLOAD

The distinction of genetically associated iron overload from secondary causes of iron overload is made based on genetic and clinical findings, but the histological changes can help guide clinical decisions. Relevant factors include whether there is a clinical history of exogenous iron intake, the degree of iron overload, the degree of liver fibrosis, and the overall pattern of iron deposits in the liver. Overall, mild to moderate but patchy iron accumulation in a liver with advanced fibrosis or cirrhosis is one of the most commonly encountered situations of increased iron deposits in the liver, but is also the least clinically relevant, as few, if any, of these cases represent genetic hemochromatosis or clinically relevant iron overload. Instead, the iron deposits in the liver result from hepcidin dysregulation as a result of the advanced liver disease. Cirrhosis in the setting of alcohol-related liver disease is particularly likely to have iron deposition, which can at times be heavy.

Classically, genetic causes of iron overload showed a hepatocyte-predominant pattern of iron deposition, with iron predominately in zone 1, while secondary causes were primarily associated with Kupffer cell iron deposits, which had a zone 3 predominance. These observations are broadly true, remembering that there is substantial iron redistribution over time. For example, in genetic hemochromatosis, occasional hepatocytes die for normal physiological reasons or because of injury due to the iron deposits, and the iron in the dead hepatocytes can be redistributed to Kupffer cells and portal macrophages. Likewise, secondary iron overload, for example, from blood transfusions, almost always has some hepatocellular iron accumulation, even when the overall pattern is that of Kupffer cell–predominant iron deposits.

FAQ: When should pathologists suggest additional testing to rule out genetic hemochromatosis?

Answer: There are no validated data to answer this question, but one reasonable approach is detailed below.

1. **Mild hepatocellular iron on Perls iron stain**
   a. This is the most common finding in liver specimens and the least specific, especially when there is liver fibrosis or other liver diseases.
   b. Recommend HFE testing: if the patient is young, the liver is noncirrhotic, and there is no other chronic liver disease on biopsy, such as chronic hepatitis or fatty liver disease.
2. **Moderate hepatocellular iron on Perls iron stain**
   a. Focally moderate iron is not uncommon, but iron that is diffusely moderate falls into this category. Diffuse means that most of the periportal regions show moderate hepatocellular iron accumulation (Fig. 12.25).
   b. Recommend HFE testing: cases where the livers are noncirrhotic, even if there is another active liver disease (e.g., fatty liver disease, chronic viral hepatitis, etc.). Patients can be of any age.
3. **Marked hepatocellular iron on Perls iron stain**
   a. Recommend HFE testing: All cases unless there is a known risk factor such as transfusion dependent anemia. Alcohol-related cirrhosis may be another exception. Patients can be of any age.
4. **Kupffer cell–predominant iron accumulation can be mild to marked. Iron can be in Kupffer cells only or be Kupffer cell predominant but also with hepatocellular iron**
   a. Test for ferroportin disease when
      i. Individuals have normal or low transferrin saturation levels but elevated ferritin levels
      ii. Or there is a family history of iron overload liver disease (because it suggests and autosomal dominant pattern of inheritance)
5. **Hepatocellular iron in young individuals (less than 40 years of age)**
   a. Consider other causes if HFE testing is negative (Fig. 12.26), such as hemojuvelin, etc.
6. **Hepatocellular iron in neonates**
   a. Suggest neonatal hemochromatosis: Any biopsy or autopsy of a neonate or stillbirth with marked liver injury/necrosis and extracellular iron deposits.

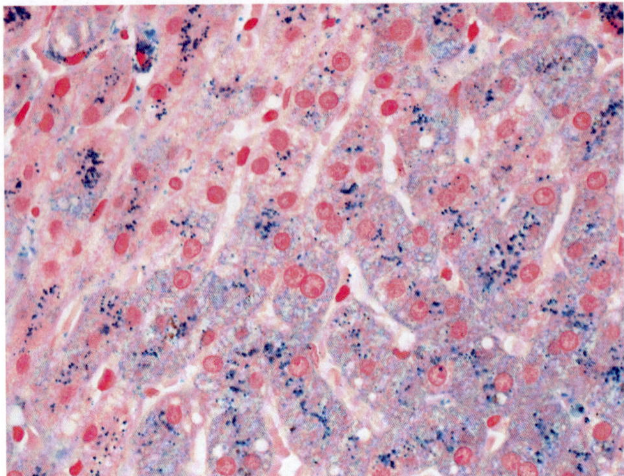

Figure 12.25. **Excess iron in a noncirrhotic liver.** In this case, the liver is noncirrhotic, and there is no significant inflammation or other disease injury patterns, but the hepatocytes show moderate iron accumulation. This type of case should be referred on for genetic testing.

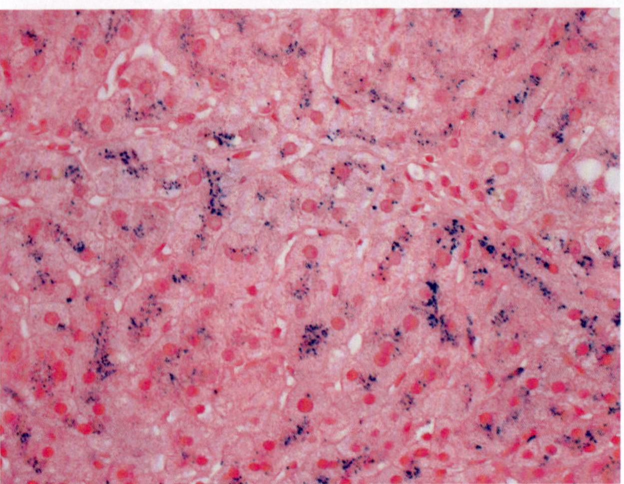

Figure 12.26. **Excess iron in a noncirrhotic liver.** In this biopsy from a young man with elevated serum blood markers, the liver is noncirrhotic and had no other disease injury patterns, but the hepatocytes show moderate iron accumulation. Testing for HFE mutations ended up being negative, so additional testing for hemojuvelin and other rare causes of genetic iron overload was suggested.

ACQUIRED/SECONDARY IRON OVERLOAD

CHECKLIST: Acquired or Secondary Overload

- ☐ Transfusion-dependent anemias
  - ○ Chronic renal dialysis
  - ○ Bone marrow transplants
- ☐ Nonspecific iron accumulation in livers with advanced fibrosis from any cause (because of impaired hepcidin synthesis). This list shows the approximate order of etiologies most likely to have iron and most likely to have more than minimal iron
  - ○ ETOH-related disease
  - ○ NASH
  - ○ Alpha-1-antitrypsin
  - ○ Chronic viral hepatitis
  - ○ Autoimmune hepatitis
  - ○ Biliary causes of cirrhosis
- ☐ Diseases with a genetic component of defective red blood cell synthesis
  - ○ Sickle cell disease
  - ○ Thalassemia
  - ○ Sideroblastic anemias
  - ○ Glucose-6-phoshphatase dehydrogenase deficiency
  - ○ Porphyria cutanea tarda

Acquired or secondary iron overload is by far the most common reason for iron accumulation in the liver (Fig. 12.27). There are many different causes, and the histology usually does not identify a specific etiology. The iron deposits occur first in the Kupffer cells (Fig. 12.28) and often have a zone 3 predominance, but in many cases, the iron appears to be somewhat randomly distributed. The iron is redistributed to hepatocytes over time, so a component of hepatocellular iron is common, especially if there is moderate or greater Kupffer cell iron.

There are a number of important genetic diseases that lead to impaired red blood cell synthesis or function. Some of these diseases require transfusions, further contributing to iron overload. The biopsies in several of these diseases can have a zone 1 predominance of hepatic iron, in addition to Kupffer cell iron deposits: sideroblastic anemia and porphyria cutanea tarda.

Sideroblastic anemia, is a heterogeneous group of disorders that can be either acquired or hereditary (Fig. 12.29). Patients have chronic anemia and bone marrow biopsies show ringed sideroblasts, which are an erythroid precursor with increased deposits of mitochondrial iron.

Other secondary iron diseases can be triggered by environmental factors. One example is patients with glucose-6-phoshphatase dehydrogenase deficiency. The disease is an X-linked recessive disorder (so only males are affected) where mutations in the glucose-6-phoshphatase dehydrogenase gene lead to a defective enzyme. This defective enzyme in turn leads to hemolytic crises when stressed by a variety of triggers such as infection and chemicals. Liver biopsies show mostly Kupffer cell iron accumulation.

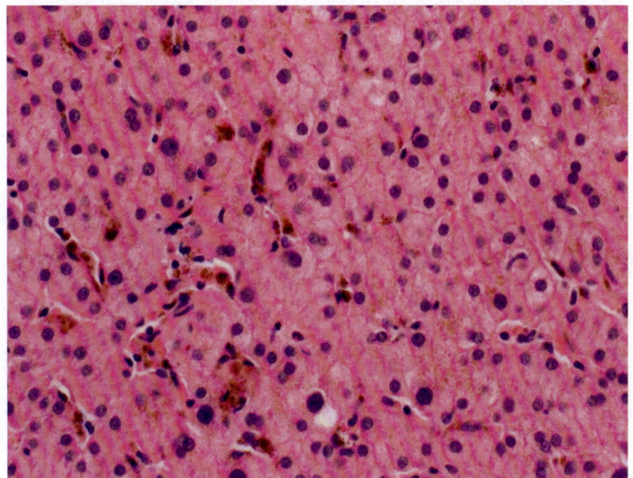

Figure 12.27. **Iron overload, secondary.** This patient had a long history of renal dialysis. There is marked Kupffer cell iron accumulation.

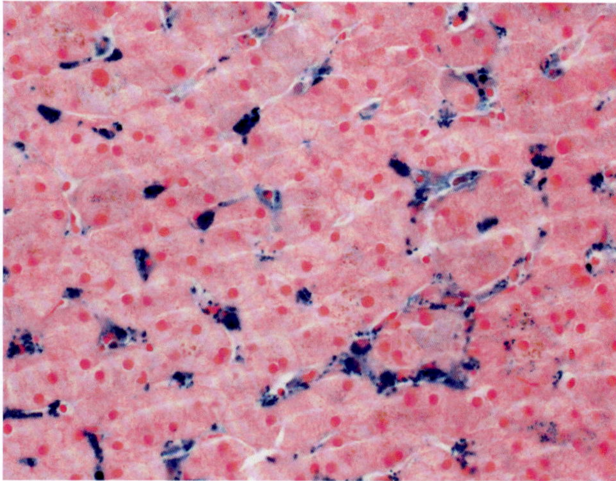

Figure 12.28. **Iron overload, secondary, Perls iron stain.** This case is another example of iron accumulation in the setting of renal dialysis. The iron is predominately found in Kupffer cells.

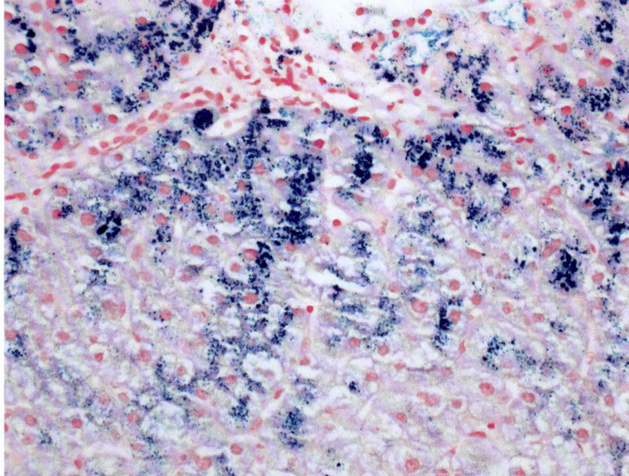

Figure 12.29. **Iron overload, sideroblastic anemia, Perls iron stain.** The iron deposits are primarily in hepatocytes and show a zone 1 gradient, but this case resulted from sideroblastic anemia and not HFE hemochromatosis.

Porphyria cutanea tarda is another example of genetic disease triggered by precipitating factors, which can include chronic hepatitis C infection or alcohol use.[46] Patients are also enriched for *HFE* gene mutations.[46] Iron deposits are seen in the zone 1 hepatocytes, Kupffer cells, and portal macrophages. In addition to the iron, the biopsy can show other findings that may have triggered the hemolysis, such as chronic hepatitis C or alcohol. In some cases, the hepatocytes can show needle-shaped crystals, but they are nearly impossible to see on H&E stains and generally require a ferric ferricyamide reduction stain.[47]

IRON IN DONOR LIVER BIOPSIES

Iron stains are performed in most academic centers on donor implant biopsies, although they are probably not necessary as up-front stains and could alternatively be performed on an as needed basis. Perls iron stains are positive in a substantial minority of cases (20% of deceased donors, 10% of living related donors) but almost always with mild and clinically insignificant levels of iron deposition.[48,49] More significant levels of iron can rarely be encountered, but in these cases, the iron is evident on the H&E, so the H&E findings will trigger an iron stain in those centers performing iron stain on an as needed basis. Low to moderate levels of iron in a donor liver do not appear to impact outcomes.[50]

Cases with moderate to marked iron deposition can represent inadvertent transplantation of livers homozygous for *HFE* mutations. Interestingly, the clinical course in these cases is surprisingly variable, reflecting other genetic polymorphisms in the allograft recipient that affect iron absorption and/or metabolism. In some cases there is progressive iron overload in the liver allograft,[51] while in other cases, iron in the liver diminishes.[52] As one example, a donor liver that was heterozygote for C282Y was transplanted into a patient with a rare R6S mutation, and the transplanted liver developed significant iron overload.[53] Overall, however, there are minimal data on the long-term consequences, if any, when donor livers with HFE mutations are transplanted. In contrast, clinical outcomes are not affected when a liver with a heterozygous mutation (C282Y/wild type or H63D/wild type) is transplanted into a patient with a wild type HFE genotype.[54]

DETERMINING IRON LEVELS IN THE LIVER

IRON-GRADING SYSTEMS

There are many different iron-grading systems that provide semiquantitative data on the extent of iron accumulation in the hepatocytes and Kupffer cells. These systems in general have taken one of three different approaches. In the first approach, the iron in hepatocytes is graded as per the zonal distribution (zone 1, zone 1 pus 2, or all three zones). In the second, the iron is graded by determining the lowest magnification that has discernable granules observable on iron stain. In the third approach, the percent of hepatocytes positive for iron is estimated to the nearest 10% or described using descriptors of mild (up to 20% of total hepatocytes in the biopsy specimen), moderate (20% to 50%), and marked (>50%). For clinical care, any of these systems work fine; hepatocellular and Kupffer cell iron should be graded separately.

QUANTITATIVE MEASUREMENT OF HEPATIC IRON CONCENTRATIONS

Quantitative iron analysis can be performed on fresh liver tissues or on paraffin-embedded tissues, with equivalent results.[55] However, paraffin-embedded tissues are generally preferred because they are easier to transport safely, and a pathologist can examine the H&E beforehand to make sure the tissue is suitable for analysis. The iron levels are not used to establish a diagnosis but are used to guide phlebotomy and other therapies to reduce organ iron accumulation. As frame of reference, results of quantitative iron analysis have been classified as mild (up to 150 µmol iron/g dry weight of liver), moderate (151 to 300), and marked (>301),[56] with the normal adult liver showing between 10 and 36 µmol iron/g dry weight of liver.

A hepatic iron index is still commonly provided by reference laboratories, but they no longer have any clinical significance. Many years ago, before the widespread availability of genetic testing, the hepatic iron index was used to separate genetic hemochromatosis from alcohol-related iron accumulation[57] and later from any cause of secondary liver iron accumulation. The premise of the hepatic iron index was that hepatic iron concentrations generally increase steadily in individuals with genetic hemochromatosis as they age, but not so in individuals who have nongenetic causes of iron overload. With this approach, a hepatic iron index greater than 1.9 was considered to be consistent with genetic hemochromatosis.

LIVER BIOPSIES IN INDIVIDUALS WITH KNOWN *HFE* MUTATIONS

Because of disease heterogeneity, patients with known *HFE* mutations need to be individually assessed for iron overload and for fibrosis. In many cases, fibrosis assessment is performed by noninvasive methods. MRI has been reported to have excellent abilities to assess iron by some radiology groups, although this assessment is not shared by all clinicians. In terms of specific management guidelines, the European Association for the Study of the Liver (EASL) recommends liver biopsies in C282Y homozygous individuals to assess the degree of fibrosis when serum ferritin levels are above 1000 µg/L, there are elevated AST levels or hepatomegaly, or patient age is over 40 years. The American association for the Study of Liver Diseases (AASLD) guidelines are similar, and biopsies are recommended to stage fibrosis when ferritin is >1000 µg/L or there are elevated serum levels of AST or ALT, for both C282Y homozygotes and compound heterozygosity for C282Y and H63D.

OTHER RARE GENETIC CAUSES OF HEMOCHROMATOSIS

CHECKLIST: Other Rare Causes of Genetic Hemochromatosis (Non-HFE Mutations)

- ☐ Ceruloplasmin mutations[58,59]
  - ○ Usually present as adults with neurological symptoms, but wide age range at presentation, from teenagers to elderly
    - ■ Younger individuals can present with anemia, mild liver enzyme elevations, and serum iron test abnormalities[60,61]
  - ○ *CP* mutations (encodes ceruloplasmin)
  - ○ Serum: elevated ferritin levels, but low iron transferrin saturation
  - ○ Iron deposits in liver, brain, and pancreas islet cells
    - ■ Iron deposits mostly in hepatocytes can be of panlobular pattern[62–66]
- ☐ DMT-1 mutations[67,68]
  - ○ Onset in late childhood, early teenage years
  - ○ *SCL11A2* mutations (encodes divalent metal transporter 1)
  - ○ Severe microcyctic anemia is common
- ☐ Ferritin mutations
  - ○ *FTL* mutations (encodes the light chain)
    - ■ Serum: high ferritin but low transferrin saturation levels
    - ■ Two disease patterns: hereditary hyperferritinemia cataract syndrome and hereditary neuroferritinopathy
    - ■ Little or no iron in the liver, but the hepatocyte nuclei can stain positive[69,70]

- *FTH* mutations (encodes the heavy chain)
  - Serum: high ferritin but low transferrin saturation levels
  - Iron accumulates in hepatocytes[71]

☐ **Juvenile hemochromatosis**

- Onset in late childhood, young adults
- Subtype 2A: *HFE2* mutations (encodes hemojuvelin)
- Subtype 2B: *HAMP* mutations (encodes hepcidin)
- Cardiomyopathy and/or hypogonadism can be prominent clinical findings
- Disease course is more aggressive than HFE mutations[72]

☐ **Transferrin mutations**[73–75]

- *TF* mutations (autosomal recessively inherited)[76]
  - homozgyous disease is called atransferrinemia
  - heterozygosity leads to iron overload only if there is another iron related gene that is mutated, such as HFE[77]
- Onset in childhood
- Very low or absent transferrin levels
- Severe hypochromic microcytic anemia
- Marked hepatic iron overload.[78]

☐ **Transferrin receptor gene 2**[79]

- Onset in adults
- *TFR2* mutations (encodes Transferrin receptor gene 2)

In all of these rare conditions, the iron deposits are primarily in hepatocytes. The iron deposition often has a zone 1 predominance, and the overall histological findings are similar to that of hemochromatosis resulting from *HFE* mutations. Kupffer cell/macrophage iron is common, generally increasing as the total amount of iron in the liver increases. Important clues to the diagnosis include mild or greater levels or hepatic iron accumulation in individuals who are young (often children, usually less than 40 years of age) and who have no other cause of liver disease, especially if there is no fibrosis or mild fibrosis. The presence of heart disease or hypogonadism can be another important clue.

FERROPORTIN DISEASE AND FERROPORTIN-ASSOCIATED HEMOCHROMATOSIS

CHECKLIST: Ferroportin Disease and Ferroportin-Associated Hemochromatosis

☐ Autosomal dominant inheritance (in contrast to other forms of genetic hemochromatosis)

☐ Adult presentation with elevated serum ferritin levels but normal or minimally elevated transferrin saturation levels

- Transferrin saturation levels can become elevated later in the course of the disease

☐ Mutations in the *SLC40A1* gene[80,81]

- Loss-of-function mutations lead to ferroportin disease, with Kupffer cell–predominant iron deposits and mild disease
- Gain of function mutations lead to ferroportin-associated hemochromatosis, with hepatocellular and Kupffer cell iron accumulation that resembles HFE-related hemochromatosis

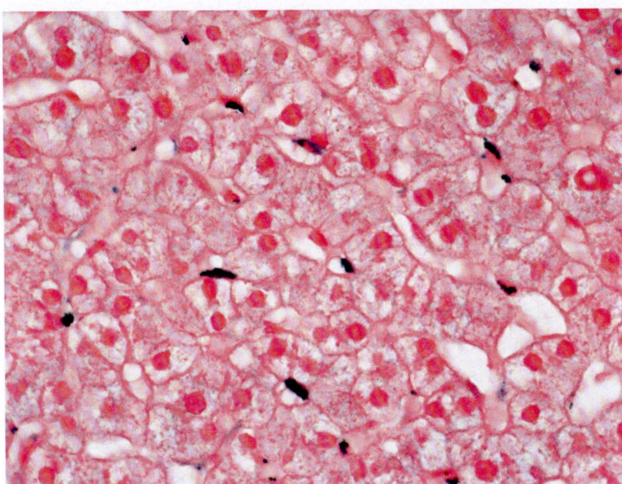

Figure 12.30. **Ferroportin disease, Perls iron stain.** This patient presented with a family history of liver disease on the father's side and mildly elevated liver enzymes. The iron deposits are exclusively in Kupffer cells.

Ferroportin disease is an inherited form of iron overload where the iron accumulates predominately in the Kupffer cells (Fig. 12.30). In contrast to other forms of genetic iron overload, ferroportin disease has an autosomal dominant pattern of inheritance.[82] Patients commonly present with mild anemia, mild elevations in liver enzymes, and sometimes with a family history of liver disease. However, ferroportin disease shows substantial phenotypic variability, which has led to the disease being subtyped into ferroportin disease (formerly called ferroportin disease type A) and ferroportin-associated hemochromatosis (formerly called ferroportin disease type B).[83] These subtypes also correlate with the type of mutations in the *SLC40A1* gene, which encodes ferroportin. Mutations in the more common ferroportin disease lead to loss of function, where the ferroportin protein is not able to export iron from Kupffer cells, leading to a Kupffer cell–predominant pattern of iron accumulation. In contrast, mutations in the less common ferroportin-associated hemochromatosis lead to gain of function, where ferroportin is less sensitive to inhibition by hepcidin, and iron accumulates in both the Kupffer cells and the hepatocytes. Overall, iron deposits are heavier in ferroportin-associated hemochromatosis than in ferroportin disease.[84] In cases of ferroportin-associated hemochromatosis, iron can also deposit in the heart and the islet cells, leading to cardiac arrhythmias and diabetes.

NEONATAL HEMOCHROMATOSIS

Neonatal hemochromatosis is an iron overload disease that likely has some genetic component but is quite different than other causes of genetic iron overload. Neonatal hemochromatosis appears to be primarily an alloimmune[85] or autoimmune[86] gestational disease, one that is caused by maternal antibodies that cross the placenta, bind to a currently unknown liver antigen, and lead to in utero liver injury.[87] Other maternal serum autoantibodies are also common. For example, serum ANA is positive in about 50% of cases.[88] However, there is no known association with autoimmune hepatitis or other autoimmune diseases in the mother.

After delivery, the prognosis is poor if the disease is not quickly recognized, but excellent for children who are successfully treated, with no medical sequelae. Treatment consists of removing the maternal antibody through plasmapheresis as well as providing supportive care. If an infant is affected by neonatal hemochromatosis, then almost all subsequent pregnancies in the mother will also be affected, regardless of the father.[85] However, the disease can be prevented in subsequent pregnancies by giving intravenous (IV) IgG from about the 18th week of gestation until delivery. Untreated pregnancies are at a high risk for late second-term and third-term fetal loss.

In newborns, clinical findings develop in the first few days after birth and consist of hypoglycemia, coagulopathy, and massive liver failure. For unclear reasons, the AST and ALT levels can be normal or only mildly elevated, even in cases of massive liver necrosis. The surviving hepatocytes can produce very high levels of AFP, typically greater than 100,000 ng/mL and as high as 800,000 ng/mL. By comparison, the healthy infant typically has values less than 80,000 ng/mL during this same time period of the first few days of life.

The liver injury pattern in most cases is that of marked hepatocyte injury, with varying amounts of inflammation, hepatocyte dropout/necrosis, and regenerative nodules (Fig. 12.31). Hepatocyte giant cell transformation and cholestasis are also common. In most cases, there is no fibrosis or mild fibrosis at presentation, but more advanced fibrosis, including cirrhosis, can develop over time. Diffuse lobular pericellular fibrosis is also common in livers with advanced fibrosis. On Perls iron stain, the hepatocytes have moderate to marked iron accumulation, although the iron deposits can be patchy and you may not see any iron if most or all of the hepatocytes are necrotic. Most of the iron will be found in the hepatocytes (Fig. 12.32), while the Kupffer cells generally have no or mild iron accumulation. In cases where specimens are obtained further in the disease course, there tends to be less iron and more fibrosis.[88]

The final diagnosis is made using a combination of clinical, laboratory, and histological findings. Extrahepatic iron deposits can be particularly helpful in confirming the diagnosis of neonatal hemochromatosis. However, extrahepatic iron is often absent in early gestational age fetuses.[88] Furthermore, multiple organs may need to be sampled, as extrahepatic iron deposits are heterogeneous from cases to case. Based on the current literature, the highest frequency of iron deposits are in these organs (in approximate order): pancreas acini, thyroid follicles, renal tubules, myocardium, minor salivary glands, and other epithelium (Brunner glands, stomach, thymus, trachea, etc.).[87] Of note, lip biopsies are often performed because of easy access to the minor salivary glands. They are helpful when positive,[89] but negative results are noninformative, both because the minor salivary glands can be missed and because the minor salivary glands can be negative for iron in bona fide cases of neonatal hemochromatosis.[88]

The massive liver injury seen with neonatal hemochromatosis can be mimicked by many other causes of acute hepatitis that lead to hepatocyte necrosis, inflammation, and cholestasis. In these cases, the proliferating bile ducts often show hemosiderin deposits on Perls iron stain, but this pattern is not specific and should not be interpreted as neonatal hemochromatosis. In contrast, in cases of neonatal hemochromatosis, there is iron deposited in hepatocytes and in extrahepatic organs. The differential for neonatal hemochromatosis also includes mitochondrial cytopathies, which can have massive liver injury, advanced fibrosis, and elevated serum iron studies. However, iron stains in the liver and extrahepatic tissues are negative.[90]

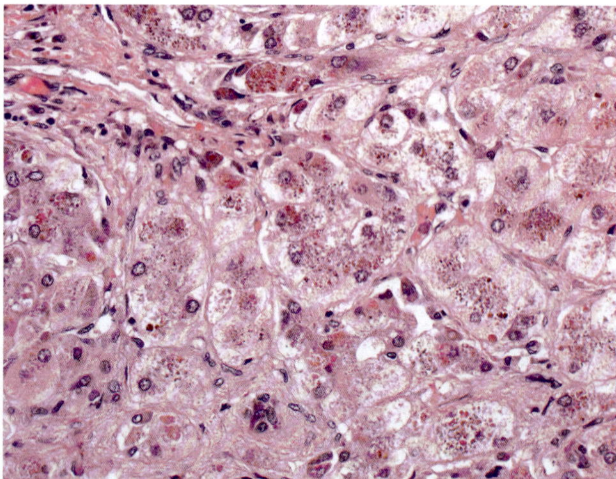

Figure 12.31. **Neonatal hemochromatosis.** The liver is cirrhotic, with cholestasis and mild nonspecific inflammation.

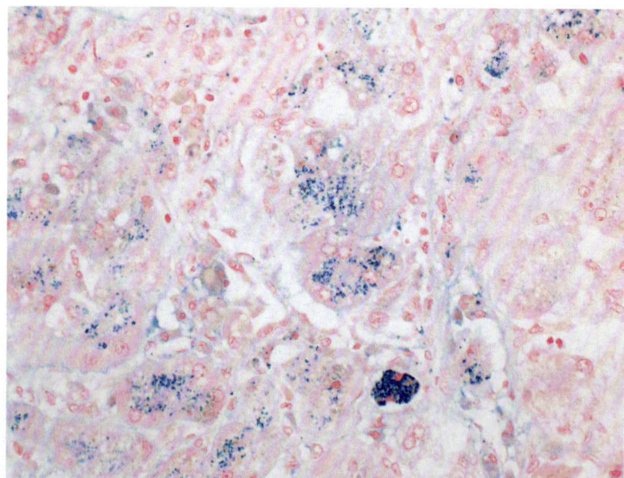

Figure 12.32. **Neonatal hemochromatosis, Perls iron stain.** There is patchy moderate hepatocellular iron accumulation (same case as preceding image).

The differential also includes the GRACILE syndrome. The GRACILE syndrome is caused by mutation in the *BCS1L* gene and is enriched in individuals of Finnish heritage.[91,92] The acronym stands for Growth Retardation, Amino aciduria, Cholestasis, Iron overload, Lactic acidosis, and Early death. In this syndrome, there can be massive liver injury, often with death in the first week of life, and massive hepatocyte iron deposits. *BCS1L* encodes a mitochondrial protein and mutations lead to defects in mitochondrial complex III. The protein may play a role in iron metabolism, but that remains unclear.

AFRICAN IRON OVERLOAD DISEASE

African iron overload, which was formerly called Bantu siderosis, is a complex iron disease of uncertain etiology. Currently it is not clear if this represents a distinct disease entity or a collection of different diseases, the latter appearing most likely. In the initial autopsy-based study that proposed this disease, marked hepatic iron overload was found predominately in men from rural sub-Saharan Africa.[93] Follow-up studies suggested the iron overload resulted from drinking beer that had been brewed in iron pots or iron drums.[94,95] However, this pattern has not held up in subsequent studies. For example, one study found similar iron deposits in the livers of individuals who did not drink beer.[96] Histologically, the liver shows a range of patterns, from predominately hepatocellular iron deposits, to predominately Kupffer cells iron deposits, to mixed patterns. Molecular studies are limited, but one case report identified novel mutations in the TFR2 gene.[97]

GLYCOGEN STORAGE DISEASES

There are many different glycogen storage diseases (Table 12.1), almost all of which develop abnormal accumulations of glucose within the hepatocytes.[98,99] In most cases, the clinical findings will include hypoglycemia (except for types II and IV), hepatomegaly, short stature, and recurrent infections. Most patients present as infants or children, but adult presentations are also well documented.

Your job as a pathologist is not to determine the exact subtype of glycogen storage disease, which will be determined instead by biochemical or genetic analysis. Rather, your job is to recognize the basic pattern of injury, look for findings that might suggest an alternative diagnosis, and determine the amount of fibrosis. Fibrosis is most commonly seen at presentation in glycogen storage disease types III and IV, but fibrosis can also be seen in types I and IX.[100]

The histological findings will vary, but in most cases, the hepatocytes show steatosis, glycogenosis, or mixed patterns with both glycogenosis and steatosis (Table 12.1) (Figs. 12.33–12.35). An exception is glycogen storage disease type IV, which has a different and distinctive pattern of injury, where hepatocytes show ground glass type inclusions (Fig. 12.36). The inclusions are PAS positive and, in most cases, are at least partially resistant to diastase digestion because they are composed of amylopectin-like material and not typical glycogen. However, many laboratories have fairly aggressive digestion, and in these cases, the inclusions can appear diastase sensitive. The histological differential includes chronic hepatitis B infection as well as drug-induced glycogen pseudo–ground glass changes, but the appropriate diagnosis is readily sorted out by correlation with clinical and serological findings.

Lafora disease can also be in the histological differential for glycogen storage disease type IV, as this disease also shows distinctive round hepatocyte inclusions, which are called polyglucosan bodies. In Lafora disease, autosomal recessive mutations in *EPM2A* (encodes laforin) or *NHLRC1* (enocodes malin) lead to glycogen molecules that are poorly soluble because they are hyperphosphorylated and insufficiently branched. This poorly soluble glycogen then precipitates out and forms inclusions in the liver (as well as the heart, muscle, and skin). Lafora disease presents in late childhood and is accompanied by rapidly fatal, progressive myoclonic epilepsy.

TABLE 12.1: Glycogen Storage Diseases

Type	Gene	Main Liver Findings	Fibrosis Risk	Hepatic Tumors
0	Glycogen synthetase	Steatosis NOT glycogenosis	Low	Not reported
Ia	Glucose-6-phoshatase	Glycogenosis Steatosis	High	Hepatic adenomas; risk for malignant transformation
Ib	Glucose-6-phoshate translocase	Glycogenosis Steatosis	High	Hepatic adenomas; risk for malignant transformation
II	Lysosomal gamma1-4 and gamma1-6 glucosidase	Cytoplasmic vacuoles	Low	Not reported
IIIa/b	Amylo-1-6 glycosidase	Steatosis Glycogenosis	High, can progress to cirrhosis	Hepatic adenomas; risk for malignant transformation
IV	Amylo-1-4 glycan6-glycoslytransferase	Hepatocyte inclusions that resemble ground glass change	High, can progress to cirrhosis	Not reported
VI	Liver phosphorylase E	Steatosis Glycogenosis	Low	Hepatic adenoma with risk of malignant transformation
IX	Liver phosphorylase kinase	Steatosis Glycogenosis	High, can progress to cirrhosis	Not reported
XI	GLUT 2 transporter	Glycogenosis	Low	Not reported

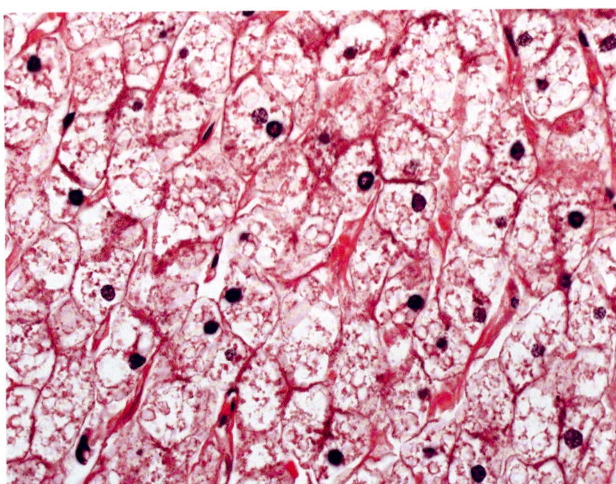

Figure 12.33. **Glycogen storage disease type 1.** The liver shows glycogenosis as the main pattern of injury.

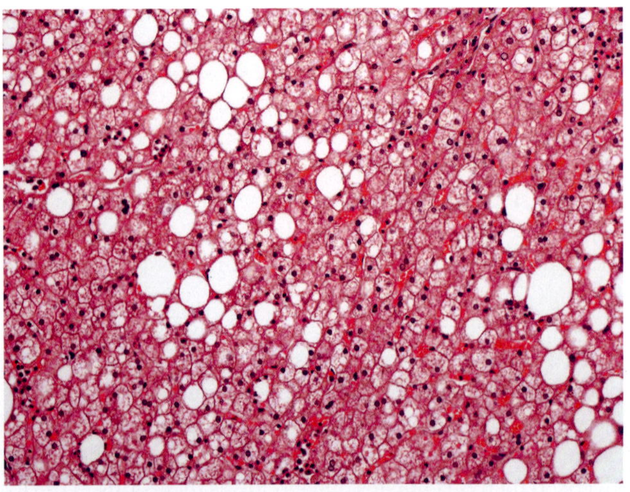

Figure 12.34. **Glycogen storage disease type 1.** In this case, from an older child, the biopsy showed mild glycogenosis and mild macrovesicular steatosis.

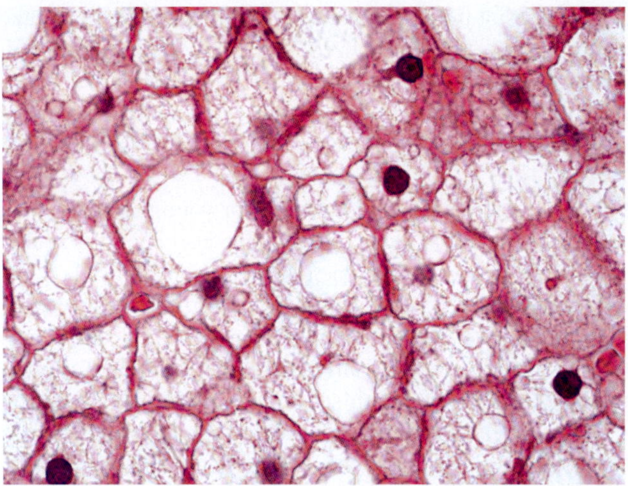

Figure 12.35. **Glycogen storage disease type 3.** The liver shows glycogenosis as the main pattern of injury, but the hepatocytes also show large dilated vacuoles in the cytoplasm.

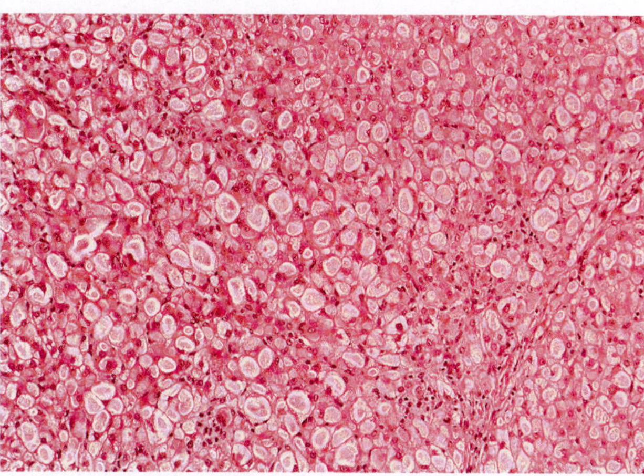

Figure 12.36. **Glycogen storage disease type 4.** The hepatocytes have distinctive round cytoplasmic inclusions.

There are several other important clinical observations for several of the glycogen storage diseases. With glycogen storage disease type IB, patients can present with severe neutropenia and have inflammatory bowel disease that resembles ulcerative colitis or Crohn disease clinically and histologically.[101,102] Several subtype of glycogen storage disease are at risk for hepatic adenomas (Fig. 12.37). The hepatic adenomas tend to develop after puberty and have a risk for malignant transformation. In type IB storage disease, the hepatic adenomas can also be associated with anemia that resolves after the adenoma is resected.[35] Molecular studies have shown that most of the adenomas are either the inflammatory subtype or unclassified.

UREA CYCLE DEFECTS

CHECKLIST: Urea Cycle Defects

- ☐ Arginase deficiency
  - ○ Mutations in *ARG1*
  - ○ Blood shows increased arginine
- ☐ Argininosuccinase acid lyase deficiency (also known as argininosuccinic aciduria)
  - ○ Mutations in *ASL*
  - ○ Blood shows increased citrulline and argininosuccinic acid
- ☐ Argininosuccinic acid synthetase deficiency (also known as citrullinemia)
  - ○ Mutations in *ASS1*
  - ○ Blood shows increased citrulline
- ☐ Carbamoyl phosphate synthetase I
  - ○ Mutations in *CPS1*
  - ○ Blood shows increased ammonia
- ☐ N-Acetylglutamate synthetase deficiency
  - ○ Mutations in *NAGS*
  - ○ Blood shows increased ammonia
- ☐ Ornithine transcarbamylase deficiency
  - ○ Blood shows high glutamine and alanine, but low citrulline and low arginine. Urine shows increased levels of orotic acid. Ammonia levels in blood also usually are elevated

Urea cycle defects are rare and most result from mutations in the 6 main genes that make up the urea cycle (see checklist). As proteins are metabolized, excess nitrogen is generated, and the function of the urea cycle is to convert nitrogen into urea, so that it can be safely excreted in the urine. If the urea cycle is not working, then nitrogen accumulates in the form of ammonia. Thus, all of the mutations in the urea cycle lead to abnormal levels of serum ammonia.

Individuals with urea cycle defects mostly present as neonates or young children with vomiting, lethargy, irritability, and seizures. Urea cycle defects have also been associated with the sudden infant death syndrome. In most cases, the diagnosis in neonates is made by clinical findings and blood work, so biopsies are relatively uncommon. Biopsies are more common in later presentations, including late childhood and adult years. Clinical findings in late presentations can include lethargy or vomiting after meals that have high protein content, intentionally avoiding meat, hyperactivity with self-injury, or other neurological or psychiatric findings. Liver enzymes are mildly elevated, and there can be hepatomegaly.

The histological findings are variable but typically show some degree of hepatic glycogenosis (Fig. 12.38), which can vary from subtle to marked. In one study of urea cycle defects, eight of eleven biopsies showed marked hepatocellular glycogen accumulation.[103] Other nonspecific findings often include megamitochondria, glycogenated nuclei, glycogen storing foci,[104] and sometimes macrovesciclar steatosis (Fig. 12.39).[105] Other subtle findings can include nodular regenerative hyperplasia (Fig. 12.40). Finally, some cases look essentially normal on H&E, with only mild nonspecific reactive changes.

One of the enzymes in the urea cycle, carbamoyl phosphate synthetase 1, is defective in cases of carbamoyl phosphate synthetase 1 deficiency. This same enzyme is the target of HepPar1, so immunostains are negative in individuals with homozygous mutations, while those with heterozygous mutations show retained staining.[106]

MUCOPOLYSACCHARIDOSIS

There are a number of mutations in genes that encode enzymes and other proteins important for glycosaminoglycans metabolism. These diseases all affect the lysosomal enzymes used to break down glycosaminoglycans. When normal metabolism is disrupted, mucopolyscacharides accumulate in the liver and other tissues. All of these disorders are very rare, but examples include Hunter syndrome, Hurler syndrome, Marquio syndrome, Marteaux–Lamy syndrome, and Sanfilippo syndrome. Disease causing mutations are mostly autosomal recessive but can also be X linked.

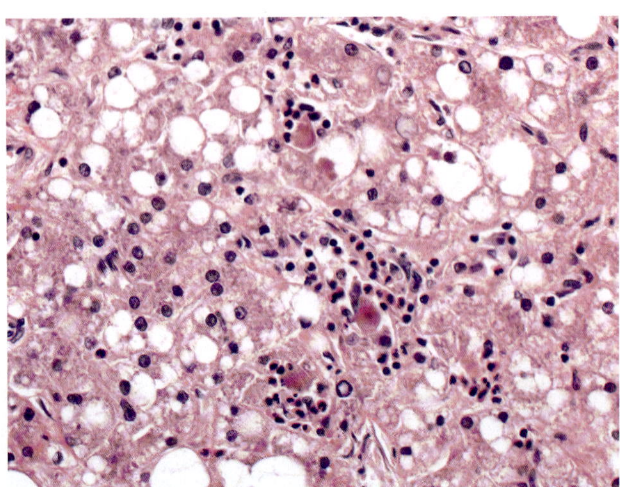

Figure 12.37. **Glycogen storage disease type 1, hepatic adenoma.** The hepatic adenoma is of the inflammatory subtype and shows a steatohepatitic-like pattern, with fat, inflammation, and balloon cells with Mallory hyaline.

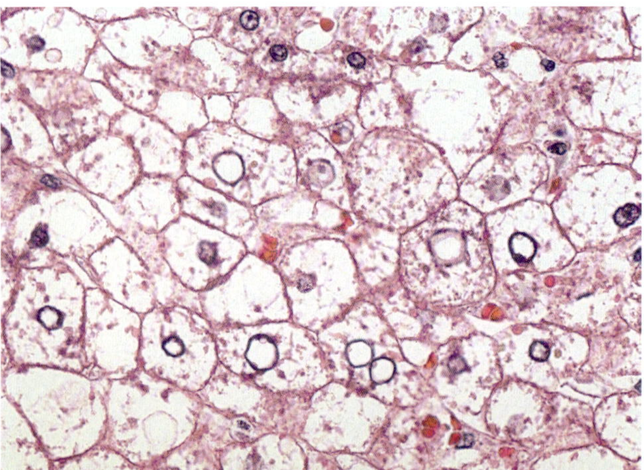

Figure 12.38. **Argininosuccinic acid synthetase deficiency.** The liver shows striking hepatic glycogenosis.

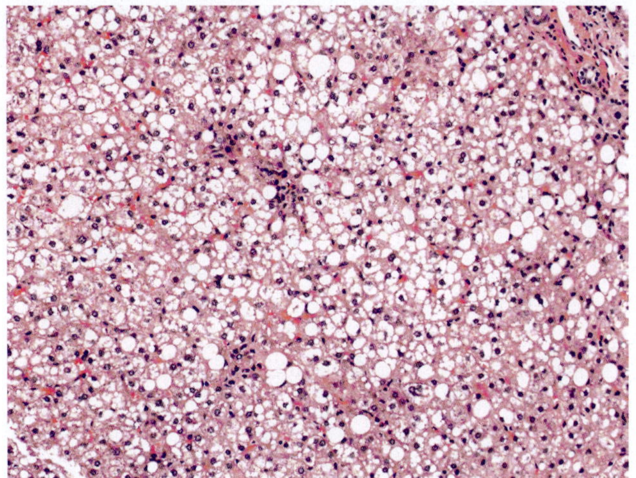

Figure 12.39. **Ornithine transcarbamylase deficiency.** The liver shows a macrovesicular steatosis pattern of injury.

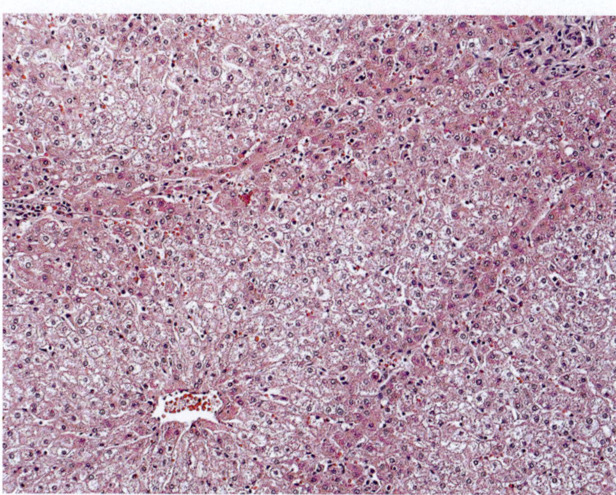

Figure 12.40. **Carbamoyl phosphate synthetase I deficiency.** At low power, a subtle pattern of nodular regenerative hyperplasia is evident.

All of these disorders can lead to mucopolyscacharide deposition in the liver. However, the morphological findings vary considerably, ranging from clear, rarified cytoplasm in hepatocytes that resembles hepatic glycogenosis but is PAS negative to showing medium- and small-sized cytoplasmic vacuoles in hepatocytes and Kupffer cells (Fig. 12.41). The mucopolysaccharides are removed by routine processing in most cases, but occasionally residual mucopolysaccharides can be highlighted by colloidal iron stains.

DISORDERS OF LIPID METABOLISM

Several lipid metabolism diseases can lead to abnormal deposits of material in the liver. All of them are rare, but the most common overall are Gaucher disease and Niemann–Pick disease. Gaucher disease results from mutations in the beta-glucosidase gene and is strongly linked to Ashkenazi Jewish ethnicity. The characteristic histological finding is the Gaucher cell, which is a Kupffer cell with abundant amphophilic cytoplasm that shows striations (Fig. 12.42).

Niemann–Pick disease also leads to deposits in the Kupffer cells/macrophages, which show foamy clumps of cells in the sinusoids and portal tracts (Fig. 12.43). The disease results from mutations in the *SMPD1* gene (types A and B) or *NPC1* or *NPC2* gene (type C), which lead to sphingomyelin deposits in the central nervous system, liver, spleen, and bone marrow. Niemann–Pick disease type A is the most common, representing 80% to 90% of cases. Niemann–Pick disease type A also has the worse prognosis, as most cases lead to death by two years of age.

Tangier disease (named after the place where the first patient was identified, Tangier Island, Virginia) is a cholesterol ester disease, where mutations in the *ABCA1* gene lead to diminished or absent levels of high-density lipoproteins, which in turn leads to cholesterol ester deposits in the liver, spleen, tongue, tonsils, and other organs. In the liver, there is Kupffer cell hyperplasia, with enlarged Kupffer cells showing foamy cytoplasm (Fig. 12.44).

Cholesteryl ester storage diseases can also result from deficient lysosomal acid lipase activity caused by mutations in the *LIPA* gene, which are autosomal recessively inherited. The lack of lysosomal acid lipase activity leads to deposits of cholesteryl esters in the liver, spleen, and macrophages. Depending on the clinical severity, which reflects the relative degree of residual gene activity, the disease is further subclassified. Wolman disease presents in infants with failure to thrive, malabsorption, and hepatosplenomegaly and has a very aggressive clinical course, with early, rapid death. In contrast, mutations that have some residual enzyme activity can present at varying ages, from childhood to adult years. The clinical findings are usually mild and nonspecific, but almost always include an element of hepatosplenomegaly.

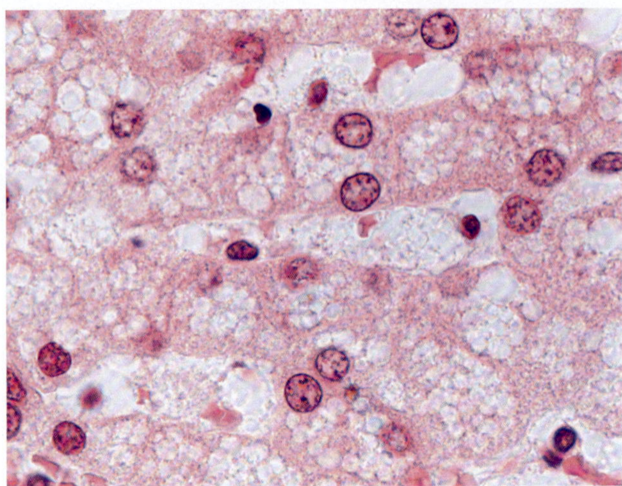

Figure 12.41. **Hunter syndrome.** The hepatocytes and Kupffer cells have numerous small vacuoles.

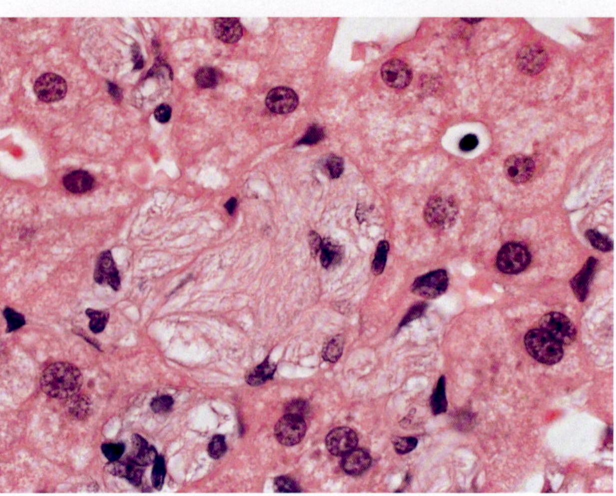

Figure 12.42. **Gaucher disease.** The lobules show a Gaucher cell, with amphophilic cytoplasm that shows striations.

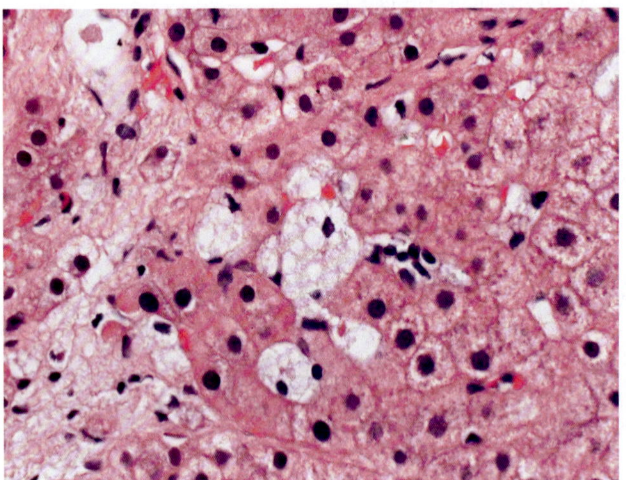

Figure 12.43. **Niemann–Pick disease.** The lobules show prominent Kupffer cells with foamy cytoplasm.

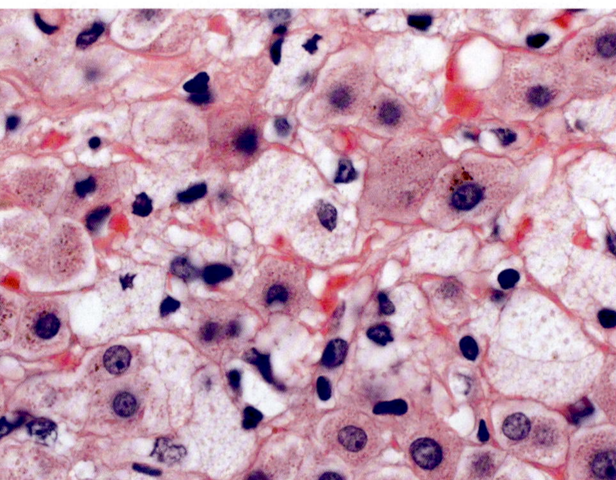

Figure 12.44. **Tangier disease.** The enlarged Kupffer cells show abundant foamy cytoplasm.

On biopsy, the Kupffer cells and portal macrophages are enlarged by foamy cytoplasm, and the hepatocytes can show microvesicular steatosis (Fig. 12.45). If frozen sections are available, then cholesteryl ester crystals can be seen under polarized light, with bright silver birefringence. The livers can become fibrotic, and some cases will progress to cirrhosis.[107]

INBORN ERRORS OF AMINO ACID METABOLISM

Normal amino acid metabolism can be disrupted by a large number of different mutations. Most lead to autosomal recessively inherited diseases that present in the early years of life. Many of these diseases lead to abnormal liver enzymes, but in general, they do not show abnormal deposits of amino acids in hepatocytes or Kupffer cells. In most cases, the biopsy findings are very mild and nonspecific, with the main finding being varying degrees of glycogen accumulation, often very subtle. Megamitochondria can be prominent. Biopsies can also show macrovesicular steatosis, especially in later disease.[108] There is no fibrosis at first clinical presentation, but fibrosis can develop if the disease is not adequately treated by dietary modifications. Tyrosinemia in particular can lead to cirrhosis and also has a high risk of hepatocellular carcinoma.[109]

PRADER–WILLI DISEASE

Prader–Willi disease is a rare disease that results from deletions of a variable number of contiguous genes on chromosome 15, genes that are paternally inherited. The precise genetic mechanism is not fully understood, but individuals are persistently hungry despite adequate food intake (hyperphagia), which can lead to the metabolic syndrome with obesity and insulin resistance.[110,111] While infants with Prader–Willi disease can be underweight, the persistent hyperphagia leads to severe obesity in older children and adults. This in turn leads to fatty liver disease, including steatosis or steatohepatitis (Fig. 12.46). Hepatic tumors have also been reported in Prader–Willi disease, including hepatoblastomas[112] and hepatic adenomas,[113] but it is not clear if Prader–Willi disease represents a significant risk factor for these tumors of if these are chance occurrences.

ERYTHROPOIETIC PROTOPORHYRIA

Erythropoietic protoporphyria results from defects in the enzyme ferrochelatase, which leads to impaired heme synthesis, with a buildup of protoporphyrin levels in the blood. Protoporphyrin is removed from the blood by the liver, where it accumulates and leads to a cholestatic pattern of liver injury. It takes some time for liver disease to develop and is generally not seen until patients are in their late teenage or adult years. Biopsies in young individuals show normal liver at the H&E level, although subtle findings are seen on electron microscopy.[114] However, even without liver disease, affected individuals typically present earlier as young children with photosensitivity, as protoporphyrin also accumulates in the skin and absorbs ultraviolet (UV) light, leading to skin irritation and injury.

Histologically, when there is liver disease, the biopsy shows dense brown black deposits of protoporphyrin in Kupffer cells, bile canaliculi, and bile ducts.[115] The protoporphyrin often appears denser and darker brown than normal bile (Fig. 12.47), but the liver can also be cholestatic, so the H&E findings alone can show overlap. However, when examined under polarized light, the protoporphyrin deposits show a red to orange birefringence. A Maltese cross pattern (Fig. 12.48) can also be seen on polarized light, although the finding can be patchy and is best seen with large biopsies or with resection specimen.

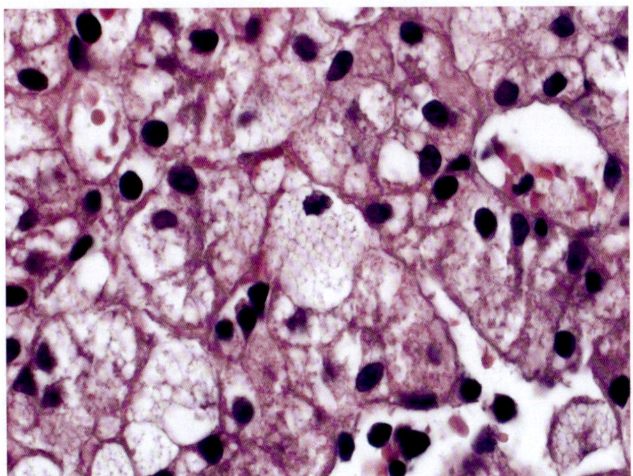

Figure 12.45. **Lysosomal acid lipase deficiency.** This adult case showed striking microvesicular steatosis.

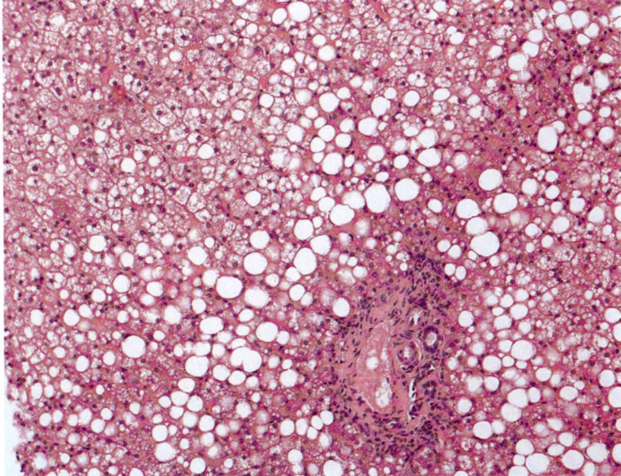

Figure 12.46. **Prader–Willi disease.** The liver shows moderate macrovesicular steatosis. The fat shows a zone 1 pattern, but not enough cases have been described to know if zone 1 fat is typical.

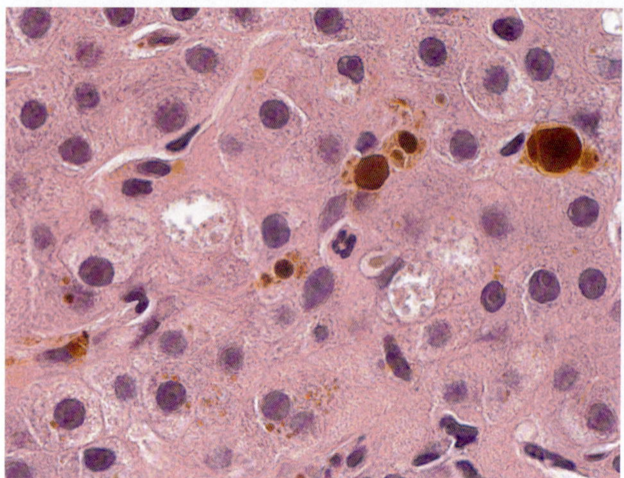

Figure 12.47. **Erthropoietic protoporphyria.** The lobules show cholestasis-like findings, with round brown plugs of protoporphyrin deposited in the sinusoidal Kupffer cells.

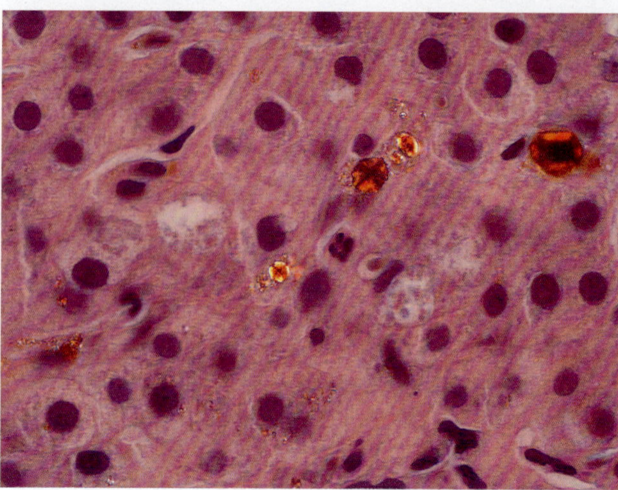

Figure 12.48. **Erthropoietic protoporphyria, polarized light.** The protoporphyrin deposits show a maltese cross configuration.

DISORDERS OF MITOCHONDRIA

Mitochondrial disease results from mutations in genes that are encoded by either mitochondrial DNA or nuclear DNA. Diseases caused by mutations in nuclear genes are inherited in an autosomal recessive fashion, while diseases caused by mutations in mitochondrial DNA are either de novo or are maternally inherited. They are all rare, but some of the more common conditions are the mitochondrial DNA depletion syndrome, Alpers syndrome, and Pearson syndrome.

Mitochondrial disease can involve many different organs, including the liver. However, not all mitochondrial diseases lead to liver disease. In general, mutations either impair the respiratory chain or other key mitochondrial functions (90% of all mitochondrial cytopathies) or impair mitochondrial function by causing depletions in the total amount of mitochondrial DNA (10% of all mitochondrial cytopathies). Clinical findings can include muscle weakness, neurological symptoms, eye disease, deafness, and intestinal pseudo-obstruction.[116] Hepatic and neurological findings tend to dominate in mitochondrial depletion syndromes. Patients can present as infants or adults.[117]

The histological findings have been described largely in case reports, with little or no comprehensive histological data published to date in a larger series of cases. Nonetheless, the most common findings appears to be steatosis,[117] which often has a prominent microvesicular steatosis component (Fig. 12.49) and sometimes has a mosaic pattern, with admixed normal appearing hepatocytes alongside those with striking microvesicular steatosis. In some cases, nodules of hepatocytes can form masslike lesions[118] that individually are similar to sporadic focal fatty change. In particular with the mitochondrial DNA depletion syndromes, the lobules can also show patches of hepatocytes with oncocytic cytoplasmic (Fig. 12.50).[119]

Other histological changes include hepatocyte ballooning,[120] cholestasis,[120] and hepatocellular iron accumulation.[118,121,122] The liver can show advanced fibrosis, even in infants, with reports of micronodular cirrhosis by 6 months of age.[122] Rare cases of hepatocellular carcinoma have been reported.[118,121]

TELOMERE SHORTENING SYNDROME

Telomere shortening syndrome results from genetic changes that lead to unusually short telomeres. Clinical presentation can include aplastic anemia, idiopathic pulmonary fibrosis, and cryptogenic liver disease.[123] The liver biopsy findings are not well described and are probably not very specific. For this reason, the best clue to the diagnosis can be a family history of unexplained lung and liver disease. In some families, there can be evidence for "genetic anticipation," where the disease develops at an earlier age in each successive generation.

The biopsy can show mild nonspecific portal chronic inflammation and mild patchy lobular hepatitis, especially when there is clinical disease involvement of the gut.[124] In addition, the portal veins are often atrophic or absent (Fig. 12.51). In response, the lobules can show aberrant arteries (Fig. 12.52) as well as nodular regenerative hyperplasia. Fibrosis can develop, with portal fibrosis and thin delicate bridging fibrosis (Fig. 12.53). Established cirrhosis has also been reported.[123,125]

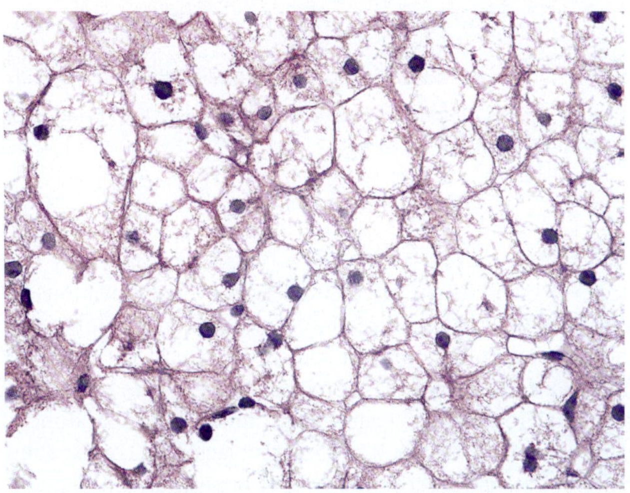

Figure 12.49. **Mitochondrial cytopathy.** The hepatocytes show microvesicular steatosis.

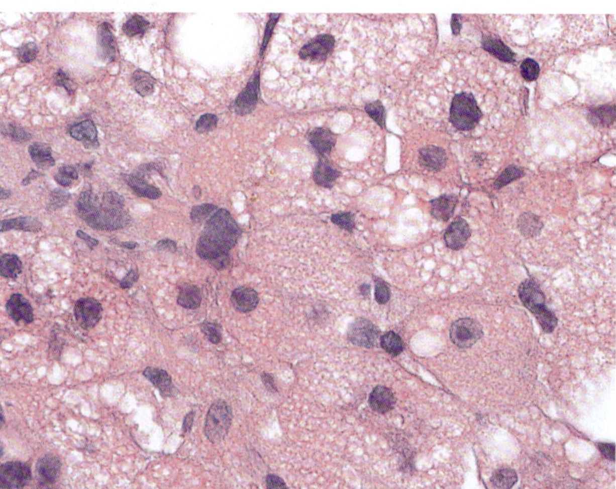

Figure 12.50. **Mitochondrial cytopathy.** The hepatocytes show oncocytic change.

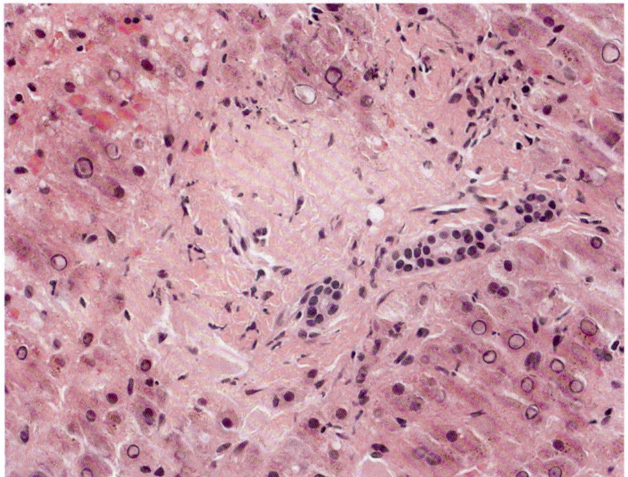

Figure 12.51. **Telomere shortening syndrome.** The portal tract shows mild fibrosis and loss of the portal vein.

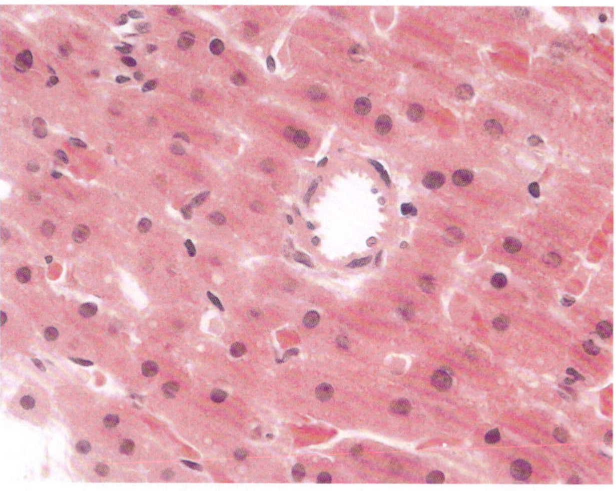

Figure 12.52. **Telomere shortening syndrome.** The lobules show aberrant arteries.

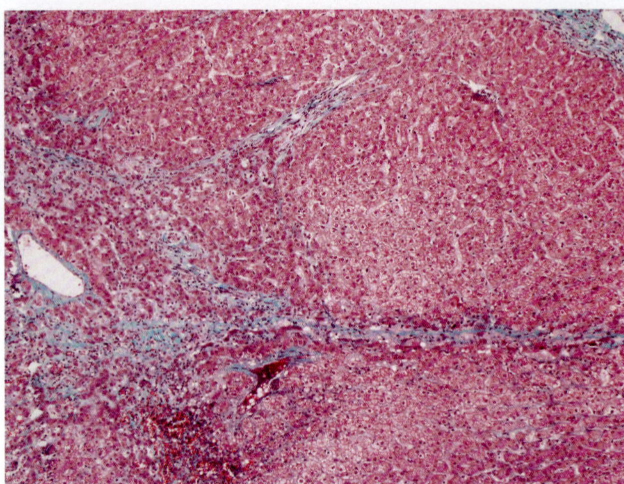

Figure 12.53. **Telomere shortening syndrome.** Thin bridges of fibrosis are present in this case.

NEAR MISSES

CASE 1. A 26-year-old woman presented with incidentally discovered elevations in her liver enzymes. An ultrasound showed fatty liver disease, but she was only mildly overweight, was not on any medications, and reported only rare social alcohol use. There was no fibrosis and no findings to suggest any additional disease process. A biopsy was performed (Fig. 12.54) and showed moderate macrovesicular steatosis with mildly active steatohepatitis. Because of the young age of the patient and lack of clear risk factors, a copper stain was performed and showed mild but extensive periportal copper deposition. Subsequent workup established a diagnosis of Wilson disease.

This case illustrates the importance of thinking of Wilson disease in young adults with otherwise unexplained fatty liver disease. A negative copper stain does not exclude Wilson disease but, when positive, can help point to the correct diagnosis. Remember that the rhodanine copper stain should be cut at 10 microns for optimal sensitively.

CASE 2. A case was presented at an interesting case conference by a young GI/liver pathologist who had signed out a biopsy as rare case of glycogen storage disease with an adult presentation. The patient was 21 years of age and had elevated liver enzymes, hepatomegaly, and elevated blood sugar levels. A biopsy showed hepatocytes with abundant diffuse glycogen accumulation (Fig. 12.55). Although this finding was evident on H&E, the young pathologist had been uncertain so he confirmed glycogen accumulation by ordering electron microscopy, before signing out the case as glycogen storage disease.

At the conference, it was pointed out that elevated blood sugar levels and the patient's age would both be unusual for glycogen storage disease and that the overall finding would be a perfect fit for glycogenic hepatopathy. Subsequent review of the medical records confirmed a history of poorly controlled type 1 diabetes mellitus.

This case illustrates the importance of interpreting histological findings in the context of clinical findings. Glycogenic hepatopathy and glycogen storage disease can indeed look similar on histology, but the clinical settings are distinct. Checking the clinical records can take some time but, in this case, established the proper diagnosis easily and would have been cheaper than electron microscopy. This case also illustrates the importance of excluding more common disease processes before considering exotic diagnoses.

CASE 3. A liver biopsy was performed in a mildly overweight but otherwise healthy young man to evaluate persistent, mild AST and ALT elevations. The biopsy shows minimal lobular inflammation, mild fatty change, no biliary tract disease, no vascular disease, and no fibrosis. An iron stain showed moderate hepatocellular iron accumulation predominately in zone 1 hepatocytes (Fig. 12.56). All of this was nicely documented in the original surgical pathology report, but the clinical team requested the case be submitted for external review.

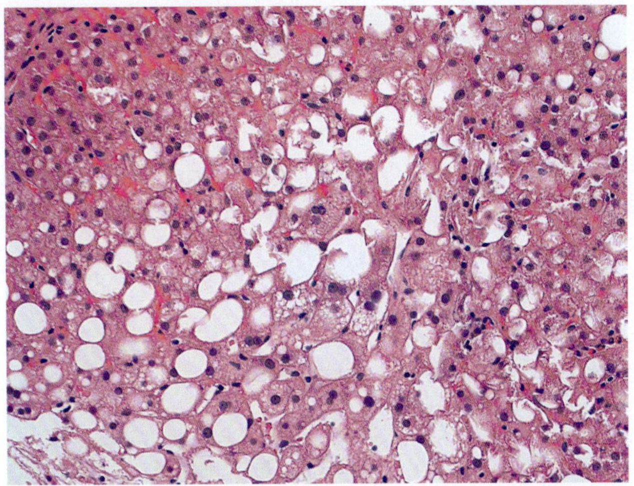

Figure 12.54. Near miss case 1, fatty liver disease. This case of fatty liver disease resulted from Wilson disease.

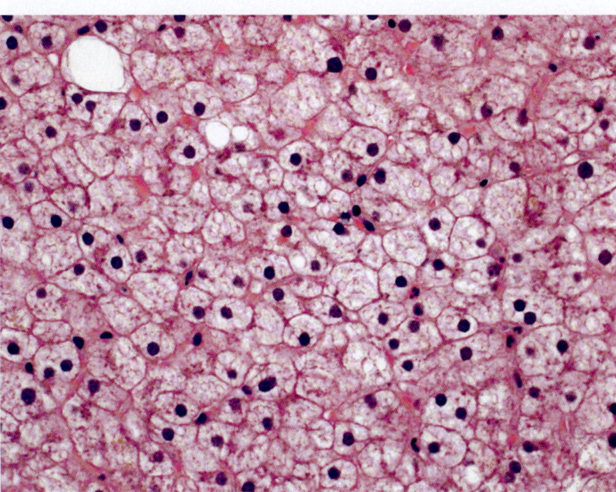

Figure 12.55. Near miss case 2, glycogen accumulation. The hepatocytes show diffuse glycogen accumulation.

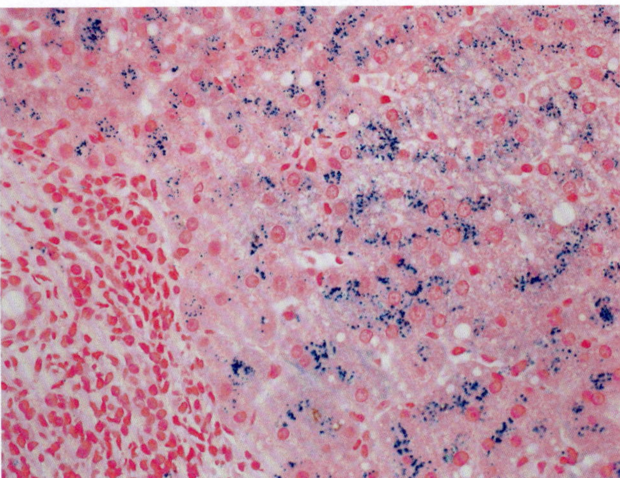

Figure 12.56. Near miss case 3, Perls iron stain. In addition to mild fatty liver, the biopsy showed moderate predominately zone 1 hepatocellular iron accumulation. Testing showed HFE hemochromatosis.

The consult report was essentially the same, except for the addition of an explanatory note about the iron. This degree of iron is too much for a nonspecific iron deposition and strongly suggests genetic hemochromatosis. Subsequent *HFE* testing showed C282Y homozygosity.

This case illustrates the importance of evaluating the iron stain in the context of the presence or absence of other active liver diseases as well as the degree of fibrosis. If this same degree of iron was found in an end-stage cirrhotic liver from chronic hepatitis C, the degree of iron would have been nonspecific. However, in the setting of no fibrosis, this degree of iron pointed to genetic hemochromatosis.

References

1. Millward-Sadler GH. Alpha-1-antitrypsin deficiency and liver disease. *Acta Med Port.* 1981:91-102.
2. Kelly JK, Taylor TV, Milford-Ward A. Alpha-1-antitrypsin Pi S phenotype and liver cell inclusion bodies in alcoholic hepatitis. *J Clin Pathol.* 1979;32:706-709.
3. Gourley MF, Gourley GR, Gilbert EF, Odell GB. Alpha 1-antitrypsin deficiency and the PiMS phenotype: case report and literature review. *J Pediatr Gastroenterol Nutr.* 1989;8:116-121.
4. Janciauskiene S, Eriksson S, Callea F, et al. Differential detection of PAS-positive inclusions formed by the Z, Siiyama, and Mmalton variants of alpha1-antitrypsin. *Hepatology.* 2004;40:1203-1210.

5. Joly P, Guillaud O, Hervieu V, Francina A, Mornex JF, Chapuis-Cellier C. Clinical heterogeneity and potential high pathogenicity of the Mmalton Alpha 1 antitrypsin allele at the homozygous, compound heterozygous and heterozygous states. *Orphanet J Rare Dis*. 2015;10:130.

6. Arroyo M, Crawford JM. Hepatitic inherited metabolic disorders. *Semin Diagn Pathol*. 2006;23:182-189.

7. Thomas RM, Schiano TD, Kueppers F, Black M. Alpha1-antichymotrypsin globules within hepatocytes in patients with chronic hepatitis C and cirrhosis. *Hum Pathol*. 2000;31:575-577.

8. Niwa K, Mimuro J, Miyata M, et al. Dysfibrinogen Kagoshima with the amino acid substitution gammaThr-314 to Ile: analyses of molecular abnormalities and thrombophilic nature of this abnormal molecule. *Thromb Res*. 2008;121:773-780.

9. Miljic P, Nedeljkov-Jancic R, Zuvela M, Subota V, Dordevic V. Coexistence of hypofibrinogenemia and factor V Leiden mutation: is the balance shifted to thrombosis? *Blood Coagul Fibrinolysis*. 2014;25:628-630.

10. Asselta R, Robusto M, Braidotti P, et al. Hepatic fibrinogen storage disease: identification of two novel mutations (p.Asp316Asn, fibrinogen Pisa and p.Gly366Ser, fibrinogen Beograd) impacting on the fibrinogen gamma-module. *J Thromb Haemost*. 2015;13:1459-1467.

11. Rubbia-Brandt L, Neerman-Arbez M, Rougemont AL, Male PJ, Spahr L. Fibrinogen gamma375 arg-->trp mutation (fibrinogen aguadilla) causes hereditary hypofibrinogenemia, hepatic endoplasmic reticulum storage disease and cirrhosis. *Am J Surg Pathol*. 2006;30:906-911.

12. Simsek Z, Ekinci O, Cindoruk M, et al. Fibrinogen storage disease without hypofibrinogenemia associated with estrogen therapy. *BMC Gastroenterol*. 2005;5:36.

13. Rosencrantz R, Schilsky M. Wilson disease: pathogenesis and clinical considerations in diagnosis and treatment. *Semin Liver Dis*. 2011;31:245-259.

14. Suvarna JC. Kayser-Fleischer ring. *J Postgrad Med* 2008;54:238-240.

15. Yang X, Tang XP, Zhang YH, et al. Prospective evaluation of the diagnostic accuracy of hepatic copper content, as determined using the entire core of a liver biopsy sample. *Hepatology*. 2015;62:1731-1741.

16. Ferenci P. Whom and how to screen for Wilson disease. *Expert Rev Gastroenterol Hepatol*. 2014;8:513-520.

17. Coffey AJ, Durkie M, Hague S, et al. A genetic study of Wilson's disease in the United Kingdom. *Brain*. 2013;136:1476-1487.

18. Usta J, Wehbeh A, Rida K, et al. Phenotype-genotype correlation in Wilson disease in a large Lebanese family: association of c.2299insC with hepatic and of p. Ala1003Thr with neurologic phenotype. *PLoS One*. 2014;9:e109727.

19. Barada K, El-Atrache M, El H, et al. Homozygous mutations in the conserved ATP hinge region of the Wilson disease gene: association with liver disease. *J Clin Gastroenterol*. 2010;44:432-439.

20. Pronicki M. Wilson disease - liver pathology. *Handb Clin Neurol*. 2017;142:71-75.

21. Liggi M, Murgia D, Civolani A, Demelia E, Sorbello O, Demelia L. The relationship between copper and steatosis in Wilson's disease. *Clin Res Hepatol Gastroenterol*. 2013;37:36-40.

22. Markiewicz-Kijewska M, Szymczak M, Ismail H, et al. Liver transplantation for fulminant Wilson's disease in children. *Ann Transplant*. 2008;13:28-31.

23. Karadag N, Tolan K, Samdanci E, Selimoglu A, Akpolat N, Yilmaz S. Effect of copper staining in Wilson disease: a liver explant study. *Exp Clin Transpl*. 2017;15:542-546.

24. Mounajjed T, Oxentenko AS, Qureshi H, Smyrk TC. Revisiting the topic of histochemically detectable copper in various liver diseases with special focus on venous outflow impairment. *Am J Clin Pathol*. 2013;139:79-86.

25. Pilloni L, Lecca S, Van Eyken P, et al. Value of histochemical stains for copper in the diagnosis of Wilson's disease. *Histopathology*. 1998;33:28-33.

26. Nemolato S, Serra S, Saccani S, Faa G. Deparaffination time: a crucial point in histochemical detection of tissue copper. *Eur J Histochem*. 2008;52:175-178.

27. Ferenci P, Steindl-Munda P, Vogel W, et al. Diagnostic value of quantitative hepatic copper determination in patients with Wilson's Disease. *Clin Gastroenterol Hepatol*. 2005;3:811-818.

28. Muller T, Schafer H, Rodeck B, et al. Familial clustering of infantile cirrhosis in Northern Germany: a clue to the etiology of idiopathic copper toxicosis. *J Pediatr*. 1999;135:189-196.

29. Muller T, Muller W, Feichtinger H. Idiopathic copper toxicosis. *Am J Clin Nutr*. 1998;67:1082S-1086S.

30. Nayak NC, Chitale AR. Indian childhood cirrhosis (ICC) & ICC-like diseases: the changing scenario of facts versus notions. *Indian J Med Res*. 2013;137:1029-1042.

31. Pietrangelo A. Hepcidin in human iron disorders: therapeutic implications. *J Hepatol*. 2011;54:173-181.

32. Pietrangelo A. Hemochromatosis: an endocrine liver disease. *Hepatology*. 2007;46:1291-1301.

33. Finberg KE, Heeney MM, Campagna DR, et al. Mutations in TMPRSS6 cause iron-refractory iron deficiency anemia (IRIDA). *Nat Genet*. 2008;40:569-571.

34. Chung A, Leo K, Wong G, Chuah K, Ren J, Lee C. Giant hepatocellular adenoma presenting with chronic iron deficiency anemia. *Am J Gastroenterol*. 2006;101:2160-2162.

35. Wang DQ, Carreras CT, Fiske LM, et al. Characterization and pathogenesis of anemia in glycogen storage disease type Ia and Ib. *Genet Med*. 2012;14:795-799.

36. Fargion S, Mandelli C, Piperno A, et al. Survival and prognostic factors in 212 Italian patients with genetic hemochromatosis. *Hepatology*. 1992;15:655-659.

37. Milman N, Pedersen P, á Steig T, Byg KE, Graudal N, Fenger K. Clinically overt hereditary hemochromatosis in Denmark 1948–1985: epidemiology, factors of significance for long-term survival, and causes of death in 179 patients. *Ann Hematol*. 2001;80:737-744.

38. Niederau C, Fischer R, Purschel A, Stremmel W, Haussinger D, Strohmeyer G. Long-term survival in patients with hereditary hemochromatosis. *Gastroenterology*. 1996;110:1107-1109.

39. Wojcik JP, Speechley MR, Kertesz AE, Chakrabarti S, Adams PC. Natural history of C282Y homozygotes for hemochromatosis. *Can J Gastroenterol*. 2002;16:297-302.

40. Hanson EH, Imperatore G, Burke W. HFE gene and hereditary hemochromatosis: a HuGE review. Human genome epidemiology. *Am J Epidemiol*. 2001;154:193-206.

41. Settin A, El-Bendary M, Abo-Al-Kassem R, El Baz R. Molecular analysis of A1AT (S and Z) and HFE (C282Y and H63D) gene mutations in Egyptian cases with HCV liver cirrhosis. *J Gastrointestin Liver Dis*. 2006;15:131-135.

42. EASL clinical practice guidelines for HFE hemochromatosis. *J Hepatol*. 2010;53:3-22.

43. Lam M, Torbenson M, Yeh MM, Vivekanandan P, Ferrell L. HFE mutations in alpha-1-antitrypsin deficiency: an examination of cirrhotic explants. *Mod Pathol*. 2010;23:637-643.

44. Mura C, Raguenes O, Ferec C. HFE mutations analysis in 711 hemochromatosis probands: evidence for S65C implication in mild form of hemochromatosis. *Blood*. 1999;93:2502-2505.

45. Pedersen P, Milman N. Genetic screening for HFE hemochromatosis in 6,020 Danish men: penetrance of C282Y, H63D, and S65C variants. *Ann Hematol*. 2009;88:775-784.

46. Cassiman D, Vannoote J, Roelandts R, et al. Porphyria cutanea tarda and liver disease. A retrospective analysis of 17 cases from a single centre and review of the literature. *Acta Gastroenterol Belg*. 2008;71:237-242.

47. Siersema PD, Rademakers LH, Cleton MI, et al. The difference in liver pathology between sporadic and familial forms of porphyria cutanea tarda: the role of iron. *J Hepatol*. 1995;23:259-267.

48. Minervini MI, Ruppert K, Fontes P, et al. Liver biopsy findings from healthy potential living liver donors: reasons for disqualification, silent diseases and correlation with liver injury tests. *J Hepatol*. 2009;50:501-510.

49. Ryan CK, Johnson LA, Germin BI, Marcos A. One hundred consecutive hepatic biopsies in the workup of living donors for right lobe liver transplantation. *Liver Transpl*. 2002;8:1114-1122.

50. Shaked O, Gonzalez A, Bahirwani R, et al. Donor hemosiderosis does not affect liver function and regeneration in the setting of living donor liver transplantation. *Am J Transplant*. 2014;14:216-220.

51. Dwyer JP, Sarwar S, Egan B, Nolan N, Hegarty J. Hepatic iron overload following liver transplantation of a C282y homozygous allograft: a case report and literature review. *Liver Int*. 2011;31:1589-1592.

52. Adams PC, McAlister V, Chakrabarti S, Levstik M, Marotta P. Is serum hepcidin causative in hemochromatosis? Novel analysis from a liver transplant with hemochromatosis. *Can J Gastroenterol*. 2008;22:851-853.

53. Wigg AJ, Harley H, Casey G. Heterozygous recipient and donor HFE mutations associated with a hereditary haemochromatosis phenotype after liver transplantation. *Gut*. 2003;52:433-435.

54. Alanen KW, Chakrabarti S, Rawlins JJ, Howson W, Jeffrey G, Adams PC. Prevalence of the C282Y mutation of the hemochromatosis gene in liver transplant recipients and donors. *Hepatology*. 1999;30:665-669.

55. Olynyk JK, O'Neill R, Britton RS, Bacon BR. Determination of hepatic iron concentration in fresh and paraffin-embedded tissue: diagnostic implications. *Gastroenterology*. 1994;106:674-677.

56. Deugnier Y, Turlin B. Pathology of hepatic iron overload. *World J Gastroenterol*. 2007;13:4755-4760.

57. Bassett ML, Halliday JW, Powell LW. Value of hepatic iron measurements in early hemochromatosis and determination of the critical iron level associated with fibrosis. *Hepatology*. 1986;6:24-29.

58. Harris ZL, Takahashi Y, Miyajima H, Serizawa M, MacGillivray RT, Gitlin JD. Aceruloplasminemia: molecular characterization of this disorder of iron metabolism. *Proc Natl Acad Sci USA*. 1995;92:2539-2543.

59. Yoshida K, Furihata K, Takeda S, et al. A mutation in the ceruloplasmin gene is associated with systemic hemosiderosis in humans. *Nat Genet*. 1995;9:267-272.

60. Meral Gunes A, Sezgin Evim M, Baytan B, Iwata A, Hida A, Avci R. Aceruloplasminemia in a Turkish adolescent with a novel mutation of ceruloplasmin gene: the first diagnosed case from Turkey. *J Pediatr Hematol Oncol*. 2014;36:e423-e425.

61. Doyle A, Rusli F, Bhathal P. Aceruloplasminaemia: a rare but important cause of iron overload. *BMJ Case Rep*. 2015;2015.

62. Kono S, Suzuki H, Takahashi K, et al. Hepatic iron overload associated with a decreased serum ceruloplasmin level in a novel clinical type of aceruloplasminemia. *Gastroenterology*. 2006;131:240-245.

63. Rusticeanu M, Zimmer V, Schleithoff L, et al. Novel ceruloplasmin mutation causing aceruloplasminemia with hepatic iron overload and diabetes without neurological symptoms. *Clin Genet*. 2014;85:300-301.

64. Bethlehem C, van Harten B, Hoogendoorn M. Central nervous system involvement in a rare genetic iron overload disorder. *Neth J Med*. 2010;68:316-318.

65. Hofmann WP, Welsch C, Takahashi Y, et al. Identification and in silico characterization of a novel compound heterozygosity associated with hereditary aceruloplasminemia. *Scand J Gastroenterol*. 2007;42:1088-1094.

66. Perez-Aguilar F, Burguera JA, Benlloch S, Berenguer M, Rayon JM. Aceruloplasminemia in an asymptomatic patient with a new mutation. Diagnosis and family genetic analysis. *J Hepatol*. 2005;42:947-949.

67. Iolascon A, Camaschella C, Pospisilova D, Piscopo C, Tchernia G, Beaumont C. Natural history of recessive inheritance of DMT1 mutations. *J Pediatr*. 2008;152:136-139.

68. Iolascon A, d'Apolito M, Servedio V, Cimmino F, Piga A, Camaschella C. Microcytic anemia and hepatic iron overload in a child with compound heterozygous mutations in DMT1 (SCL11A2). *Blood*. 2006;107:349-354.

69. Wong K, Barbin Y, Chakrabarti S, Adams P. A point mutation in the iron-responsive element of the L-ferritin in a family with hereditary hyperferritinemia cataract syndrome. *Can J Gastroenterol*. 2005;19:253-255.

70. Mancuso M, Davidzon G, Kurlan RM, et al Hereditary ferritinopathy: a novel mutation, its cellular pathology, and pathogenetic insights. *J Neuropathol Exp Neurol*. 2005;64:280-294.

71. Kato J, Fujikawa K, Kanda M, et al. A mutation, in the iron-responsive element of H ferritin mRNA, causing autosomal dominant iron overload. *Am J Hum Genet*. 2001;69:191-197.

72. Pietrangelo A. Hereditary hemochromatosis: pathogenesis, diagnosis, and treatment. *Gastroenterology*. 2010;139:393-408, e1-2.

73. Knisely AS, Gelbart T, Beutler E. Molecular characterization of a third case of human atransferrinemia. *Blood*. 2004;104:2607.

74. Beutler E, Gelbart T, Lee P, Trevino R, Fernandez MA, Fairbanks VF. Molecular characterization of a case of atransferrinemia. *Blood*. 2000;96:4071-4074.

75. Aslan D, Crain K, Beutler E. A new case of human atransferrinemia with a previously undescribed mutation in the transferrin gene. *Acta Haematol*. 2007;118:244-247.

76. Athiyarath R, Arora N, Fuster F, et al. Two novel missense mutations in iron transport protein transferrin causing hypochromic microcytic anaemia and haemosiderosis: molecular characterization and structural implications. *Br J Haematol*. 2013;163:404-407.

77. Beaumont-Epinette MP, Delobel JB, Ropert M, et al. Hereditary hypotransferrinemia can lead to elevated transferrin saturation and, when associated to HFE or HAMP mutations, to iron overload. *Blood Cell Mol Dis*. 2015;54:151-154.

78. Hamill RL, Woods JC, Cook BA. Congenital atransferrinemia. A case report and review of the literature. *Am J Clin Pathol*. 1991;96:215-218.

79. Camaschella C, Fargion S, Sampietro M, et al. Inherited HFE-unrelated hemochromatosis in Italian families. *Hepatology*. 1999;29:1563-1564.

80. Montosi G, Donovan A, Totaro A, et al. Autosomal-dominant hemochromatosis is associated with a mutation in the ferroportin (SLC11A3) gene. *J Clin Invest*. 2001;108:619-623.

81. Njajou OT, Vaessen N, Joosse M, et al. A mutation in SLC11A3 is associated with autosomal dominant hemochromatosis. *Nat Genet*. 2001;28:213-214.

82. Pietrangelo A, Montosi G, Totaro A, et al. Hereditary hemochromatosis in adults without pathogenic mutations in the hemochromatosis gene. *N Engl J Med*. 1999;341:725-732.

83. Pietrangelo A. Ferroportin disease: pathogenesis, diagnosis and treatment. *Haematologica*. 2017;102:1972-1984.

84. Girelli D, De Domenico I, Bozzini C, et al. Clinical, pathological, and molecular correlates in ferroportin disease: a study of two novel mutations. *J Hepatol*. 2008;49:664-671.

85. Lopriore E, Mearin ML, Oepkes D, Devlieger R, Whitington PF. Neonatal hemochromatosis: management, outcome, and prevention. *Prenat Diagn*. 2013;33:1221-1225.

86. Smyk DS, Mytilinaiou MG, Grammatikopoulos T, et al. Primary biliary cirrhosis-specific antimitochondrial antibodies in neonatal haemochromatosis. *Clin Dev Immunol*. 2013;2013:642643.

87. Whitington PF. Neonatal hemochromatosis: a congenital alloimmune hepatitis. *Semin Liver Dis*. 2007;27:243-250.

88. Collardeau-Frachon S, Heissat S, Bouvier R, et al. French retrospective multicentric study of neonatal hemochromatosis: importance of autopsy and autoimmune maternal manifestations. *Pediatr Dev Pathol*. 2012;15:450-470.

89. Smith SR, Shneider BL, Magid M, Martin G, Rothschild M. Minor salivary gland biopsy in neonatal hemochromatosis. *Arch Otolaryngol Head Neck Surg*. 2004;130:760-763.

90. Pronicka E, Weglewska-Jurkiewicz A, Taybert J, et al. Post mortem identification of deoxyguanosine kinase (DGUOK) gene mutations combined with impaired glucose homeostasis and iron overload features in four infants with severe progressive liver failure. *J Appl Genet*. 2011;52:61-66.

91. Fellman V. The GRACILE syndrome, a neonatal lethal metabolic disorder with iron overload. *Blood Cell Mol Dis*. 2002;29:444-450.

92. Visapaa I, Fellman V, Vesa J, et al. GRACILE syndrome, a lethal metabolic disorder with iron overload, is caused by a point mutation in BCS1L. *Am J Hum Genet*. 2002;71:863-876.

93. Gordeuk VR, McLaren CE, MacPhail AP, Deichsel G, Bothwell TH. Associations of iron overload in Africa with hepatocellular carcinoma and tuberculosis: Strachan's 1929 thesis revisited. *Blood*. 1996;87:3470-3476.

94. Walker AR, Arvidsson UB. Iron overload in the South African Bantu. *Trans R Soc Trop Med Hyg*. 1953;47:536-548.

95. Bothwell TH, Bradlow BA. Siderosis in the Bantu. A combined histopathological and chemical study. *Arch Pathol*. 1960;70:279-292.

96. Moyo VM, Gangaidzo IT, Gomo ZA, et al. Traditional beer consumption and the iron status of spouse pairs from a rural community in Zimbabwe. *Blood*. 1997;89:2159-2166.

97. Majore S, Ricerca BM, Radio FC, et al. Type 3 hereditary hemochromatosis in a patient from sub-Saharan Africa: is there a link between African iron overload and TFR2 dysfunction? *Blood Cell Mol Dis*. 2013;50:31-32.

98. McAdams AJ, Hug G, Bove KE. Glycogen storage disease, types I to X: criteria for morphologic diagnosis. *Hum Pathol*. 1974;5:463-487.

99. Jevon GP, Finegold MJ. Reliability of histological criteria in glycogen storage disease of the liver. *Pediatr Pathol*. 1994;14:709-721.

100. Gogus S, Kocak N, Ciliv G, et al. Histologic features of the liver in type Ia glycogen storage disease: comparative study between different age groups and consecutive biopsies. *Pediatr Dev Pathol*. 2002;5:299-304.

101. Yamaguchi T, Ihara K, Matsumoto T, et al. Inflammatory bowel disease-like colitis in glycogen storage disease type 1b. *Inflamm Bowel Dis*. 2001;7:128-132.

102. Couper R, Kapelushnik J, Griffiths AM. Neutrophil dysfunction in glycogen storage disease Ib: association with Crohn's-like colitis. *Gastroenterology*. 1991;100:549-554.

103. Miles L, Heubi JE, Bove KE. Hepatocyte glycogen accumulation in patients undergoing dietary management of urea cycle defects mimics storage disease. *J Pediatr Gastroenterol Nutr*. 2005;40:471-476.

104. Badizadegan K, Perez-Atayde AR. Focal glycogenosis of the liver in disorders of ureagenesis: its occurrence and diagnostic significance. *Hepatology*. 1997;26:365-373.

105. Yaplito-Lee J, Chow CW, Boneh A. Histopathological findings in livers of patients with urea cycle disorders. *Mol Genet Metab*. 2013;108:161-165.

106. Yamaguchi M, Kataoka TR, Shibayama T, et al. Loss of Hep Par 1 immunoreactivity in the livers of patients with carbamoyl phosphate synthetase 1 deficiency. *Pathol Int*. 2016;66:333-336.

107. Bernstein DL, Hulkova H, Bialer MG, Desnick RJ. Cholesteryl ester storage disease: review of the findings in 135 reported patients with an underdiagnosed disease. *J Hepatol*. 2013;58:1230-1243.

108. McManus DT, Moore R, Hill CM, Rodgers C, Carson DJ, Love AH. Necropsy findings in lysinuric protein intolerance. *J Clin Pathol*. 1996;49:345-357.

109. Seda Neto J, Leite KM, Porta A, et al. HCC prevalence and histopathological findings in liver explants of patients with hereditary tyrosinemia type 1. *Pediatr Blood Cancer*. 2014;61:1584-1589.

110. Haqq AM, Muehlbauer MJ, Newgard CB, Grambow S, Freemark M. The metabolic phenotype of Prader-Willi syndrome (PWS) in childhood: heightened insulin sensitivity relative to body mass index. *J Clin Endocrinol Metab*. 2011;96:E225-E232.

111. Brambilla P, Crino A, Bedogni G, et al. Metabolic syndrome in children with Prader-Willi syndrome: the effect of obesity. *Nutr Metab Cardiovasc Dis*. 2011;21:269-276.

112. Hashizume K, Nakajo T, Kawarasaki H, et al. Prader-Willi syndrome with del(15)(q11,q13) associated with hepatoblastoma. *Acta Paediatr Jpn*. 1991;33:718-722.

113. Takayasu H, Motoi T, Kanamori Y, et al. Two case reports of childhood liver cell adenomas harboring beta-catenin abnormalities. *Hum Pathol*. 2002;33:852-855.

114. Rademakers LH, Cleton MI, Kooijman C, Baart de la Faille H, van Hattum J. Early involvement of hepatic parenchymal cells in erythrohepatic protoporphyria? An ultrastructural study of patients with and without overt liver disease and the effect of chenodeoxycholic acid treatment. *Hepatology*. 1990;11:449-457.

115. MacDonald DM, Germain D, Perrot H. The histopathology and ultrastructure of liver disease in erythropoietic protoporphyria. *Br J Dermatol*. 1981;104:7-17.

116. Oztas E, Ozin Y, Onder F, Onal IK, Oguz D, Kocaefe C. Chronic intestinal pseudo-obstruction and neurological manifestations in early adulthood: considering MNGIE syndrome in differential diagnosis. *J Gastrointestin Liver Dis*. 2010;19:195-197.

117. Cloots K, Verbeek J, Orlent H, Meersseman W, Cassiman D. Mitochondrial hepatopathy in adults: a case series and review of the literature. *Eur J Gastroenterol Hepatol*. 2013;25:892-898.

118. Teraoka M, Yokoyama Y, Ichimura K, Mori R, Seino Y. Fatal neonatal mitochondrial cytopathy with disseminated fatty nodules in the liver. *Pediatr Int*. 2003;45:570-573.

119. Mandel H, Hartman C, Berkowitz D, Elpeleg ON, Manov I, Iancu TC. The hepatic mitochondrial DNA depletion syndrome: ultrastructural changes in liver biopsies. *Hepatology*. 2001;34:776-784.

120. Al-Hussaini A, Faqeih E, El-Hattab AW, et al. Clinical and molecular characteristics of mitochondrial DNA depletion syndrome associated with neonatal cholestasis and liver failure. *J Pediatr*. 2014;164:553-559.e1-e2.

121. Scheers I, Bachy V, Stephenne X, Sokal EM. Risk of hepatocellular carcinoma in liver mitochondrial respiratory chain disorders. *J Pediatr*. 2005;146:414-417.

122. Bioulac-Sage P, Parrot-Roulaud F, Mazat JP, et al. Fatal neonatal liver failure and mitochondrial cytopathy (oxidative phosphorylation deficiency): a light and electron microscopic study of the liver. *Hepatology*. 1993;18:839-846.

123. Alder JK, Chen JJ, Lancaster L, et al. Short telomeres are a risk factor for idiopathic pulmonary fibrosis. *Proc Natl Acad Sci USA*. 2008;105:13051-13056.

124. Jonassaint NL, Guo N, Califano JA, Montgomery EA, Armanios M. The gastrointestinal manifestations of telomere-mediated disease. *Aging Cell*. 2013;12:319-323.

125. Speckmann C, Sahoo SS, Rizzi M, et al. Clinical and molecular heterogeneity of RTEL1 deficiency. *Front Immunol*. 2017;8:449.

PEDIATRIC BENIGN AND MALIGNANT TUMORS 13

CHAPTER OUTLINE

HEPATOBLASTOMA

CHECKLIST: Hepatoblastoma

- ☐ Young age, most cases in children less than 2 years of age
- ☐ Markedly elevated serum alpha-fetoprotein (AFP) levels
- ☐ Tumors show hepatic differentiation that recapitulates normal hepatic development
  - ○ Small cell undifferentiated (hepatic differentiation evident only on immunostains)
  - ○ Embryonal
  - ○ Fetal
- ☐ About 40% of cases also have a mesenchymal component
  - ○ Mostly composed of undifferentiated spindled cells

Hepatoblastomas are malignant hepatic tumors. They show a wide range of hepatocellular differentiation. Most cases are composed of tumor cells with definite hepatic differentiation in at least some areas, while rare tumors are composed of undifferentiated cells where hepatic differentiation is evident only on immunostains. About 40% of hepatoblastomas will also have a mesenchymal component.

Clinically, hepatoblastomas generally present with an abdominal mass, failure to thrive, jaundice, or gastrointestinal (GI) symptoms such as vomiting or diarrhea. Up to 20% of individuals with hepatoblastomas will have metastatic disease at the time of presentation, most commonly involving the lungs.[1,2] The male to female ratio is about 2:1 with an average age at presentation of about 18 months. About 2/3 of cases present before the age of 2 years and greater than 90% of all cases present before the age of 5 years.[3] Rare cases are identified in utero.[4] Hepatoblastomas can occur in children past the age of 5 years, but they are exceptionally rare, and conventional hepatocellular carcinoma should be carefully excluded. Cases past the age of 12 years are essentially nonexistent. Hepatoblastomas have been reported in adults,[5] but many reported cases are not very convincing and seem likely to have a better diagnosis.

Serum AFP levels are markedly elevated in almost all cases of hepatoblastoma. One exception is a rare variant of hepatoblastoma that is composed of very primitive cells, called the small cell undifferentiated variant, where AFP can be normal or only mildly elevated. Elevated serum AFP levels are not specific for hepatoblastoma, also being increased in mesenchymal hamartomas[6] and conventional hepatocellular carcinomas. However, the serum AFP results are helpful diagnostically in some cases, as tumors that show definite hepatic differentiation on H&E, but do not have elevated serum AFP, are not hepatoblastomas.

Low birth weight is the best documented risk factor for hepatoblastoma, especially with birth weights less than 1500 g.[7] Hepatoblastomas can arise in the setting of a number of inherited diseases and/or other congenital anomalies. The most common inherited diseases associated with hepatoblastaomas are familial adenomatous polyposis[8] and the Beckwith–Wiedemann syndrome.[9] In terms of other congenital abnormalities, the most common are structural abnormalities of the kidney and bladder.[10]

Resected specimens are processed in essentially the same way as conventional hepatocellular carcinomas. Histological sampling for hepatoblastomas is similar to that for hepatocellular carcinomas, with current guidelines calling for at least one section per cm of tumor diameter.[11] Many cases will have tumor and nontumor tissues snap frozen as part of research protocols. The background livers are noncirrhotic but can show various nonspecific mass effect changes in those sections obtained from immediately adjacent to the tumor. If the tumor has been treated before surgery, then the percent necrosis should be estimated to the nearest 10%.

The prognosis for hepatoblastoma has dramatically improved over the past several decades, with five-year-survival rates improving from 30% to 90%.[12–17] A number of pathology findings are relevant to prognosis. Multifocal hepatoblastomas have a worse prognosis[14,18] as do cases with small cell undifferentiated morphology. The subtype with the best prognosis is a pure fetal hepatoblastoma with low mitotic activity.

HISTOLOGICAL TYPES

CHECKLIST: Hepatoblastoma, Pure Epithelial Subtypes

1. Small cell undifferentiated
   a. Normal or mildly elevated serum AFP (<100)
   b. Small undifferentiated tumor cells
   c. Perform INI-1 to rule out INI-1 loss tumors
2. Embryonal
3. Pure fetal with low mitotic activity
4. Fetal with mitotic activity
5. Fetal, pleomorphic
6. Macrotrabecular
7. Cholangioblastic

Mesenchymal components will also be present in about 40% of cases, but an epithelial component is required for the diagnosis of hepatoblastoma. Epithelial hepatoblastomas are further classified into 7 different subtypes to help guide therapy. The most common subtypes are the embryonal and fetal patterns. Overall, at least some component of the fetal pattern is seen in about 80% of cases and some component of embryonal in 30% of cases. Each of the rest of the patterns is seen in 5% or less of cases. In terms of clinical care, the most important patterns are the pure fetal pattern with low mitotic activity (because resection alone can be curative) and the small cell undifferentiated pattern (more aggressive chemotherapy is often used).

Also of note, any given case often has multiple different epithelial patterns. However, hepatoblastomas that do show single patterns (about 20% of cases) usually show one of the fetal variants.[19,20] Cases with mixed epithelial patterns are diagnosed as such, for example: mixed fetal and embryonal hepatoblastoma. The pure fetal pattern, as indicated by the name, requires a pure fetal pattern of epithelium.

Small Cell Undifferentiated (Table 13.1)

The tumor cell in the small cell undifferentiated pattern are small (5 to 10 microns) with scant, pale to amphophilic cytoplasm and grow in discohesive nests and sheets (Fig. 13.1). They do not have well-defined acini, psuedoglands, or trabeculae and can sometimes mimic blastemal mesenchymal cells. In most cases, the small cell undifferentiated pattern is a minor component of the total hepatoblastoma, usually less than 10%,[21,22] but any degree of small cell undifferentiated growth should be mentioned in the report. In rare cases, the tumor is made up mostly or exclusively of small cell undifferentiated tumor cells. In these cases in particular, an INI-1 stain should be performed to rule out INI-1 loss.[23] The potential role for other stains in that pathway, such as BRG1, remains unclear.

If there is INI-1 loss, then the tumor has a worse prognosis and a traditional rhabdoid tumor should be carefully excluded. In some cases of rhabdoid tumors, the INI-1 loss can be germline, so testing for germline mutations in the SMARCB1/INI1 gene in the rest of the family is important. In the small cell undifferentiated pattern of hepatoblastoma, immunostains for hepar-1[24] and arginase are negative but glypican 3 is positive,[25] although it can be focal. Beta-catenin is usually negative, or only very focally positive, for abnormal beta-catenin nuclear or cytoplasmic staining. The normal staining for beta-catenin, seen in the background liver, is membranous.

Embryonal Pattern (Table 13.1)

In the embryonal pattern, the tumor cells have angulated nuclei with high N:C ratios and basophilic cytoplasm (Fig. 13.2). At low power, the cytology can look even more primitive and basophilic than the small cell undifferentiated pattern, but this pattern is more clearly epithelial, with tumor cells growing in solid sheets, often with pseudoglands or tumor rosettes (Fig. 13.3). This pattern is almost never pure, at least in resection specimens, being admixed in most cases with the fetal growth pattern. Immunostains are positive for Hepar-1, arginase, and glypican 3.[25] Beta-catenin shows abnormal nuclear and or cytoplasmic staining (Fig. 13.4).

TABLE 13.1: Most Common Epithelial Cell Types in Hepatoblastomas

Feature	Small Cell Undifferentiated	Embryonal	Fetal
Cell size	Small cells (5 to 10 microns)	Medium-sized cells (10 to 15 microns)	Larger cells (10 to 20 microns in size)
Cytoplasm	Scant, pale to amphophilic	Basophilic, high N:C ratio	Moderate amounts of eosinophilic to clear cytoplasm
Nucleus	Fine chromatin Inconspicuous nucleoli	Angulated Small nucleoli	Clumpy chromatin Variably prominent nucleoli
Architecture	• Often discohesive • Solid or nested growth pattern • Never show well-defined trabeculae, acini, or psuedoglands	• Solid growth pattern • Pseudoglands	• Solid growth pattern • Trabecular growth pattern • Alternating "light and dark"
Immustains	• Glypican 3 positive • HepPar negative	• Glypican 3 positive • HepPar positive	• Glypican 3 positive • HepPar positive

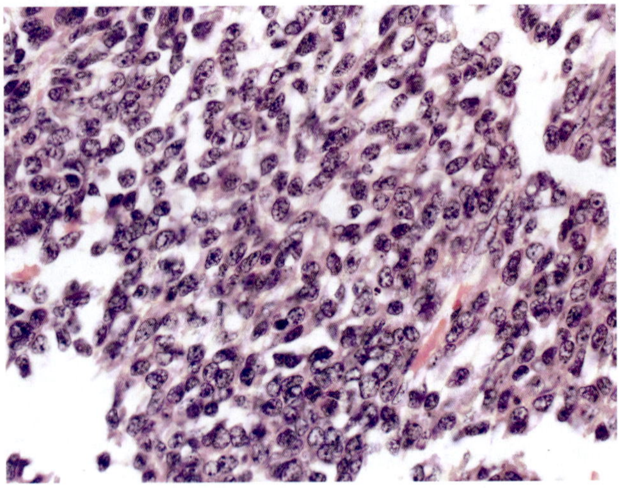

Figure 13.1. **Hepatoblastoma, small cell undifferentiated pattern.** The tumor cells are small, undifferentiated, and growing in discohesive sheets.

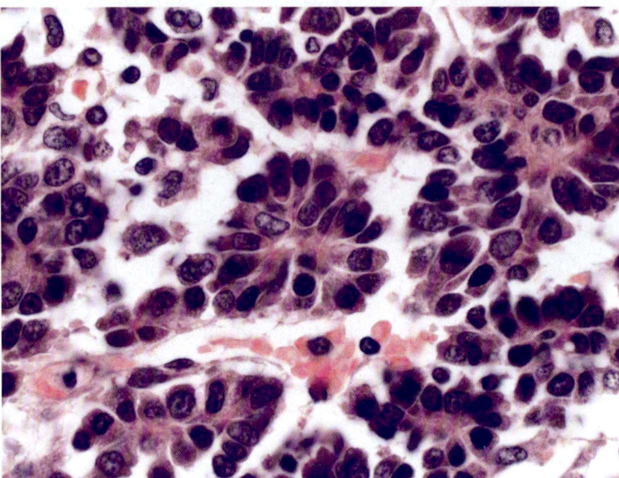

Figure 13.2. **Hepatoblastoma, embryonal pattern.** The cells have angulated nuclei with high N:C ratios and basophilic cytoplasm.

Fetal Pattern (Table 13.1)

In this pattern, the tumor cells are recognizable on H&E as showing hepatic differentiation. They are larger than embryonal pattern tumor cells, with moderate amounts of cytoplasm. The cytoplasm can be clear in areas of glycogen accumulation (Fig. 13.5). Sometimes, irregular patches of glycogen accumulation can lead to alternating areas of "light and dark" tumor cells at low power (Fig. 13.6). The tumor cells grow have a solid or trabeculae architecture. There can be cholestasis (Fig. 13.7).

The fetal growth pattern is the most common growth pattern in hepatoblastomas and is further subdivided based on mitotic counts and on cytological atypia. Tumors that show only the fetal growth pattern and have 1 or fewer mitotic figures in 10 high-power fields are called *pure fetal hepatoblastoma with low mitotic activity*. These tumors have an excellent prognosis, and complete resection alone is curative in most cases. If the tumor shows a pure fetal

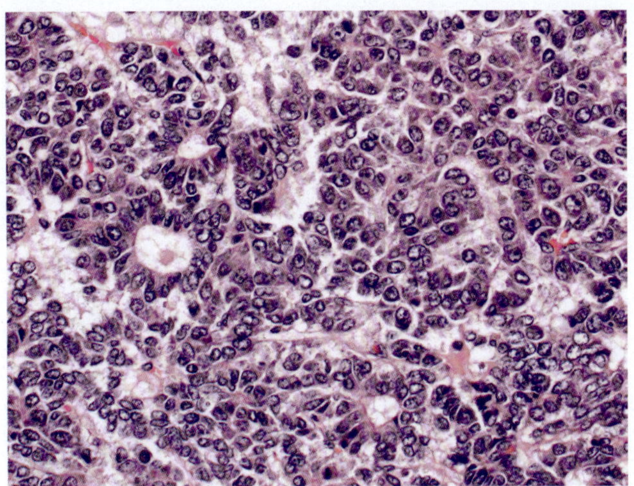

Figure 13.3. **Hepatoblastoma, embryonal pattern.** At low power, pseudoglands or tumor rosettes can be appreciated.

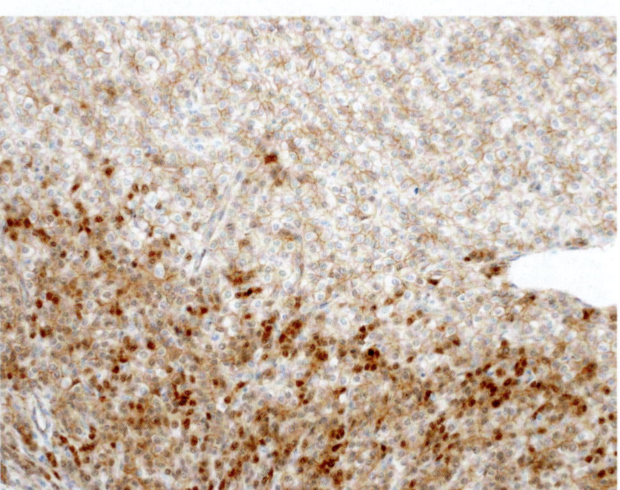

Figure 13.4. **Hepatoblastoma, embryonal and fetal patterns, beta-catenin.** Beta-catenin shows abnormal nuclear accumulation in the embryonal pattern (lower part of image) but not the fetal pattern (upper part of image). The fetal pattern shows membranous staining.

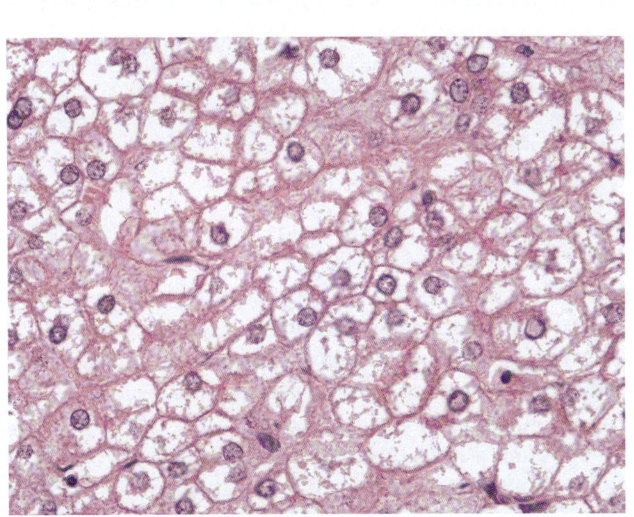

Figure 13.5. **Hepatoblastoma, fetal pattern.** The tumor cytoplasm is clear because of glycogen accumulation.

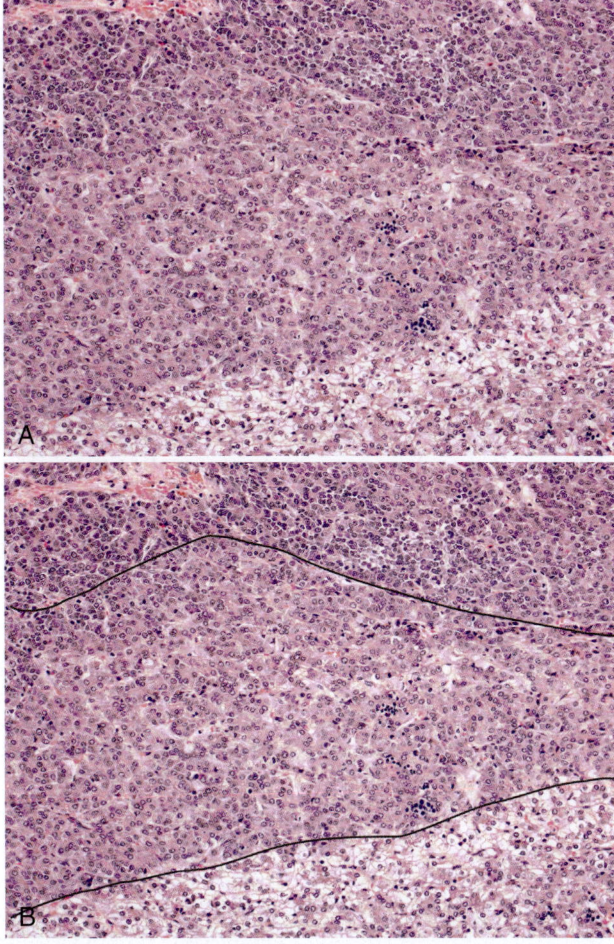

Figure 13.6. **Hepatoblastoma, fetal pattern.** A, At low power, the fetal pattern is seen composed of alternating areas of "light and dark" tumor cells. At the very top, a component of fetal pattern is also present. B, Thin lines have been added to separate the different components.

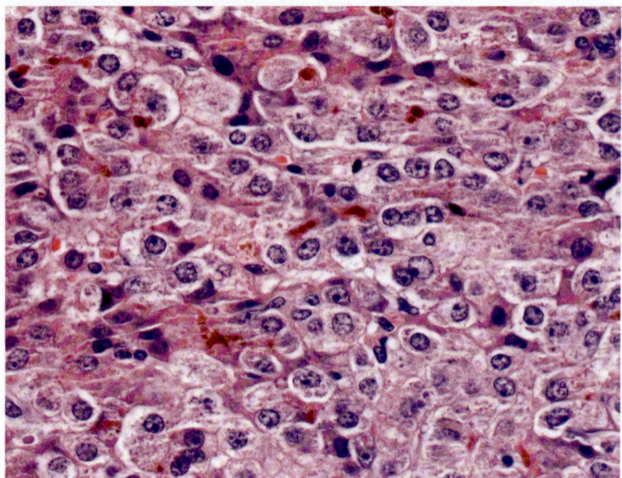

Figure 13.7. **Hepatoblastoma, fetal pattern.** The tumor cells show cholestasis.

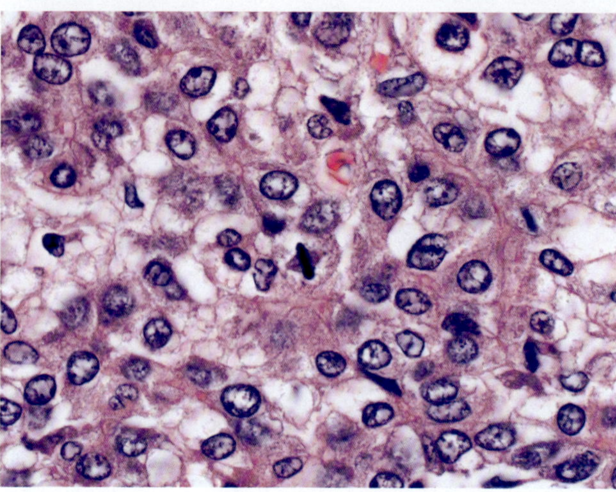

Figure 13.8. **Hepatoblastoma, mitotically active fetal pattern.** This hepatoblastoma was of the pure fetal type and showed 4 mitoses in 10 high-power fields.

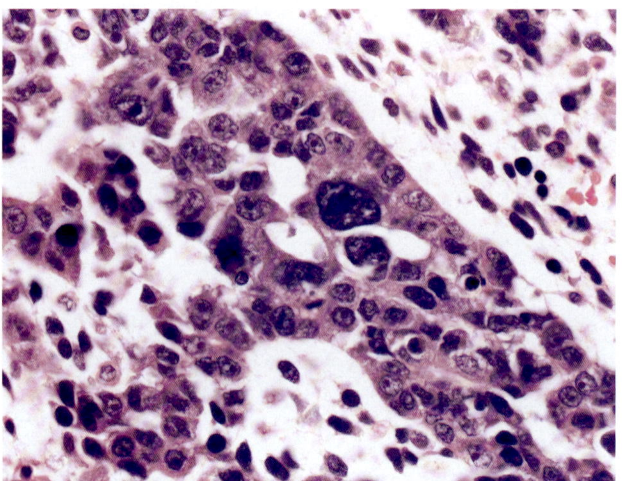

Figure 13.9. **Hepatoblastoma, pleomorphic fetal pattern.** This hepatoblastoma showed a mixed epithelial and mesenchymal pattern. The epithelial component was mostly fetal with a small amount of the embryonal pattern. The fetal pattern had focal areas of more significant nuclear pleomorphism.

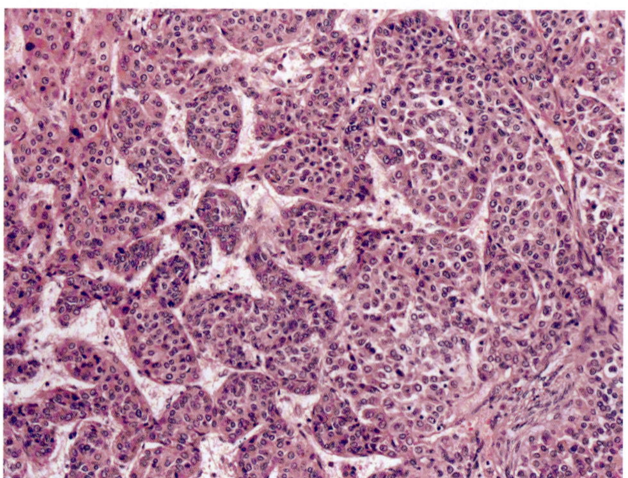

Figure 13.10. **Hepatoblastoma, macrotrabecular fetal pattern.** The tumor cells in this image show a fetal morphology but are organized into thick trabecula. This pattern was multifocal in a hepatoblastoma that showed mostly a typical fetal pattern, admixed with embryonal areas.

growth pattern but has 2 or more mitoses in 10 high-power fields (40X), then it is classified as a *mitotically active fetal hepatoblastoma* (Fig. 13.8). If the hepatoblastoma shows a fetal growth pattern with more cytological atypia (Fig. 13.9), then the pattern is called a *pleomorphic fetal hepatoblastoma*. This pattern is rare, and in many ways, the cytology is reminiscent of a conventional hepatocellular carcinoma. Hepatoblastomas with the pleomorphic fetal pattern generally contain areas with other hepatoblastoma patterns, such as embryonal, which help differentiate these cases from conventional hepatocellular carcinoma.

In all of the fetal patterns, immunostains are positive for Hepar-1, arginase, and glypican 3. Beta-catenin commonly shows a membranous staining pattern, with rare nuclear and/or cytoplasmic staining seen in most cases.

Macrotrabecular Pattern

This pattern shows fetal-type cells, but they are organized into thick macrotrabecula (Fig. 13.10), which should be at least 10 cells thick but commonly are more than 20 cells thick. Although not necessary for diagnosis, an immunostain for CD34 highlights the thick trabeculae. The immunostain profile for markers of hepatic differentiation has not been well described in the literature, but cases are positive for Hepar-1 and, in most cases, glypican 3. Beta-catenin usually shows a membranous staining pattern. In most cases, the macrotrabecular growth pattern is a minor component of the hepatoblastoma.

A very similar growth pattern can be seen in a small subset of conventional hepatocellular carcinomas. AFP levels are elevated in both entities, so other findings are used to distinguish these two types of tumor. The most useful finding is other patterns of typical hepatoblastoma growth (indicates the tumor is a hepatoblastoma) or other areas of conventional hepatocellular carcinoma growth (which would argue against a hepatoblastoma). A tumor that shows a pure macrotrabecular growth pattern is more likely to be a conventional hepatocellular carcinoma than a hepatoblastoma. Correlation with clinical findings such as age and underling liver disease is also important.

Cholangiocellular Pattern

The cholangiocellular pattern is very rare and usually a focal finding. This pattern can be somewhat more common if the tumor was previously treated. The cholangiocellular pattern shows small, hyperchromatic cells that form ductlike structures, usually embedded in a mesenchymal component. The histological differential can sometimes include a benign ductular proliferation, but the cholangiocellular pattern shows significant cytological atypia, can have mitotic activity, lacks the organization found in many ductular reactions, and is not limited to the tumor–nontumor interface, as would be the case for a benign ductular reaction. Beta-catenin can sometimes be helpful if there is nuclear accumulation, which would indicate the cells are malignant.

Mesenchymal Component

A mesenchymal component is present in about 40% of fully resected hepatoblastomas. The mesenchymal component is composed of nondescript spindle cells that can vary in their cellularity from loose and myxoid to more dense and cellular (Fig. 13.11). Rare cases have other elements including skeletal muscle, cartilage, or osteoid material (Fig. 13.12). Of these, osteoid is the most common. If the tumor shows other elements of mesenchymal or epithelial differentiation, then it is called a *teratoid hepatoblasoma*. These cases can show primitive neural cells, glial cells, melanin-containing cells, neuroendocrine differentiation, gland formation, or mucinous or squamous differentiation (Fig. 13.13).

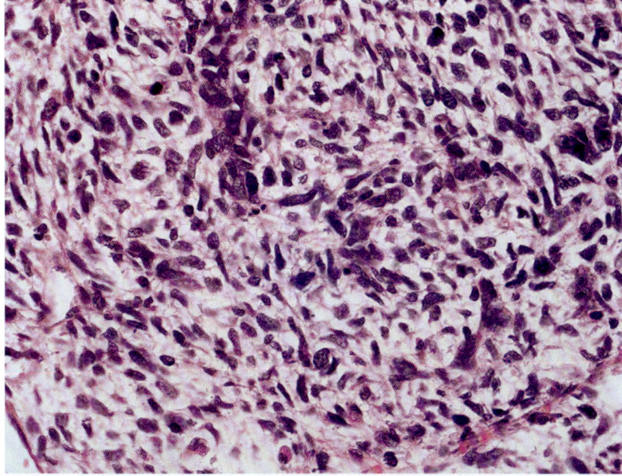

Figure 13.11. **Hepatoblastoma, mesenchymal component.** The mesenchymal component in this case is composed of rather nondescript but fairly cellular spindle cells.

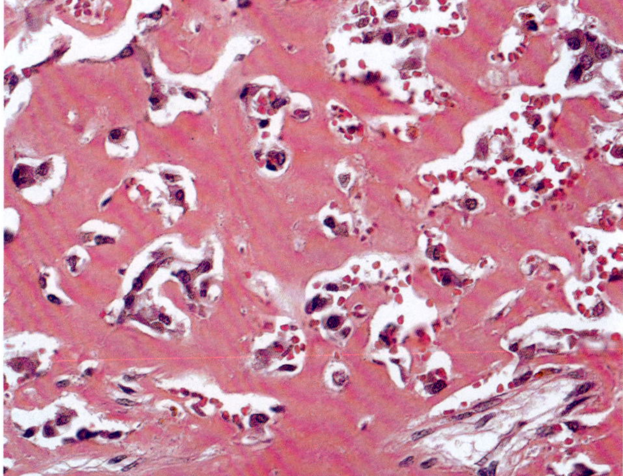

Figure 13.12. **Hepatoblastoma, osteoid component.** This case has a lot of osteoid material in the mesenchymal component.

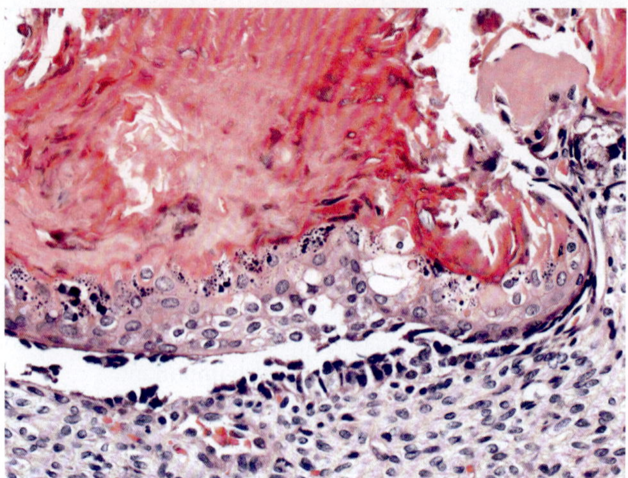

Figure 13.13. **Hepatoblastoma, teratoid features.** Focal squamous differentiation was present in this hepatoblastoma.

HEPATOBLASTOMA STAGING

There are several different methods used for staging hepatoblastomas, with usage depending largely on the country. In the United States, the Children's Oncology Group (COG) staging system is commonly used for pathology findings (Table 13.2). In addition, a more comprehensive risk assessment approach is commonly used to help guide clinical management (Table 13.3). In contrast, in most of Europe, hepatoblastomas are staged using a system called the pretreatment extent of disease (PRETEXT), which is based on imaging. Information from both systems can be combined to provide risk assessment.

The PRETEXT system divides the liver into four segments, and the stage of the hepatoblastoma is determined by the number of segments involved by tumor (Fig. 13.14). In this system, high-risk hepatoblastomas are defined by any of these findings: PRETEXT IV, serum AFP levels <100 IU/mL at diagnosis, metastatic disease at diagnosis, or small cell undifferentiated histology. In contrast, hepatoblastomas that have AFP levels >100, do not have metastatic disease, have no small cell undifferentiated histology, and are PRETEXT stages I, II, or III are considered to have standard-risk disease.

The PRETEXT staging system further annotates the stage with additional potentially important findings:

- (V). A case is scored as V positive or V negative depending on whether there is tumor involving the inferior vena cava or hepatic veins. This finding, when present, is further scored on a scale of 1 to 3 as follows: V1 = tumor touching the vein; V2 = tumor compressing the vein or distorting; and V3 = tumor ingrowth, encasement, or thrombus of the vein.
- (P). A case is scored as P positive or P negative depending on whether there is tumor involving the main portal vein or if there is tumor involving both the right and left branches of the portal vein (both branches are needed). This finding, when present, is further scored on a scale of 1 to 3 as follows: P1 = tumor touching the vein; P2 = tumor compressing the vein or distorting; and P3 = tumor ingrowth, encasement, or thrombus of the vein.
- (E). A case is scored as E positive or E negative depending on whether there is extrahepatic disease by direct extension into another organ. This finding, when present, is further scored on a scale of 1 to 3 as follows: E1 = direct extension into adjacent organs or into the diaphragm; E2 = peritoneal nodules; and E3 = peritoneal nodules with ascites.
- (C). A case is scored as positive if disease involves the caudate lobe (C+).

- (N). A case is scored as N positive if there is nodal disease. This finding, when present, is further scored on a scale of 1 to 2 as follows: N1 = abdominal lymph node disease only and N2 = extra-abdominal lymph node disease.
- (M). A case is scored as M positive if there is metastatic disease.

HEPATOBLASTOMA VERSUS HEPATOCELLULAR CARCINOMA

In most cases, a tumor is readily classified as hepatoblastoma versus conventional hepatocellular carcinoma, but rare cases can be challenging to classify when they show pure fetal type epithelium, as the fetal epithelium can be fairly well differentiated and resemble tumor cells of conventional hepatocellular carcinoma. This is particularly a challenge if the patient is 5 or more years old.

Overall, immunostain findings do not help much, and the distinction is made on clinical, serological, and histological grounds. Clinical and serological findings that would support a diagnosis of conventional hepatocellular carcinoma are the following: underlying chronic liver disease and serum AFP <100 in a case without small cell undifferentiated morphology. These histological findings would support a diagnosis of hepatoblastoma: a mesenchymal component or a distinct second population of embryonal cells. Do not over interpret "light and dark" areas in a tumor, as they can also be seen in typical conventional hepatocellular carcinoma.

TABLE 13.2: Children's Oncology Group (COG) Staging System

Stage	Description
I	The tumor is entirely resected with negative margins.
II	The tumor is grossly entirely resected, but there is microscopic tumor cells close at the margin.
III	There is grossly visible tumor that could not be resected.
IV	Metastatic disease is present.

TABLE 13.3: Current Children's Oncology Group (COG) Risk Category

Risk Category	Description
Very low risk	PRETEXT (pretreatment extent of disease) stage I or II with pure fetal histology and successful primary resection
Low risk	PRETEXT stage I or II with no small cell undifferentiated histology and successful primary resection
Intermediate risk	PRETEXT stage II, III, or IV that is unresectable at presentation or has any of the following: small cell undifferentiated histology, V+, P+, E+
High risk	Any PRETEXT that is M+ and/or AFP (alpha-fetoprotein) <100 ng/mL at diagnosis

Data from http://www.cancer.gov/types/liver/hp/child-liver-treatment-pdq#link/_740_toc. Accessed 1, 2018.

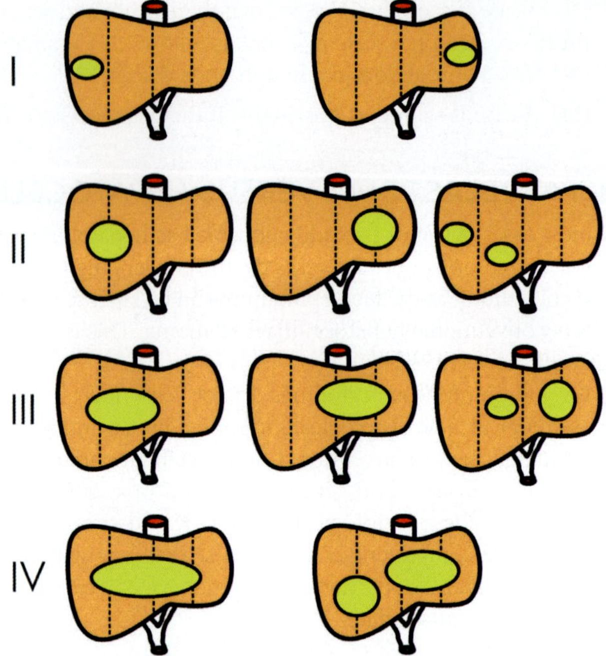

Figure 13.14. **PRETEXT (pretreatment extent of disease) staging system.** In this approach, the liver is divided into four sections based on imaging, with the boundaries being the right and middle hepatic veins and the umbilical fissure. Stage I tumors are defined by 3 contiguous sections of the liver that are uninvolved by hepatoblastoma. Stage II tumors are defined by 2 contiguous sections of the liver that are uninvolved by hepatoblastoma. Stage III tumors are defined by 1 section that is free of disease. In stage IV, there are no sections that are free of disease. When hepatoblastomas are multifocal, then additional combinations are possible for stages II and III (not all possible combinations are illustrated). This system is also applied after therapy and is then called the POST-TEXT.

CALCIFYING NESTED STROMAL–EPITHELIAL TUMOR

CHECKLIST: Calcifying Nested Stromal–Epithelial Tumors

- □ Rare
- □ Most but not all cases behave in an indolent manner
- □ 20% present with Cushing syndrome
- □ Histology
  - ○ Nests of spindled to epithelioid keratin-positive tumor cells that are surrounded by a desmoplastic response
  - ○ No hepatic differentiation
  - ○ Can stain with a wide variety of different markers, which can lead to diagnostic confusion

Calcifying nested stromal–epithelial tumors are very rare primary tumors of the liver. They show both epithelial and stromal elements, so in times past were often classified as hepatoblastomas, but it is now clear that they are not hepatoblastomas, as the epithelial elements do not show hepatic differentiation and the stromal elements are not neoplastic. The tumor was first described in the 2001 edition of the Armed Forces Institute of Pathology (AFIP) fascicle, using the term "ossifying stromal–epithelial tumor."[26]

To date, all calcifying nested stromal–epithelial tumors have been reported in children and young adults, with an age range of 2 to 33 years.[27] There is a female predominance.

Most cases are identified as incidental tumors,[28] but some patients have clinical symptoms. The most common clinical finding is Cushing syndrome, which is present in 10% to 20% of reported cases and can resolve once the tumor is resected.[27–32] Several cases have been reported in the setting of Beckwith–Wiedemann syndrome.[33,34] Patients, especially those with the Cushing syndrome, can have elevated serum adrenocorticotropic (ACTH) levels, but serum AFP levels are normal and there are no serum tumor markers helpful for diagnosis. Most patients have a favorable clinical course, but tumors can recur, can metastasize (usually to lymph nodes and lungs), and can lead to patient death.[30,35–37]

Calcified nested stromal–epithelial tumors are mostly unifocal, but rarely can be multifocal. Some cases are composed of an aggregate of separate but adjacent nodules. Histologically, calcified nested stromal–epithelial tumors show rounded to irregular nests of epithelial cells surrounded by bands of desmoplastic stroma (Figs. 13.15 and 13.16). The centers of the individual epithelial nests can show necrosis (Fig. 13.17), while the center of the entire tumor is often densely fibrotic and calcified (Fig. 13.18). Vascular invasion can be seen occasionally.

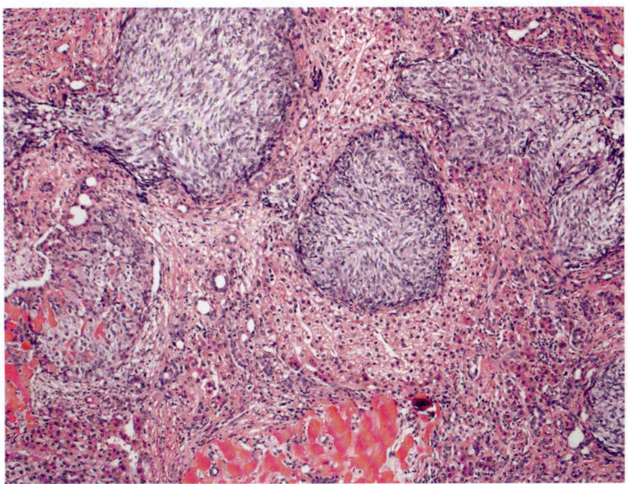

Figure 13.15. **Calcifying nested stromal–epithelial tumor.** At low power, the tumor cells are growing in discrete nests.

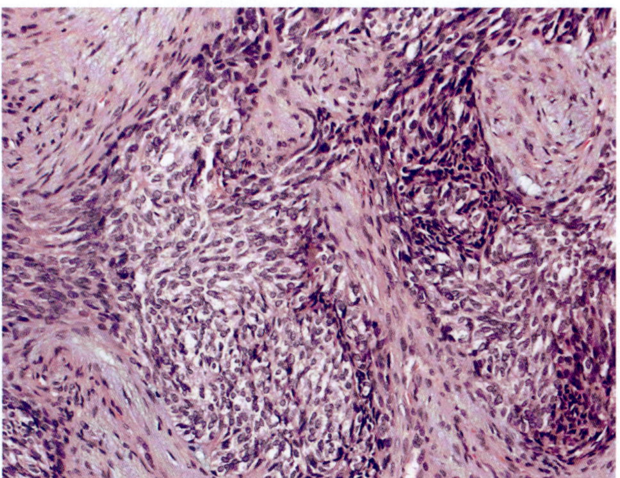

Figure 13.16. **Calcifying nested stromal–epithelial tumor.** The tumor cells are short, plump, and spindled. They show no recognizable line of differentiation.

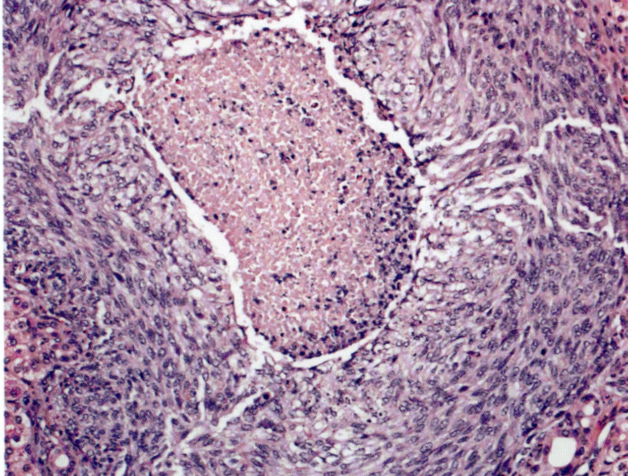

Figure 13.17. **Calcifying nested stromal–epithelial tumor.** The center of this tumor nest shows necrosis.

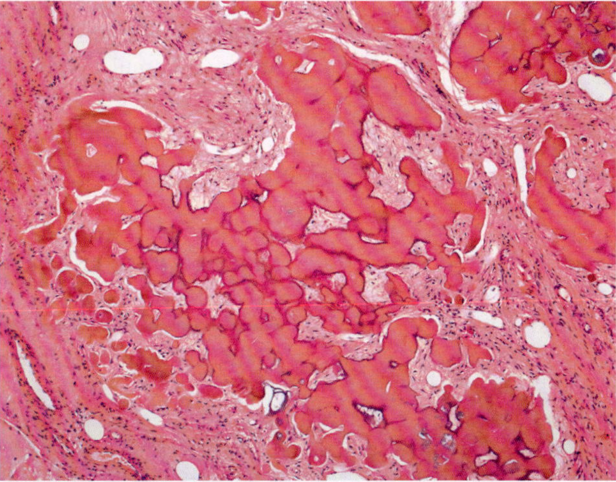

Figure 13.18. **Calcifying nested stromal–epithelial tumor.** The center of this tumor was essentially acellular, replaced by fibrosis and calcifications.

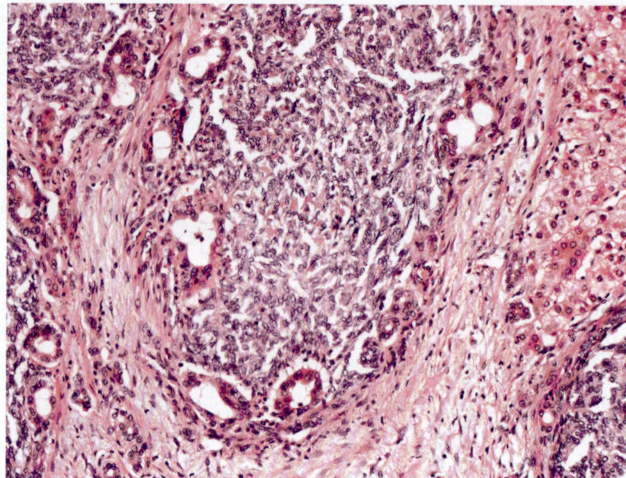

Figure 13.19. **Calcifying nested stromal–epithelial tumor.** The edges of many of the tumor nests show a ductular-like reaction.

The epithelial cells grow in broad sheets without trabecular or glandular growth patterns. Scattered nests can show calcifications and/or ossification. The edges of the tumor nests often have a bile ductular reaction (Fig. 13.19), which appears to be a reactive process and not neoplastic. The individual tumor cells show scant to moderate amounts of clear to amphophilic cytoplasm. The tumor cells can be epithelioid or short, stubby spindle cells. The nuclear chromatin is vesiculated, and nucleoli are inconspicuous. The mitotic activity usually ranges from 1 to 5 mitoses per 10 high-power fields. Rarely, tumors can show areas of dedifferentiation, where the tumor cells show more nuclear atypia, have an increased N:C ration, and often lose their nested growth pattern, instead growing as large irregular sheets and ribbons of tumor cells.

The epithelial cells are keratin positive, with cytokeratin AE1/3 and CAM5.2 positive in the vast majority of cases.[27,28,38,39] Other keratins such as CK7, CK8, and CK19 are positive in a variable number of cases, while CK20 is typically negative. Beta-catenin nuclear accumulation is found in all case,[33,40] while markers of hepatic differentiation are negative,[27,28,38,39] including polyclonal CEA, HepPar1, arginase, and albumin in situ hybridization. ACTH is positive in about a fourth of cases,[27,28] correlating with serum findings and clinical findings of Cushing syndrome. Interestingly, NSE, WT-1, and vimentin are also positive in nearly 100% of cases,[27,28,38] which can often lead to confusion, especially on small biopsies. CD56 is routinely positive, but there is no evidence of neuroenodocrine differentiation and chromogranin, and synaptophysin are consistently negative.[27,28,38,41]

Molecular studies on calcifying nested stromal–epithelial tumors show that they have consistent deletions in exon 3 of the beta-catenin gene, which explains the beta-catenin nuclear accumulation by immunohistochemistry.[40] There is no evidence for the EWS-WT1 fusion gene (found in desmoplastic small round cell tumors),[27,38,41] for the SYT-SSX fusion gene (found in synovial sarcomas),[38] for FGFR2 translocations (found in some cholangiocarcinomas), or for the DNAJB1-PRKACA fusion gene (found in fibrolamellar carcinoma).

INFANTILE HEMANGIOMA

CHECKLIST: Infantile Hemangioma

- ☐ 90% present before 6 months of age
- ☐ 90% of cases limited to liver
- ☐ Cytologically bland vascular tumor-forming medium-sized vessels in a fibrous background
- ☐ Most will involute on their own; others are treated by medication (such as propanol) or by embolization to induce involution
- ☐ Benign, but small risk of malignant transformation

Infantile hemangiomas are very rare tumors that were previously called *infantile hemangioendothelioma*. They can be either limited to the liver or part of a more diffuse hemangiomatosis that affects multiple organs, most commonly the skin, lungs, GI tract, and adrenal gland. About 90% of cases occur before 6 months of age, although rare cases have been reported in teenagers and young adults. The female to male ratio is about 2:1. Affected patients can have numerous congenital anomalies that vary considerably by organ, without any strong patterns.

The tumors are neoplastic, but they are benign, with only a very low risk of malignant degeneration. In general, the tumors tend to grow rapidly for a short time after birth but then slowly involute during childhood. However, a small percent of tumors can cause heart failure or liver failure when they affect most of the liver. Most that come to medical attention are large in size, usually greater than 5 cm. Most (about 60%) of infantile hemangiomas are single lesions, but larger lesions in particular can be multifocal. The current management approach for larger and symptomatic tumors is to use drug therapy such as propanol to enhance tumor involution, followed by arterial embolization, and/or resection if needed.

Histologically, infantile hemangiomas are vasoformative, with well-defined blood vessels in a fibrous background (Fig. 13.20). The tumor vessels are dilated, irregularly shaped and medium sized. The center of the lesion can have larger, rounded vessels that resemble a cavernous hemangioma. The center can also have areas of thrombosis, infarction, fibrosis, and calcification. The endothelial cells have no cytological atypia, but mitotic figures are common, with areas of >10 mitoses per 10 hpf. However, this does not impact diagnosis or prognosis, instead being a reflection of their rapid, but transient, postnatal growth. Those rare cases diagnosed in older children typically do not have a high proliferative rate.

At the tumor's interface with the background liver, there are areas of admixed tumor and normal liver. Entrapped bile ducts are particularly common at the periphery. In about 1/3 of cases, infantile hemangiomas show more extensive parenchymal infiltration at the margins, and entrapped hepatocytes often undergo a ductular transformation. Of note, the hepatocytes at the tumor interface can produce large amounts of AFP,[42,43] which can sometimes lead to clinical and pathological concern for a hepatic malignancy, but the AFP-producing hepatocytes appear to be reactive.

Infantile hemangiomas have a small but well-documented risk of malignant transformation. Areas of concern will show high-grade cytology and architectural atypia, such as papillary tufts, solid areas of growth (Fig. 13.21), or Kaposiform-like areas. In most cases, these foci are small and scattered, and patients are cured when the entire infantile hemangioma is completely resected. Overall, the presence or absence of atypia does not affect the clinical outcome in fully resected cases. Nonetheless, the very small subset of cases

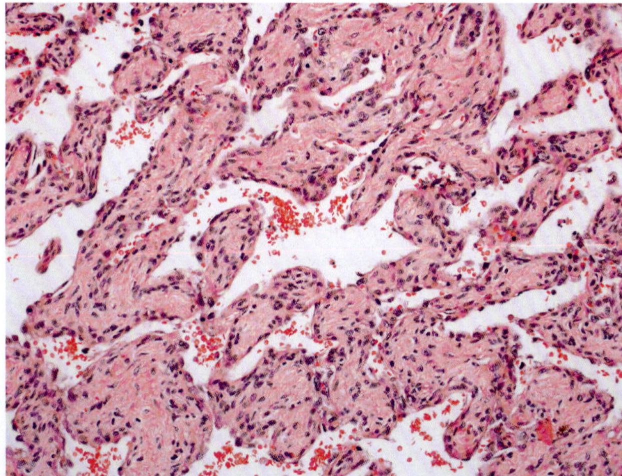

Figure 13.20. **Infantile hemangioma.** The tumor is composed of medium-sized vessels lined by cytologically bland tumor cells. The intervening stroma is collagenized.

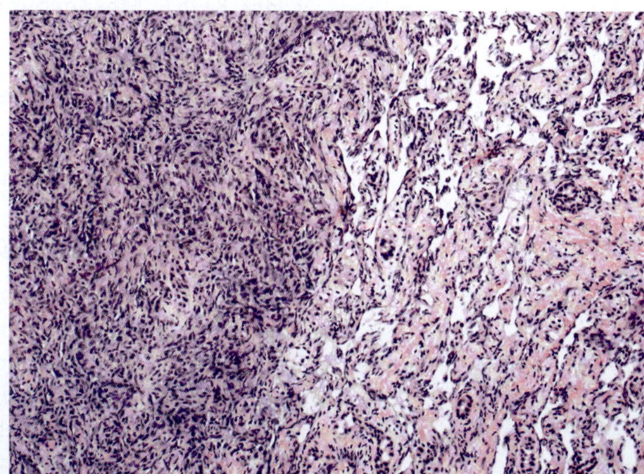

Figure 13.21. **Infantile hemangioma with angiosarcoma.** An angiosarcoma with a solid growth pattern (left half of image) developed in the center of this infantile hemangioma (right half of image).

that show aggressive behavior (tumor recurrence is more common than metastases) have histologically atypical areas. In particular, larger areas of atypia are concerning, especially if there is a grossly visible subnodule.

The diagnosis of infantile hemangioma is made on H&E, and immunostains are not necessary. Nonetheless, infantile hemangiomas stain with typical vascular markers such as ERG, FLI-1, CD31, and C34. The differential is primarily that of a vascular malformation (see also section below). Infantile hemangiomas are usually GLUT-1 positive, while vascular malformations are GLUT-1 negative.[44]

VASCULAR MALFORMATION

CHECKLIST: Vascular Malformation

- ☐ Rare cause of liver mass
- ☐ Vascular shunt leads to a central area of vascular proliferation, congestions, and fibrosis, with an outer rim of reactive hepatocytes
    - ○ Actual vascular shunting is seen on resection specimens, usually not on biopsies

Vascular malformations can form mass lesions with a central cystic areas of malformed vessels (shunt vessels) surrounded by a thick rim if reactive smaller sized blood vessels, and sometimes a final layer of benign nodules of hepatocytes that resemble a focal nodular hyperplasia. Most cases are symptomatic at birth or within the first few weeks after birth.[44] Imaging findings are usually adequate for diagnosis, so the lesions are generally not biopsied. The histological differential is largely that of an infantile hemangioma. They can have some histological overlap, but infantile hemangiomas tend to look more uniform and organized throughout the lesion, while the vessels in vascular malformations are generally located in a reactive cuff around a central zone that has thicker walled shunt vessels and often has large, dilated blood-filled spaces with areas of organizing thrombi and fibrosis. GLUT-1 is either negative or shows focal staining, but lacks the strong and diffuse staining seen in infantile hemangiomas.[44]

MESENCHYMAL HAMARTOMA

CHECKLIST: Mesenchymal Hamartoma

- ☐ Rare
- ☐ Benign but can dedifferentiate into an embryonal sarcoma
- ☐ Histology
    - ○ Mostly composed of loose edematous mesenchymal tissue
    - ○ Scattered clusters of bile ducts and islands of hepatocytes

This rare pediatric tumor is benign and is composed mostly of loose connective tissue admixed with a few benign bile ducts and occasional small islands or cords of hepatocytes. The loose connective tissue often shows cystic type changes. The etiology for mesenchymal hamartoma is unclear, but the tumors can arise in the setting of the Beckwith–Wiedemann syndrome.[45,46] Mesenchymal hamartomas have frequent genetic alterations of chromosome 19 involving a gene-poor region called *MHLB1*.[47,48] Translocations have been reported between MHLB1 and multiple partners, including *MALAT1* and *AK023515*.[49]

Clinically, most cases present before the age of 3 years with mild nonspecific findings such as an abdominal mass. Rare cases are even detected by prenatal ultrasound.

Mesenchymal hamartomas have also been linked to placental mesenchymal dysplasia (also seen with Beckwith–Wiedemann syndrome).[50] In placental mesenchymal dysplasia, the placenta is enlarged and shows dilated, thick-walled chorionic plate vessels along with stem villi that are hydropic, enlarged, hypervascular, and can have central cystlike spaces lined by lymphatic endothelium. Most mesenchymal hamartomas are unifocal, bur rare multifocal tumors have been reported.[51] Serum levels of AFP can be elevated.[51,52] Rare cases have been reported in adults,[53] but such a diagnosis should be approached very cautiously as a good proportion of cases appear to be other tumors mimicking mesenchymal hamartomas.

Mesenchymal hamartomas are composed mostly of rather nondescript, loose connective tissue (Fig. 13.22). Within this connective tissue are recognizable but somewhat unorganized bits of normal liver, including scattered benign bile ducts (Fig. 13.23) and occasional small islands of ordinary appearing hepatocytes (Fig. 13.24). The bile duct epithelium and the hepatocytes are cytologically bland with no atypia or mitotic activity. They stain as expected, with various cytokeratins (CK7 and CK19 in the ductal areas) and markers of hepatic differentiation (HepPar1 in the hepatic areas). Also, the islands of hepatocytes can be AFP[52] and glypican 3 positive,[54] but this should not be mistaken for malignancy. The ducts can look like ordinary adult bile ducts, or can show changes that suggest a bile duct plate malformation, or in some cases form small biliary cysts. The connective tissue,

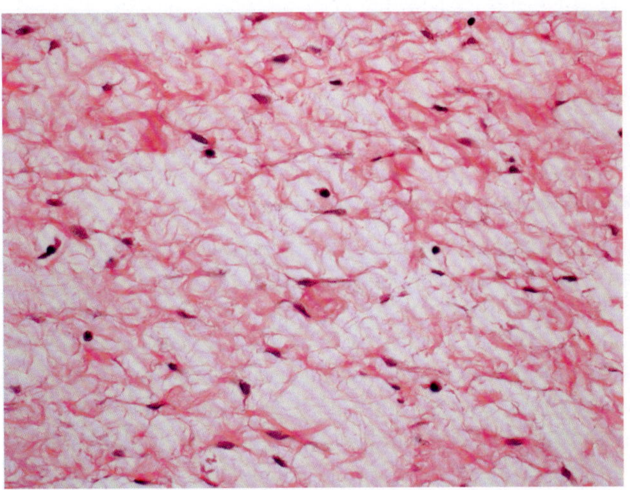

Figure 13.22. Mesenchymal hamartoma. The tumor is composed mostly of loose, nondescript spindle cells.

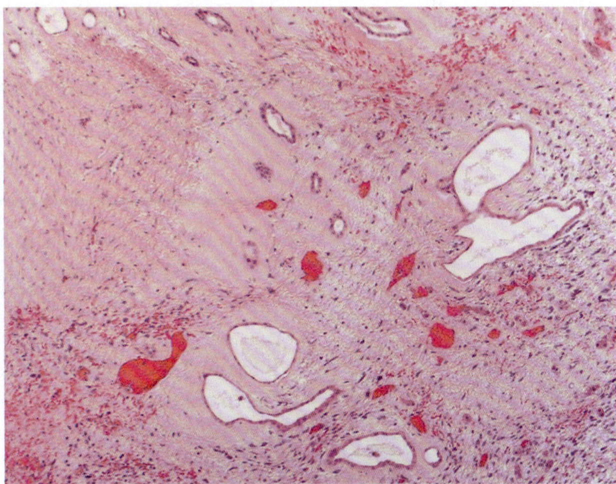

Figure 13.23. Mesenchymal hamartoma. A small cluster of somewhat disorganized, but still recognizable, bile ducts are seen. This case had undergone transformation to an embryonal sarcoma, but a small remnant of residual mesenchymal hamartoma was evident.

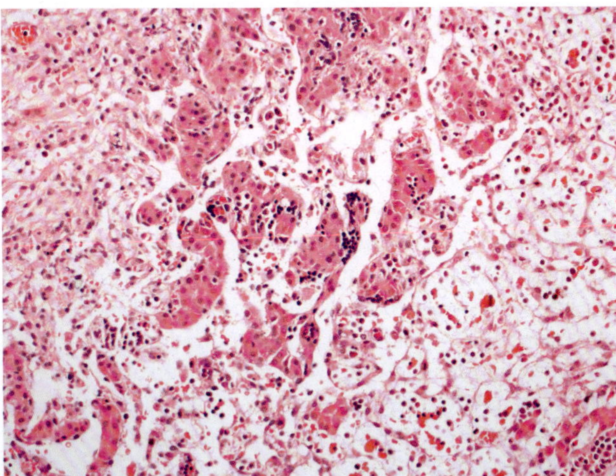

Figure 13.24. Mesenchymal hamartoma. A small cluster of unremarkable hepatocytes is present.

which makes up most of the tumor, is of low cellularity but also shows some variation in appearance, with areas that are myxoid and edematous and other areas that are more densely collagenized. As with the epithelial elements, the mesenchymal components have no cytological atypia and no mitotic activity. Immunostains are not necessary, but the loose connective tissue is typically vimentin positive and can also be smooth muscle actin positive,[55,56] usually with weak and patchy staining.

In general, the tumors have no real organization, but overall the epithelial elements are best seen with sampling of the edges of the tumor. Small vascular proliferations have also been reported at the periphery.[57] The tumor center often shows cystic degeneration of the connective tissue. The lesion commonly shows extramedullary hematopoiesis. Rare mesenchymal hamartomas undergo malignant transformation to embryonal sarcoma.

EMBRYONAL SARCOMA

CHECKLIST: Embryonal Sarcoma

- ☐ Rare
- ☐ Can be sporadic or arise from dedifferentiation of an embryonal sarcoma
- ☐ Histology
  - ○ Primitive, usually cellar, mesenchymal cells
  - ○ Diffuse cytological atypia
  - ○ Tumor cells can have PAS positive cytoplasmic globules

Embryonal sarcoma is an undifferentiated sarcoma that is most commonly found in the pediatric population. Another term used in the literature is *undifferentiated embryonal sarcoma*. They are all undifferentiated, so the terms are equivalent. Embryonal sarcomas are rare, but they are equally common in both genders, with an average age at presentation of about 10 years.[58] Rare cases also present in adults, but metastatic sarcomas from other sites have to be carefully excluded. In the teenage population, some embryonal sarcomas arise out of mesenchymal hamartomas,[59] but in most cases no precursor is evident and the etiology is unknown.

Embryonal sarcomas are composed of undifferentiated spindled cells (Fig. 13.25). The tumor cellularity varies, but most cases show moderate cellularity. The spindle cells are medium to large in size, show significant cytological atypia, and often have scattered areas of giant cell transformation (Fig. 13.26). Tumor cells often have hyaline globules, but the globules can be sparse and may not be present on biopsy specimens. A PASD stain can highlight the globules. The background stroma is usually loose and myxoid but can be more dense and fibrotic. Irregular pseudocysts are common, and in some cases there can be marked cystic degeneration.[60,61]

Immunostains are not needed for the diagnosis and can be more confusing than helpful. The tumor cells can show patchy positive staining for kertains, including cytokeratin AE1/3 and Cam5.2.[62–64] A perinuclear dotlike positivity for cytokeratins AE1/3 and Cam5.2 has been reported.[62] The tumor cells show no evidence for a consistent line of differentiation, but vimentin and CD68 are routinely positive,[64,65] and most tumors will be positive for alpha-1-antitrypsin and alpha-1-antichymotrypsin.[63,64] Tumors also show patchy positivity for desmin and alpha-smooth muscle in about 50% of cases.[63,64,66] Tumor cells can be positive for CD56 and focally for CD10 (membranous staining).[62] Markers of hepatic differentiation are negative, though glypican 3 can be positive.[54] Markers of muscle differentiation are generally negative but sometimes show rare focal positive staining.[58,63,64] Markers of melanocytic, vascular, endocrine, and neural differentiation are negative, as are CKIT and DOG1. Similar translocations have been reported in both mesenchymal hamartomas and embryonal sarcomas (see discussion on mesenchymal hamartomas).

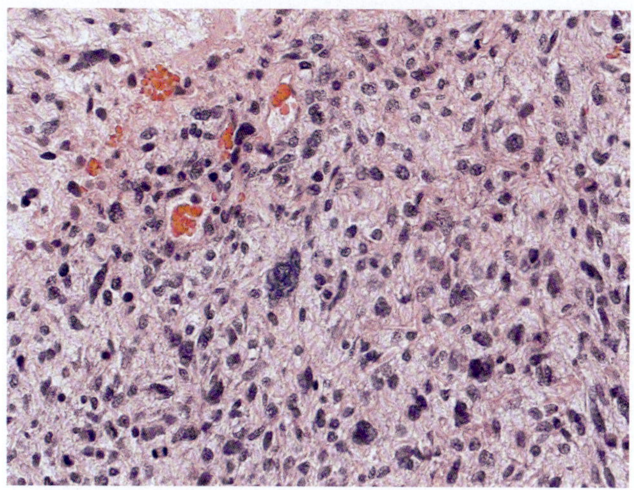

Figure 13.25. **Embryonal sarcoma.** The tumor is composed of malignant but undifferentiated spindled cells. There is diffuse anaplasia.

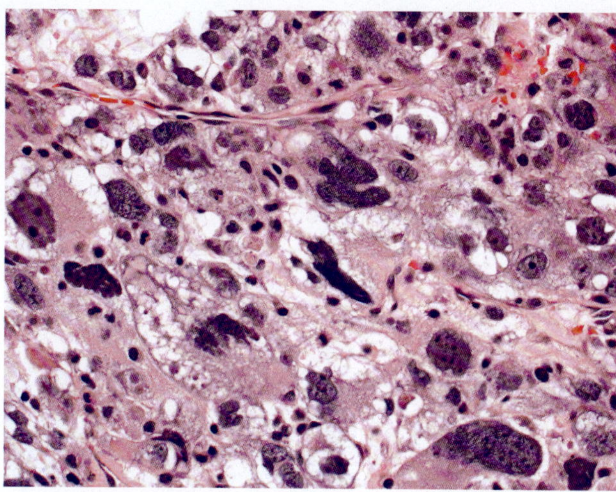

Figure 13.26. **Embryonal sarcoma.** The tumor cells show striking cytological atypia and nuclear anaplasia.

RHABDOID TUMORS

CHECKLIST: Rhabdoid Tumors

- ☐ Rare
- ☐ Defined by loss of INI-1 on immunostain, or genetic testing
- ☐ Large rhabdoid cells growing in discohesive sheets

Primary malignant rhabdoid tumors of the liver are very rare and are defined by compatible histological findings plus either loss of nuclear INI-1 expression by immunohistochemistry or molecular testing that shows mutations/deletions in the SMARCB1/INI-1 gene on chromosome 22q11.2 gene. The mutations in the SMARCB1 gene are germline in about 30% of cases.[67] No other risk factors or etiologically associations are known for malignant rhabdoid tumors of the liver. The SMARCB1 encodes a protein that is part of the SWI/SNF complex. The SWI/SNF protein complex is a tumor suppressor that is composed of many proteins and plays a central role in chromatin remodeling. Mutations in other proteins of the SWI/SNF complex are less common but have also been reported in other organs, including SMARCA2, PBRM1, SMARCA4, and ARID1a.[68] Mutations/deletions in SMARCA4 can be detected with immunostains by the loss of BRG1 nuclear expression. To date, these less common mutations of the SWI/SNF complex have not been reported in rhabdoid tumors primary to the liver.

Most cases present with nonspecific findings such as lethargy, anorexia, or hepatomegaly. There is no gender predilection.[69] Uncommonly, cases can present with spontaneous tumor rupture.[67,70–72] Serum AFP levels are usually normal or mildly elevated but rarely can be markedly elevated. One case was reported with serum AFP levels of 13,000 ng/mL.[67] The average age at presentation is 2 years,[73] with most cases occurring before 5 years.[67,69] However, individuals can also present in teenage years[69] and rare cases have been reported in adults.[74,75] Regardless of the age at presentation, the prognosis is poor, with a median survival in one study of 1.5 months.[69] There is metastatic disease at presentation in about 2/3 of cases.[67]

Malignant rhabdoid tumors can be multifocal and tend to be very large at presentation, often replacing most of the liver. Tumors often show hemorrhage, necrosis, and cystic degeneration. The tumor cells are epithelioid with abundant eosinophilic cytoplasm (Fig. 13.27). The tumor cells can have a plasmacytoid or rhabdoid appearance, with an eccentrically located nucleus, but this finding is not prominent in all cases. In some areas, the tumor cells can look more spindled. The tumor cells show vesicular chromatin and prominent nucleoli. The cells mostly grow in discohesive sheets, often with admixed inflammation

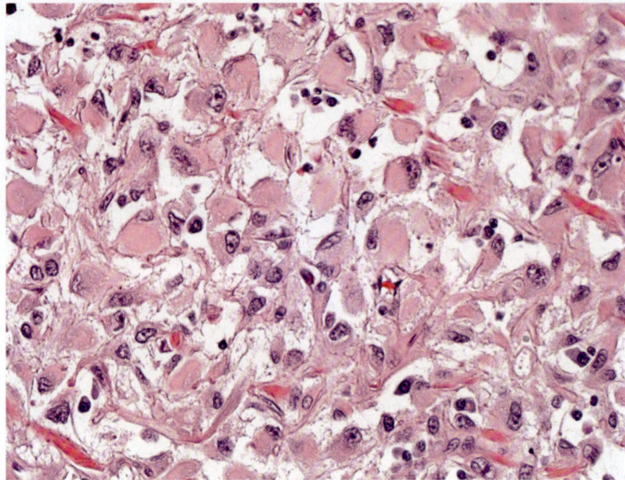

Figure 13.27. **Rhabdoid tumor.** The tumor cells are epithelioid and show abundant cytoplasm with eccentrically located nuclei.

and patchy necrosis. Occasionally tumor cells will grow with trabecular or nested growth patterns. Intratumoral necrosis, hemorrhage, and inflammation can sometimes be very prominent and obscure the tumor cells.

The tumor cells show loss of INI-1 or BRG-1 nuclear expression by immunohistochemistry (Fig. 13.25). PAS-positive perinuclear inclusions can be seen in some cases. Tumor cells are strongly positive for vimentin (90% of cases) and usually positive with pankeratin markers (60% of cases).[76–79] Immunostains for makers of hepatic differentiation (e.g., HepPar1 and arginase) are negative. However, glypican 3 is positive in about 2/3 of cases,[80,81] which can be an important diagnostic pitfall, leading to a misdiagnosis of hepatoblastoma or hepatocellular carcinoma. There is a high proliferative rate on Ki-67.

A very long list of other stains can be positive in some cases, often leading to diagnostic confusion. These stains include chromogranin, CD34, EGFR, CD-99, S-100 (usually cytoplasmic), HMB-45, GFAP, NSE, synaptophysin, polyclonal CEA, and smooth muscle actin. However, immunostains are negative for markers of skeletal muscle differentiation (myogenin, myo-D1).

RHABDOMYOSARCOMA (ALSO CALLED EMBRYONAL RHABDOMYOSARCOMA)

CHECKLIST: Rhabdomyosarcomas

- ☐ Rare
- ☐ Infants and children
- ☐ Tumor grows around bile ducts
  - ○ Spindle cell neoplasm with strap cells
  - ○ Cambium layer

Rhabdomyosarcomas of the liver are very rare and are almost always pediatric tumors, with a median age at presentation of about 3 years,[58] but rare cases can be seen in adults.[82,83] They most commonly affect the extrahepatic bile ducts and but can also form intrahepatic mass lesions.[84] Most patients present with obstructive jaundice.[85]

Rhabdomyosarcoma tumor cells can be spindled (Fig. 13.28), rounded, and somewhat epithelioid or have intermediate, racquet-shaped cells. The neoplastic cells typically cuff larger bile ducts and can lead to biliary obstruction. The tumor cells located immediately beneath the bile ducts are often smaller and more cellular, a finding referred to as a cambium layer (Fig. 13.29). Mitotic figures are easily seen within the tumor and larger tumors commonly show areas of necrosis and hemorrhage.

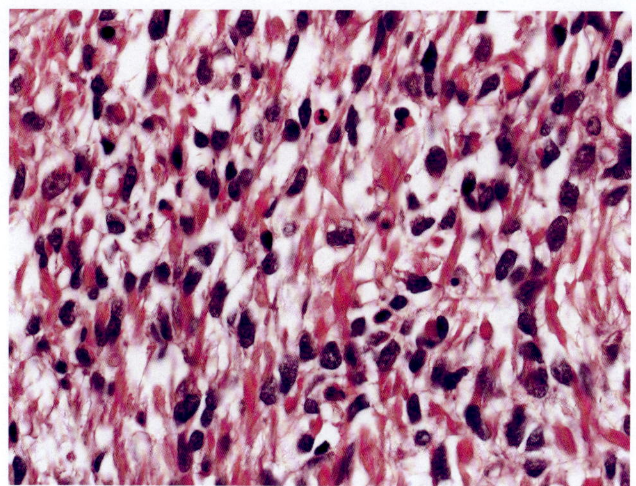

Figure 13.28. **Rhabdomyosarcoma.** The tumor cells in this case are spindled and showed an area of strap cells, with densely eosinophilic cytoplasm and equivocal cytoplasmic striations.

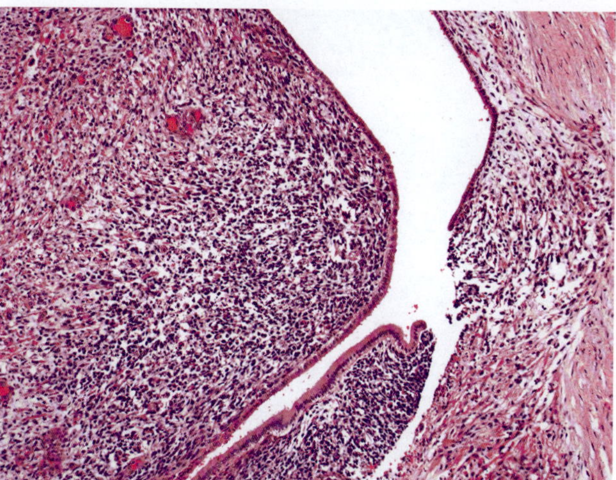

Figure 13.29. **Rhabdomyosarcoma.** The tumor grew as a cuff around the bile ducts. The tumor cells immediately beneath the bile ducts show a cambium layer, being composed of smaller more cellular tumor cells.

The main differential is with an embryonal sarcoma. The individual tumor cells in rhabdomyosarcomas tend to look fairly monotonous, without the anaplasia typically seen in embryonal sarcomas. In addition, hyaline globules are less frequently present in rhabdomyosarcomas than in embryonal sarcomas. Cross-striations in tumor cells would support a diagnosis of rhabdomyosarcoma, but they are often hard to find, so immunostains are important in confirming the diagnosis. Rhabdomyosarcomas are positive in most cases for either or both myogenin and myogenic regulatory protein D1 (MyoD1).[58] Of note, glypican 3 is positive in about 25% of cases[86] and represents an important diagnostic pitfall in cases that look more epithelioid. In some cases, the differential can also include rhabdoid tumors, but INI-1 is retained in rhabdomyosarcomas.

NEAR MISSES

CASE 1. A 13-year-old boy underwent a liver biopsy for a large liver tumor. The serum AFP was normal, and there was no background liver disease. The tumor was initially signed out as fibrolamellar carcinoma. On reviewing the case, the tumor was clearly malignant and showed hepatic differentiation by H&E and immunostains. However, the histological findings were that of typical hepatocellular carcinoma and not a fibrolamellar carcinoma (Fig. 13.30). In discussing the case with the referring pathologist, it was evident that the primary reason for the submitted diagnosis of fibrolamellar carcinoma was the patient's young age and lack of underlying liver disease.

This case illustrates the important finding that conventional hepatocellular carcinomas also rarely occur in children and teenagers, so young age alone does not establish the diagnosis of fibrolamellar carcinoma. Likewise, the presence of background liver disease makes fibrolamellar carcinoma unlikely, but a normal background liver can be seen with both conventional hepatocellular carcinoma and fibrolamellar carcinoma.

CASE 2. A 17-year-old male had history of Wilm tumor as a child, which had been successfully treated. During follow-up imaging studies a new 4-cm mass lesion was noted. The lesion was biopsied to rule out recurrent Wilm tumor. The biopsy was small but showed mature hepatocytes with a lack of normal portal tracts. There was no loss of reticulin, a low ki-67 proliferative rate, and glypican 3 was negative. There was retained LFABP expression and negative staining for CRP and SAA. Beta-catenin was negative for nuclear accumulation, but glutamine synthetase was strong and diffuse. The biopsy was interpreted as showing a hepatic adenoma, beta-catenin activated type because there was strong and diffuse glutamine synthetase staining (Fig. 13.31).

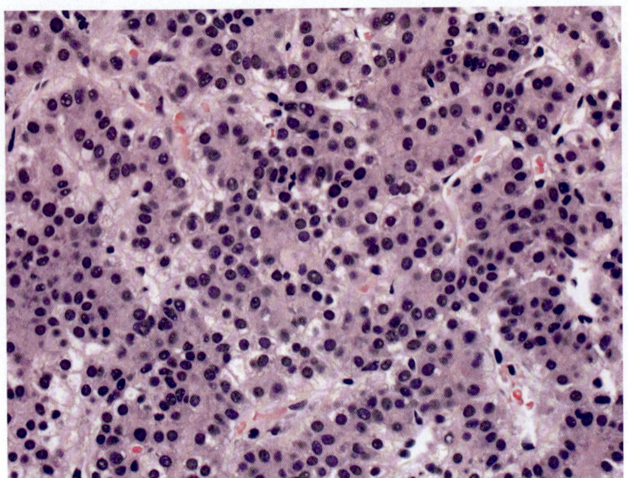

Figure 13.30. **Near miss case 1, hepatocellular carcinoma in a young person.** This hepatocellular carcinoma does not look like a fibrolamellar carcinoma, but the young age and lack of underlying liver disease led to a near miss by suggesting fibrolamellar carcinoma.

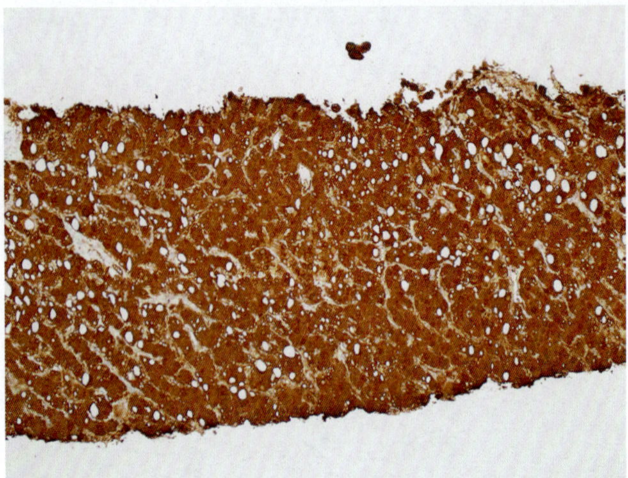

Figure 13.31. **Near miss case 2, glutamine synthetase staining.** This small biopsy showed strong and diffuse glutamine synthetase staining but ended up being a focal nodular hyperplasia, one that mimicks a beta-catenin active hepatic adenoma.

The decision was made to resect the tumor which was submitted for external consultation. On review, the lesion showed classic morphological findings of a focal nodular hyperplasia, confirmed by immunostaining.

This case illustrates an important pitfall for interpreting glutamine synthetase when biopsies are small. The large blotches of staining seen on glutamine synthetase with focal nodular hyperplasias can be over interpreted as beta-catenin activation if the biopsy is small enough to capture only the stained area.

References

1. Feusner JH, Krailo MD, Haas JE, Campbell JR, Lloyd DA, Ablin AR. Treatment of pulmonary metastases of initial stage I hepatoblastoma in childhood. Report from the Childrens Cancer Group. *Cancer*. 1993;71:859-864.
2. Brown J, Perilongo G, Shafford E, et al. Pretreatment prognostic factors for children with hepatoblastoma– results from the International Society of Paediatric Oncology (SIOP) study SIOPEL 1. *Eur J Cancer*. 2000;36:1418-1425.
3. Lack EE, Neave C, Vawter GF. Hepatoblastoma. A clinical and pathologic study of 54 cases. *Am J Surg Pathol*. 1982;6:693-705.
4. Shih JC, Tsao PN, Huang SF, et al. Antenatal diagnosis of congenital hepatoblastoma in utero. *Ultrasound Obstet Gynecol*. 2000;16:94-97.
5. Duan XF, Zhao Q. Adult hepatoblastoma: a review of 47 cases. *ANZ J Surg*. 2018;88:E50-E54.
6. Unal E, Koksal Y, Akcoren Z, Tavl L, Gunel E, Kerimoglu U. Mesenchymal hamartoma of the liver mimicking hepatoblastoma. *J Pediatr Hematol Oncol*. 2008;30:458-460.
7. de Fine Licht S, Schmidt LS, Rod NH, et al. Hepatoblastoma in the Nordic countries. *Int J Cancer*. 2012;131:E555-E561.
8. Giardiello FM, Petersen GM, Brensinger JD, et al. Hepatoblastoma and APC gene mutation in familial adenomatous polyposis. *Gut*. 1996;39:867-869.
9. DeBaun MR, Tucker MA. Risk of cancer during the first four years of life in children from The Beckwith-Wiedemann Syndrome Registry. *J Pediatr*. 1998;132:398-400.
10. Venkatramani R, Spector LG, Georgieff M, et al. Congenital abnormalities and hepatoblastoma: a report from the Children's Oncology Group (COG) and the Utah Population Database (UPDB). *Am J Med Genet A*. 2014;164A:2250-2255.
11. Lopez-Terrada D, Alaggio R, de Davila MT, et al. Towards an international pediatric liver tumor consensus classification: proceedings of the Los Angeles COG liver tumors symposium. *Mod Pathol*. 2014;27:472-491.

12. Hishiki T, Matsunaga T, Sasaki F, et al. Outcome of hepatoblastomas treated using the Japanese Study Group for Pediatric Liver Tumor (JPLT) protocol-2: report from the JPLT. *Pediatr Surg Int.* 2011;27:1-8.

13. Tannuri AC, Cristofani LM, Teixeira RA, Odone Filho V, Tannuri U. New concepts and outcomes for children with hepatoblastoma based on the experience of a tertiary center over the last 21 years. *Clinics (Sao Paulo).* 2015;70:387-392.

14. Saettini F, Conter V, Provenzi M, et al. Is multifocality a prognostic factor in childhood hepatoblastoma? *Pediatr Blood Cancer.* 2014;61:1593-1597.

15. Hiyama E, Ueda Y, Onitake Y, et al. A cisplatin plus pirarubicin-based JPLT2 chemotherapy for hepatoblastoma: experience and future of the Japanese Study Group for Pediatric Liver Tumor (JPLT). *Pediatr Surg Int.* 2013;29:1071-1075.

16. Haeberle B, Schweinitz D. Treatment of hepatoblastoma in the German cooperative pediatric liver tumor studies. *Front Biosci (Elite Ed).* 2012;4:493-498.

17. Meyers RL, Rowland JR, Krailo M, Chen Z, Katzenstein HM, Malogolowkin MH. Predictive power of pretreatment prognostic factors in children with hepatoblastoma: a report from the Children's Oncology Group. *Pediatr Blood Cancer.* 2009;53:1016-1022.

18. Maibach R, Roebuck D, Brugieres L, et al. Prognostic stratification for children with hepatoblastoma: the SIOPEL experience. *Eur J Cancer.* 2012;48:1543-1549.

19. Czauderna P, Lopez-Terrada D, Hiyama E, Haberle B, Malogolowkin MH, Meyers RL. Hepatoblastoma state of the art: pathology, genetics, risk stratification, and chemotherapy. *Curr Opin Pediatr.* 2014;26:19-28.

20. Ishak KG, Goodman ZD, Stocker JT. *Tumors of the Liver and Intrahepatic Bile Ducts.* Washington, DC: Armed Forces Institute of Pathology; 1999.

21. Zhou S, Gomulia E, Mascarenhas L, Wang L. Is INI1-retained small cell undifferentiated histology in hepatoblastoma unfavorable? *Hum Pathol.* 2015;46:620-624.

22. Haas JE, Muczynski KA, Krailo M, et al. Histopathology and prognosis in childhood hepatoblastoma and hepatocarcinoma. *Cancer.* 1989;64:1082-1095.

23. Trobaugh-Lotrario AD, Tomlinson GE, Finegold MJ, Gore L, Feusner JH. Small cell undifferentiated variant of hepatoblastoma: adverse clinical and molecular features similar to rhabdoid tumors. *Pediatr Blood Cancer.* 2009;52:328-334.

24. Badve S, Logdberg L, Lal A, et al. Small cells in hepatoblastoma lack "oval" cell phenotype. *Mod Pathol.* 2003;16:930-936.

25. Zynger DL, Gupta A, Luan C, Chou PM, Yang GY, Yang XJ. Expression of glypican 3 in hepatoblastoma: an immunohistochemical study of 65 cases. *Hum Pathol.* 2008;39:224-230.

26. Ishak KG, Goodman ZD, Stocker JT, Armed Forces Institute of Pathology (U.S.), Universities Associated for Research and Education in Pathology. *Tumors of the Liver and Intrahepatic Bile Ducts.* Washington, DC: Armed Forces Institute of Pathology; 2001. 356p.

27. Makhlouf HR, Abdul-Al HM, Wang G, Goodman ZD. Calcifying nested stromal-epithelial tumors of the liver: a clinicopathologic, immunohistochemical, and molecular genetic study of 9 cases with a long-term follow-up. *Am J Surg Pathol.* 2009;33:976-983.

28. Heerema-McKenney A, Leuschner I, Smith N, Sennesh J, Finegold MJ. Nested stromal epithelial tumor of the liver: six cases of a distinctive pediatric neoplasm with frequent calcifications and association with cushing syndrome. *Am J Surg Pathol.* 2005;29:10-20.

29. Geramizadeh B, Foroutan H, Foroutan A, Bordbar M. Nested stromal epithelial tumor of liver presenting with cushing syndrome: a rare case report. *Indian J Pathol Microbiol* 2012;55:253-255.

30. Brodsky SV, Sandoval C, Sharma N, et al. Recurrent nested stromal epithelial tumor of the liver with extrahepatic metastasis: case report and review of literature. *Pediatr Dev Pathol.* 2008;11:469-473.

31. Rod A, Voicu M, Chiche L, et al. Cushing's syndrome associated with a nested stromal epithelial tumor of the liver: hormonal, immunohistochemical, and molecular studies. *Eur J Endocrinol.* 2009;161:805-810.

32. Weeda VB, de Reuver PR, Bras H, Zsiros J, Lamers WH, Aronson DC. Cushing syndrome as presenting symptom of calcifying nested stromal-epithelial tumor of the liver in an adolescent boy: a case report. *J Med Case Rep.* 2016;10:160.

33. Malowany JI, Merritt NH, Chan NG, Ngan BY. Nested stromal epithelial tumor of the liver in Beckwith-Wiedemann syndrome. *Pediatr Dev Pathol.* 2013;16:312-317.

34. Khoshnam N, Robinson H, Clay MR, Schaffer LR, Gillespie SE, Shehata BM. Calcifying nested stromal-epithelial tumor (CNSET) of the liver in Beckwith-Wiedemann syndrome. *Eur J Med Genet*. 2017;60:136-139.

35. Hommann M, Kaemmerer D, Daffner W, et al. Nested stromal epithelial tumor of the liver–liver transplantation and follow-up. *J Gastrointest Cancer*. 2011;42:292-295.

36. Heywood G, Burgart LJ, Nagorney DM. Ossifying malignant mixed epithelial and stromal tumor of the liver: a case report of a previously undescribed tumor. *Cancer*. 2002;94:1018-1022.

37. Meletani T, Cantini L, Lanese A, et al. Are liver nested stromal epithelial tumors always low aggressive? *World J Gastroenterol*. 2017;23:8248-8255.

38. Hill DA, Swanson PE, Anderson K, et al. Desmoplastic nested spindle cell tumor of liver: report of four cases of a proposed new entity. *Am J Surg Pathol*. 2005;29:1-9.

39. Grazi GL, Vetrone G, d'Errico A, et al. Nested stromal-epithelial tumor (NSET) of the liver: a case report of an extremely rare tumor. *Pathol Res Pract*. 2010;206:282-286.

40. Assmann G, Kappler R, Zeindl-Eberhart E, et al. Beta-catenin mutations in 2 nested stromal epithelial tumors of the liver–a neoplasia with defective mesenchymal-epithelial transition. *Hum Pathol*. 2012;43:1815-1827.

41. Oviedo Ramirez MI, Bas Bernal A, Ortiz Ruiz E, Bermejo J, De Alava E, Hernandez T. Desmoplastic nested spindle cell tumor of the liver in an adult. *Ann Diagn Pathol*. 2010;14:44-49.

42. Han SJ, Tsai CC, Tsai HM, Chen YJ. Infantile hemangioendothelioma with a highly elevated serum alpha-fetoprotein level. *Hepatogastroenterology*. 1998;45:459-461.

43. Sari N, Yalcin B, Akyuz C, Haliloglu M, Buyukpamukcu M. Infantile hepatic hemangioendothelioma with elevated serum alpha-fetoprotein. *Pediatr Hematol Oncol*. 2006;23:639-647.

44. Mo JQ, Dimashkieh HH, Bove KE. GLUT1 endothelial reactivity distinguishes hepatic infantile hemangioma from congenital hepatic vascular malformation with associated capillary proliferation. *Hum Pathol*. 2004;35:200-209.

45. Abrahao-Machado LF, de Macedo FC, Dalence C, et al. Mesenchymal hamartoma of the liver in an infant with Beckwith-Wiedemann syndrome: a rare condition mimicking hepatoblastoma. *ACG Case Rep J*. 2015;2:258-260.

46. Cajaiba MM, Sarita-Reyes C, Zambrano E, Reyes-Mugica M. Mesenchymal hamartoma of the liver associated with features of Beckwith-Wiedemann syndrome and high serum alpha-fetoprotein levels. *Pediatr Dev Pathol*. 2007;10:233-238.

47. Speleman F, De Telder V, De Potter KR, et al. Cytogenetic analysis of a mesenchymal hamartoma of the liver. *Cancer Genet Cytogenet*. 1989;40:29-32.

48. Rakheja D, Margraf LR, Tomlinson GE, Schneider NR. Hepatic mesenchymal hamartoma with translocation involving chromosome band 19q13.4: a recurrent abnormality. *Cancer Genet Cytogenet*. 2004;153:60-63.

49. Mathews J, Duncavage EJ, Pfeifer JD. Characterization of translocations in mesenchymal hamartoma and undifferentiated embryonal sarcoma of the liver. *Exp Mol Pathol*. 2013;95:319-324.

50. Mack-Detlefsen B, Boemers TM, Groneck P, Bald R. Multiple hepatic mesenchymal hamartomas in a premature associated with placental mesenchymal dysplasia. *J Pediatr Surg*. 2011;46:e23-e25.

51. Fretzayas A, Moustaki M, Kitsiou S, Nychtari G, Alexopoulou E. Long-term follow-up of a multifocal hepatic mesenchymal hamartoma producing a-fetoprotein. *Pediatr Surg Int*. 2009;25:381-384.

52. Ito H, Kishikawa T, Toda T, Arai M, Muro H. Hepatic mensenchymal hamartoma of an infant. *J Pediatr Surg*. 1984;19:315-317.

53. Papastratis G, Margaris H, Zografos GN, Korkolis D, Mannika Z. Mesenchymal hamartoma of the liver in an adult: a review of the literature. *Int J Clin Pract*. 2000;54:552-554.

54. Levy M, Trivedi A, Zhang J, et al. Expression of glypican-3 in undifferentiated embryonal sarcoma and mesenchymal hamartoma of the liver. *Hum Pathol*. 2012;43:695-701.

55. Shintaku M, Watanabe K. Mesenchymal hamartoma of the liver: a proliferative lesion of possible hepatic stellate cell (Ito cell) origin. *Pathol Res Pract*. 2010;206:532-536.

56. Yesim G, Gupse T, Zafer U, Ahmet A. Mesenchymal hamartoma of the liver in adulthood: immunohistochemical profiles, clinical and histopathological features in two patients. *J Hepatobiliary Pancreat Surg*. 2005;12:502-507.

57. Stringer MD, Alizai NK. Mesenchymal hamartoma of the liver: a systematic review. *J Pediatr Surg*. 2005;40:1681-1690.

58. Nicol K, Savell V, Moore J, Teot L, Spunt SL, Qualman S. Distinguishing undifferentiated embryonal sarcoma of the liver from biliary tract rhabdomyosarcoma: a Children's Oncology Group study. *Pediatr Dev Pathol*. 2007;10:89-97.

59. Lauwers GY, Grant LD, Donnelly WH, et al. Hepatic undifferentiated (embryonal) sarcoma arising in a mesenchymal hamartoma. *Am J Surg Pathol*. 1997;21:1248-1254.

60. Buetow PC, Buck JL, Pantongrag-Brown L, et al. Undifferentiated (embryonal) sarcoma of the liver: pathologic basis of imaging findings in 28 cases. *Radiology*. 1997;203:779-783.

61. Yoon JY, Lee JM, Kim do Y, et al. A case of embryonal sarcoma of the liver mimicking a hydatid cyst in an adult. *Gut Liver*. 2010;4:245-249.

62. Perez-Gomez RM, Soria-Cespedes D, de Leon-Bojorge B, Ortiz-Hidalgo C. Diffuse membranous immunoreactivity of CD56 and paranuclear dot-like staining pattern of cytokeratins AE1/3, CAM5.2, and OSCAR in undifferentiated (embryonal) sarcoma of the liver. *Appl Immunohistochem Mol Morphol*. 2010;18:195-198.

63. Kiani B, Ferrell LD, Qualman S, Frankel WL. Immunohistochemical analysis of embryonal sarcoma of the liver. *Appl Immunohistochem Mol Morphol*. 2006;14:193-197.

64. Zheng JM, Tao X, Xu AM, Chen XF, Wu MC, Zhang SH. Primary and recurrent embryonal sarcoma of the liver: clinicopathological and immunohistochemical analysis. *Histopathology*. 2007;51:195-203.

65. Nishio J, Iwasaki H, Sakashita N, et al. Undifferentiated (embryonal) sarcoma of the liver in middle-aged adults: smooth muscle differentiation determined by immunohistochemistry and electron microscopy. *Hum Pathol*. 2003;34:246-252.

66. Lepreux S, Rebouissou S, Le Bail B, et al. Mutation of TP53 gene is involved in carcinogenesis of hepatic undifferentiated (embryonal) sarcoma of the adult, in contrast with Wnt or telomerase pathways: an immunohistochemical study of three cases with genomic relation in two cases. *J Hepatol*. 2005;42:424-429.

67. Trobaugh-Lotrario AD, Finegold MJ, Feusner JH. Rhabdoid tumors of the liver: rare, aggressive, and poorly responsive to standard cytotoxic chemotherapy. *Pediatr Blood Cancer*. 2011;57:423-428.

68. Rao Q, Xia QY, Wang ZY, et al. Frequent co-inactivation of the SWI/SNF subunits SMARCB1, SMARCA2 and PBRM1 in malignant rhabdoid tumours. *Histopathology*. 2015;67:121-129.

69. Oita S, Terui K, Komatsu S, et al. Malignant rhabdoid tumor of the liver: a case report and literature review. *Pediatr Rep*. 2015;7:5578.

70. Kachanov D, Teleshova M, Kim E, et al. Malignant rhabdoid tumor of the liver presented with initial tumor rupture. *Cancer Genet*. 2014;207:412-414.

71. Clairotte A, Ringenbach F, Laithier V, Aubert D, Kantelip B. Malignant rhabdoid tumor of the liver with spontaneous rupture: a case report. *Ann Pathol*. 2006;26:122-125.

72. Ravindra KV, Cullinane C, Lewis IJ, Squire BR, Stringer MD. Long-term survival after spontaneous rupture of a malignant rhabdoid tumor of the liver. *J Pediatr Surg*. 2002;37:1488-1490.

73. Martelli MG, Liu C. Malignant rhabdoid tumour of the liver in a seven-month-old female infant: a case report and literature review. *Afr J Paediatr Surg*. 2013;10:50-54.

74. Sibileau E, Moroch J, Teyssedou C, Aube C. Malignant rhabdoid tumors of the liver: an exceptional tumor in adults - a case report and literature review. *Eur J Gastroenterol Hepatol*. 2011;23:104-108.

75. Marzano E, Lermite E, Nobili C, et al. Malignant rhabdoid tumour of the liver in the young adult: report of first two cases. *HPB Surg*. 2009;2009:628206.

76. Yuri T, Danbara N, Shikata N, et al. Malignant rhabdoid tumor of the liver: case report and literature review. *Pathol Int*. 2004;54:623-629.

77. Scheimberg I, Cullinane C, Kelsey A, Malone M. Primary hepatic malignant tumor with rhabdoid features. A histological, immunocytochemical, and electron microscopic study of four cases and a review of the literature. *Am J Surg Pathol*. 1996;20:1394-1400.

78. Foschini MP, Van Eyken P, Brock PR, et al. Malignant rhabdoid tumour of the liver. A case report. *Histopathology*. 1992;20:157-165.

79. Hunt SJ, Anderson WD. Malignant rhabdoid tumor of the liver. A distinct clinicopathologic entity. *Am J Clin Pathol*. 1990;94:645-648.

80. Kohashi K, Nakatsura T, Kinoshita Y, et al. Glypican 3 expression in tumors with loss of SMARCB1/INI1 protein expression. *Hum Pathol*. 2013;44:526-533.

81. Chan ES, Pawel BR, Corao DA, et al. Immunohistochemical expression of glypican-3 in pediatric tumors: an analysis of 414 cases. *Pediatr Dev Pathol*. 2013;16:272-277.

82. Li H, Zhang Y, Pan Y, Hui D, Chen J, Jin Y. Clinicopathological analysis of concomitant hepatic embryonal rhabdomyosarcoma and hepatocellular carcinoma. *Pathol Res Pract*. 2017;213:1014-1018.

83. Arora A, Jaiswal R, Anand N, Husain N. Primary embryonal rhabdomyosarcoma of the liver. *BMJ Case Rep*. 2016;2016.

84. Kebudi R, Gorgun O, Ayan I, Cosar R, Bilgic B. Rhabdomyosarcoma of the biliary tree. *Pediatr Int*. 2003;45:469-471.

85. Perruccio K, Cecinati V, Scagnellato A, et al. Biliary tract rhabdomyosarcoma: a report from the Soft Tissue Sarcoma Committee of the Associazione Italiana Ematologia Oncologia Pediatrica. *Tumori*. 2018;104:232-237.

86. Kinoshita Y, Tanaka S, Souzaki R, et al. Glypican 3 expression in pediatric malignant solid tumors. *Eur J Pediatr Surg*. 2015;25:138-144.

14 HEPATOCELLULAR TUMORS

CHAPTER OUTLINE

FOCAL FATTY NODULE

CHECKLIST: Focal Fatty Nodules

- ☐ Rare
- ☐ Reactive lesion; not a tumor
- ☐ Focal well-circumscribed area of fat that resembles a tumor on imaging
- ☐ Histologically, looks like ordinary macrovesicular steatosis
- ☐ Main differential: hepatic adenoma, angiomyolipoma

Focal fatty nodules are benign reactive lesions and do not represent precursors to benign or malignant tumors. They are composed of nodular aggregates of hepatocytes with macrovesicular steatosis, but no other changes. Their main clinical significance is that they can mimic neoplasms on imaging studies, although a rare case of bleeding following trauma has also been reported.[1]

Focal fatty nodules are also called *focal fatty change* or *focal fatty liver*. Sometimes, there can be an aggregate of separate small nodules, which is called *multifocal nodular fatty change*.[2] The literature on focal fatty nodules in the liver is sparse, but one imaging study found they were typically subcapsular and were more common in the porta hepatis, gallbladder fossa, and the medial segment of the liver near the falciform ligament.[3] Histologically, they are well-demarcated nodules of hepatocytes with macrovesicular steatosis. The nodularity results only from the focal fatty change, and there are no other architectural changes (Fig. 14.1). Portal tracts and central veins are present in normal numbers and distribution. The lesions are not encapsulated. Rarely, the focal fatty nodule can show changes of steatohepatitis, with inflammation, balloon cells, and fibrosis.[2] The background liver shows no or minimal fatty change and no or minimal fibrosis. The etiology is thought to be focal changes in the blood flow.[4,5] Interestingly, the opposite can also occur, where the liver shows diffuse steatosis, but with focal fat sparing that mimics a tumor on imaging.[6]

The differential includes angiomyolipomas with a fatty morphology and hepatic adenomas. Usually, the morphological findings are distinctive, but immunostains can be helpful on biopsies or if there is uncertainty after reviewing the H&E findings.

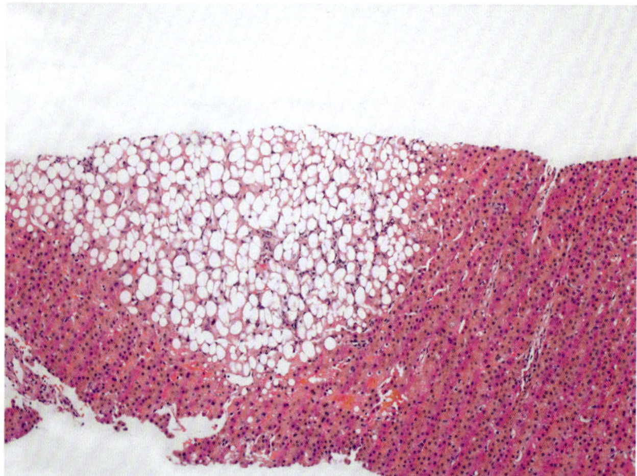

Figure 14.1. **Focal nodular hyperplasia.** There is a distinct, well-circumscribed focus of macrovesicular steatosis that mimicked a tumor by imaging.

FOCAL NODULAR HYPERPLASIA

CHECKLIST: Focal Nodular Hyperplasia

- ☐ Noncirrhotic livers
- ☐ Benign, no malignant potential
- ☐ Benign nodules of hepatocytes surrounded by bands of fibrosis
- ☐ Bands of fibrosis have bile ductular proliferation and sometimes thick-walled vessels
- ☐ Diagnosis is based on morphology; maplike staining for glutamine synthetase can supplement H&E findings
- ☐ Main differential: hepatic adenomas, in particular inflammatory adenomas

Focal nodular hyperplasia is a benign nodular lesion of the liver that results from focal vascular shunting in a noncirrhotic liver. Focal nodular hyperplasias have no malignant potential. Sometimes, similar lesions can develop in a cirrhotic liver, which is not terribly surprising as cirrhotic livers often have vascular shunting. What should such lesions be called? The current name in common usage is *focal nodular hyperplasia-like lesion,* which is appropriately descriptive but otherwise unattractive in that it seems to confuse a lot of clinicians. From a pathology perspective, one important pearl is to avoid making that diagnosis on a needle biopsy directed toward a mass lesion in a cirrhotic liver, as the histological changes can look similar to the peritumoral mass effect adjacent to an unsampled tumor.

The female to male ratio for focal nodular hyperplasia is about 10:1, and the most common age at presentation is in the late 30s and early 40s.[7,8] Most focal nodular hyperplasias in adults are without a clear cause, but well-recognized risk factors include vascular flow abnormalities such as Budd–Chiari.[9] In contrast, oral contraception is not an important risk factor.[10] Focal nodular hyperplasias also can occur in children or teenagers who had solid tumors previously treated with chemotherapy or radiation therapy that included the liver in the radiation field.[11,12] Children with hematopoietic stem cell transplantation also seem to be at increased risk.[13]

Overall, about 80% of focal nodular hyperplasias are single lesions. Multiple lesions are almost always limited to three or less. Cases with greater numbers of focal nodular hyperplasia almost always occur in the setting of recognized risk factors such as vascular disease or chemotherapy.[9,14]

Focal nodular hyperplasias form distinct lesions in the liver that are usually well circumscribed grossly but lack a fibrous capsule. They are composed of nodules of benign hepatocytes with intralesional bands of fibrosis that surround the nodules—giving the appearance of focal cirrhosis (Figs. 14.2–14.4). The fibrous bands have mild chronic inflammation and show bile ductular proliferation (Fig. 14.5). Medium to large caliber vessels can also be seen in the fibrous bands, either in the periphery or the center of the lesion (Fig. 14.6). The vessels can have muscular walls that can be eccentrically thickened. In focal nodular hyperplasias larger than 4 cm, the fibrous bands within the tumor often coalesce into a central scar. In contrast, smaller lesions are less likely to have a central scar and are less likely to have well-developed bands of fibrosis. Overall, central scars are present in 60% to 80% of resected focal nodular hyperplasias, being more common in larger lesions.

Within the lesion, the hepatocytes look about the same as hepatocytes in the background liver. They have normal N:C ratios and no nuclear atypia. When the background liver shows fatty liver disease, the focal nodular hyperplasia will often do the same (Fig. 14.7). There can be areas of mild patchy sinusoidal dilation or congestion (Fig. 14.8). Aberrant lobular arteries are also found in many cases (Fig. 14.9). Focal nodular hyperplasias lack true portal tracts and normal bile ducts. While they usually do not show cholestasis, there is impaired bile drainage, so cholate stasis is common in the hepatocytes lining the fibrous bands. These same hepatocytes also commonly show copper accumulation (Fig. 14.10).[15] Copper accumulation, however, is not diagnostically specific, as inflammatory adenomas are the main lesion in the differential, and they can also be copper positive.[16] Reticulin stains show a normal reticulin network in focal nodular hyperplasia and Ki-67 shows a proliferative rate that matches the background liver. Glypican 3 is negative.

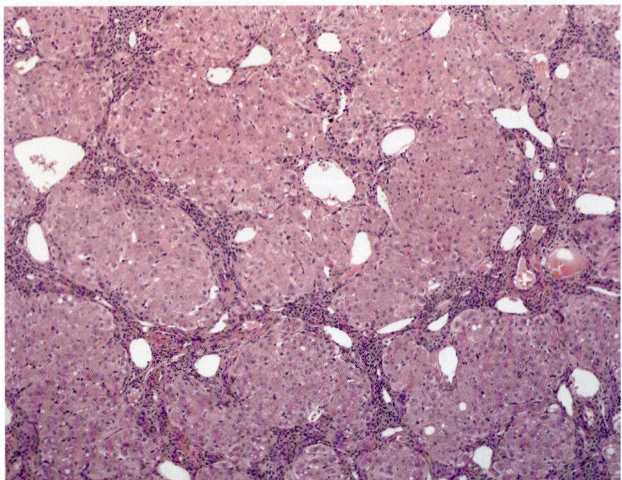

Figure 14.2. **Focal nodular hyperplasia.** The lesion shows nodules of hepatocytes surrounded by inflamed bands of fibrosis, giving a cirrhosis-like appearance at low power.

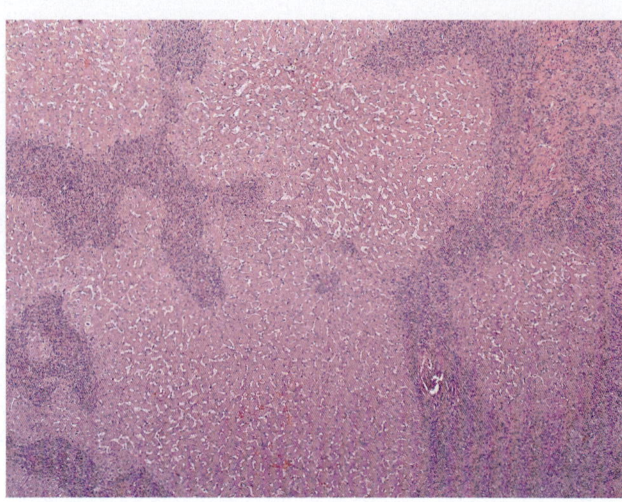

Figure 14.3. **Focal nodular hyperplasia.** In this case, nodularity is still evident, but it is less pronounced than in the case showed in Figure 14.1.

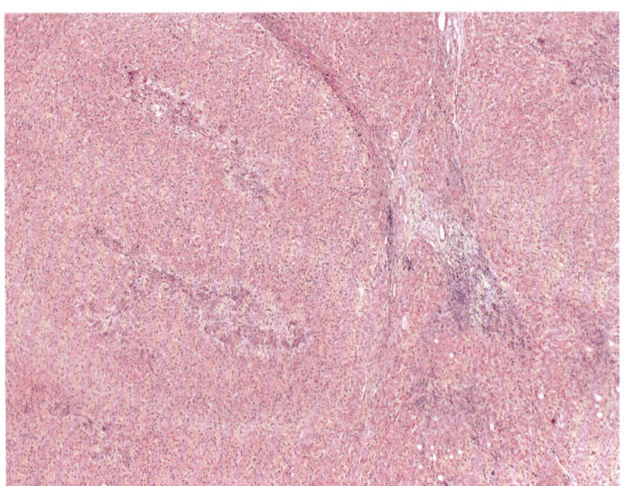

Figure 14.4. **Focal nodular hyperplasia.** In this example, there is even less parenchymal nodularity, compared with Figures 14.1 and 14.2, and less well-developed bands of fibrosis.

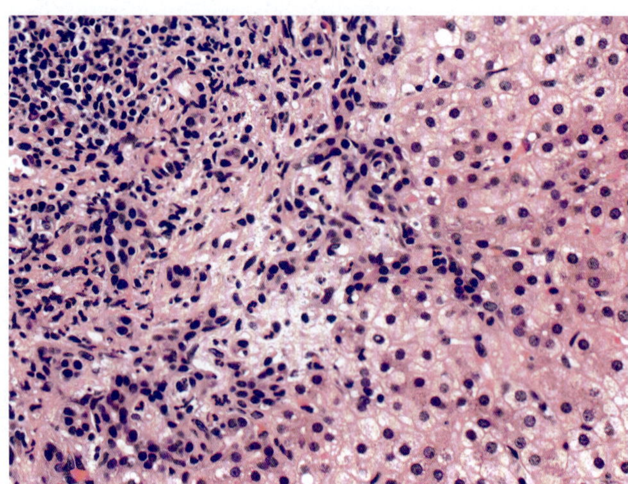

Figure 14.5. **Focal nodular hyperplasia.** The bands of fibrosis show a ductular proliferation and nonspecific chronic inflammation.

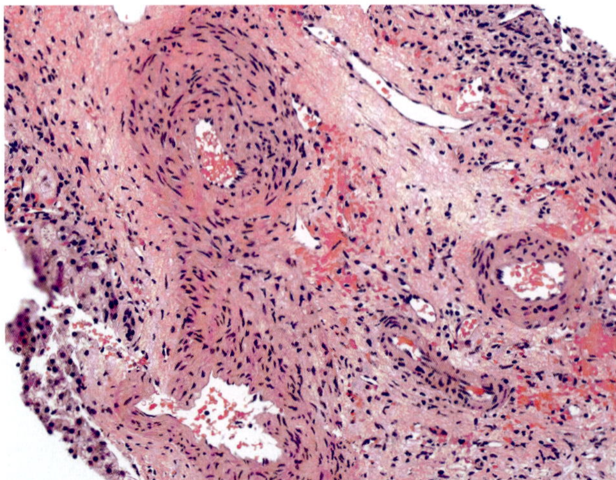

Figure 14.6. **Focal nodular hyperplasia.** The center of this lesion has a fibrous scar that contains thick-walled abnormal vessels.

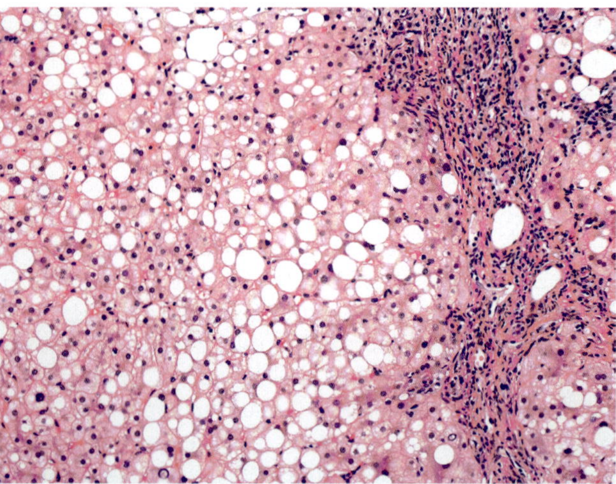

Figure 14.7. **Focal nodular hyperplasia, steatosis.** The background liver and the focal nodular hyperplasia both showed steatosis.

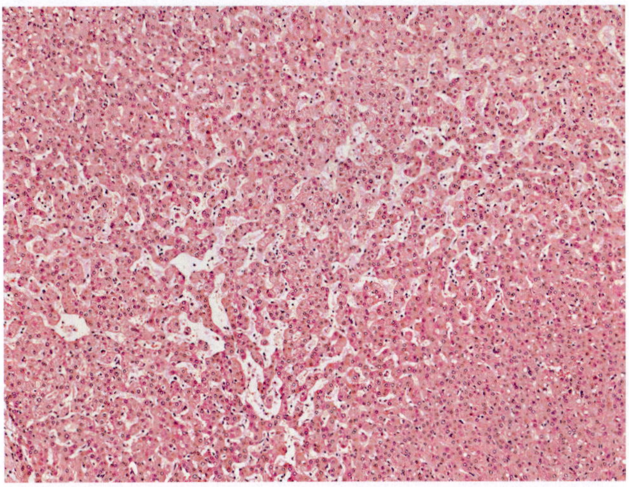

Figure 14.8. **Focal nodular hyperplasia.** An area of sinusoidal dilatation is seen.

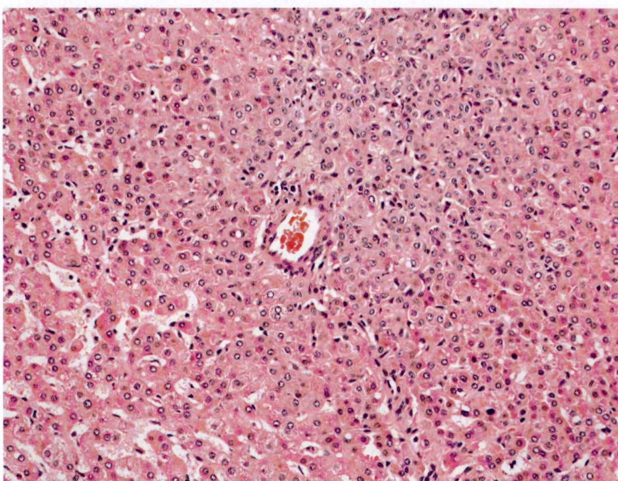

Figure 14.9. **Focal nodular hyperplasia.** An aberrant, or naked, artery is seen in the lobules.

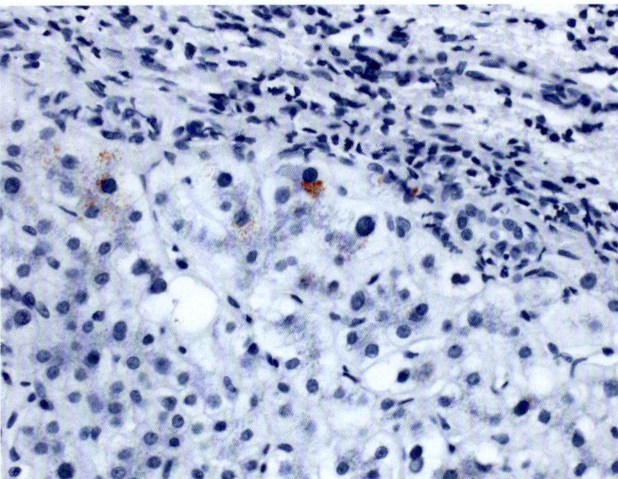

Figure 14.10. **Focal nodular hyperplasia, rhodanine copper stain.** Focal copper deposition is present next to the bands of fibrosis.

Immunostains for glutamine synthetase show a maplike staining pattern in focal nodular hyperplasia (Fig. 14.11). There are large irregular blotches of strong staining with relative sparing of the hepatocytes that line the fibrous bands (Fig. 14.12). In cases with classic morphology, the stain works particularly well, and it is these cases that authors like myself prefer to photograph for books and papers. When cases are more challenging because of small sample size or because the focal nodular hyperplasia itself is unusual, then its more of a toss-up as to whether the glutamine synthetase stain will help you or mislead you. In these difficult cases, adding C-reactive protein (CRP) and serum amyloid A (SAA) immunostains is often like doubling down on a doubtful bet—you frequently regret it. However, if you are careful you can avoid the two most common pitfalls.

First pitfall: biopsies that sample only a small portion of a focal nodular hyperplasia can easily be mistaken for a beta-catenin–activated adenoma because CRP and SAA are often dirty stains and glutamine synthetase can be "strong and diffuse" in small areas of a focal nodular hyperplasia (Fig. 14.13). Second pitfall: some adenomas can develop a psuedo-map-like staining pattern that seems to result from vascular shunting in the adenoma—the morphological correlate is often a nodular regenerative hyperplasia-like appearance within the adenoma—and this staining pattern is easily misinterpreted as the maplike staining pattern seen with FNH (Fig. 14.14). With CRP and SAA, the stains are most helpful when there is adjacent nonlesional tissue so that you can assess the degree of background staining and

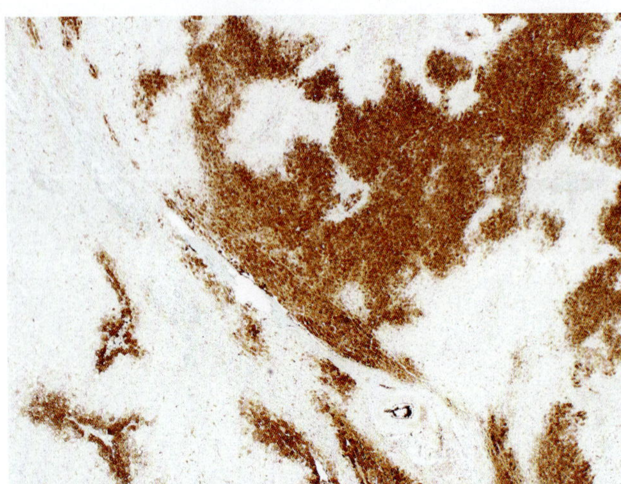

Figure 14.11. **Focal nodular hyperplasia, glutamine synthetase stain.** At low power, the staining suggests a map. The normal liver, located in the lower left of this image, shows staining of the hepatocytes in zone 3.

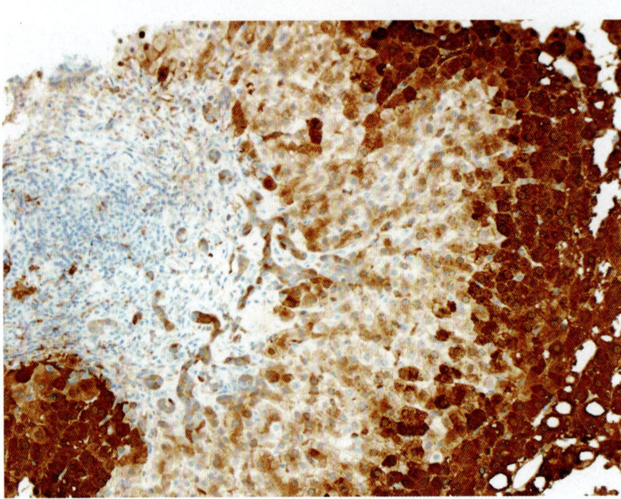

Figure 14.12. **Focal nodular hyperplasia, glutamine synthetase stain.** At high power, the areas of absent or less intense staining are typically located next to the fibrosis bands.

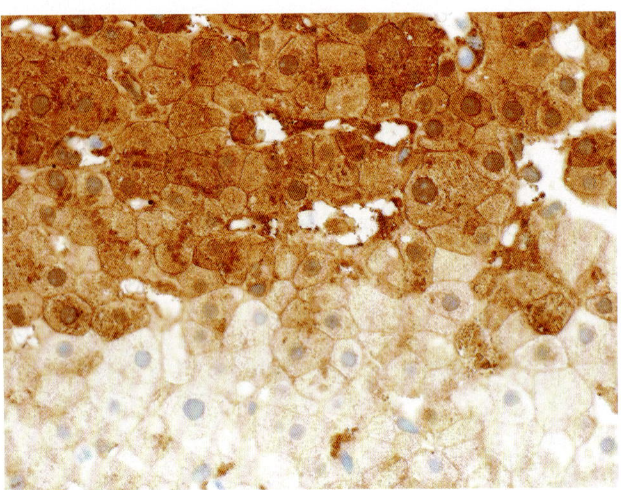

Figure 14.13. **Focal nodular hyperplasia, glutamine synthetase stain.** On this small biopsy, strong staining within the lesion (upper part of image) was mistaken as evidence for a beta-catenin–activated adenoma.

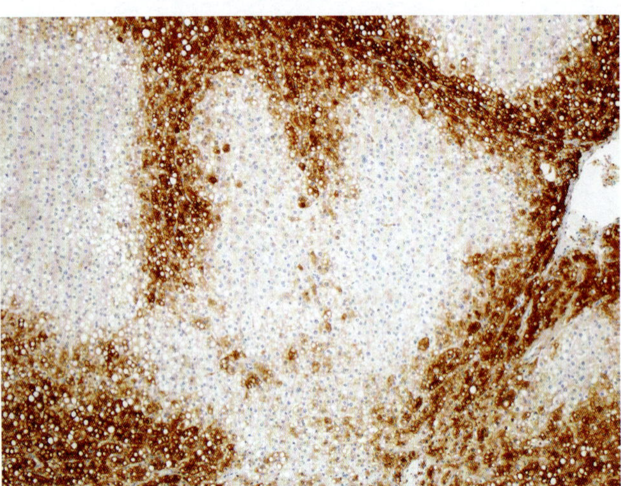

Figure 14.14. **Hepatic adenoma, glutamine synthetase stain.** This hepatic adenoma shows a pseudomap-like staining pattern, but note that the staining does not spare the areas around bands of fibrosis, but instead there is no intratumoral fibrosis.

make sure that any positivity is strong, diffuse, and clearly above that of the background liver. The best solution to these challenges is to make sure your diagnosis is first built on compatible H&E findings. If the H&E findings are not there, it is imprudent to make a diagnosis of focal nodular hyperplasia solely based on immunostain results.

The differential for focal nodular hyperplasia is mostly that of hepatic adenomas, in particular inflammatory adenomas, because they also can have bile duct–like structures. Histological findings that favor focal nodular hyperplasia include well-defined bands of fibrosis, well-formed bile ductular proliferation, and thick-walled vessels in the bands of fibrosis. The bile duct–like structures in inflammatory adenomas are located in pseudoportal tracts (*faux* portal tracts), and not in bands of fibrosis. On the other hand, the lack of intralesional bands of fibrosis and finding faux portal tracts favor an inflammatory adenoma. Stains are helpful but have to be interpreted with care. As discussed above, a maplike staining pattern on glutamine synthetase supports a diagnosis of focal nodular hyperplasia. In contrast, strong and diffuse staining for CRP and/or SAA supports a diagnosis of inflammatory adenoma but be aware that both of these stains can have high background staining, in particular CRP, so strong and diffuse staining is needed.

Rarely, neoplasms can develop a focal nodular hyperplasia–like response in the adjacent nontumoral liver, as part of mass effect changes.[17] Biopsies in this setting typically sample at least some of the actual tumor, but in very rare cases, the tumor proper can be missed, sampling only the adjacent focal nodular hyperplasia–like changes. Immunostains are not helpful in this setting, and you must rely on your judgment. If the biopsy is small and the imaging findings unusual, then rebiopsy can be helpful.

HEPATIC ADENOMA

CHECKLIST: Hepatic Adenomas

- ☐ Arise in noncirrhotic livers
- ☐ Risk factors: excess estrogen, excess androgen, chronic vascular disease, glycogen storage disease, and other rare genetic metabolic diseases
- ☐ Benign, but well-established risk of malignant transformation
- ☐ Risk of bleeding
- ☐ Hepatic adenomas are subtyped by immunostains and morphology
- ☐ Subtyping is performed to identify risk for malignancy and for bleeding

Hepatic adenomas are benign neoplasms composed of phenotypically mature hepatocytes. Overall, the term *hepatic adenoma* tends to be more commonly used in the United States and Canada, while *hepatocellular adenoma* tends to be more commonly used in Europe. However, these terms are synonyms and can be used interchangeably. I try to use both when writing to avoid offending anyone.

Most hepatic adenomas (80% to 90%) occur in one of these settings[18]: (1) young to middle-aged women with exogenous estrogen exposure, most commonly oral contraception or (2) young to middle-aged women with fatty liver disease. Of note, fatty liver disease increases endogenous estrogen levels, so is likely working through the same biological mechanism. The remaining adenomas either have no risk factors or have rare risk factors including excess androgen exposure, genetic metabolic diseases such as glycogen storage disease,[19] or the McCune Albright syndrome,[20] or abnormal hepatic blood blow such as the Abernathy syndrome or Budd–Chiari.[21,22] Of the different glycogen storage diseases, most hepatic adenomas have been identified in type 1 glycogen storage disease.[19]

Hepatic adenomas develop in noncirrhotic livers. The background liver can show fatty liver disease but is otherwise histologically normal. Fatty liver disease is a well-established risk factor for inflammatory adenomas in particular. When hepatocellular adenomas develop in the setting of glycogen storage diseases, other rare metabolic liver diseases, or vascular disease such as Budd–Chiari, the background liver will show changes of the underlying liver disease.

Histologically, hepatic adenomas have essentially no cytological atypia, although mild patchy large cell change is acceptable for inflammatory adenomas. There is no architectural atypia. By molecular analysis, they are clonal and driven by mutations but have many fewer mutations than hepatocellular carcinomas. By definition, the term hepatic adenomatosis is used if there are 10 or greater hepatic adenomas.

HEPATIC ADENOMA–LIKE NODULES IN CIRRHOTIC LIVERS

Several recent papers[23–26] have reported SAA-positive nodules in cirrhotic livers with alcohol as the underlying disease. While these data are interesting, less helpful was the suggestion by some authors that these should be called *hepatocellular adenomas*. While these nodules look somewhat like adenomas by light microscopy, they also look just as much like macroregnerative nodules. It's also true that a subset of these nodules stain with SAA and/or CRP, but so do a subset of ordinary cirrhotic nodules, so the data do not indicate that their proper classification is hepatic adenoma. Also, clonality within the lesion is not informative, as macroregenerative nodules in cirrhotic livers are frequently clonal.[27]

It is theoretically possible that an inflammatory hepatic adenoma could have developed in a noncirrhotic liver secondary to fatty liver disease (a recognized risk factor) and still be evident after the liver became cirrhotic. However, even if this were the case, the greater truth is that the biological behavior of these lesions is not known. This stands in contrast to hepatic adenomas, where the natural is well-established, and risk factors for malignant transformation and hemorrhage, while not fully known, are at least well-enough established to guide patient management. Thus, it is hard to see how calling these lesions *hepatocellar adenoma* is in the best interest of patients. This is particularly true in a biopsy of a nodule in a cirrhotic liver, where the use of the term *hepatocellular adenoma* is very strongly discouraged. Perhaps the landscape will change in the future, but at this point, the term *hepatocellular adenoma* is not justified for lesions in cirrhotic livers.

FAQ: What role does subtyping play in the management of hepatic adenomas?

Answer: Guidelines for managing hepatic adenomas have been published by both the European Association for Study of the Liver (EASL)[28] and the American College of Gastroenterology (ACG).[29] These societies currently do not recommend the use of liver biopsies for the routine diagnosis or management of hepatic adenomas. Biopsies are recommended only if imaging findings or clinical findings are not typical for a hepatic adenoma. Instead, they recommend that hepatic adenomas be diagnosed by imaging. Following an image based diagnosis, cases are managed by the risk factors of gender, size, and interval growth. Surgery is recommended in most cases when adenomas are in men, >5 cm, or show interval growth during follow-up. This approach is based on a series of paper that reported excellent sensitivity and specificity for diagnosing adenomas based on magnetic resonance imaging (MRI). In many cases, the MRI findings are indeed classic, but the overall published experience does not always match the experience of physicians in their own practice, so biopsies are still obtained on a fairly regular basis.

HISTOLOGICAL FINDINGS, OVERVIEW

Hepatic adenomas are composed of phenotypically mature hepatocytes. At the cytological level, the individual tumor cells look about the same as they do in the background liver, with little or no atypia (Fig. 14.15). There are two exceptions to the "no cytological atypia" rule. First, inflammatory adenomas can have mild cytological atypia, with a few scattered cells showing large cell change (Fig. 14.16), but there should not be anything more than that. Secondly, androgen-related adenomas can also show cytological atypia, again in the form of large cell type changes. Other atypical findings include numerous Mallory bodies or hyaline bodies. As an exception, hepatic adenomas in the setting of glycogen storage disease type 1 can sometimes show a steatohepatitic morphology with Mallory hyaline (Fig. 14.17).[30,31]

Adenomas should have no architectural atypia, with no small cell change, nodule-within-nodule growth, and no thickened trabeculae. While pseudorosettes are acceptable in androgen-related adenomas, they are an atypical finding in other adenomas. The reticulin framework should be within normal limits, remembering that there can be physiological reduction in reticulin in areas of fatty change.[32] The proliferative rate within the hepatic adenoma, as indicated by a Ki-67 immunostain, should be similar to the background nonneoplastic liver, with no difference detected by visual examination. Overall, most hepatic adenomas have a proliferative rate of less than 2% to 3%, but a higher rate is acceptable if it matches that of the background liver. Immunostains are positive for arginase and HepPar1, although HepPar1 can show patchy loss, especially in inflammatory hepatic adenomas.[33] Immunostains are negative for glypican 3 and AFP. CD34 can show either a strong diffuse staining pattern (Fig. 14.18) or a patchier staining pattern and does not reliably separate an adenoma from hepatocellular carcinoma. Finally, the immunostains used to subtype hepatic adenomas are relevant only after the diagnosis of hepatic adenoma is made, as they are not useful to determine if a neoplasm is a hepatic adenoma versus a hepatocellular carcinoma and are not useful to determine if a hepatocellular carcinoma arose from a hepatic adenoma.[34]

PEARLS & PITFALLS

In rare cases, the histological findings do not allow confident distinction between a hepatic adenoma and focal nodular hyperplasia. In almost all of these cases, this results from a small and fragmented biopsy. In these cases, immunostains are worth trying, but often there is little that can be done, other than rebiopsy the lesion.

The most common error is to mistake a focal nodular hyperplasia for an inflammatory adenoma based on CRP and/or SAA positivity. This error can happen because patchy but strong staining, for CRP in particular, is common in focal nodular hyperplasia, and depending on sampling, stains can show strong and diffuse staining on small biopsies of focal nodular hyperplasia, leading to a mistaken diagnosis of inflammatory adenoma.

A similar error can occur with glutamine synthetase stains. If there is a small biopsy of a focal nodular hyperplasia, chance sampling can show strong and diffuse glutamine synthesis staining of a small tissue fragment, which can lead to a mistaken diagnosis of inflammatory adenoma with beta-catenin activation.

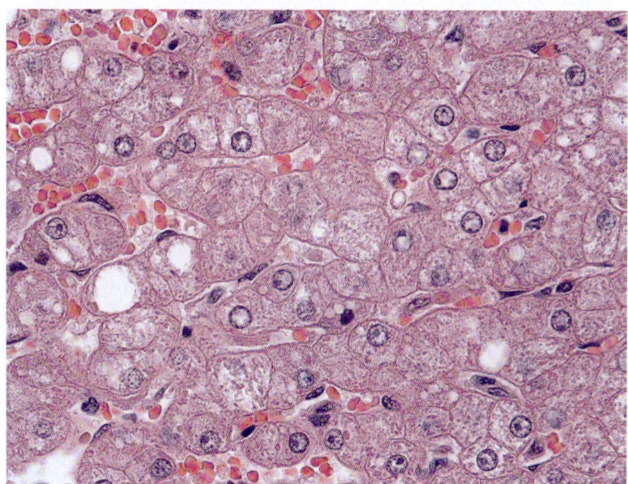

Figure 14.15. **Hepatic adenoma.** There is no cytological atypia.

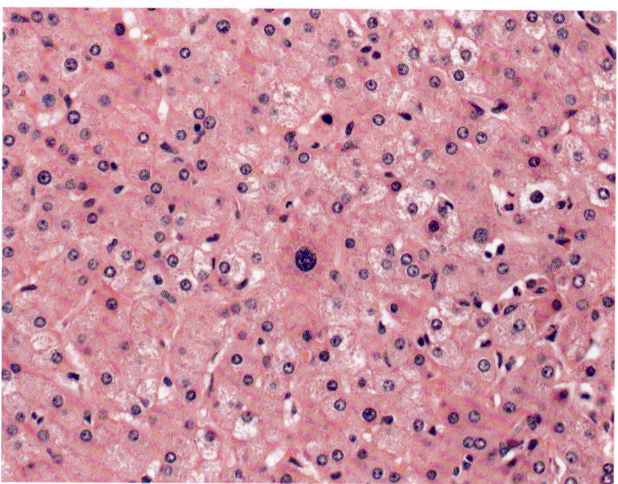

Figure 14.16. **Hepatic adenoma, inflammatory subtype.** Mild cytological atypia is seen in the form of large cell change, where scattered tumor cells have enlarged hyperchromatic nuclei, but have relatively preserved N:C ratios.

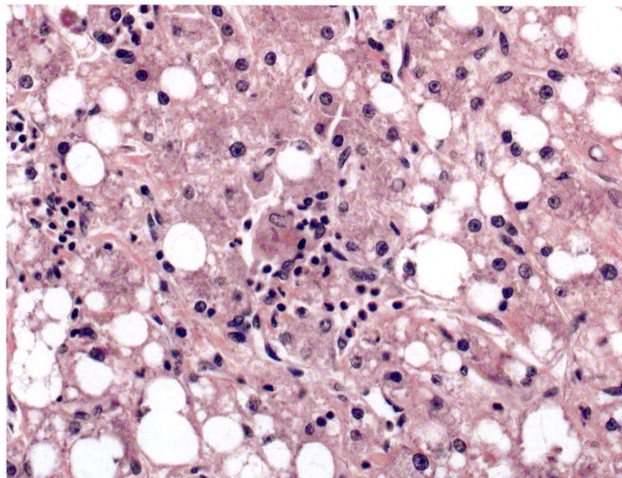

Figure 14.17. **Hepatic adenoma, glycogen storage disease type 1.** This hepatic adenoma shows a steatohepatitic morphology, a finding that is rare in hepatic adenomas outside the setting of glycogen storage disease type 1.

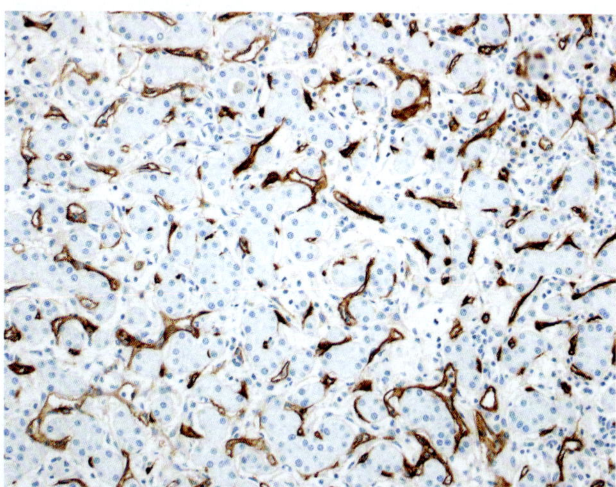

Figure 14.18. **Hepatic adenoma, CD34.** This hepatic adenoma has a strong and diffuse CD34 staining pattern. CD34 does not reliably distinguish between FNH, hepatic adenomas, or hepatocellular carcinomas.

ATYPICAL HEPATIC ADENOMAS

CHECKLIST: Atypical Adenomas

- ☐ Clinical findings
  - ○ Men
  - ○ Postmenopausal women
- ☐ H&E findings
  - ○ Cytological atypia
  - ○ Architectural atypia such as pseudoglands
- ☐ Histochemical findings
  - ○ Equivocal reticulin loss
  - ○ Ki-67 that is low but clearly above the background liver

In rare cases, the histological findings do not permit a confident diagnosis of hepatic adenoma or of hepatocellular carcinoma, typically because a biopsy is small and fragmented. This situation arises most commonly when there is no definite architectural atypia that would allow a confident diagnosis of hepatocellular carcinoma, but too much cytological atypia to permit a confident diagnosis of hepatic adenoma. In other cases, there can be small biopsies that show equivocal reticulin loss or a Ki-67 proliferative rate that appears to be greater than the adjacent nonneoplastic liver. In these cases, the terms used in the diagnostic line of your surgical pathology report will vary depending on your degree of suspicion for hepatocellular carcinoma, but some helpful terms include *atypical adenoma*, *well-differentiated hepatic neoplasm of uncertain malignant potential*,[35] or *well-differentiated hepatic neoplasm, see note*. Regardless of the terminology in your diagnostic line, the note should go on to indicate your overall degree of concern for malignancy, as well as what finding made the tumor difficult to classify. Rebiopsy can be suggested if the first biopsy has inadequate size or excess fragmentation. If the biopsy is adequate in size, but the histological findings are still challenging, then it can be helpful to share the case with local or outside colleagues who have experience with these types of cases. If the lesion still cannot be properly classified, then resection should be strongly considered, even if the tumor is less than 5 cm.

SAMPLE REPORT 1

Well-differentiated hepatic neoplasm, favor hepatic adenoma. Please see note.

Note: This biopsy is from a 5 cm liver tumor in a 31-year-old woman. There is no history of underlying liver disease, and by report the patient has a 7-year history of oral contraceptive use.

The small size of the biopsy limits evaluation, but there are several small fragments of a well-differentiated hepatocellular neoplasm composed of mature hepatocytes with mild fatty change and no cytological atypia. While I favor this to be a hepatic adenoma, there is focal equivocal reticulin loss and there appears to be a mildly increased proliferative rate on Ki-67. Unfortunately, only a very small fragment of the tumor remained on the Ki-67 stain and reticulin stains, and there was no remaining background nonneoplastic liver, making interpretation of these stains challenging. There also was no tissue remaining in the block to do additional studies. Because of the limited tissue, a definite diagnosis cannot be made, but the overall findings favor a hepatic adenoma. Careful correlation with clinical and imaging findings is recommended. A rebiopsy should be considered if there are concerning clinical or imaging findings.

There is insufficient background liver tissue to comment on underlying liver disease or fibrosis.

SAMPLE REPORT 2

Well-differentiated hepatic neoplasm. Please see note.

Note: This biopsy is from a 7 cm liver tumor in a 51-year-old woman. There is no history of underlying liver disease, and by report no risk factors for hepatic adenomas.

The biopsy is adequate in size and shows a well-differentiated hepatic neoplasm. The tumor cells show abundant eosinophilic cytoplasm with a near-normal N:C ratio. There is mild but definite nuclear atypia and scattered hepatic pseudorosettes. A Ki-67 immunostain shows an equivocally increased proliferative rate compared with the background liver. There is no reticulin loss, and a glypican 3 stain is negative. The background liver shows minimal macrovesicular steatosis (less than 5%) and no fibrosis.

While the histological findings do not reach the threshold of definite hepatocellular carcinoma, there is more cytological atypia than is typical for hepatic adenomas and a hepatocellular carcinoma cannot be completely excluded. Given the tumor size and the histological findings, resection should be considered.

HEPATIC ADENOMA SUBTYPES

CHECKLIST: Hepatic Adenoma Subtypes

- □ Immunostain classification
  - ○ HNF1-alpha–inactivated hepatic adenoma
  - ○ Inflammatory hepatic adenoma
  - ○ Beta-catenin–activated hepatic adenoma
  - ○ Unclassified hepatic adenoma
- □ Additional subtypes
  - ○ Androgen-related hepatic adenoma
  - ○ Pigmented hepatic adenoma
  - ○ Myxoid hepatic adenoma
  - ○ Provisional: hedgehog-activated hepatic adenomas and hepatic adenomas positive for argininosuccinate synthase

Hepatic adenomas are subtyped to predict risk for malignant transformation and for bleeding. The tumors at highest risk for malignant transformation are these: beta-catenin–activated adenomas, androgen adenomas, pigmented adenomas, and myxoid adenomas. The subtypes of hepatic adenomas at highest risk for clinical bleeding are the following: beta-catenin–activated adenomas, inflammatory adenomas, and potentially hedgehog-activated adenomas and adenomas positive for argininosuccinate synthase. As noted previously, the histological diagnosis and subclassification of hepatic adenomas are not a mandatory part of current clinical guidelines, but histology can still play a central role in guiding management decisions, especially when there are ambiguous imaging findings, inadequate access to MRI to assess for interval changes, or patient reluctance for surgery in adenomas that are >5 cm. High-risk adenomas will push toward definitive therapy, while low-risk adenomas support a wait-and-watch approach.

HNF1-Alpha–Inactivated Adenoma

CHECKLIST: HNF1-Alpha–Inactivated Adenoma

- □ Frequency: 35%
- □ Risk factors: Exogenous estrogen

- Genetic changes: *HNF1A* mutations—most mutations are sporadic but rare germline mutations can be found, also being associated with mature onset diabetes of the young (MODY3)
- Morphology: Many adenomas will have macrovesicular steatosis
- Immunohistochemistry definition: Loss of LFABP staining in hepatic adenomas
- Beta-catenin activation by immunohistochemistry: less than 1%

Risk factors for HNF1-alpha–inactivated adenomas include excess estrogen exposure and germline HNF1A mutations, which can also lead to mature onset diabetes (MODY3).[36] HNF1-alpha–inactivated adenomas typically have macrovesicular steatosis (Fig. 14.19) that can range from mild and patchy to marked and diffuse. Some hepatic adenomas will completely lack steatosis. They have no other distinguishing histological features and are defined by compatible morphology plus the loss of LFABP by immunohistochemistry (Fig. 14.20). The stain works very well overall, but it is still prudent to stain a block with both tumor and nontumor whenever possible. The background liver will show strong diffuse staining, while the adenoma is negative. Right at the interface of the background liver and the tumor, the tumor cells can show weak blurry staining.

Resected specimens will also frequently have microadenomas in the background liver. Microadenomas are small tumors that are not seen grossly but are evident on microscopic examination. Some of them can be quite tiny and are picked up better by LFABP loss than by H&E findings. Neither steatosis nor microadenomas is specific for HNF1-alpha–inactivated adenomas, so immunostains (or molecular studies) are needed to identify this subtype. Overall, this subtype has the lowest risk for hemorrhage and for malignant transformation, but malignancy is well documented in both sporadic HNF1-alpha–inactivated adenomas[18] and in those arising in the setting of MODY3.[36,37] When these adenomas do undergo malignant transformation, they are less likely than inflammatory adenomas to do so by activating the Wnt signaling pathway through beta-catenin mutations.

Other high-risk adenomas, such as pigmented adenomas, can also show loss of LFABP. In this situation the adenoma is classified as a pigmented adenoma and not an HNF1-alpha–inactivated adenoma, to better convey clinical risk for malignant transformation.

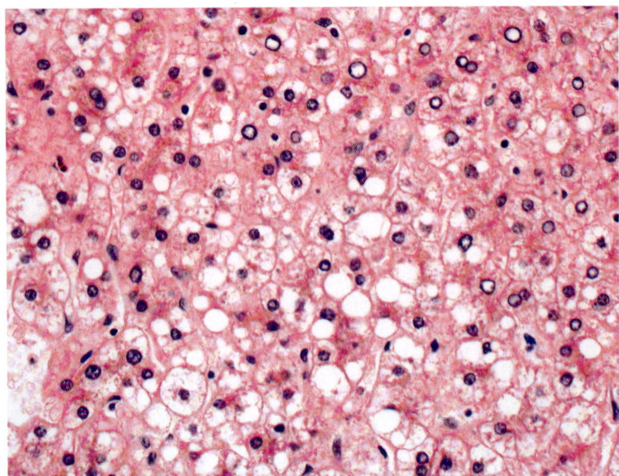

Figure 14.19. Hepatic adenoma, HNF1-alpha–inactivated subtype. The adenoma shows mild macrovescicular steatosis.

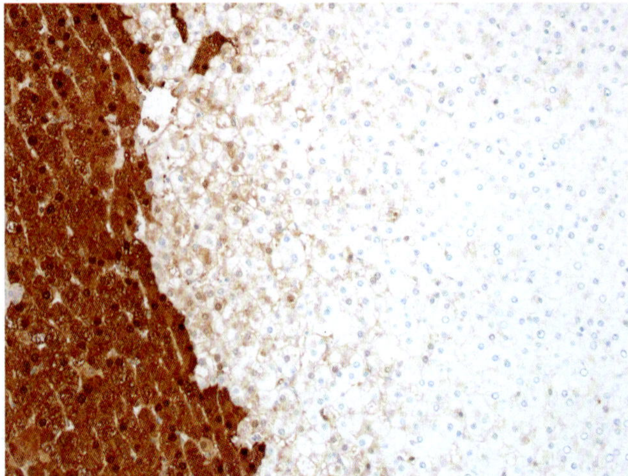

Figure 14.20. Hepatic adenoma, HNF1-alpha–inactivated subtype, LFABP stain. The adenoma shows loss of staining, while there is strong diffuse staining in the background liver.

Inflammatory Adenoma

CHECKLIST: Inflammatory Hepatocellular Adenoma

- □ Frequency: 50%
- □ Risk factors: Exogenous estrogen, fatty liver disease
- □ Genetic changes: JAK/STAT pathway activation via mutations in *IL6ST, STAT3, FRK, JAK1*, or *GNAS*
- □ Morphology: inflammation, congestion, *faux* portal tracts
- □ Immunohistochemistry definition: Positive for CRP/SAA and retained LFABP staining
- □ Beta-catenin activation by immunohistochemistry: ~10%

Risk factors for inflammatory adenomas include exogenous estrogen exposure, as well as fatty liver disease.[38,39] The fatty liver disease can be from either the metabolic syndrome or from alcohol use. Of course, most women with fatty liver disease do not get hepatic adenomas, so there are still major risk factors that we do not understand.

Inflammatory adenomas are associated with a variety of mutations that active the JAK/STAT pathway and lead to upregulation of SAA and CRP, which in turn are used to help make the diagnosis. Morphologically, these adenomas tend to show more inflammation than other adenomas—although the inflammation is still generally mild and patchy (Fig. 14.21). The inflammation is predominately lymphocytic and located somewhat haphazardly within the tumor. In addition, the tumor tends to show patchy sinusoidal dilation and congestion (Fig. 14.22). In most cases, the sinusoidal dilatation is mild and patchy, but it can range from absent to marked. The third morphological finding is that of pseudoportal tracts (or faux portal tracts) that show an artery in a sleeve of connective tissue with a bile ductular–like proliferation at the edges (Figs. 14.23 and 14.24). These faux portal tracts can mimic true portal tracts at first glance, but they lack a proper bile duct, and the ductular-like reaction tends to be less well formed and composed of plumper cells, compared with a true bile ductular reaction. This constellation of findings (inflammation, sinusoidal congestion, faux portal tracts) is not complete in every case, and in some cases, none of these features are well represented. This morphological variability has not been correlated with the underlying genetic changes to date, but it may be that different mutations are associated with differences in morphologies. In any case, immunostains for SAA and/or CRP are needed to make the diagnosis in many cases (Figs. 14.25 and 14.26).

Microadenomas can also be seen, but they are not as common as they are in cases of HNF1-alpha–inactivated hepatic adenomas. Both the background liver and the inflammatory adenoma often show steatosis or steatohepatitis, but it is unusual to find fat in the adenoma but not the background liver, a finding more common in either HNF1-alpha or unclassified adenomas. Inflammatory adenomas also commonly show mild cytological atypia in the form of scattered tumor cells with large cell changes (Fig. 14.16).

Overall, SAA tends to be a cleaner stain than CRP, but both can show significant staining in adjacent nontumor liver, especially if there is inflammation. Thus, to avoid over calling these stains, it is best to use sections that have both the background liver and the tumor and to hold out for staining that is clearly strong and diffuse compared with the background liver. If the inflammatory adenoma also shows nuclear accumulation on beta-catenin immunostain, or strong and diffuse glutamine synthetase staining, then the term *inflammatory adenoma with beta-catenin activation* is used.

The main diagnostic challenge with this type of adenoma is distinguishing it from a focal nodular hyperplasia. In fact, before inflammatory adenomas were recognized as a hepatic adenoma subtype,[40] they were initially classified as telangiectatic focal nodular hyperplasias. Nonetheless, in cases with adequate sampling, the distinction is now readily made. Focal nodular hyperplasias have bands of fibrosis, intralesional nodularity, a true ductular proliferation in the fibrous bands, and often have large vessels with eccentrically thickened walls. In smaller focal nodular hyperplasias, intralesional nodularity can be less well developed, while larger ones will also commonly have central scars. Sinusoidal dilatation can be present in both inflammatory hepatocellular adenomas and focal nodular hyperplasia.

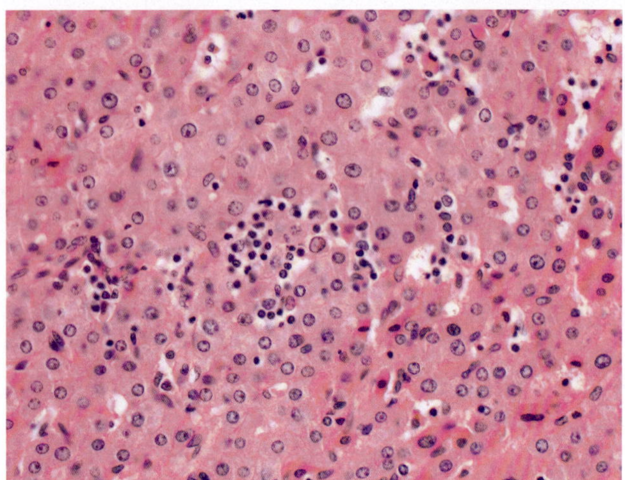

Figure 14.21. **Hepatic adenoma, inflammatory subtype.** The tumor showed patchy lobular inflammation, without any injury to the tumor cells.

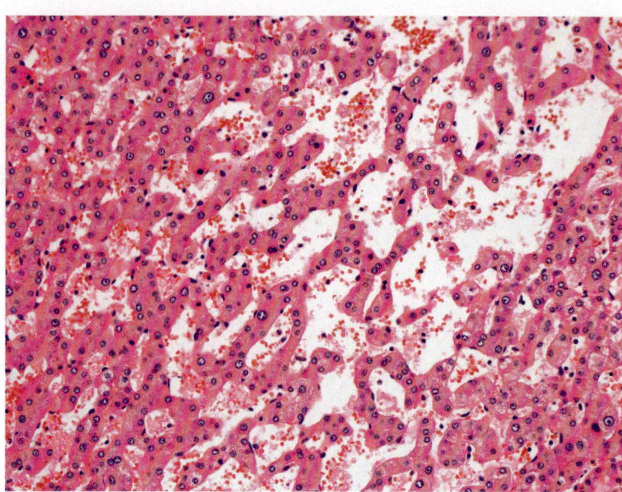

Figure 14.22. **Hepatic adenoma, inflammatory subtype.** Patchy sinusoidal congestion is seen.

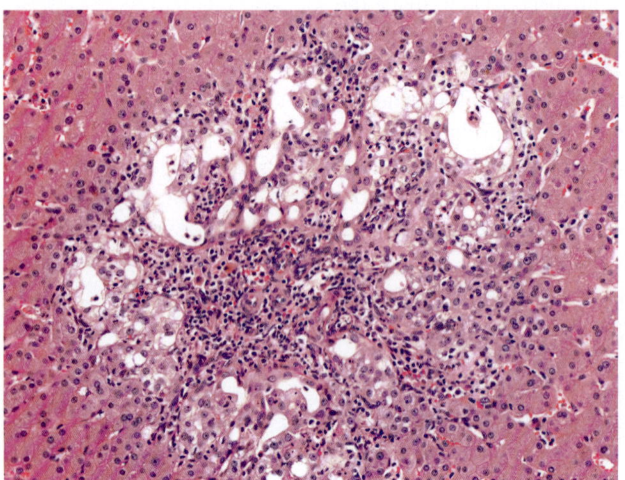

Figure 14.23. **Hepatic adenoma, inflammatory subtype.** This faux portal tract is made of a sleeve of connective tissue with an artery, mild mixed inflammation, and a ductular-like reaction at the edges.

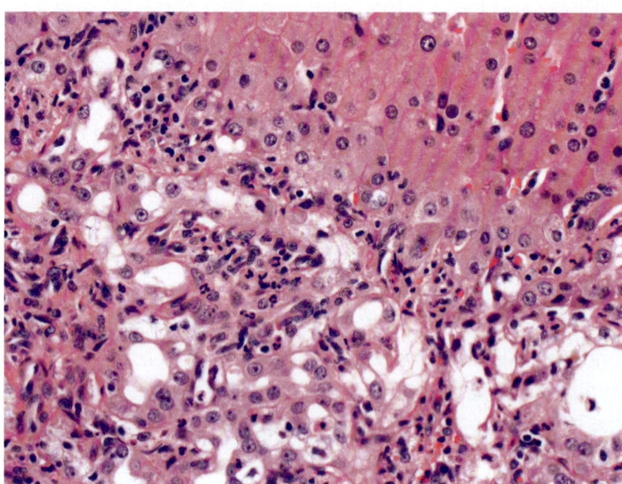

Figure 14.24. **Hepatic adenoma, inflammatory subtype.** At higher power, the bile ductular–like proliferation is composed of tumor hepatocytes that show cholate stasis and ductular metaplasia (same cases as preceding).

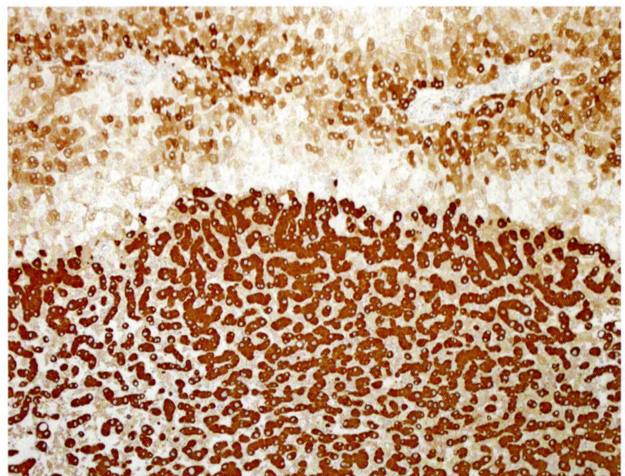

Figure 14.25. **Hepatic adenoma, inflammatory subtype, C-reactive protein (CRP) immunostain.** The adenoma in the bottom half of the image is strongly positive, but note the background staining.

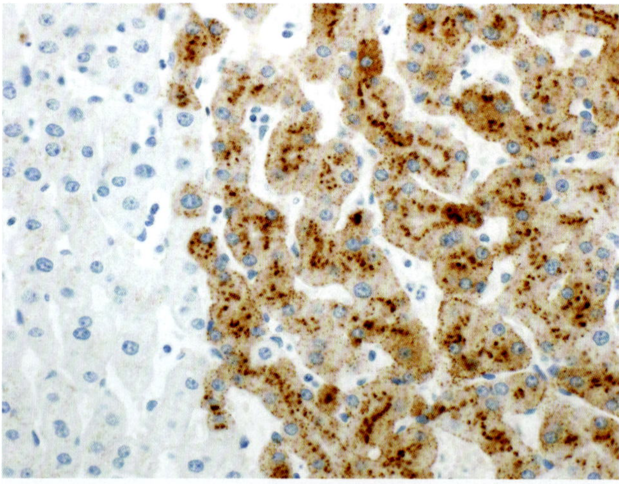

Figure 14.26. **Hepatic adenoma, inflammatory subtype, serum amyloid A (SAA) immunostain.** The tumor (right side of image) is positive, while the background liver is not.

Likewise, both inflammatory adenomas and focal nodular hyperplasia can have steatosis or steatohepatitis, if the background liver also has fatty change. Aberrant lobular arteries are common in both and play no role in distinguishing adenomas (of any type) from focal nodular hyperplasia. A maplike staining pattern for glutamine synthetase will support a diagnosis of focal nodular hyperplasia, while strong and diffuse staining for CRP or SAA will support a diagnosis of inflammatory adenoma. Copper accumulation is not a distinguishing feature, as both tumors can be positive.[16]

Do not forget to compare the results of special stains with the H&E. Most diagnostic errors result from over interpretation of very small biopsies. On small biopsies, if the H&E morphology and the immunostain findings are perfect for an entity, then make the diagnosis. If either the H&E morphology or the immunostain findings are not perfect, then it is often best to make a diagnosis of a benign liver lesion and indicate your prioritized differential in a note, along with the limitations of the biopsy (e.g., small, fragmented, bad stains, etc.).

FAQ: Which stain is better, CRP or SAA?

Answer: There is no correct answer but here are some general considerations. CRP definitely has more background staining than SAA. On the other hand, staining with CRP tends to be stronger and brighter. There are little or no data on their performance in a head-to-head comparison, but my personal experience is that CRP tends to be more sensitive than SAA, although I have had cases that are CRP negative, SAA positive, and vice versa.

Beta-Catenin–Activated Adenoma

CHECKLIST: Beta-Catenin–Activated Adenoma

- ☐ Frequency: 1% to 30%
- ☐ Risk factors: unknown
- ☐ Genetic changes: *CTNNB1* (beta-catenin) mutations
- ☐ Morphology: no distinctive morphology
- ☐ Immunohistochemistry definition: nuclear positivity for beta-catenin, or strong and diffuse staining with glutamine synthetase
- ☐ HNF1-alpha–inactivated adenomas and inflammatory adenomas can also be beta-catenin activated, showing either nuclear positivity for beta-catenin or strong and diffuse glutamine synthetase staining

This subtype of adenoma has no distinct morphological findings. By definition, there has to be nuclear positivity on a beta-catenin immunostain, strong and diffuse glutamine synthetase staining, or sequencing data showing a beta-catenin mutation. In the context of hepatic adenomas, the terms *beta-catenin activation* and *Wnt signaling activation* or *Wnt pathway activation* are often used interchangeably. The Wnt pathway is the name of the overall signaling pathway, and beta-catenin protein plays a central role by activing the pathway when it translocates to the nucleus.

In the most common approach to diagnosis, beta-catenin–activated adenomas show retained expression of LFABP and negative staining for SAA and CRP. If an adenoma shows beta-catenin activation plus evidence for HNF1-alpha inactivation or CRP/SAA staining, then it is called *HNF1-alpha–inactived adenoma with beta-catenin activation* or an *inflammatory adenoma with beta-catenin activation*, respectively. Recent proposals have suggested using the specific beta-catenin mutation to subgroup hepatic adenomas,[18] which is probably not widely implementable, as most centers do not routinely sequence adenomas. In most centers, the immunostain approach for identifying beta-catenin activation is still the most widely used and works well for clinical care. The high-risk adenomas (pigmented adenoma, androgen adenoma, myxoid adenoma) can also be beta-catenin activated but are primarily classified as pigmented, androgen, or myxoid adenomas, with an additional statement on whether they are also beta-catenin activated.

The frequency of isolated beta-catenin–activated adenomas, that is without cooccurring loss of LFABP or positive staining for CRP/SAA, varies a lot in the literature, with a range from about 1% to 25% in the literature, although more recent studies are essentially always at the lower end, usually less than 5%. It is not entirely clear why the range is so large or why there has been a shift toward a lower frequency, but it seems to reflect both how strongly the beta-catenin immunostain is titrated as well as the inclusion of some tumors in earlier studies that many pathologists would have classified as well-differentiated hepatocellular carcinomas. In addition, immunostains for glutamine synthetase can be challenging to interpret, as there can be equivocal staining that is not clearly negative or positive. In my experience, the frequency of beta-catenin–activated adenomas (with retained staining of LFABP and negative staining for CRP and/or SAA) is less than 5% when using standard pathology laboratory immunostains.

Identification of Beta-Catenin Activation

Immunostains for beta-catenin and glutamine synthetase are used to identify beta-catenin activation at most centers. When using the beta-catenin immunostain, even a single clearly positive tumor nucleus is scored as positive. There is a reasonable correlation with the number of beta-catenin positive nuclei and the underlying mutation,[41] so one reasonable approach is to report out the number of positive nuclei as rare (single or a few, always less than 1%) or many (>1%) (Figs. 14.27 and 14.28). In cases with many positive nuclei, make sure you carefully exclude hepatocellular carcinoma.

The glutamine synthetase stain is consistent with Wnt signaling activation when there is strong and diffuse staining (Fig. 14.29). In early papers, *strong and diffuse* was defined as greater than 50% of tumor cells. However, in most cases with strong Wnt signaling activation, the staining will be greater than 90% of tumor cells. In the end, Wnt signaling activation identified by immunostains does not correlate perfectly with molecular studies,[42] but importantly, it does appear to capture most cases with mutations that lead to the highest levels of Wnt pathway activation (Table 14.1).

PEARLS & PITFALLS WITH THE BETA-CATENIN STAIN

- Look carefully, because even a single positive tumor nucleus is scored as positive.
- When positive, most hepatic adenomas have only a few positive tumor nuclei. One exception is androgen-related adenomas, which can have many positive tumor nuclei. Outside of this setting, finding many beta-catenin–positive tumor nuclei is unusual and hepatocellular carcinoma should be carefully excluded.

PEARLS & PITFALLS WITH THE GLUTAMINE SYNTHETASE STAIN

- The glutamine synthetase stain tends to be dirty (Figs. 14.30 and 14.31), so use as a guide the degree of positivity in zone 3 hepatocytes in the background liver. To be informative, the staining intensity in the tumor should at least reach the intensity of zone 3 hepatocytes in the normal liver.
- Adenomas that are not beta-catenin activated commonly show a rim of staining in tumor cells that surround veins within the adenoma.
- Some adenomas will have a nodular regenerative hyperplasia look to their parenchyma when examined at low power. Some of these adenomas will show a pseudomap-like staining pattern that can be mistaken for focal nodular hyperplasia.
- A reasonable approach is to report out the results as follows:
  - Negative or nonspecific staining patterns.
  - *Positive with a heterogeneous staining pattern.* Staining is seen in most but not all tumor cells, usually ~50% to 90%.
  - *Positive with a homogenous staining pattern.* In these cases, almost all of the tumor cells are positive.

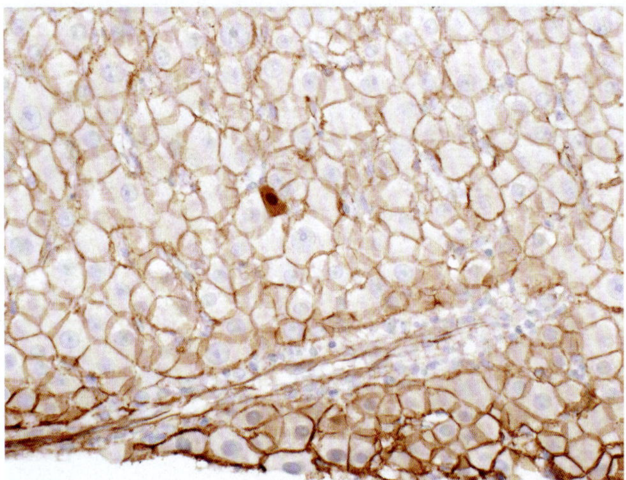

Figure 14.27. **Hepatic adenoma, inflammatory subtype, beta-catenin immunostain.** A rare tumor cell shows strong nuclear staining.

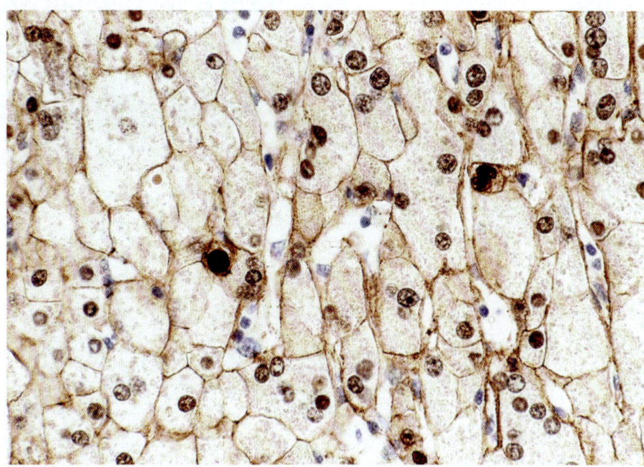

Figure 14.28. **Hepatic adenoma, inflammatory subtype, beta-catenin immunostain.** Many nuclei are positive in this case.

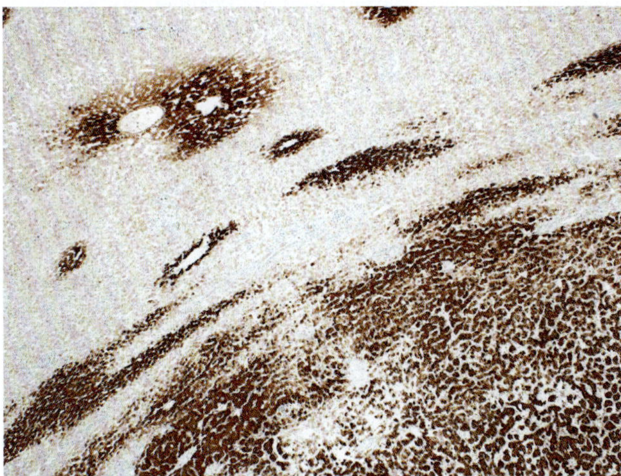

Figure 14.29. **Hepatic adenoma, beta-catenin activated, glutamine synthetase.** This case showed strong and diffuse staining within the adenoma. The background liver (upper left) shows the expected zone 3 staining of hepatocytes.

Unclassified Adenomas

This group of adenomas makes up about 10% of all hepatic adenomas, and as the name indicates, they cannot be classified into any of the other categories of hepatic adenoma. Morphologically, mild steatosis and mild glycogen accumulation is common, but overall they do not have any distinctive findings (Fig. 14.32).

Newly Reported Subtypes

Two potentially new subtypes of hepatic adenomas have been recently reported based on molecular analysis of the unclassified group of hepatic adenomas: sonic hedgehog–activated adenoma (~4% of all adenomas)[18] and argininosuccinate synthase–positive adenoma (~7% adenomas).[43] For both of these potential subtypes, there is overlap (some cases are positive for both markers), and the main clinical correlate is a high risk for bleeding. The morphological correlates, if any, have not been described to date. The sonic hedgehog adenoma is associated with a mutation leading to the fusion of the *INHBE* and *GLI1* genes. The argininosuccinate synthase subtype was identified by increased expression of argininosuccinate synthase and arginosuccinate lyase, but this may be a secondarily acquired phenotype, as the protein overexpression does not appear to be restricted to a morphologically distinct group of adenomas.[43]

TABLE 14.1: Beta-Catenin Mutations in Hepatic Adenomas

Mutation	Strength of Wnt Pathway Activation	Beta-Catenin Nuclear Accumulation	Glutamine Synthetase Staining Pattern and Interpretation	Relative Risk of HCC
Large exon 3 deletions	Strong	>1% of nuclei	Intensity: Strong Distribution: Diffuse (usually >90%) Surgical pathology interpretation: Positive	High
Exon 3 deletion D32-37	Strong	>1% of nuclei	Intensity: Strong Distribution: Diffuse (usually >90%) Surgical pathology interpretation: Positive	High
Exon 3, T41	Moderate	>1% of nuclei	Intensity: Strong Distribution: Diffuse (usually 50% to 90%) Surgical pathology interpretation: Positive	High
Exon 3, S45	Weak	<1%, with absent to rare positive nuclei	Intensity: Moderate to strong Distribution: Patchy Surgical pathology interpretation: Positive or negative depending on stain results	Low
Exon 7, K335	Weak	Absent	Intensity: Weak to strong Distribution: Patchy or perivenular Surgical pathology interpretation: Negative	Low
Exon 8, N387	Weak	Absent	Intensity: Weak to strong Distribution: Patchy or perivenular Surgical pathology interpretation: Negative	Low

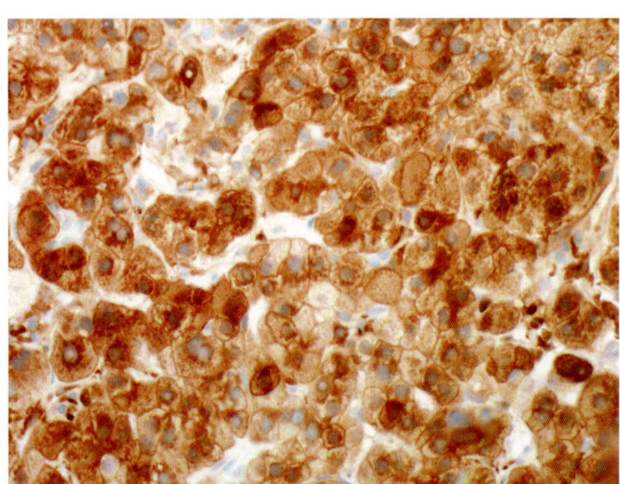

Figure 14.30. **Hepatic adenoma, uninterpretable glutamine synthetase immunostain.** In this biopsy specimen, the adenoma is strongly positive for glutamine synthetase, but see the next image.

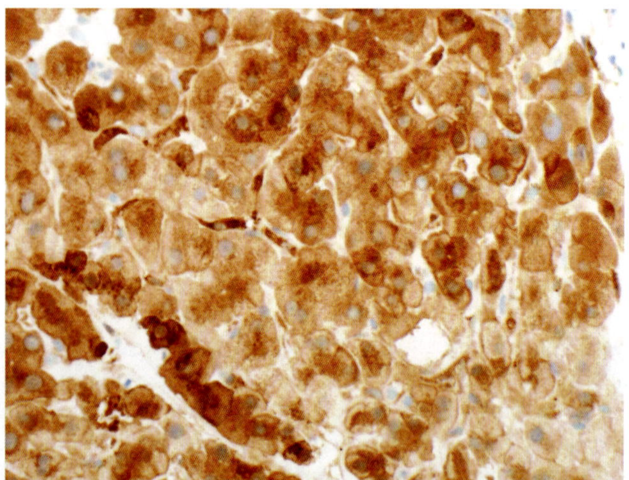

Figure 14.31. **Hepatic adenoma, uninterpretable glutamine synthetase immunostain.** The background liver in the biopsy is just as strong as the tumor, so the glutamine synthetase stain is not informative.

SPECIAL HIGH-RISK SUBTYPES OF HEPATIC ADENOMAS

CHECKLIST: Special Adenomas With a High Risk of Malignant Transformation

- ☐ Androgen adenomas
- ☐ Pigmented adenomas
- ☐ Myxoid adenomas

There are three additional subtypes of hepatic adenomas that do not fit well into the traditional classification schema: androgen adenomas, pigmented adenomas, and myxoid adenomas. Overall, these three adenoma subtypes are rare, but they are clinically important because each has an increased risk of malignancy.

Androgen adenomas by definition occur in the setting of exogenous androgen exposure, which can result from medical therapy or recreational uses. Histologically, they are frequently cholestatic, have small psuedoglands (Fig. 14.33), and have patchy but significant cytological atypia in the form or large cell change (Fig. 14.34). When they are subtyped by immunostains, androgen adenomas can be HNF1-alpha inactivated, inflammatory, or unclassified.[44] The majority of androgen adenomas are beta-catenin activated,[44] and they are more likely than other adenomas to show numerous beta-catenin nuclear positive cells.

Pigmented adenomas have diffuse moderate to heavy lipofuschin within the tumor cells (Fig. 14.35). The pigment is sufficiently heavy that it can be seen by gross examination in many cases. By immunostain analysis, pigmented adenomas can be also be classified as HNF1-alpha–inactivated or inflammatory adenomas. While data are limited, there appears to an enrichment for the HNF1-alpha subtype.[45] In any case, it is important to indicate the presence of heavy pigmentation within the report, as these adenomas are more likely to have cytological atypia, beta-catenin activation, and malignant transformation.[45–47]

The last special subtype of hepatic adenoma is the myxoid hepatic adenoma, which is appropriately named because they are characterized by striking myxoid material dissecting through the tumor trabecula (Fig. 14.36).[48] They can be single or multiple, with some cases having a hepatic adenomatosis pattern with greater than 10 adenomas. The adenomatosis cases can also have microadenomas, and even the microadenomas will show the distinctive myxoid change.

Myxoid hepatocellular adenomas have a sticky, tacky, mucoid feel by gross examination and also have distinctive imaging findings.[49] The nature of the myxoid material is unclear (Fig. 14.37), but it seems to be produced by the tumor cells and has some features of

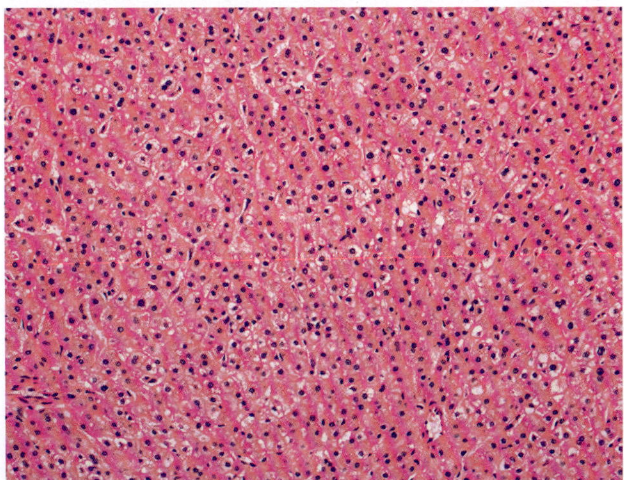

Figure 14.32. **Hepatic adenoma, unclassified subtype.** The adenoma shows no distinguishing features.

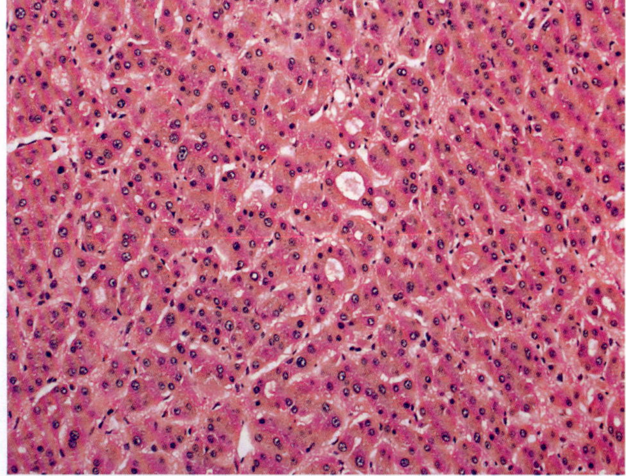

Figure 14.33. **Hepatic adenoma, androgen subtype.** This adenoma developed in the setting of androgens used for body building. Scattered psuedoglands can be seen.

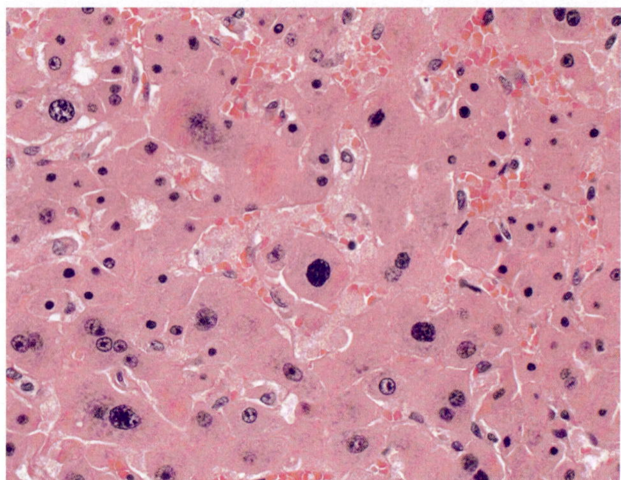

Figure 14.34. **Hepatic adenoma, androgen subtype.** The adenoma shows patchy cytological atypia in the form of large cell change.

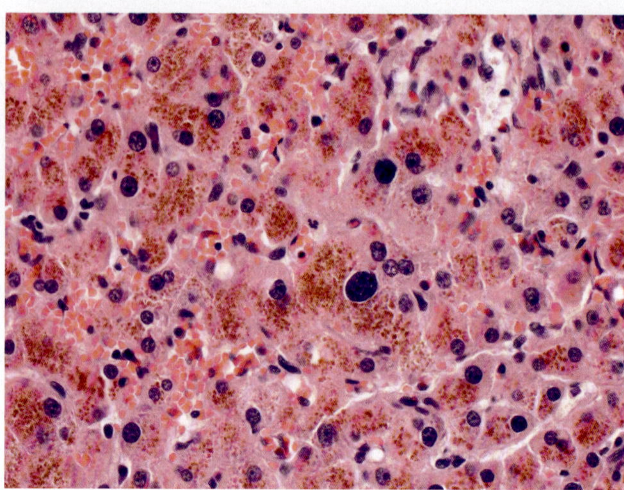

Figure 14.35. **Hepatic adenoma, pigmented subtype.** This adenoma showed diffuse, striking deposits of lipofuschin.

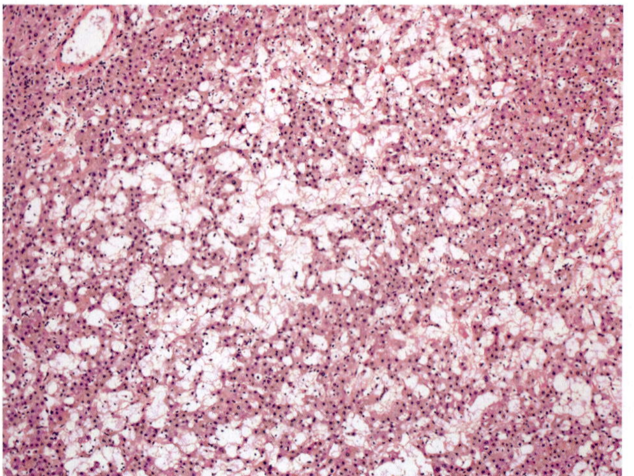

Figure 14.36. **Hepatic adenoma, myxoid subtype.** Myxoid material is seen dissecting through the tumor trabecula.

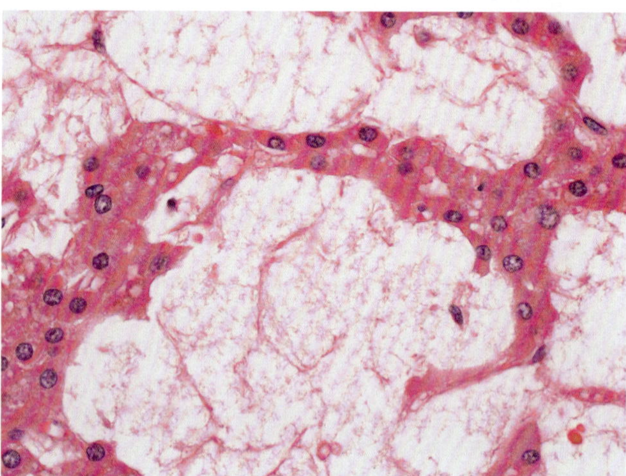

Figure 14.37. **Hepatic adenoma, myxoid subtype.** At high power, the myxoid material is loose and flocculent.

tissue/stromal mucin. The myxoid material is weakly Alcian blue positive, and sometimes weakly mucicarmine positive, but is not the true mucin of glandular differentiation. The material appears to dissect through the sinusoids on H&E, but endothelial stains suggest the material is mostly within a greatly expanded space of Disse or in other non-sinusoidal spaces (Fig. 14.38). By immunostain analysis, they have LFABP loss and can have HNF1A mutations. One of the earliest cases was described in the setting of the Carney complex,[50] so activation of protein kinase A pathways may be relevant to the pathogenesis, but at this point the molecular data underlying this tumor's distinctive morphology is unclear. In any case, they have a high risk for malignant transformation.

CONTROVERSY: Beta-Catenin Activation—a Secondary Event?

- Currently, beta-catenin–activated adenomas are given a separate subtype
- Another way to look at the data is that beta-catenin activation is not a separate subtype per se but instead a secondary event that can happen in any subtype of adenoma
    - The current data also support this alternative approach
- The same can be said for pigmented adenomas—probably a secondary event that can occur in any hepatic adenoma

CONTROVERSY: Should Clinical Etiology Plus Molecular Changes Be Used to Classify Adenomas, and Not Just Molecular Changes?

- The major etiologies for adenomas are excess estrogen, excess androgen, vascular diseases, glycogen storage disease, and other inherited metabolic diseases.
- Malignant potential may depend on both the underlying etiology and the molecular subtype, not just the molecular subtype.

MALIGNANT TRANSFORMATION

CHECKLIST: Risk Factors for Malignant Transformation of a Hepatic Adenoma

- ☐ Male gender
- ☐ Interval growth during follow-up by MRI
- ☐ Size >5 cm
- ☐ Beta-catenin activation
- ☐ Androgen as the underlying risk factor
- ☐ Pigmented adenoma
- ☐ Myxoid adenoma

Hepatic adenomas can undergo malignant transformation. The overall frequency of malignancy arising in an adenoma is hard to precisely determine but is probably less than 1%. However, in larger adenomas that undergo surgical resection, the frequency is close to 5%.[51] A diagnosis of malignancy is made in the same fashion as when there is no adenoma, using morphological findings and immunohistochemical stains. Overall, the histological findings for hepatocellular carcinomas that develop in hepatic adenomas are the same as they are for ordinary sporadic hepatocellular carciomas.[52]

There are two basic patterns of malignant transformation. In the first, a distinctive nodule of hepatocellular carcinoma is found within the adenoma itself (Fig. 14.39). The nodule of hepatocellular carcinoma shows higher grade cytology, increased proliferation, and reticulin loss. In the second pattern, there is patchy but definite reticulin loss, but with more diffuse and mild cytological atypia and no nodule-in-nodule growth. This latter pattern is more subtle and challenging to diagnosis and requires definite reticulin loss.

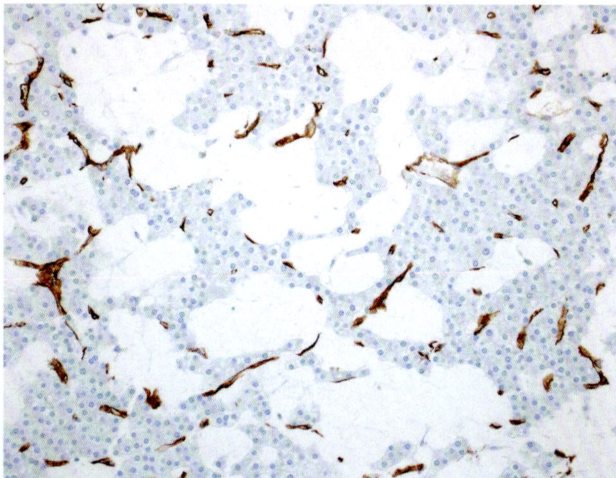

Figure 14.38. Hepatic adenoma, myxoid subtype, CD34 immunostain. The myxoid material does not seem to be in tumor sinusoids but instead may be in greatly expanded and distorted spaces of Disse.

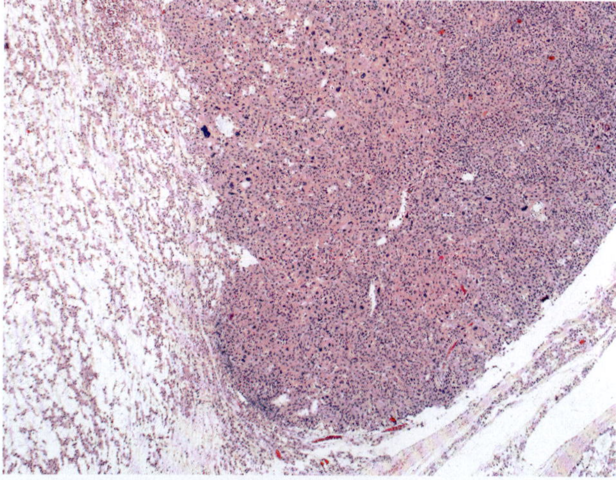

Figure 14.39. Hepatic adenoma, myxoid subtype, hepatocellular carcinoma. A large focus of hepatocellular carcinoma developed within this myxoid hepatic adenoma.

On resection specimens, if there is equivocal reticulin loss, it is helpful to stain several additional blocks. In biopsy specimens, it is helpful to repeat the reticulin stain and use additional stains such as Ki-67 and glypican 3. Glypican 3 is only helpful if it is positive, as well-differentiated hepatocellular carcinomas are frequently negative. Also, make sure to cross check with the H&E, as lipofuscin can also stain with glypican 3. When evaluating the reticulin stain, avoid areas with marked macrovesicular steatosis, as these areas can have patchy but striking physiological reticulin loss.

FAQ: How do you know for sure an adenoma underwent malignant transformation, when complete resection is curative in essentially all cases?

Answer:

- It is true that a complete resection is curative in essentially all cases of hepatic adenomas, including those adenomas that are thought to have underwent malignant transformation, so follow-up studies are largely noninformative on which tumors had the ability to behave aggressively.
- For the reason above, the approach is to follow the same criteria used for conventional hepatocellular carcinomas, where cytological, architectural, and immunohistochemical criteria of malignancy are better validated as evidence of malignancy.

NEAR MISSES

CASE 1. A 34-year-old woman had >10 liver tumors, one of which was biopsied because it was 7 cm. The biopsy was signed out as a hepatic adenoma by a young academic pathologist. Because of the size, the 7 cm tumor was resected, where it was evaluated by a different young academic pathologist and signed out as a focal nodular hyperplasia because of what was perceived as a maplike staining pattern on glutamine synthetase (Fig. 14.40). The case was subsequently reviewed at a radiology–pathology QA conference where the proper diagnosis of a hepatocellular adenoma was made.

This case illustrates several classic diagnostic pitfalls, all made by the pathologist who saw the resected specimen. First, the morphology in both the biopsy and the resected specimen was that of that of a hepatocellular adenoma (Fig. 14.41) and not a focal nodular hyperplasia, but this was ignored and the incorrect diagnosis of focal nodular hyperplasia

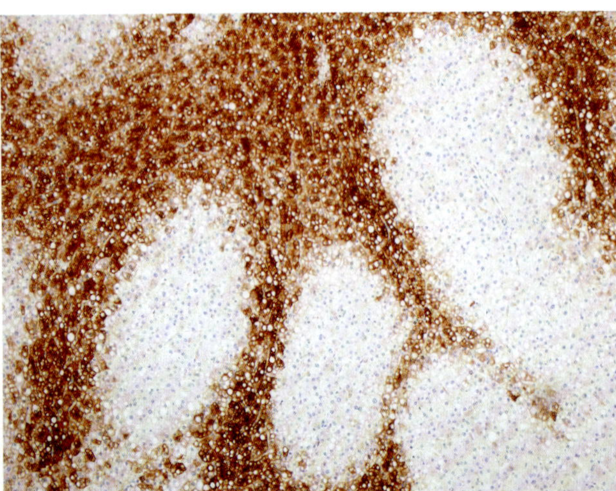

Figure 14.40. **Near miss case 1, glutamine synthetase with a pseudomap-like staining pattern in an hepatic adenoma.** This pseudomap-like staining pattern can mimic the maplike staining pattern of focal nodular hyperplasia.

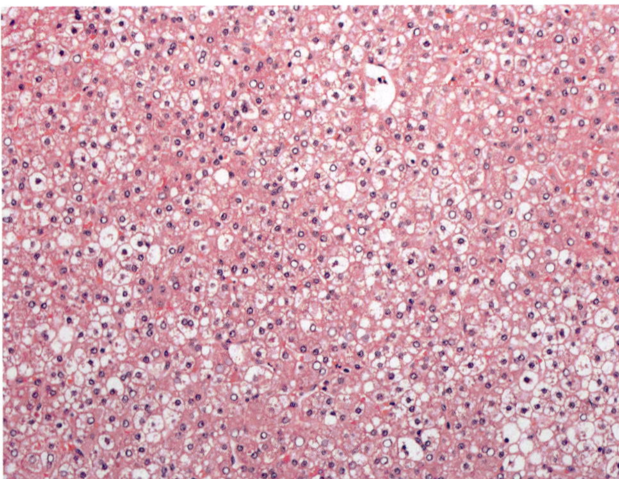

Figure 14.41. **Near miss case 1, hepatic adenoma.** This hepatic adenoma is unclassified, with no loss of LFABP and negative staining for C-reactive protein (CRP), serum amyloid A (SAA), and beta-catenin.

was rendered based on the glutamine immunostain alone. A diagnosis should never be based on immunostains alone and, in many cases, not on morphology alone. Instead, difficult cases are best approached using both together. If there are discrepancies, additional studies should be used to break the tie. To make matters worse, the glutamine synthetase stain was incorrectly interpreted, as it showed a psuedomap-like staining pattern and not a true maplike staining pattern. With a true maplike staining pattern, the areas that do not stain are the areas of scaring, ductular proliferation, and the hepatocytes immediately adjacent to the fibrous band. In this case, the areas of negative staining did not have those features.

Second, the pathologist who got the diagnosis wrong had shared it with a more senior gastrointestinal (GI) pathologist, but one who was largely unfamiliar with the subtleties of liver tumor pathology. This illustrates the importance of choosing who to seek consultation with for difficult cases. Depending on your practice, your options may be limited, but as much as possible it is best to share difficult cases with the pathologist in your group who is most experienced in that area, even if you would prefer to share cases with individuals with whom you are friendlier or whose office is closer. Sharing a case with a colleague on the basis of convenience, with the primary goal of documenting that it was a difficult case and having a second name on the report, can seem disingenuous when there are demonstrably greater experts in the group who could have been shown the case but were not. Such a practice should be avoided because it can lead to errors, as seen by this case.

Third, the clinical/imaging findings were known but were ignored. More than 10 focal nodular hyperplasias would be exceedingly rare, yet more than 10 hepatic adenomas are well known to occur in the setting of hepatic adenomatosis.

References

1. Marmorale C, Romiti M, Bearzi I, Giovagnoni A, Landi E. Traumatic rupture of nodular focal fatty infiltration of the liver: case report. *Ann Ital Chir*. 2003;74:217-221.
2. Berkelhammer C, Cuadros H, Blumstein A, Mesleh G, Patel M. Multifocal nodular nonalcoholic steatohepatitis: resolution with rosiglitazone. *Gastroenterol Hepatol (NY)*. 2007;3:196-198.
3. Karcaaltincaba M, Akhan O. Imaging of hepatic steatosis and fatty sparing. *Eur J Radiol*. 2007;61:33-43.
4. Osame A, Mitsufuji T, Kora S, Yoshimitsu K, Morihara D, Kunimoto H. Focal fatty change in the liver that developed after cholecystectomy. *World J Radiol*. 2014;6:932-936.
5. Tani M, Yamaue H, Oka M, et al. Focal fatty liver after pancreaticoduodenectomy: a case report of a rare entity of intrahepatic tumor. *Hepatogastroenterology*. 2002;49:1087-1089.
6. Zezos P, Tatsi P, Nakos A, et al. Focal fatty liver sparing lesion presenting as a "pseudotumour": case report. *Acta Gastroenterol Belg*. 2006;69:323-326.
7. Luciani A, Kobeiter H, Maison P, et al. Focal nodular hyperplasia of the liver in men: is presentation the same in men and women? *Gut*. 2002;50:877-880.
8. Nguyen BN, Flejou JF, Terris B, Belghiti J, Degott C. Focal nodular hyperplasia of the liver: a comprehensive pathologic study of 305 lesions and recognition of new histologic forms. *Am J Surg Pathol*. 1999;23:1441-1454.
9. Ibarrola C, Castellano VM, Colina F. Focal hyperplastic hepatocellular nodules in hepatic venous outflow obstruction: a clinicopathological study of four patients and 24 nodules. *Histopathology*. 2004;44:172-179.
10. Mathieu D, Kobeiter H, Maison P, et al. Oral contraceptive use and focal nodular hyperplasia of the liver. *Gastroenterology*. 2000;118:560-564.
11. Bouyn CI, Leclere J, Raimondo G, et al. Hepatic focal nodular hyperplasia in children previously treated for a solid tumor. Incidence, risk factors, and outcome. *Cancer*. 2003;97:3107-3113.
12. Freidl T, Lackner H, Huber J, et al. Focal nodular hyperplasia in children following treatment of hemato-oncologic diseases. *Klin Padiatr*. 2008;220:384-387.
13. Pillon M, Carucci NS, Mainardi C, et al. Focal nodular hyperplasia of the liver: an emerging complication of hematopoietic SCT in children. *Bone Marrow Transpl*. 2015;50:414-419.
14. Donadon M, Di Tommaso L, Roncalli M, Torzilli G. Multiple focal nodular hyperplasias induced by oxaliplatin-based chemotherapy. *World J Hepatol*. 2013;5:340-344.
15. Makhlouf HR, Abdul-Al HM, Goodman ZD. Diagnosis of focal nodular hyperplasia of the liver by needle biopsy. *Hum Pathol*. 2005;36:1210-1216.

16. Chandan VS, Shah SS, Mounajjed T, Torbenson MS, Wu TT. Copper deposition in focal nodular hyperplasia and inflammatory hepatocellular adenoma. *J Clin Pathol*. 2017;71.

17. Saxena R, Humphreys S, Williams R, Portmann B. Nodular hyperplasia surrounding fibrolamellar carcinoma: a zone of arterialized liver parenchyma. *Histopathology*. 1994;25:275-278.

18. Nault JC, Couchy G, Balabaud C, et al. Molecular classification of hepatocellular adenoma associates with risk factors, bleeding, and malignant transformation. *Gastroenterology*. 2017;152:880-894 e6.

19. Sakellariou S, Al-Hussaini H, Scalori A, et al. Hepatocellular adenoma in glycogen storage disorder type I: a clinicopathological and molecular study. *Histopathology*. 2012;60:E58-E65.

20. Nault JC, Fabre M, Couchy G, et al. GNAS-activating mutations define a rare subgroup of inflammatory liver tumors characterized by STAT3 activation. *J Hepatol*. 2012;56:184-191.

21. Sempoux C, Paradis V, Komuta M, et al. Hepatocellular nodules expressing markers of hepatocellular adenomas in Budd-Chiari syndrome and other rare hepatic vascular disorders. *J Hepatol*. 2015;63:1173-1180.

22. Chira RI, Calauz A, Manole S, Valean S, Mircea PA. Unusual discovery after an examination for abdominal pain: Abernethy 1b malformation and liver adenomatosis. A case report. *J Gastrointestin Liver Dis*. 2017;26:85-88.

23. Calderaro J, Nault JC, Balabaud C, et al. Inflammatory hepatocellular adenomas developed in the setting of chronic liver disease and cirrhosis. *Mod Pathol*. 2016;29:43-50.

24. Kumagawa M, Matsumoto N, Watanabe Y, et al. Contrast-enhanced ultrasonographic findings of serum amyloid A-positive hepatocellular neoplasm: does hepatocellular adenoma arise in cirrhotic liver? *World J Hepatol*. 2016;8:1110-1115.

25. Sasaki M, Yoneda N, Sawai Y, et al. Clinicopathological characteristics of serum amyloid A-positive hepatocellular neoplasms/nodules arising in alcoholic cirrhosis. *Histopathology*. 2015;66:836-845.

26. Sasaki M, Yoneda N, Kitamura S, Sato Y, Nakanuma Y. A serum amyloid A-positive hepatocellular neoplasm arising in alcoholic cirrhosis: a previously unrecognized type of inflammatory hepatocellular tumor. *Mod Pathol*. 2012;25:1584-1593.

27. Paradis V, Laurendeau I, Vidaud M, Bedossa P. Clonal analysis of macronodules in cirrhosis. *Hepatology*. 1998;28:953-958.

28. European Association for the Study of the L. EASL clinical practice guidelines on the management of benign liver tumours. *J Hepatol*. 2016;65:386-398.

29. Marrero JA, Ahn J, Rajender Reddy K, Americal College of G. ACG clinical guideline: the diagnosis and management of focal liver lesions. *Am J Gastroenterol*. 2014;109:1328-1347; quiz 48.

30. Volmar KE, Burchette JL, Creager AJ. Hepatic adenomatosis in glycogen storage disease type Ia: report of a case with unusual histology. *Arch Pathol Lab Med*. 2003;127:e402-e405.

31. Bianchi L. Glycogen storage disease I and hepatocellular tumours. *Eur J Pediatr*. 1993;152 suppl 1:S63-S70.

32. Singhi AD, Jain D, Kakar S, Wu TT, Yeh MM, Torbenson M. Reticulin loss in benign fatty liver: an important diagnostic pitfall when considering a diagnosis of hepatocellular carcinoma. *Am J Surg Pathol*. 2012;36:710-715.

33. Jones A, Mounajjed T, Torbenson M, Moreira R. Hepar-1 loss in telangiectatic/inflammatory hepatic adenomas – a novel observation with potential tumor biology implications. In: *Abstract 1665, Presented at the 2016 United States and Canadian Academy of Pathology*. 2016;413-429. Modern Pathology; vol. 29.

34. Liu L, Shah SS, Naini BV, et al. Immunostains used to subtype hepatic adenomas do not distinguish hepatic adenomas from hepatocellular carcinomas. *Am J Surg Pathol*. 2016;40:1062-1069.

35. Bedossa P, Burt AD, Brunt EM, et al. Well-differentiated hepatocellular neoplasm of uncertain malignant potential: proposal for a new diagnostic category. *Hum Pathol*. 2014;45:658-660.

36. Bluteau O, Jeannot E, Bioulac-Sage P, et al. Bi-allelic inactivation of TCF1 in hepatic adenomas. *Nat Genet*. 2002;32:312-315.

37. Stueck AE, Qu Z, Huang MA, Camprecios G, Ferrell LD, Thung SN. Hepatocellular carcinoma arising in an HNF-1alpha-mutated adenoma in a 23-year-old woman with maturity-onset diabetes of the young: a case report. *Semin Liver Dis*. 2015;35:444-449.

38. Bioulac-Sage P, Rebouissou S, Thomas C, et al. Hepatocellular adenoma subtype classification using molecular markers and immunohistochemistry. *Hepatology*. 2007;46:740-748.

39. Paradis V, Champault A, Ronot M, et al. Telangiectatic adenoma: an entity associated with increased body mass index and inflammation. *Hepatology*. 2007;46:140-146.

40. Bioulac-Sage P, Rebouissou S, Sa Cunha A, et al. Clinical, morphologic, and molecular features defining so-called telangiectatic focal nodular hyperplasias of the liver. *Gastroenterology*. 2005;128:1211-1218.

41. Rebouissou S, Franconi A, Calderaro J, et al. Genotype-phenotype correlation of CTNNB1 mutations reveals different ss-catenin activity associated with liver tumor progression. *Hepatology*. 2016;64:2047-2061.

42. Hale G, Liu X, Hu J, et al. Correlation of exon 3 beta-catenin mutations with glutamine synthetase staining patterns in hepatocellular adenoma and hepatocellular carcinoma. *Mod Pathol*. 2016;29:1370-1380.

43. Henriet E, Hammoud AA, Dupuy JW, et al. Argininosuccinate synthase 1 (ASS1): a marker of unclassified hepatocellular adenoma and high bleeding risk. *Hepatology*. 2017;66.

44. Gupta S, Naini BV, Munoz R, et al. Hepatocellular neoplasms arising in association with androgen use. *Am J Surg Pathol*. 2016;40:454-461.

45. Mounajjed T, Yasir S, Aleff PA, Torbenson MS. Pigmented hepatocellular adenomas have a high risk of atypia and malignancy. *Mod Pathol*. 2015;28:1265-1274.

46. Souza LN, de Martino RB, Thompson R, Strautnieks S, Heaton ND, Quaglia A. Pigmented well-differentiated hepatocellular neoplasm with beta-catenin mutation. *Hepatobiliary Pancreat Dis Int*. 2015;14:660-664.

47. Hechtman JF, Raoufi M, Fiel MI, et al. Hepatocellular carcinoma arising in a pigmented telangiectatic adenoma with nuclear beta-catenin and glutamine synthetase positivity: case report and review of the literature. *Am J Surg Pathol*. 2011;35:927-932.

48. Salaria SN, Graham RP, Aishima S, Mounajjed T, Yeh MM, Torbenson MS. Primary hepatic tumors with myxoid change: morphologically unique hepatic adenomas and hepatocellular carcinomas. *Am J Surg Pathol*. 2015;39:318-324.

49. Young JT, Kurup AN, Graham RP, Torbenson MS, Venkatesh SK. Myxoid hepatocellular neoplasms: imaging appearance of a unique mucinous tumor variant. *Abdom Radiol (NY)*. 2016;41.

50. Terracciano LM, Tornillo L, Avoledo P, Von Schweinitz D, Kuhne T, Bruder E. Fibrolamellar hepatocellular carcinoma occurring 5 years after hepatocellular adenoma in a 14-year-old girl: a case report with comparative genomic hybridization analysis. *Arch Pathol Lab Med*. 2004;128:222-226.

51. Stoot JH, Coelen RJ, De Jong MC, Dejong CH. Malignant transformation of hepatocellular adenomas into hepatocellular carcinomas: a systematic review including more than 1600 adenoma cases. *HPB (Oxford)*. 2010;12:509-522.

52. Micchelli ST, Vivekanandan P, Boitnott JK, Pawlik TM, Choti MA, Torbenson M. Malignant transformation of hepatic adenomas. *Mod Pathol*. 2008;21:491-497.

MALIGNANT HEPATOCELLULAR TUMORS AND PRECUSORS 15

CHAPTER OUTLINE

MACROREGENERATIVE NODULE

CHECKLIST: Macroregenerative Nodules

- ☐ Benign
- ☐ Stand out from background liver by size (>10 mm) and often by gross appearance
- ☐ Three big No's: No more cytological than seen in the background liver, No reticulin loss, No increased proliferation
- ☐ Can be challenging to separate from ordinary cirrhotic nodule on liver biopsy

Macroregenerative nodules occur in two settings: following massive liver necrosis[1] and in cirrhosis. In both cases, larger nodules develop that stand out from the background liver (Fig. 15.1). In cirrhotic livers, they stand out from the background nodular parenchyma because they are larger than adjacent nodules. Macroregenerative nodules average about 15 mm in size. They can also stand out from the background liver because of differences in color or texture. The overall frequency in cirrhotic livers is about 25%,[2,3] but the frequency varies a lot depending on what criteria are used. Most are between 10 and 20 mm,[2,3] but sometimes they can be several cm. They are single (1/3 of cases) or multifocal (2/3 of cases). When multifocal, most cases show less than 5 macroregenerative nodules, but rarely there can be more. A definite diagnosis of macroregenerative nodule is usually made on a wedge biopsy or resection specimen; a definite diagnosis is not confidently made on needle biopsy in most cases because of concerns that the lesion may not have been adequately sampled.

On histological examination, the hepatocytes in the nodule should look the same as the hepatocytes in the background liver, with no cytological atypia beyond that seen in the background liver. The N:C ratio is preserved (Fig. 15.2). Macroregenerative nodules can show large cell change when the background liver does so, but there should be no small cell change and no nodule-within-nodule architecture. They have portal tracts within the nodule (Fig. 15.2), often with mild nonspecific inflammation. They have an intact reticulin framework, are negative for glypican 3, and have a proliferation rate similar to that of the background liver.

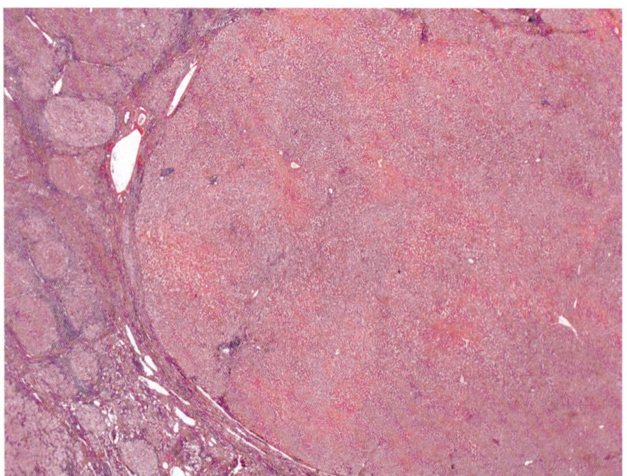

Figure 15.1. Macroregenerative nodule. At low power, a nodule stands out from the background cirrhotic liver.

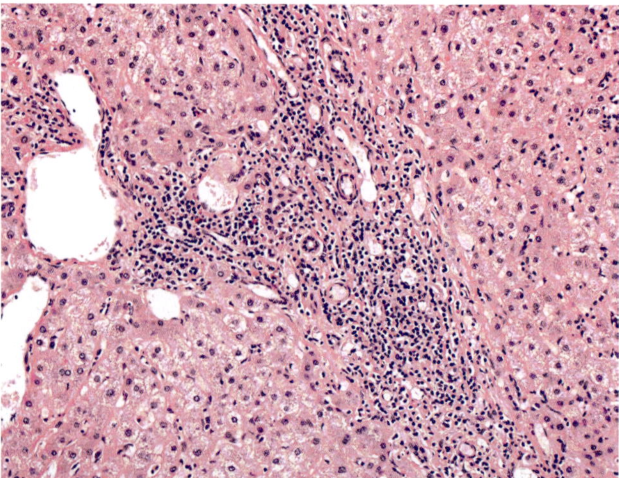

Figure 15.2. Macroregenerative nodule. There is no cytological atypia. A portal tract is present.

DYSPLASTIC NODULE

CHECKLIST: Dysplastic Nodule

- ☐ Nodules in cirrhotic livers that have more atypia than the background liver but do not reach the full criteria for hepatocellular carcinoma
- ☐ Classified as low grade or high grade depending on the degree of atypia
- ☐ Some dysplastic nodules will progress to hepatocellular carcinoma, high-grade dysplastic nodules in particular

A diagnosis of a dysplastic nodule is made for the most part on fully removed lesions. In a biopsy specimen, the findings can of course be consistent with a dysplastic nodule, but a firm diagnosis depends on adequate sampling of the lesion to fully exclude hepatocellular carcinoma. Although data are limited largely to dysplastic nodules in the setting of chronic viral hepatitis, there is good evidence that dysplastic nodules are precursors to hepatocellular carcinoma, with approximately 10% of low-grade nodules and 30% of high-grade nodules progressing to hepatocellular carcinoma within 2 to 3 years.[4–6]

Dysplastic nodules show more atypia than the background liver but do not have the full criteria for hepatocellular carcinoma. Dysplastic nodules are further divided based on their degree of atypia into low-grade and high-grade dysplastic nodules. The line that divides a macrorogenerative nodule from a low-grade dysplastic nodule, or a low-grade dysplastic nodule from a high-grade dysplastic nodule, is not always sharp and bright, so there tends to be fair amount of subjectivity in certain cases, but the overall approach works reasonably well. Low-grade dysplastic nodules show mild cytological atypia but more than the background liver. The cytological atypia can include mild nuclear pleomorphism, mild changes in the N:C ratio, and pseudoglands (Fig. 15.3). Low-grade dysplastic nodules frequently have portal tracts within the nodule and have occasional aberrant lobular arteries. They often have large cell change but do not have small cell change. High-grade dysplastic nodules may or may not have more cytological atypia than low-grade nodules but have only rare residual portal tracts and more frequent aberrant arteries and may have either small cell or large cell change. Psuedoglands are also common.

In both low-grade and high-grade dysplastic nodules, the Ki-67 proliferative rate is similar to the background liver, and there is no reticulin loss. Both are negative for AFP and for beta-catenin nuclear accumulation. Glypican 3 is usually negative but can show patchy or focal staining in high-grade dysplastic nodules (Fig. 15.4). Strong and diffuse glypican 3 staining strongly suggests hepatocellular carcinoma. Strong and diffuse staining

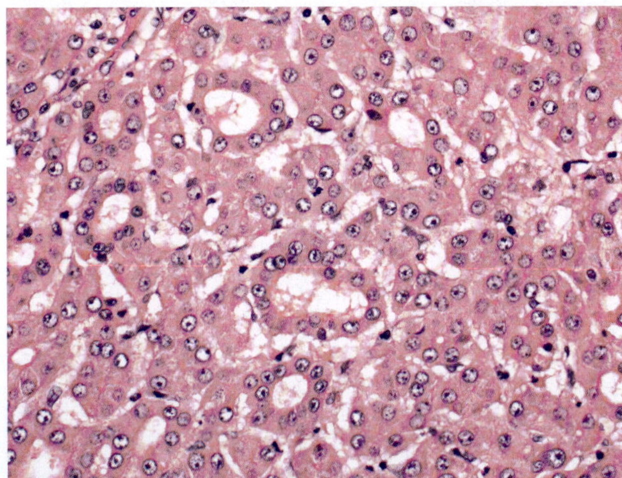

Figure 15.3. **Dysplastic nodule, high grade.** This nodule showed mild cytological atypia and scattered foci of psuedoglands. There was not cytological atypia, and the Ki-67 was similar to the background liver.

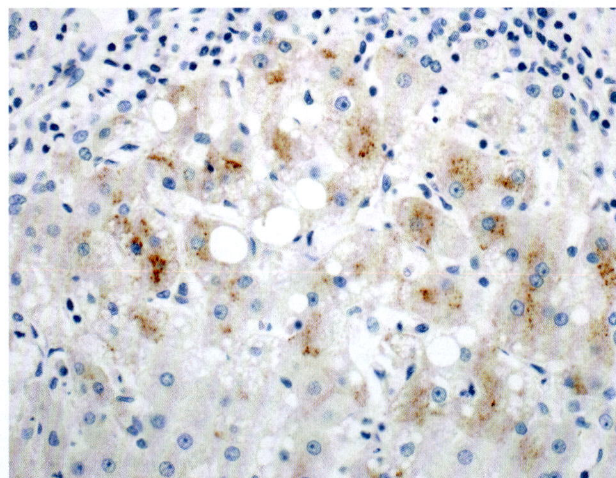

Figure 15.4. **Dysplastic nodule, glypican 3.** This high-grade dysplastic nodule showed focal glypican 3 staining.

for glutamine synthetase would also favor hepatocellular carcinoma over a dysplastic nodule. Finally, the finding called *stromal invasion* strongly suggests hepatocellular carcinoma.[7–9] Stromal invasion was initially defined as malignant cells invading the stroma of the portal tracts or fibrous bands surrounding a nodule (Fig. 15.5). In practice, stromal invasion is rarely evident on H&E in well-differentiated hepatocellular carcinomas, so the definition of stromal invasion has been expanded to include the lack of a bile ductular proliferation at the edges of a nodule. In cirrhotic livers, the fibrous bands surrounding cirrhotic nodules invariably have a subtle bile ductular proliferation, which can be highlighted by either CK7 or CK19 immunostains (Fig. 15.6). Dysplastic nodules retain this finding, while hepatocellular carcinomas do not (Fig. 15.7), and CK7 or CK19 stains will demonstrate an absence of bile ductules.[10] The use of these stains on biopsies is not as reliable because of sampling issues, especially with the smaller needles used today at most centers. This approach also has not been validated in biopsy specimens. For this reason, these stains should not be the sole basis, or even the major reason, for either confirming or excluding a diagnosis of hepatocellular carcinoma on biopsies. Nonetheless, they work very well with resections, wedge biopsies, and even sometimes in biopsies with lots of tissue.

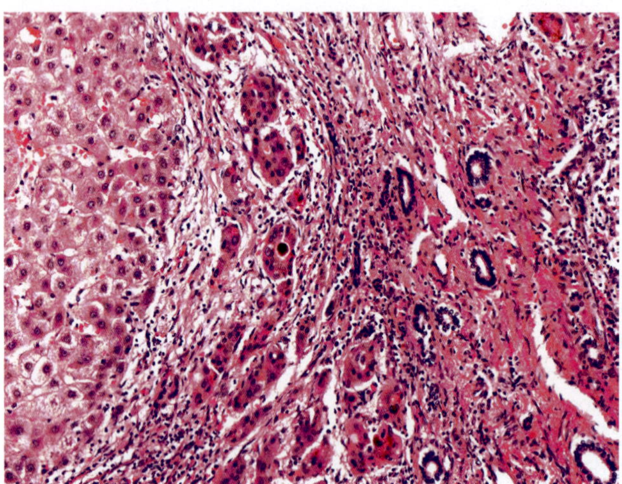

Figure 15.5. **Hepatocellular carcinoma, stromal invasion.** There are malignant tumor cells extending along the portal tracts and septal spaces. The main tumor mass was located immediately below this image.

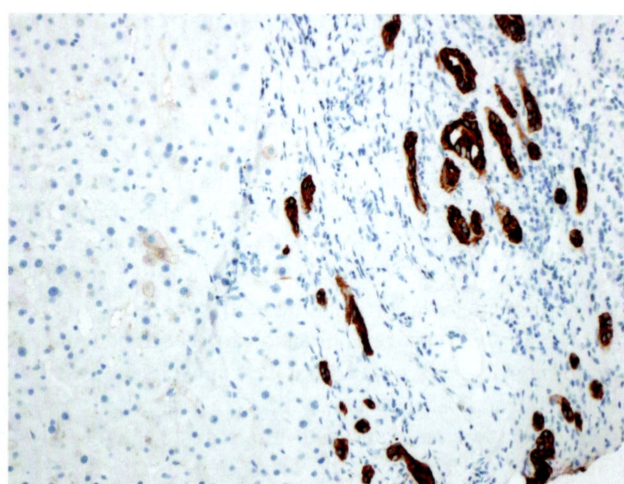

Figure 15.6. **Negative for stromal invasion, CK7.** In this biopsy, a ductular proliferation is seen next to benign cirrhotic nodules.

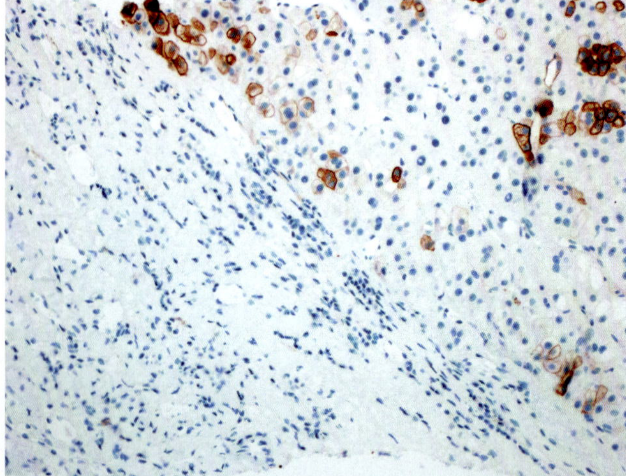

Figure 15.7. **Stromal invasion, CK7.** In this biopsy, a focus of well-differentiated hepatocellular carcinoma shows occasional positive tumor cells, but a ductular reaction is absent.

HEPATOCELLULAR CARCINOMA

CHECKLIST: Hepatocellular Carcinoma Overview

- ☐ Male predominance
- ☐ Average age 65 years
- ☐ Risk factor: cirrhosis from any cause, but common etiologies include alcohol, chronic viral hepatitis B and C, and nonalcohol fatty liver disease
- ☐ Cirrhosis is present in about 80% of cases
- ☐ Diagnosis is based on histological findings plus immunohistochemical stains

Hepatocellular carcinomas have identifiable risk factors in about 80% of cases, but having one of these risk factors, and even having advanced fibrosis, do not prove a specific tumor is hepatocellular carcinoma. For example, metastatic carcinomas, especially from the gastrointestinal (GI) tract are not rare in cirrhotic livers (Fig. 15.8).[11] On the other hand, about 20% of hepatocellular carcinomas arise in livers without advanced fibrosis or cirrhosis. Some of these tumors will have identifiable risk factors, the most common being chronic viral hepatitis B,[12] viral hepatitis C,[13] or fatty liver disease,[14,15] but about half will not.

HOW TO MAKE THE DIAGNOSIS OF HEPATOCELLULAR CARCINOMA

The first step is to find the tumor. This is usually the easiest step but can be challenging with well-differentiated tumors. For well-differentiated tumors, start by identifying the background liver and then look for areas of the biopsy that have loss of the normal portal tracts (Fig. 15.9) and cytological differences with the background liver, such as greater nuclear atypia, prominent nucleoli, increased N:C ratio, or changes in the cytoplasmic appearance, such as clear cell change, more or less fat than the background liver, or more or less lipofuscin than the background liver (Fig. 15.10). Aberrant or naked arteries (arteries located in the lobules) are common in hepatocellular carcinoma in many cases (Fig. 15.11). However, they are not specific for a neoplasm, also being found in diseased but nontumor liver, so should not be used in isolation.

PEARLS & PITFALLS

There are a couple of important pitfalls to know about, ones that are somewhat underappreciated by many pathologists.

- First, aberrant arteries are not specific for a tumor and can be found in a variety of liver diseases that do not have tumors. The most common situation, but by no means the only the one, is livers with steatohepatitis and advanced fibrosis, where aberrant lobular arteries are common. Vascular disease is another important setting (Fig. 15.12).
- A second pitfall is that aberrant arteries say nothing about the nature of the hepatic tumor, being present in focal nodular hyperplasia, adenomas, macroregenerative nodules, dysplastic nodules, and hepatocellular carcinomas.

Although these pitfalls remain stubbornly persistent points of confusion, the good thing is that you can readily verify the two points above yourself, probably over the next few weeks to months of sign-out, if you care to, and have enough liver specimens in your practice. If not, then at least these observations are well published in both books and the peer-reviewed literature and hopefully will help pathologists avoid these pitfalls.

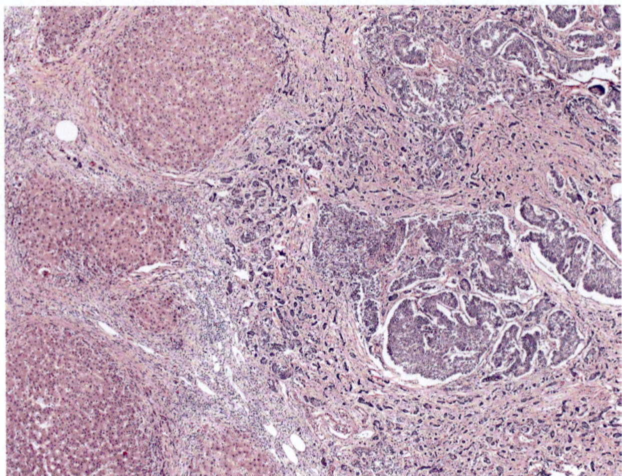

Figure 15.8. **Metastatic carcinoma to a cirrhotic liver.** A neuroendocrine carcinoma metastasized to a cirrhotic liver.

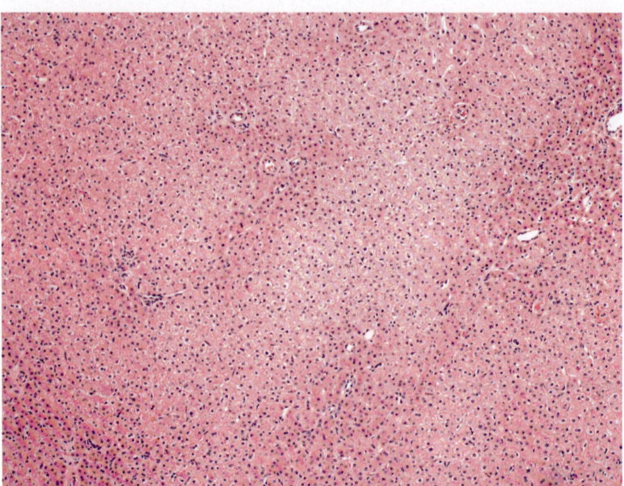

Figure 15.9. **Absence of portal tracts.** The lack of portal tracts helps identify this area as being part of the tumor.

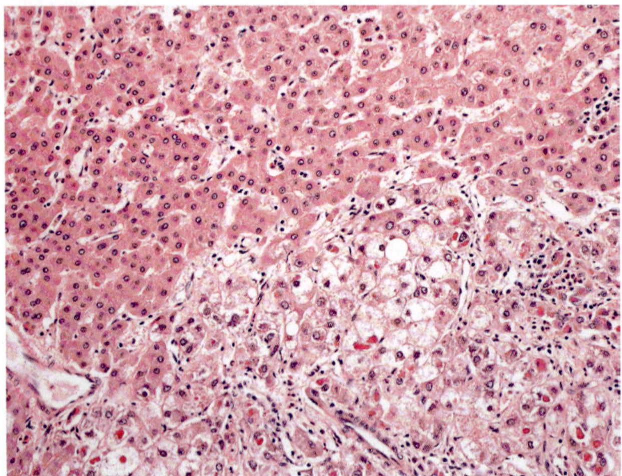

Figure 15.10. **Differences in morphology.** At low power, the hepatocellular carcinoma, but not the background liver, shows cell swelling and Mallory hyaline.

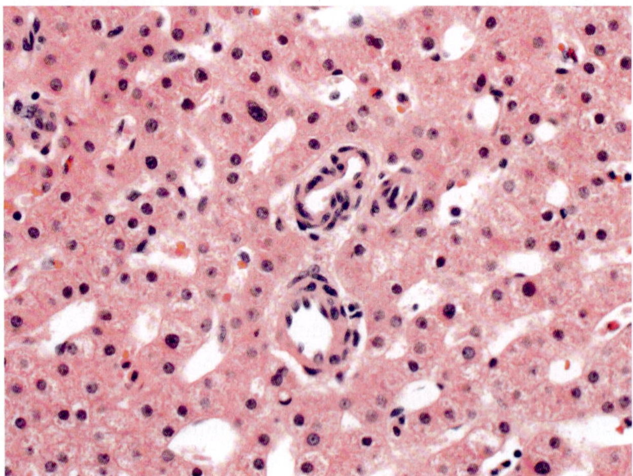

Figure 15.11. **Hepatocellular carcinoma, naked artery.** This finding is not specific for a tumor but can be helpful when parts of the biopsy have naked arteries and other parts do not. Naked arteries can be found in all benign and malignant hepatic proliferations including focal nodular hyperplasia, hepatic adenomas, macroregenerative nodules, dysplastic nodules, and hepatocellular carcinomas.

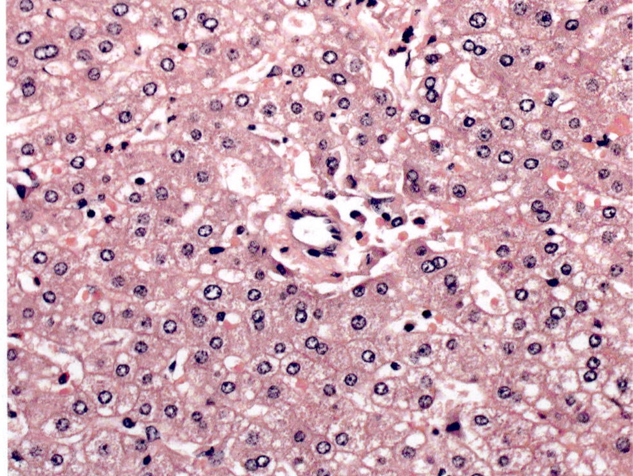

Figure 15.12. **Portal vein thrombosis with hepatoportal sclerosis and naked artery.** Scattered small lobular arterioles were present, even though there was no tumor.

Sometimes stains can help identify the tumor, such as keratin stains that will highlight the bile ducts in the background liver but not the tumor, CD34, which can show a normal zone 1 staining pattern in the background liver but an abnormal diffuse or patchy cytoplasmic staining in the tumor, or a glutamine synthetase that normally shows a zone 3 staining pattern in the background liver but can show abnormal patchy or diffuse staining patterns in tumors. These stains will not distinguish an adenoma from a hepatocellular carcinoma but can help identify the tumor itself in difficult cases that show very well-differentiated morophology.

Once you know where the tumor is on the biopsy, then stains can be used to (1) confirm hepatic differentiation (Table 15.1) (2) distinguish hepatocellular carcinoma from benign liver lesions (Table 15.2). Stains for hepatic differentiation are not always needed, but some tumors can closely mimic hepatocellular carcinomas (Fig. 15.13), such as metastatic neuroendocrine tumors, metastatic paragangliomas, adrenal cortical carcinomas, and renal oncocytic neoplasms, so markers of hepatic differentiation are important to perform in most cases. The best of these stains are HepPar and Arginase, with the caveat that arginase can be negative in approximately 5% of well-differentiated hepatocellular carcinomas,[16] especially if your laboratory is using a monoclonal antibody.

TABLE 15.1: Stains Used for Demonstrating Hepatic Differentiation

Stains	Comment
Arginase 1	• Stains benign and malignant hepatocytes • Staining pattern: cytoplasmic or nuclear staining • Staining distribution: can be patchy or diffuse • Staining intensity: strong and bright • Positive in 90% of hepatocellular carcinomas • Arginase can be negative at both ends of the differentiation spectrum: well or poorly differentiated
HepPar1	• Stains benign and malignant hepatocytes • Staining pattern: cytoplasmic • Staining distribution: can be patchy or diffuse • Staining intensity: strong and bright • Positive in 80% to 90% of hepatocellular carcinomas • Negative cases are usually poorly differentiated

Glypican 3	• Stains malignant hepatocytes
	  • Benign hepatocytes can rarely show focal staining when there is lots of inflammation
	  • High-grade dysplastic nodules can show focal staining
	• Staining pattern: cytoplasmic
	• Staining distribution: can be patchy or diffuse
	• Staining intensity: strong and bright
	• Positive in 70% to 90% of hepatocellular carcinomas
	• 50% of well-differentiated hepatocellular carcinomas are negative
	• Major pitfall 1: can also stain lipofuscin
	• Major pitfall 2: rarely benign hepatocytes can be positive when there is marked inflammation

In situ hybridization for albumin	• Stains benign and malignant hepatocytes • Staining pattern: cytoplasmic • Staining distribution: usually diffuse • Staining intensity: strong and bright • Positive in >95% of hepatocellular carcinomas • Major pitfall: positive in 80% to 95% of cholangiocarcinomas

(Continued)

TABLE 15.1: Stains Used for Demonstrating Hepatic Differentiation (Continued)

Stains	Comment
Polyclonal CEA and CD10	• Stains benign and malignant hepatocytes • Staining pattern: canalicular, cytoplasmic, membranous • Only the canalicular pattern supports hepatic differentiation; other patterns are fine for HCC, but not specific • Staining distribution: diffuse in well-differentiated tumors, patchy to focal to negative in poorly differentiated tumors • Staining intensity: strong to weak • Positive in 60% to 80% of hepatocellular carcinomas

Alpha-fetoprotein	• Stains malignant hepatocytes
	• Staining pattern: cytoplasmic
	• Staining distribution: more often patchy than diffuse
	• Staining intensity: strong and bright
	• Positive in about one-third of hepatocellular carcinomas
	  • Not very sensitive, but can still be helpful in poorly differentiated tumors negative for other hepatic markers
	  • Positive in all cases of the macrotrabecular variant of hepatocellular carcinoma
	• Major pitfall 1: background staining is common and can make stains hard to interpret, if background liver is not present
	• Major pitfall 2: yolk sac tumors

TABLE 15.2: Stains Used to Distinguish Benign From Malignant Hepatic Lesions

Stain	Comment
Reticulin	• This is the most important stain, but there are several caveats. First, avoid fatty areas, which can have physiological reticulin loss. Second, there are rare well-differentiated hepatocellular carcinomas (<1%) that do not have definite reticulin loss.
Ki-67	• To use this stain, compare the background liver with the tumor. To be informative, the tumor staining should be significantly higher than the background liver staining. • Not all hepatocellular carcinomas have a proliferative rate higher than the background liver (at least on visual examination), so the diagnosis can be made based on other findings, even if Ki-67 is not elevated.
Glypican 3	• The stain is positive in about 50% of well-differentiated hepatocellular carcinomas, so is not informative if it is negative. There can also be focal staining in some high-grade dysplastic nodules. • Lipofuschin can also stain positive. Lipofuschin can be found in both benign and malignant tumors, so correlation with the H&E findings is important.
Alpha-fetoprotein	• One-third of hepatocellular carcinomas are positive, with a greater frequency of positivity in hepatocellular carcinomas that develop in cirrhotic livers and in hepatocellular carcinomas that are poorly differentiated.

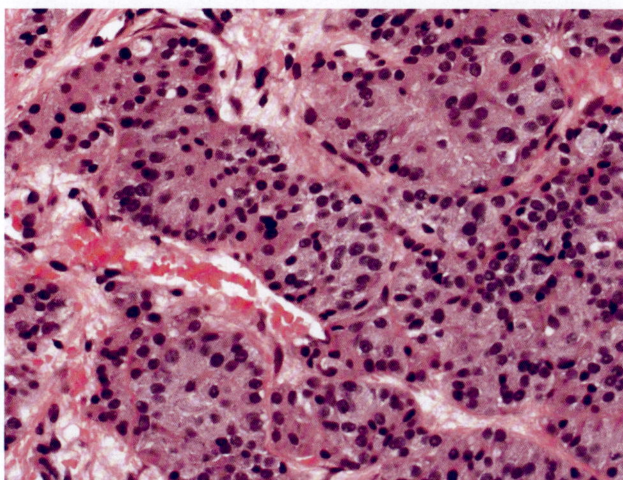

Figure 15.13. **Metastatic neuroendocrine tumor, mimicking hepatocellular carcinoma.** The tumor cells have abundant eosinophilic cytoplasm and are growing in trabeculae.

Once you have found the tumor and are sure it shows hepatic differentiation, then the next step is to distinguish benign tumors from hepatocellular carcinoma. In noncirrhotic livers, the differential might include focal nodular hyperplasia and hepatic adenomas. In cirrhotic livers, the differential can include macroregenerative nodules and dysplastic nodules. A useful starting panel of stains is the reticulin stain, Ki-67, and glypican 3. If these stains exclude hepatocellular carcinoma, then proceed to distinguish an adenoma from a focal nodular hyperplasia in noncirrhotic livers and a macroregenerative nodule from a dysplastic nodule in cirrhotic livers.

The starting panel of stains (reticulin stain, Ki-67, and glypican 3) will confirm hepatocellular carcinoma if there is convincing loss of reticulin. Strong and diffuse glypican 3 staining also indicates hepatocellular carcinoma. A Ki-67 that is significantly above the background liver also favors malignancy. Stains are best interpreted in association with the H&E findings, so it can be useful to flip back and forth between the H&E and the special stains on a regular basis when evaluating difficult cases. In those biopsies with many tiny fragments, it is often helpful to use an ink pen and mark the tumor on the H&E slide and then transfer those same marks to the special stain slides.

In contrast to the discussion above, in many cases, the tumor is obviously carcinoma by H&E and stains are needed to decide between hepatocellular carcinoma, cholangiocarcinoma, and metastatic disease. In these cases, stains for hepatic differentiation are used to rule in hepatocellular carcinoma (Table 15.1). Reticulin and Ki-67 stains will not be needed.

EVALUATING THE RETICULIN STAIN

Hepatocellular carcinomas are characterized by reticulin loss. Although the biology behind this observation is not clear, it has been the backbone of morphology-based diagnosis for decades. In the normal liver, in focal nodular hyperplasia, and in hepatic adenomas, the reticulin stain outlines hepatic trabecula that are about one or two hepatocytes thick (Fig. 15.14), with each hepatocyte touching the reticulin fibers on at least one of their membranes. In rapidly regenerating livers, the trabeculae can be focally thicker, up to three to four cells (Fig. 15.15). However, in hepatocellular carcinomas there is a definite reduction in the reticulin network (Figs. 15.16 and 15.17). While the reticulin network is almost never entirely absent, there will be numerous areas of reduced reticulin, leaving scattered clusters of tumor cells or large areas of tumor cells that are not in contact with reticulin fibers. An additional abnormal pattern can be present in both benign and malignant tumor cells, with tumor cells in some areas being individually surrounded by reticulin fibers—a pattern that seems to be somewhat more common in areas of tumor congestion.

PEARLS & PITFALLS: On Using the Reticulin Stain

There are several important pitfalls when using the reticulin stain. First, the reticulin stain can be technically suboptimal, so it is very important to examine the normal liver and make sure it has a strongly staining intact reticulin framework, whenever there is normal tissue on the biopsy. A clue that the stain is not working is if the edges of the biopsy show reticulin loss that is not evident in the middle of the biopsy. In addition, complete absence of reticulin staining is unusual, even for poorly differentiated hepatocellular carcinomas, and the stain should be repeated.

Second, there is physiological, normal reticulin reduction in areas of fatty change, even in the nontumor liver (Fig. 15.18).[17] This reticulin reduction tends to be focal but can complicate interpretation of reticulin stains in well-differentiated tumors. In these cases, it is best to examine the reticulin in areas of the tumor that do not have steatosis or to hold out for reasonably extensive reticulin loss.

Third, well-differentiated hepatocellular carcinomas (less than 1%) will rarely have a normal reticulin staining pattern on liver biopsy, often those with significant intratumoral fibrosis. In these cases, the diagnosis of hepatocellular carcinoma is made by the presence of more cytological atypia than is acceptable for a benign tumor, a proliferative rate that is significantly above the background liver, and/or abnormal staining for glypican 3 or AFP.

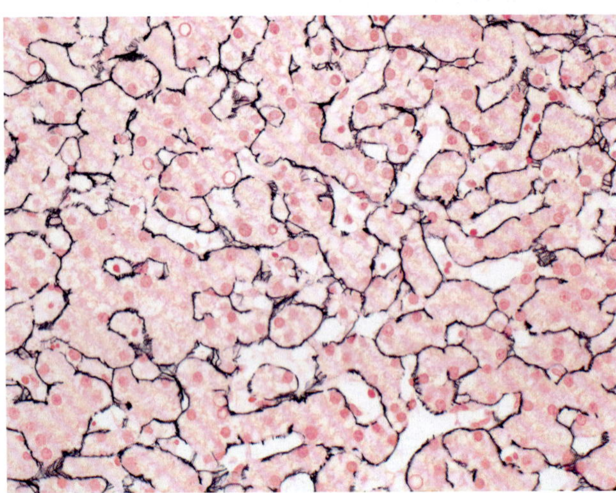

Figure 15.14. **Hepatic adenoma, reticulin stain.** There is mild variation in the thickness of the cell plates, but there is no loss of reticulin.

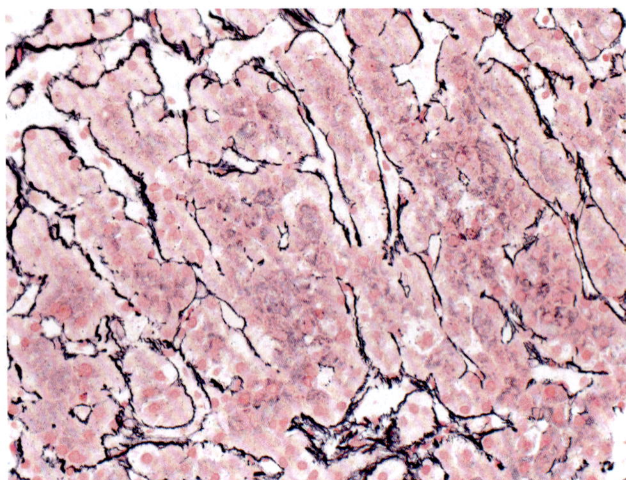

Figure 15.15. **Benign liver, reticulin stain.** This liver had rapid regeneration after an episode of acute hepatic vein thrombosis (Budd–Chiari). The hepatic plates were focally thickened 2-3 cells in thickness.

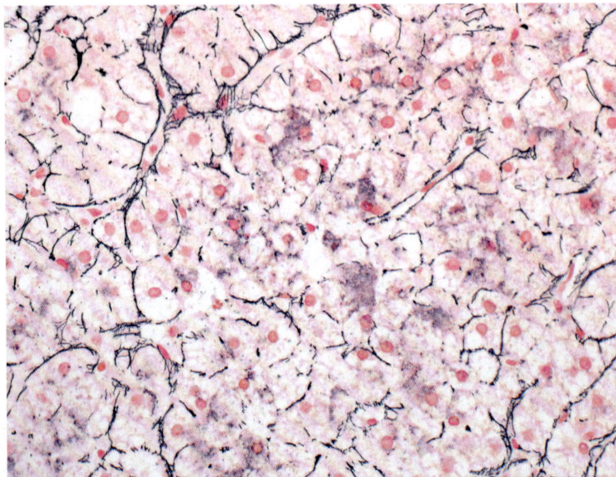

Figure 15.16. **Hepatocellular carcinoma, reticulin stain.** There is loss of reticulin, with many tumor cells not touching the reticulin framework on any of their sides.

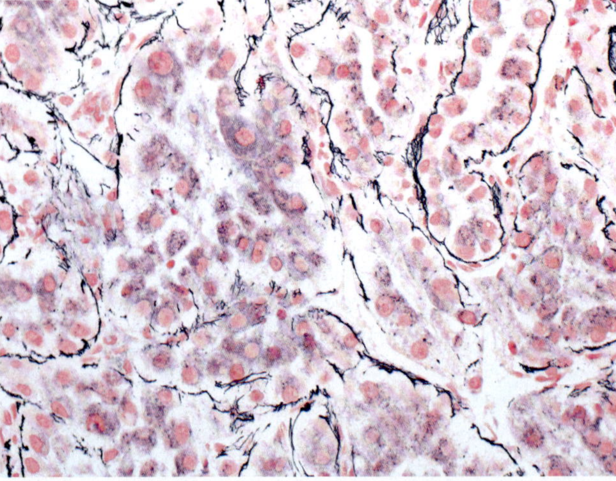

Figure 15.17. **Hepatocellular carcinoma, reticulin stain.** Another example of reticulin loss in hepatocellular carcinoma.

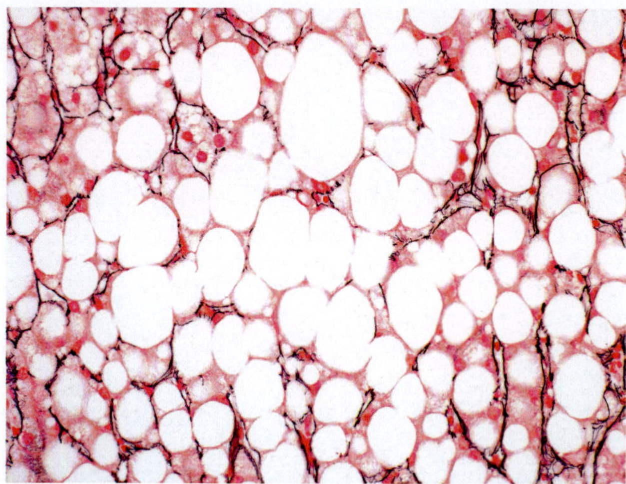

Figure 15.18. **Benign liver with macrovesicular steatosis, reticulin stain.** This is a medical biopsy performed to grade and stage fatty liver disease. There is no mass lesion or tumor. Note that the reticulin loss can focally reach the levels seen in hepatocellular carcinoma.

GROWTH PATTERNS

CHECKLIST: H&E Tumor Findings

- ☐ Four major histological growth patterns for hepatocellular carcinoma: trabecular (70%), solid (20%), pseudoglandular (10%), and macrotrabecular (1%)
- ☐ About 12 recognized histological variants
- ☐ Other findings
  - ○ Nodule-within-nodule growth
  - ○ Peliosis
  - ○ Bile production
  - ○ Clusters of foamy macrophages in tumor sinusoids
  - ○ Hyaline bodies
  - ○ Pale bodies
  - ○ Intratumoral inflammation and/or fibrosis
  - ○ Fat or glycogen accumulation in tumor cells

Hepatocellular carcinomas have four major histological growth patterns (Figs. 15.19–15.23): trabecular (70%), solid (also known as compact, 20%), pseudoglandular (also known as pseudoacinar, 10%), and macrotrabecular (1%). These growth patterns are defined by H&E findings without the use of special stains. Multiple growth patterns are common within any given tumor, with about ½ of resected hepatocellular carcinomas showing two or more growth patterns. In most studies, a minimum cutoff of 5% is used to classify a growth pattern as present. The distinction of solid from trabecular growth patterns tends to be fairly subjective, but the other two patterns (psuedoacni and macrotrabecular) are more robustly identifiable. Of note, growth patterns are not the same as hepatocellular carcinoma subtypes, which are described in their own section below. In fact, any of the growth patterns can be found in any of the hepatocellular carcinoma subtypes.

The solid growth pattern is defined as solid sheets of tumor cells with no definite areas of trabecular, pseudoacinar, or macrotrabecular growth. In the trabecular variant, the trabeculae of tumor cells should be well defined on H&E. The trabeculae will be of variable thickness but usually are less than 5 cells wide. In contrast, if the tumor trabeculae are at least 10 cells in thickness on average, then the growth pattern is classified as macrotrabecular. Finally, the pseudoglandular pattern shows glandlike or rosettelike structures. Their sizes can vary considerably, and when large, they are often filled with a thin, eosinophilic, flocculent material. Tumors with very large pseudocysts are sometimes described as have folliclelike growth (Fig. 15.22).

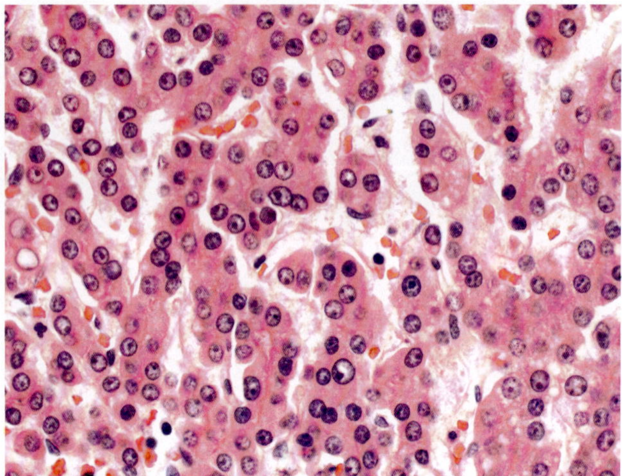

Figure 15.19. Hepatocellular carcinoma, growth patterns. This case shows a trabecular growth pattern, which is the most common growth pattern.

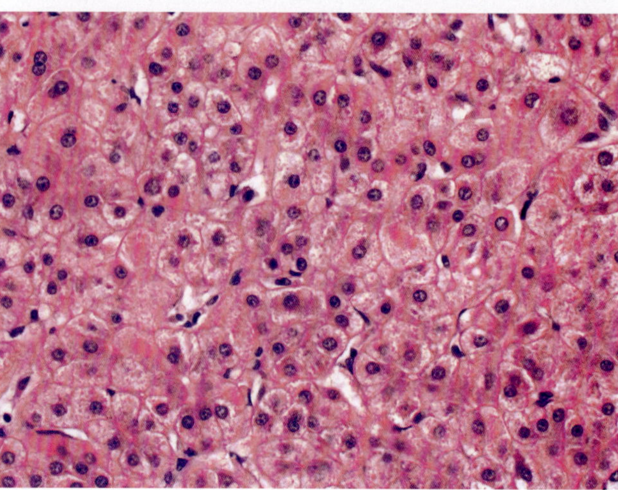

Figure 15.20. Hepatocellular carcinoma, growth patterns. This case shows a solid or compact growth pattern.

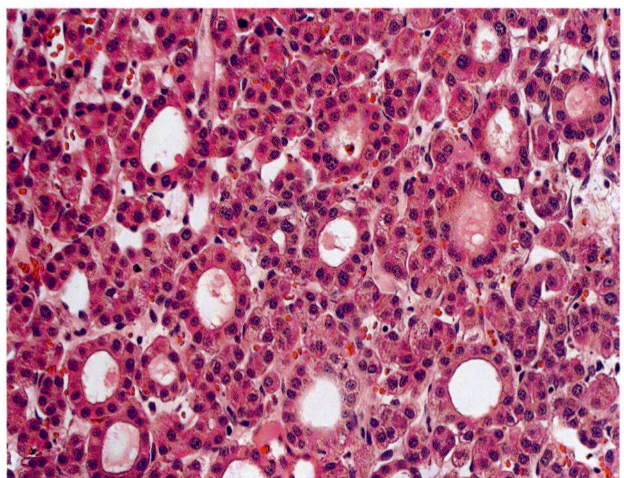

Figure 15.21. Hepatocellular carcinoma, pseudoglandular growth pattern. This case shows a pseudoglandular or pseudoacinar growth pattern.

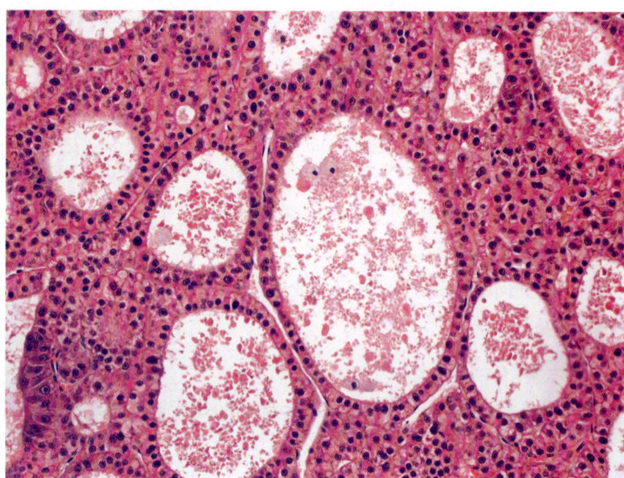

Figure 15.22. Hepatocellular carcinoma, pseudoglandular growth pattern. In this case, the pseudoglands are very large, a pattern sometimes called follicle like.

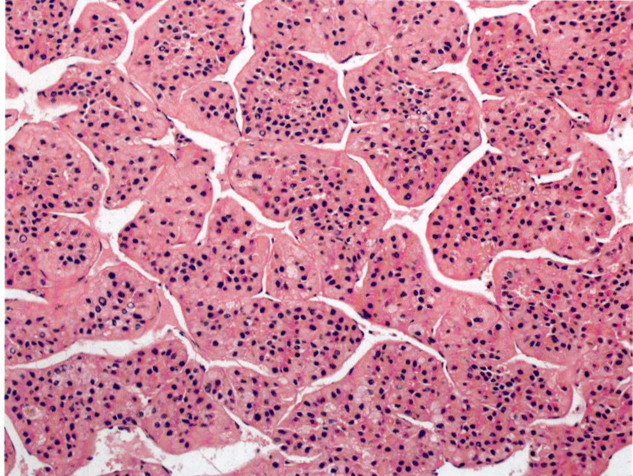

Figure 15.23. Hepatocellular carcinoma, macrotrabecular growth pattern. This case shows a macrotrabecular growth pattern, which is the least common growth pattern.

OTHER FINDINGS

Hepatocellular carcinomas can have a variety of other findings at the cytological and architectural levels. Cytological changes include bile production, which can be helpful when present, as it proves hepatic differentiation (Fig. 15.24). Some tumors can have dilated and congested sinusoids (Fig. 15.25). Cluster of foamy macrophages can rarely be found in the sinusoids of hepatocellular carcinomas (Fig. 15.26). Other hepatocellular carcinomas can have numerous Mallory Denk bodies (Fig. 15.27) or numerous hyaline bodies (Fig. 15.28). Hyaline bodies, in contrast to Mallory Denk bodies, are round and inclusion like. When present, hyaline bodies are associated with a worse prognosis.[18] They are also more common after TACE therapy.[19] Pale bodies are often found in fibrolamellar carcinoma and less commonly in conventional hepatocellular carcinoma (Fig. 15.29). Well-differentiated hepatocellular carcinomas can rarely show adaptive changes in response to medications, including smooth endoplasmic reticulum proliferation, giving the tumor cells an induced appearance (Fig. 15.30).

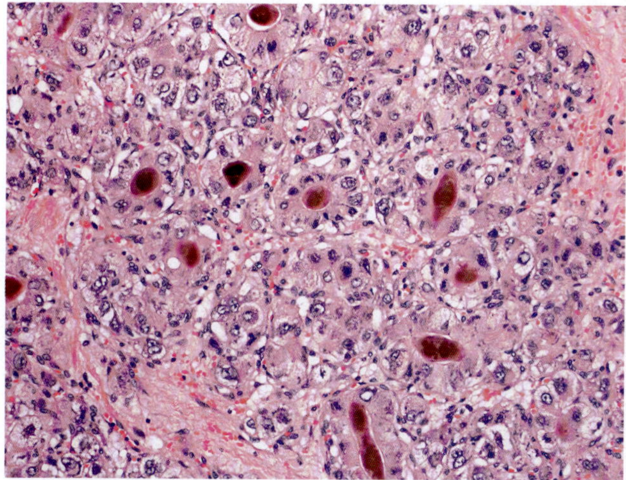

Figure 15.24. Hepatocellular carcinoma, bile production. The tumor shows definite bile production. While bile production is specific for hepatic differentiation, care is warranted, as sometimes secretions in adenocarcinomas can become bile stained and resemble bile.

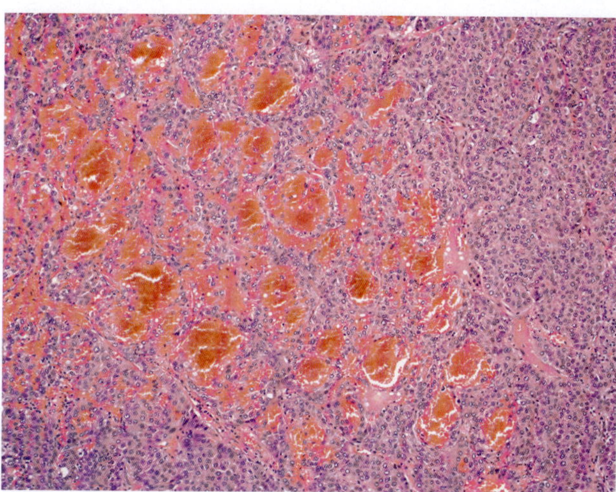

Figure 15.25. Hepatocellular carcinoma, sinusoidal congestion. In this case, the hepatocellular carcinoma shows marked sinusoidal congestion, forming peliotic like areas.

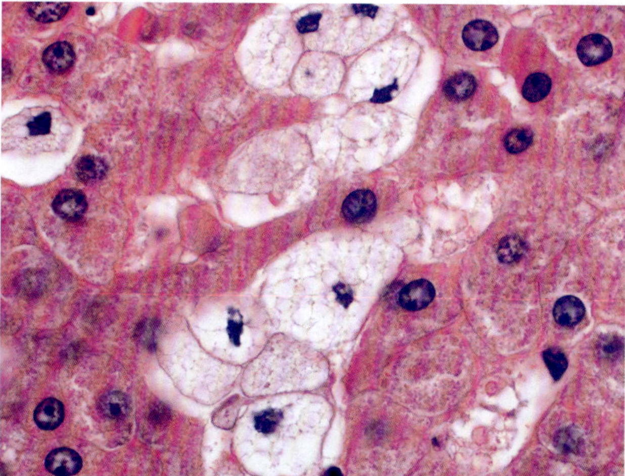

Figure 15.26. Hepatocellular carcinoma, foamy macrophages in sinusoids. The sinusoids in this hepatocellular carcinoma showed distinctive clusters of foamy macrophages.

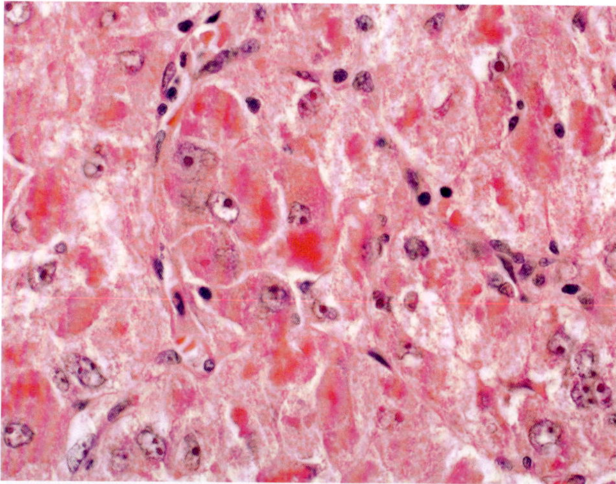

Figure 15.27. Hepatocellular carcinoma, Mallory Denk bodies. This hepatocellular carcinoma did not have fat but had abundant Mallory Denk bodies.

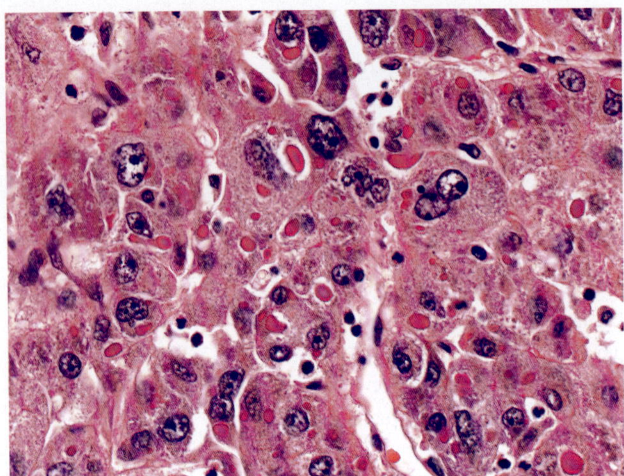

Figure 15.28. **Hepatocellular carcinoma, hyaline bodies.** This hepatocellular carcinoma has numerous round hyaline bodies in the tumor cytoplasm.

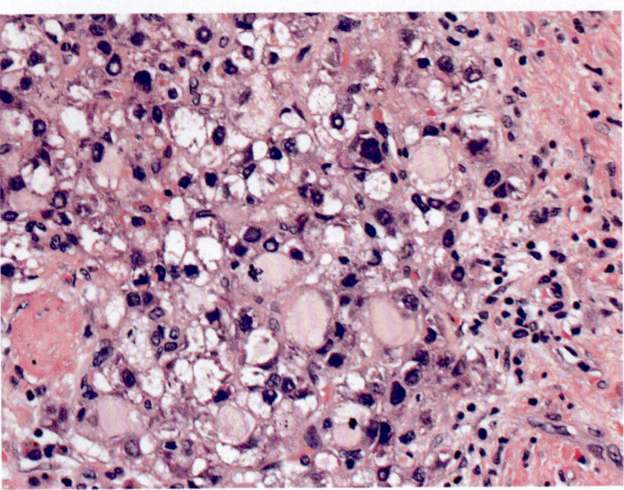

Figure 15.29. **Hepatocellular carcinoma, pale bodies.** This conventional hepatocellular carcinoma (not a case of fibrolamellar carcinoma) had occasional pale bodies.

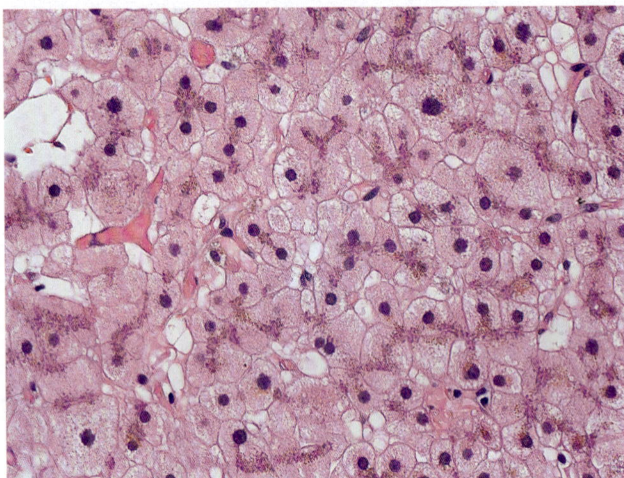

Figure 15.30. **Hepatocellular carcinoma, induced tumor cells.** This patient was on numerous medications, and one of the medications led to cytoplasmic changes in the tumor cells that resembled induced hepatocytes.

Hepatocellular carcinomas can be encapsulated (Fig. 15.31), partially encapsulated, or unencapsulated. Encapsulated tumors have a somewhat better prognosis, but this finding in general does not provide prognostic information independent of stage, grade, and angiolymphatic invasion. The presence or absence of a capsule on histology does not correlate very well with the presence or absence of a capsule on imaging studies. Hepatocellular carcinomas frequently show multiple different morphologies. In some cases hepatocellular carcinomas show tumor progression (nodule in nodule), with a focus of less well-differentiated hepatocellular carcinoma (Fig. 15.32). In other cases, hepatocellular carcinomas have distinct nodules that seem to be similar in differentiation (multinodular pattern), suggesting genomic instability more than tumor progression (Fig. 15.33).

ANGIOLYMPHATIC INVASION

The specimen should be carefully examined for macrovascular invasion, which is present in 5% to 30% of cases on imaging, but is less common on gross examination of surgical specimens because it is typically a contraindication to surgery when seen by imaging. Microscopic angiolymphatic invasion is best seen near the tumor–nontumor interface, so that area should be well sampled. The overall frequency of microvascular invasion is between 15% and 60%.[20] Portal vein invasion (Fig. 15.34) is at least 10X more common than central vein invasion,[21] while arterial invasion is very rare. The diagnosis of angiolymphatic invasion is made by H&E examination. Retraction artifact around small invasive foci of tumor at the tumor, nontumor junction can mimic invasion, but these foci will lack an endothelial lining. If you are not sure about a focus, then it is usually best to keep looking for a more definitive foci of vascular invasion, as special stains are only rarely helpful. Often, the vascular invasion distends the vessel, leading to the vessel wall being molded around the tumor thrombus. In some cases, there can be an organized blood clot associated with the tumor invasion. Sectioning artifact, especially in poorly differentiated tumors, often leads to rare isolated tumor cells or small clusters of tumor cells floating freely in a vascular lumen, but these foci are not considered to be vascular invasion.

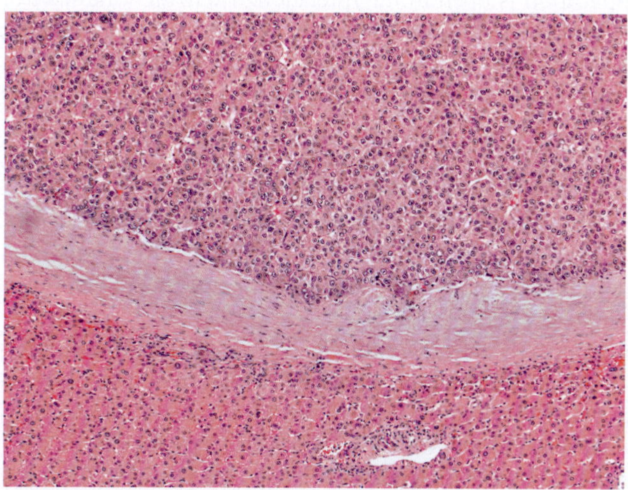

Figure 15.31. **Hepatocellular carcinoma, capsule.** This tumor is surrounded by a well-formed fibrous capsule.

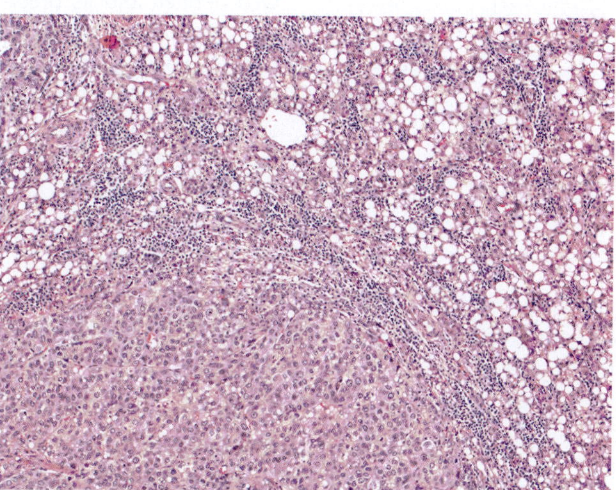

Figure 15.32. **Hepatocellular carcinoma, nodule in nodule.** Most of the hepatocellular carcinoma was well differentiated with a steatohepatitic morphology (upper part of image), but there was nodule within the main tumor that showed a poorly differentiated morphology (lower part of image).

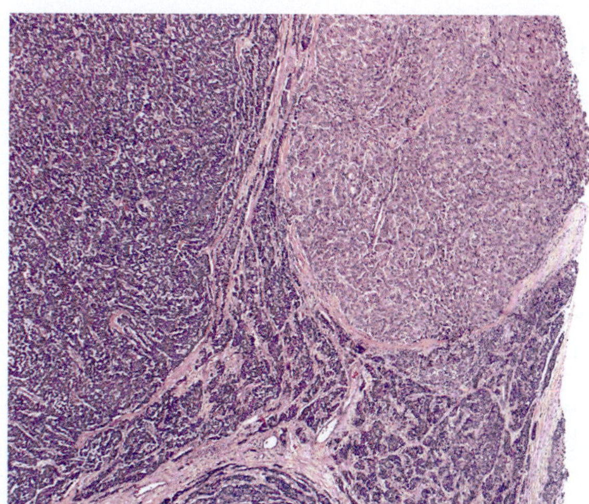

Figure 15.33. **Hepatocellular carcinoma, multinodular pattern.** The tumor was composed of several different morphologies that were all about the same degree of differentiation and did not seem to have any clear evidence that one morphology had led to the others.

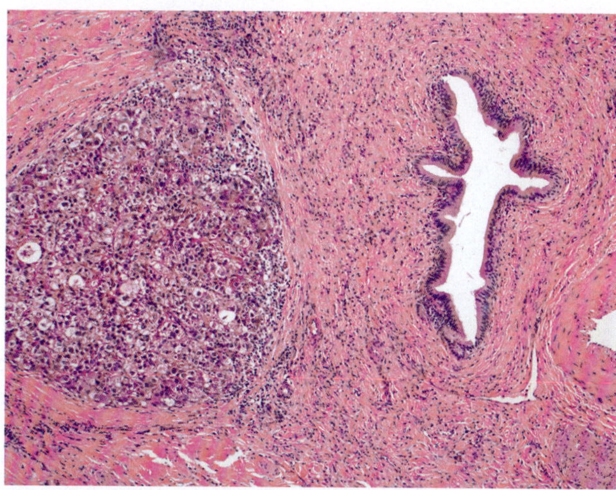

Figure 15.34. **Hepatocellular carcinoma, vascular invasion.** There is invasion into the portal vein of a portal tract at the edge of the main mass lesion.

GRADING HEPATOCELLULAR CARCINOMA

A tumor grade should be provided for cases of hepatocellular carcinoma, as tumor grade provides important prognostic information, predicting tumor recurrence in cirrhotic livers,[22,23] in noncirrhotic livers,[24] and after liver transplantation.[22,25] Tumor grade correlates with tumor size and with angiolymphatic invasion, both of which are also important prognostic findings, but in multivariate analysis, tumor grade consistently has independent prognostic value. In general, as hepatocellular carcinomas become less well differentiated, they tend to have increasing degrees of nuclear atypia as well as less abundant cytoplasm, increasingly basophilic cytoplasm, and are less likely to show clear cell change or steatosis. These basic observations have been incorporated into formal grading systems.

There are several research grade systems, such as the modified Edmonson–Steiner grading system (Table 15.3),[26] but they have not been widely adopted for clinical care. The 2010 WHO blue book also provides a brief section on grading, but the criteria are not well defined and its precise application is open to interpretation. There are a number of other barriers to consistent tumor grading. Most of the grading systems use a combination of nuclear atypia and cytoplasmic changes that include the amount of tumor cytoplasm and whether the cytoplasm is eosinophilic versus basophilic. Often, these types of changes are hard to reliably score in isolation, that is, when you have not seen other hepatocellular carcinomas for some time, so it's good practice to flip through the images in a book chapter or review article before grading the tumor. Another barrier to grading is that it is not always clear what to do when the nuclear and cytoplasmic changes are discordant (for example high-grade nuclear cytology in tumor cells with abundant eosinophilic cytoplasm or low-grade nuclear cytology in tumor cells with moderate to scant amounts of basophilic cytoplasm).

For clinical care, a common approach is as follows (Table 15.4). **Well differentiated** (Fig. 15.35): the tissue is clearly hepatocellular, and stains are necessary to make sure its cancer, as a benign liver tumor could reasonably be in the H&E differential; **moderately differentiated** (Fig. 15.36): the tumor is clearly cancer on H&E, *and* hepatocellular differentiation is morphologically evident; **poorly differentiated** (Figs. 15.37 and 15.38): the tumor is clearly cancer on H&E, *but* hepatocellular differentiation is not confidently seen on H&E, only on special stains. When using this approach, the goal is to put the tumor into the best overall category using low- to medium-power examination.

It is not uncommon for hepatocellular carcinomas to have a nodule-in-nodule growth pattern, with multiple distinct morphologies. In this case, the tumor is classified according to the least well-differentiated areas.

IMMUNOHISTOCHEMICAL PATTERNS

Immunohistochemical stains are important tools in evaluating liver tumors and are used to do the following: (1) distinguish between a benign or malignant liver tumor (Table 15.2); (2) subclassify hepatic adenomas after a diagnosis of hepatic adenoma is made; and (3) in a clearly malignant tumor, distinguish between hepatocellular carcinoma, cholangiocarcinoma, and metastatic disease using markers of hepatic differentiation (Table 15.1).

TABLE 15.3: Modified Edmondson–Steiner Grading System for Hepatocellular Carcinoma

Grade	Criteria
1	Abundant cytoplasm; minimal nuclear atypia
2	Mild nuclear atypia with prominent nucleoli, hyperchromasia, and nuclear irregularity
3	Moderate nuclear atypia with greater hyperchromasia and nuclear irregularity
4	Marked nuclear pleomorphism, marked hyperchromasia, and anaplastic giant cells

TABLE 15.4: Clinical Grading Schema for Hepatocellular Carcinomas

Grade	Criteria
Well-differentiated	• On H&E, tumor could be benign or malignant (i.e., differential would include a benign hepatic lesion/tumor) • Hepatic differentiation is clearly seen on H&E • Minimal to mild nuclear atypia • Cytoplasm typically eosinophilic • N:C ratio is normal or very slightly increased
Moderately differentiated	• Tumor is clearly malignant on H&E • Overall morphology strongly suggests hepatocellular origin, but stains are helpful in confirming hepatocyte differentiation (i.e., differential would include other carcinomas such as renal, adrenal, etc.) • Moderate nuclear atypia • Cytoplasm ranges from eosinophilic to basophilic • N:C ratio increased

Poorly differentiated	• Tumor is clearly malignant on H&E
	• H&E morphology is consistent with a range of poorly differentiated carcinomas, and immunostains are needed to confirm hepatic differentiation
	• Nuclear atypia
	  • Marked
	  • Moderate but the tumor has a very high N:C ratio
	• Cytoplasm usually basophilic
	• N:C ratio increased

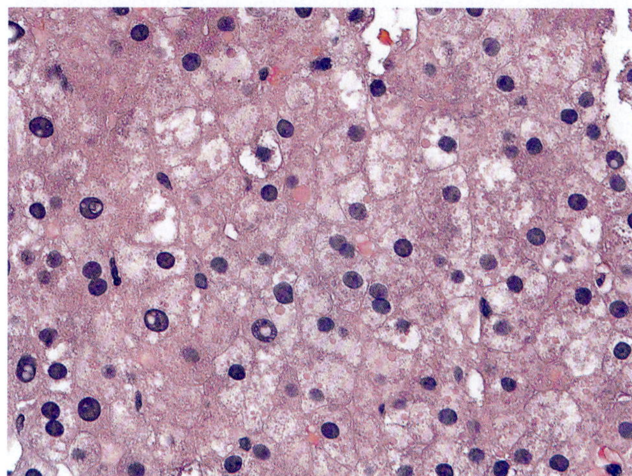

Figure 15.35. **Hepatocellular carcinoma, well differentiated.** The tissue is clearly hepatic in differentiation, and stains are necessary to make sure it is cancer, as a benign liver tumor could reasonably be in the H&E differential.

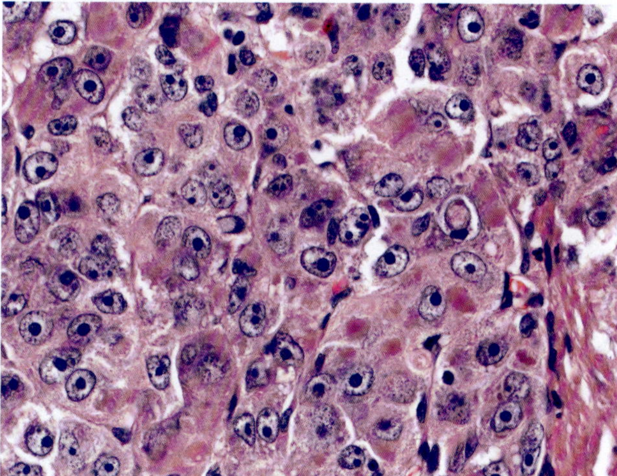

Figure 15.36. **Hepatocellular carcinoma, moderately differentiated.** The tumor is clearly cancer on H&E, and hepatocellular differentiation is morphologically evident. Note that this case also has hyaline bodies.

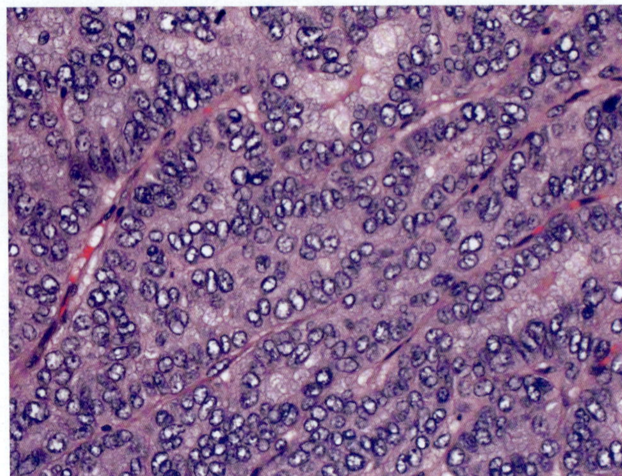

Figure 15.37. **Hepatocellular carcinoma, poorly differentiated.** The tumor is clearly cancer on H&E, but special stains are needed to demonstrate hepatocellular differentiation.

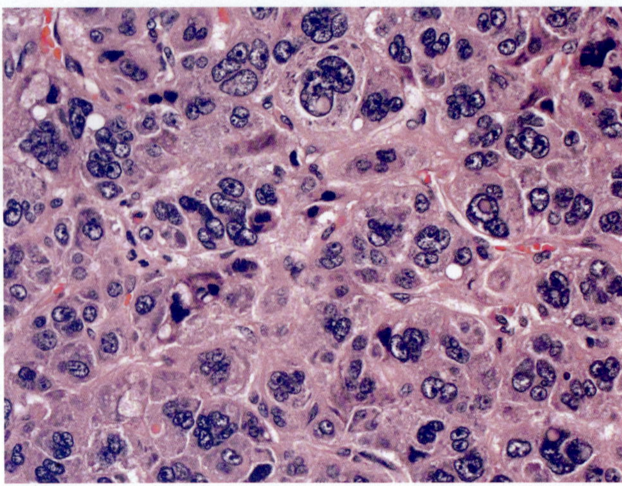

Figure 15.38. **Hepatocellular carcinoma, poorly differentiated.** Another example of a poorly differentiated hepatocellular carcinoma; this one with more nuclear pleomorphism.

PEARLS & PITFALLS WHEN USING IMMUNOHISTOCHEMICAL STAINS

Using immunostains requires training, experience, and common sense, but mostly common sense. To aide in their interpretation, it can be helpful to remember that there are four fundamental, immutable laws that govern the use of immunohistochemistry in liver tumors.

Law 1. *No special stains should be interpreted in isolation; all require correlation with the H&E findings.* This is very important and solves many problems. For example, none of the stains for hepatic differentiation are entirely specific, but when combined with morphology, the specificity approaches its maximum. For example HepPar, arginase, glypican 3, and albumin in situ hybridization can all be positive in other tumors, but most of these tumors do not look like hepatocellular carcinoma on H&E and were mostly discovered during comprehensive surveys of expression in various tumors.

Law 2. *The sensitivity and specificity of immunostains gets worse in time, until it reaches its true test characteristics.* This is true for all tests in the literature. The first set of papers always show the best sensitivity and specificity, which drops off as the test is used in more primary and metastatic liver tumors. Eventually, a very solid understanding of the sensitivity and specificity emerge, but this can take up to 5 years, sometimes longer.

Law 3. *If there is a discrepancy between the morphology and immunohistochemical findings, additional studies must be performed.* This seems a bit obvious but can be a point of confusion. As one example, it almost always turns out to be an error to diagnose hepatocellular carcinoma based only on stains for hepatic differentiation, when the H&E morphology is not a good fit for hepatocellular carcinoma. If the morphology and immunostain findings are discrepant, resolve with additional sections (on resection specimens) or additional stains as needed.

Law 4. *A difficult case is the wrong time to first use a stain you are not familiar with.* When your laboratory sets up a new stain, it takes some time to develop enough experience to use the stain wisely. During that initial time period, it can be tempting to base a diagnosis for a difficult case primarily on the exciting new stain—but this often leads to regret the next morning. Take the time to fully understand the strengths and weaknesses of a stain before fully integrating it into your practice.

Cytokeratin Stains

Cytokeratin stains are used to identify epithelial lineage and mostly come into play in poorly differentiated tumors. Hepatocellular carcinomas are positive CK8, CK18, and CAM5.2 as well as many pankeratins. Hepatocellular carcinomas are less commonly positive for CK7 (about 30% are positive, in particular cholestatic tumors),[27,28] CK AE1/3 (15% are positive),[29] CK19 (15% are positive, also indicates a worse prognosis),[27,28,30] and CK20 (5% are positive). In contrast, CK 5/6 is negative in almost all hepatocellular carcinomas.[31] Most hepatocellular carcinomas that show CK20 or CK19 positivity are also positive for CK7.[27,28]

Hepatocellular Carcinoma Versus Adenocarcinoma

MOC31 is a useful marker of adenocarcinomas. MOC31 is positive in >90% of cholangiocarcinomas and positive in about 30% of hepatocellular carcinomas. MOC31 tends to be more strong and diffuse in adenocarcinomas than it is in hepatocellular carcinoma, but this distinction is most evident in cases where its not needed, being best seen in cases that are obviously adenocarcinoma or hepatocellular carcinoma on the H&E. In poorly differentiated adenocarcinomas, MOC31 staining can be patchier and show overlap with the changes seen in poorly differentiated hepatocellular carcinomas. Nonetheless, strong and diffuse staining would favor an adenocarcinoma. Mucicarmine staining also proves a tumor is an adenocarcinoma, with the caveat that many peripheral cholangiocarcinomas are mucicarmine negative. Strong and diffuse CDX2 staining favors metastasis from the GI tract, but about 5% of poorly differentiated hepatocellular carcinomas can show focal CDX2 staining.[32] If the tumor is definitely an adenocarcinoma, then positivity for albumin in situ hybridization favors it to be a cholangiocarcinoma,[33] although the test is not entirely specific and adenocarcinoma from other sites can rarely be positive.

Hepatocellular Carcinoma Versus Cholangiocarcinoma

Some cholangiocarcinomas can show significant overlap with hepatocellular carcinoma (Fig. 15.39). Useful stains include markers of hepatic differentiation, with HepPar and arginase being more specific for hepatic differentiation than glypican 3. Albumin in situ hybridization is positive in both hepatocellular carcinomas and in most cholangiocarcinomas, so it does not help in this situation. Mucicarmine staining indicates glandular differentiation, but many peripheral cholangiocarcinomas are negative. There are no positive, affirmative markers of biliary differentiation, but a tumor that is negative for hepatic markers and positive for CK19, CK7, MOC31, and albumin in situ hybridization would favor a cholangiocarcinoma. If the albumin in situ hybridization is negative, then the tumor could still be a cholangiocarcinoma, but metastatic disease needs to be carefully excluded.

Hepatocellular Carcinoma Versus Metastatic Disease

A subset of metastatic neoplasms can closely mimic hepatocellular carcinoma at the cytological level (Fig. 15.40), with tumor cells showing abundant eosinophilic cytoplasm, prominent nucleoli, and tumor cells growing in trabeculae. These include (in approximate order of frequency in surgical pathology specimens) neuroendocrine tumors, renal oncocytic tumors, acinar cell carcinoma of the pancreas, paragangliomas, and adrenal cortical carcinoma. The diagnosis is made using stains to show the lack of hepatic differentiation and positivity for other relevant markers, such as synaptophysin and chromogranin in neuroendocrine tumors.

Undifferentiated Carcinoma

In rare cases, the imaging and clinical findings show no tumor except for in the liver, but biopsies of the tumor show a poorly differentiated neoplasm that stains only for keratins. After other malignancies that can sometimes show aberrant keratin expression have been excluded, then the tumor is classified as an undifferentiated carcinoma.

BACKGROUND LIVER

The background liver should be evaluated for underlying liver disease and for fibrosis stage in resection specimens. It is important to take sections at least 1 cm away from the tumor, to avoid secondary mass effect changes. Mass effect changes vary considerably from case

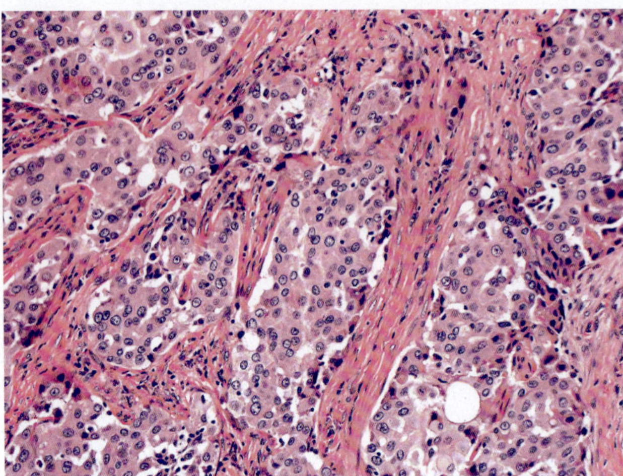

Figure 15.39. **Cholangiocarcinoma mimicking hepatocellular carcinoma.** This cholangiocarcinoma was initially misdiagnosed as a hepatocellular carcinoma.

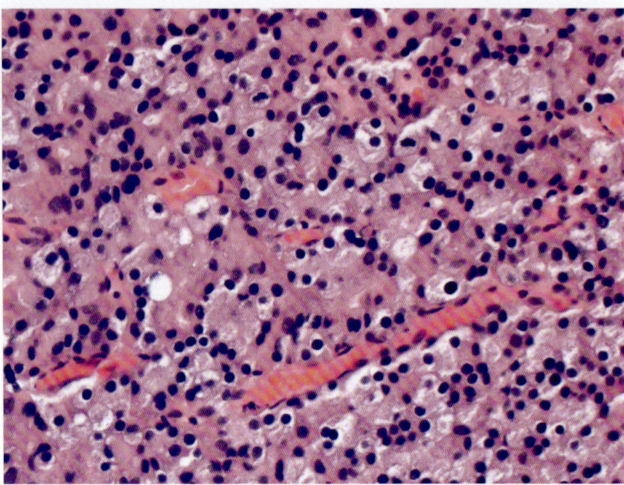

Figure 15.40. **Metastatic oncocytic renal cell carcinoma mimicking hepatocellular carcinoma.** The histological findings are reminiscent of a well-differentiated hepatocellular carcinoma. In this case, the patient also had a renal mass and immunostain evaluation on the liver metastasis confirmed a renal origin.

to case, but there can be substantial fibrosis next to the tumor, while sections away from the mass showing little or no fibrosis (which can lead to over staging). Mass effect also commonly leads to more inflammation and less fatty change than the background liver.

CHANGES AFTER CHEMOEMBOLIZATION THERAPY

Hepatocellular carcinomas are staged in the same way, regardless of whether they have been treated. The percent of tumor necrosis should be estimated to the nearest 10% using the gross and/or the histological findings. After TACE, the percent of tumor necrosis ranges from 0% to 100%. There is no reliable way to distinguish treatment-related necrosis from spontaneous necrosis, so all necrosis is included in the estimate. Tumors with necrosis average about 60% necrosis, with about 1/3 of tumors found to be completely necrotic.[34–36] Interestingly, hepatocellular carcinomas with strong and diffuse CD34 staining appear to be more resistant to TACE.[37]

In addition to necrosis, treatment can also affect the grade, with one study showing that hepatocellular carcinomas had higher tumor grades after TACE therapy.[19] Treated tumors are also more likely to express CK19 and have areas with spindled cell morphology.[38,39] Other changes can include lymphocytic or neutrophilic inflammation and fibrosis within the tumors. After TACE, embolic beads can be found in the tumor (Fig. 15.41) and the adjacent nontumor liver. In some cases, the beads can escape the liver and damage other organs, in particular the stomach (Fig. 15.42) and gallbladder.[40]

HISTOLOGICAL SUBTYPES

Most hepatocellular carcinomas show no distinctive features and are classified as hepatocellular carcinomas not otherwise specified, but about 35% of cases can be classified as unique subtypes or variants (Table 15.5). The histological subtypes are defined by four main features (see FAQ box),[41] but it is important to note that these features will not be equally well developed when a subtype is first identified, as each of the features can take some time to be fully developed.

FAQ: How are subtypes of hepatocellular carcinoma defined?

Answer: There are four elements that are used to define a variant/subtype of hepatocellular carcinoma.

The following are the four elements of a hepatocellular carcinoma variant.

1. Unique H&E histological findings. These findings need to be consistently and reproducibly present.
2. Unique test results that confirm the H&E morphological impression. These may be immunostains or molecular tests.
3. Unique clinical correlates. These correlates can include age, gender, risk factors, and prognosis.
4. Unique molecular findings. These in turn are often used to develop more accurate tests for step 2 above, a case in point being fibrolamellar carcinoma. Note that this approach to determining subtypes is different than that of defining subtypes based solely on the basis of mutation patterns, epigenetic changes, or patterns of gene expression, without regard to morphology.

Finally, note that subtypes of hepatocellular carcinoma are different than growth patterns in hepatocellular carcinomas. The four main growth patterns (trabecular, solid, pseudoglandular, and macrotrabecular) are defined solely by the H&E architectural patterns and can be found to vary degrees in many of the different hepatocellular carcinoma subtypes.

Subtypes of hepatocellular carcinoma are important for several reasons. First, they improve diagnosis in surgical pathology, as the morphological findings in hepatocellular carcinomas are organized into meaningful patterns, each with its own challenges and diagnostic pitfalls. Second, the variants provide prognostic information (Table 15.5). Third, they add to our understanding of the biology of hepatocellular carcinomas, in part by allowing clinical, pathological, and molecular studies to focus on homogenous groups of tumor. Finally, they can affect clinical management. At this time, the last reason is relevant only for fibrolamellar carcinomas, mixed hepatocellular carcinoma–cholangiocarcinoma, and mixed hepatocellular carcinoma–neuroendocrine carcinoma, but it seems likely to become more relevant as research leads to improved therapy. In the section that follows, key points are summarized and illustrated for each recognized hepatocellular carcinoma variant, as well as proposed variants.

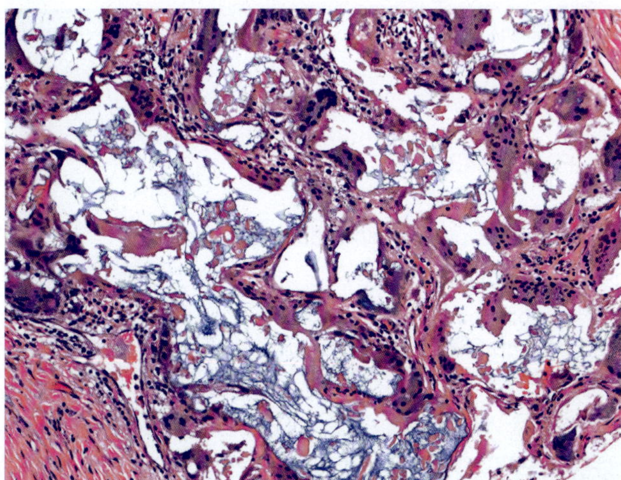

Figure 15.41. **TACE material.** Degenerating foreign material with a giant cell reaction was present in proximity to the hepatocellular carcinoma.

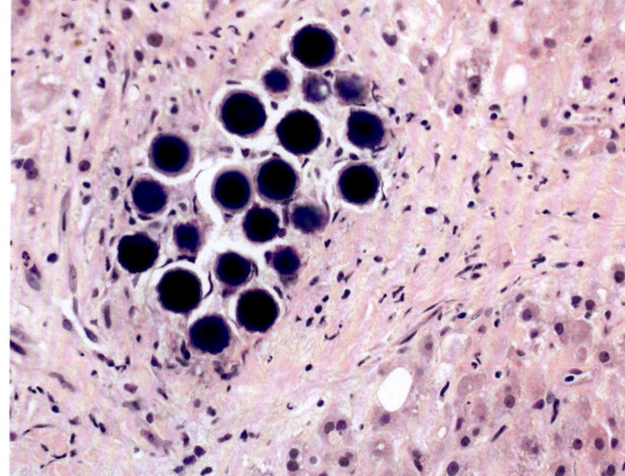

Figure 15.42. **Y90 beads.** These beads can also escape the liver and cause disease in other organs, including cholecystitis and gastritis.

TABLE 15.5: Hepatocellular Carcinoma Subtypes

Subtype	Frequency[a]	Prognosis[b]	Major Tumor Findings
Steatohepatitic	20%	similar	Fat, inflammation, and fibrosis
Clear cell	7%	better	Glycogen accumulation
Scirrhous	4%	similar to better	Dense diffuse intratumoral fibrosis
Cirrhotomimetic	1%	worse	Defined by gross findings: numerous small nodules (typically >30) that resemble cirrhotic nodules in size
Combined hepatocellular-cholangiocarcinoma	1%	worse	Two distinct morphologies: hepatocellular carcinoma and cholangiocarcinoma
Fibrolamellar carcinoma	1%	Similar to better	Tumor cell with abundant eosinophilic cytoplasm, vesiculated nuclear chromatin with prominent nucleoli, and intratumoral fibrosis
Combined hepatocellular and neuroendocrine	<1%	worse	Two distinct morphologies: hepatocellular carcinoma and neuroendocrine carcinoma
Granulocyte colony-stimulating factor–producing	<1%	worse	Poorly differentiated with moderate to marked intratumoral neutrophils
Sarcomatoid	<1%	worse	Spindle cell growth
Carcinosarcoma	<1%	worse	Two distinct morphologies: hepatocellular carcinoma and sarcoma
Lymphocyte rich	<1%	better	Marked intratumoral lymphocytes

[a]The frequencies of the more aggressive subtypes are routinely higher in autopsy studies.
[b]Compared with conventional hepatocellular carcinoma.

KEY POINTS: Carcinosarcoma (Figs. 15.43 and 15.44)

- Frequency: <1%.
- Prognosis: worse (compared with conventional hepatocellular carcinomas).
- Molecular correlates: no consistent findings to date.
- Morphology: malignant epithelial component (hepatocellular carcinoma, cholangiocarcinoma, or undifferentiated carcinoma) plus a distinctly different component of sarcoma.
- Both components are diagnosed in the usual way.
- The most common sarcomas are leiomyosarcoma, rhabdomyosarcoma, chondrosarcoma, fibrosarcoma, or osteosarcoma.[42–44]
- Differential is sarcomatoid hepatocellular carcinoma. In sarcomatoid hepatocellular carcinoma, the spindle cell component retains keratin staining and is negative for definite, specific mesenchymal differentiation by morphology and immunostains. The opposite is true for the sarcoma component in carcinosarcomas, which are routinely keratin negative, do not stain with hepatic markers, and instead can be positive for markers of specific mesenchymal differentiation.

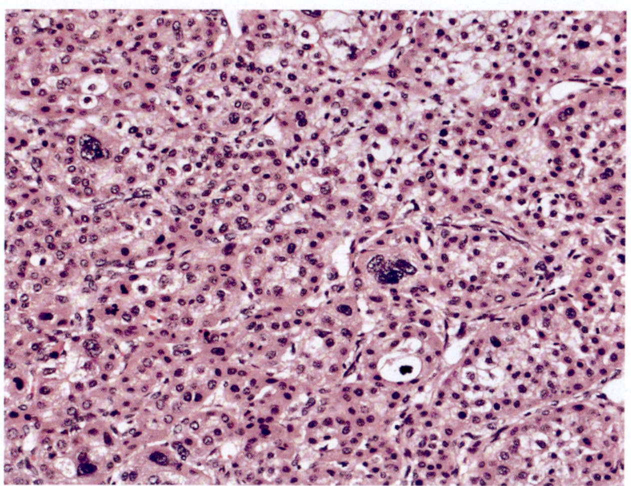

Figure 15.43. **Carcinosarcoma, hepatocellular carcinoma component.** The hepatocellular carcinoma component in this case showed chromophobe morphology (see also section below) and was ALT FISH positive.

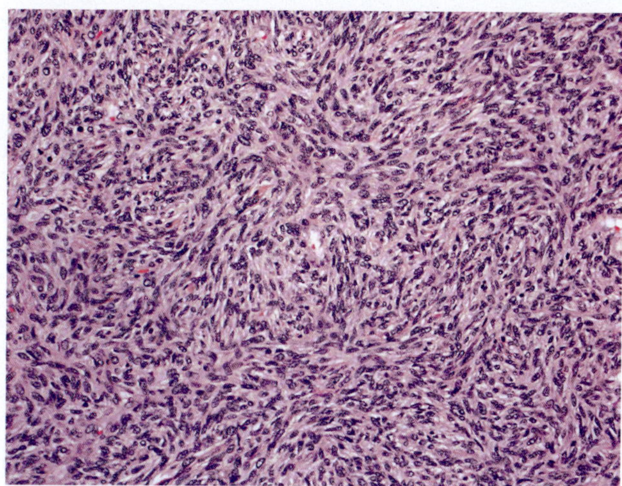

Figure 15.44. **Carcinosarcoma, sarcoma component.** The sarcoma component was an undifferentiated fibrosarcoma and was also ALT positive.

KEY POINTS: Carcinosarcoma With Osteoclast-Like Giant Cells

- Frequency: <1%.
- Prognosis: worse.
- Molecular correlates: no consistent findings to date.
- Morphology: malignant epithelial component (hepatocellular carcinoma, cholangiocarcinoma, or undifferentiated carcinoma) plus a distinctly different component of sarcoma that shows the following features[45–49]:
  - Sheets of mononuclear tumor cells that are plump to spindled and are negative for markers of hepatic differentiation. The mononuclear cells are usually negative for keratins (focal staining can be seen) and for other lineage markers, including those of mesenchymal differentiation.
  - Benign osteoclast-like giant cells are found scattered throughout the tumor. They stain strongly for CD68 and other markers of osteoclast-like differentiation.[45,46,50]
  - There is extensive intratumoral necrosis, hemorrhage, and cystic change, although this is not always evident on biopsies owing to sampling. Hemosiderin-laden macrophages are common.
- Sometimes the epithelial component is minimal or absent even in resection specimens, in which case the tumor is called an *undifferentiated carcinoma with osteoclast-like giant cells.*
- Correlation with imaging findings is important when there is no hepatocellular carcinoma component, as undifferentiated carcinomas with osteoclast-like giant cells can arise in other organs and metastasize to the liver.

KEY POINTS: Cirrhotomimetic Hepatocellular Carcinoma (Fig. 15.45)

- Also called diffuse hepatocellular carcinoma.
- Frequency: <1%.
- Prognosis: worse.
- Molecular correlates: no consistent findings to date.
- Morphology: defined solely by gross findings.
  - Numerous small nodules of hepatocellular carcinoma, usually >30, that are about the same size as the cirrhotic nodules in the background liver.
  - Tumor burden is invariably underestimated by imaging and gross examination.
  - Nodules can coalesce to form a grossly evident mass.

- Differential is convention hepatocellular carcinoma with satellite nodules. With conventional hepatocellular carcinomas, the number of satellite nodules is less than 5 in 90% of cases and less than 10 in essentially 100% of cases. Moreover, satellite nodules are found in close proximity to the main tumor mass, usually a cm or two, in contrast to the more diffuse and widespread disease of cirrhotomimetic hepatocellular carcinoma.

KEY POINTS: Clear Cell Hepatocellular Carcinoma (Figs. 15.46 and 15.47)

- Frequency: 5% to 10%.
- Prognosis: better.
- Molecular correlates: no consistent findings to date.
- Morphology: tumor cells have abundant clear cytoplasm.
  - A cutoff of 50% has been used in some papers; a better cutoff is 90%, providing a purer group of tumors.
  - Mild patchy macrovesicular steatosis is also common.
- Differential is metastatic clear cell carcinomas.
  - 35% of clear cell carcinomas of the ovary are HepPar1 positive,[51] so additional/other markers of hepatic differentiation should be considered if ovarian clear cell carcinoma is in your differential.
  - Clear cell carcinomas of the kidney are HepPar1 negative.[52]

KEY POINTS: Combined Hepatocellular Carcinoma–Cholangiocarcinoma (Figs. 15.48 and 15.49)

- Frequency: 1%.
- Prognosis: worse.
- Molecular correlates: no consistent findings to date.
- Serologies: serum CA19-9 and AFP levels are both elevated in about 50% of cases.[53]
- Morphology: must have two distinct morphologies.
  - One that looks like hepatocellular carcinoma on H&E and on immunostains.
  - One that looks like cholangiocarcinoma on H&E and on immunostains.
  - **Both** morphological and immunohistochemical evidence are necessary for both components.

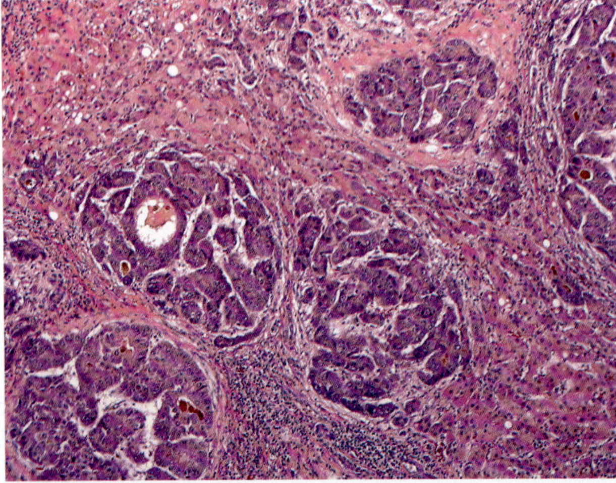

Figure 15.45. **Diffuse hepatocellular carcinoma.** This hepatocellular carcinoma was composed of numerous small nodules about the size of an ordinary cirrhotic nodule.

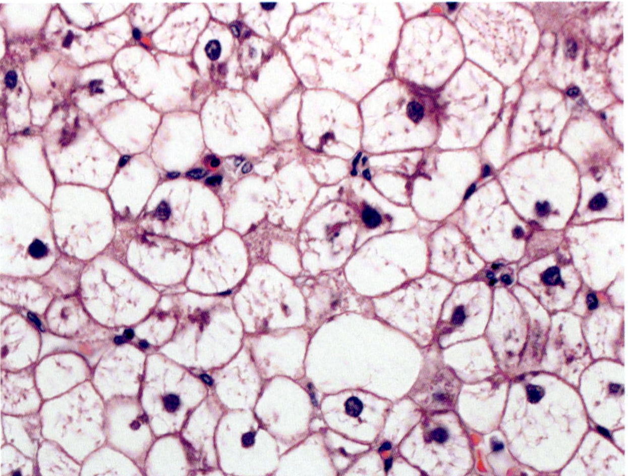

Figure 15.46. **Clear cell hepatocellular carcinoma.** The tumor cells have abundant clear cytoplasm that results from glycogen accumulation. The nuclear cytology in this case is low grade.

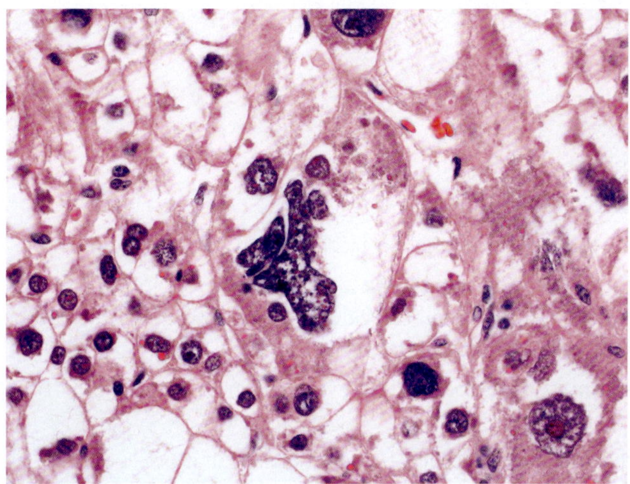

Figure 15.47. **Clear cell hepatocellular carcinoma.** In this example, the tumor shows high grade cytology.

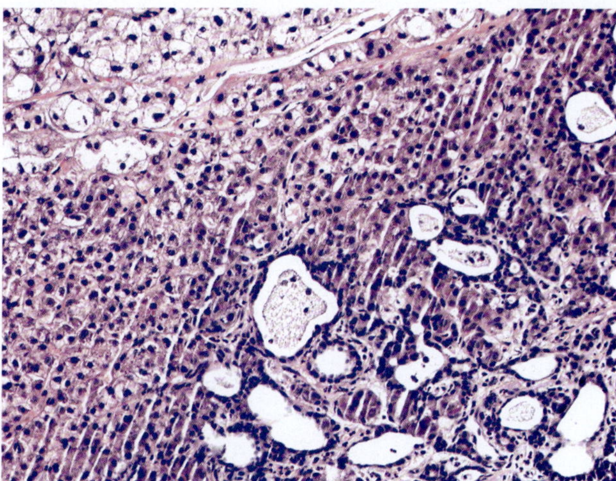

Figure 15.48. **Combined hepatocellular carcinoma–cholangiocarcinoma.** The hepatocellular carcinoma is on the left and top of the image. The cholangiocarcinoma is in the right corner of the image.

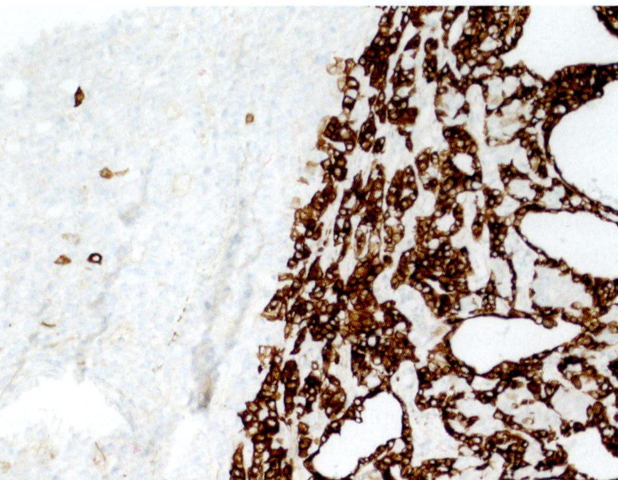

Figure 15.49. **Combined hepatocellular carcinoma–cholangiocarcinoma, CK7 immunostain.** Same case as Figure 15.48. The cholangiocarcinoma component is strongly positive, while the hepatocellular carcinoma component is negative.

- Other findings: hilar lymph node metastatic disease is more common than in hepatocellular carcinoma.
- Other findings: metastatic disease is usually the cholangiocarcinoma component.
- Differential: do not mistake combined hepatocellular carcinoma–cholangiocarcinomas for double primaries of hepatocellular carcinoma and cholangiocarcinoma, where the liver shows separate nodules of cholangiocarcinoma and hepatocellular carcinoma but has nonneoplastic liver between the two separate nodules of tumor.
- Common pitfall: diagnosing combined hepatocellular carcinoma–cholangiocarcinoma for a tumor that morphologically is either all hepatocellular carcinoma or all cholangiocarcinoma but has aberrant expression of proteins by immunostaining. Examples including cholangiocarcinoma with patchy glypican 3 staining or hepatocellular carcinoma with CK19 or MOC31 staining.

KEY POINTS: Combined Hepatocellular and Neuroendocrine Carcinoma (Figs. 15.50 and 15.51)

- Frequency: <1%.
- Prognosis: worse.
- Molecular correlates: no consistent findings to date.
- Morphology: must have two distinct morphologies
  - One that looks like hepatocellular carcinoma on H&E and on immunostains.
  - One that looks like neuroendocrine carcinoma on H&E and on immunostains. Neuroendocrine component is usually small cell carcinoma and is often found in the sinusoids of the hepatocellular carcinoma component.
  - **Both** morphological and immunohistochemical evidence are necessary for both components.
- Other findings: metastatic disease is usually the neuroendocrine carcinoma component.
- Common pitfall: diagnosing combined hepatocellular and neuroendocrine carcinoma in a hepatocellular carcinoma that shows aberrant staining for synaptophysin or CD56.

KEY POINTS: Fibrolamellar Carcinoma (Figs. 15.52–15.58)

- Frequency: 1%.
- Clinical correlates:
  - Young individuals (median age 22 years).[54]
  - No underlying liver disease.[55,56]
  - Almost all cases are sporadic but rare cases occur in the Carney complex.[57]
- Serologies: AFP levels always normal or mild nonspecific elevations.[54]
- Prognosis: similar to convention hepatocellular carcinomas in noncirrhotic livers.[54]
- Molecular correlates: microdeletion on Chr. 19 leading to DNAJB1-PRKACA fusion.
  - This molecular change is very sensitive and specific for fibrolamellar carcinoma.
  - Can be detected in formalin fixed paraffin embedded tissues by FISH.[58]
- Morphology: tumor cells have abundant eosinophilic cytoplasm, vesiculated nuclear chromatin with prominent nucleoli, and intratumoral fibrosis (Figs. 15.52 and 15.53).

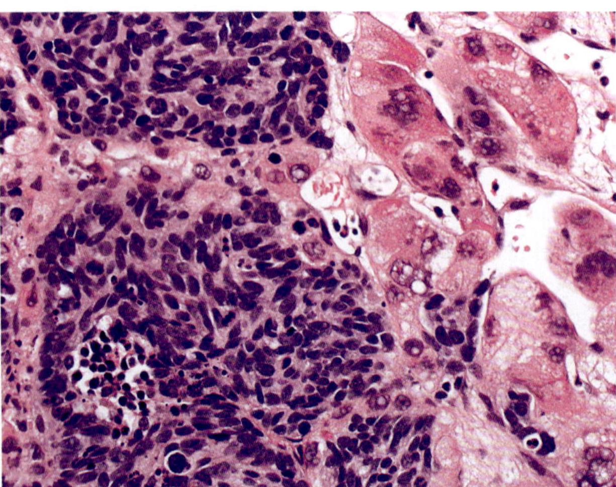

Figure 15.50. **Combined hepatocellular and neuroendocrine carcinoma.** The hepatocellular carcinoma has a small cell neuroendocrine component that is growing within the sinusoids.

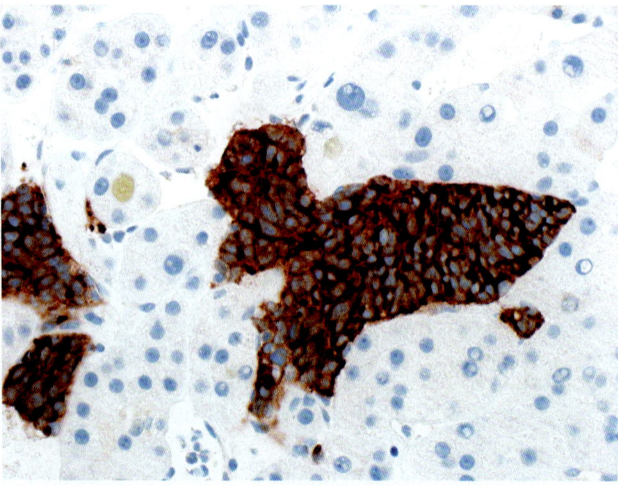

Figure 15.51. **Combined hepatocellular and neuroendocrine carcinoma, synaptophysin.** The small cell neuroendocrine is strongly positive.

- Some areas of the tumor may have minimal or absent intratumoral fibrosis; this is still acceptable as fibrolamellar carcinoma and is not a combined hepatocellular carcinoma–fibrolamellar carcinoma.
- Other findings:
  - Pseudoglands (Fig. 15.54).
  - Pale bodies, hyaline bodies (Figs. 15.55 and 15.56); neither are sensitive or specific for fibrolamellar carcinoma.
- Immunostain findings (Figs. 15.57 and 15.58): positive for CK7 and CD68 (KP1 clone) as CD68 cross-reacts with tumor lysosomes; neither stain is specific in isolation, but when there is consistent morphology and coexpression of both CK7 and CD68, then essentially all cases are fibrolamellar carcinomas.[59]
- Common pitfall: overdiagnosing fibrolamellar carcinoma when conventional hepatocellular carcinomas occur in young individuals with noncirrhotic livers.
- Differential diagnosis: scirrhous hepatocellular carcinoma. Morphological findings can be very similar, so testing to prove fibrolamellar carcinoma is strongly recommended.

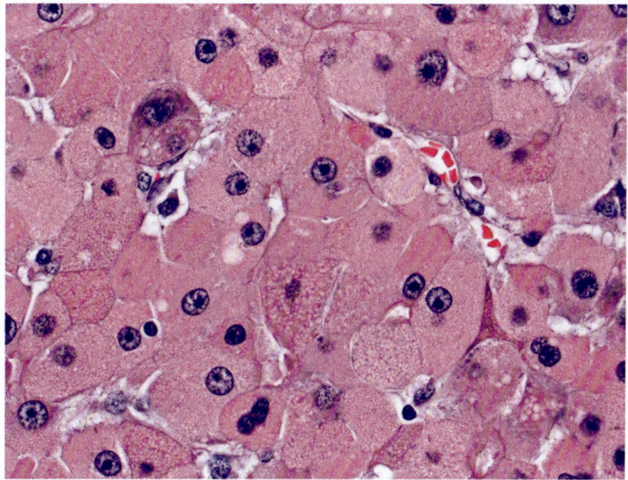

Figure 15.52. **Fibrolamellar carcinoma, cytology.** The tumor cells have abundant eosinophilic cytoplasm and prominent nucleoli.

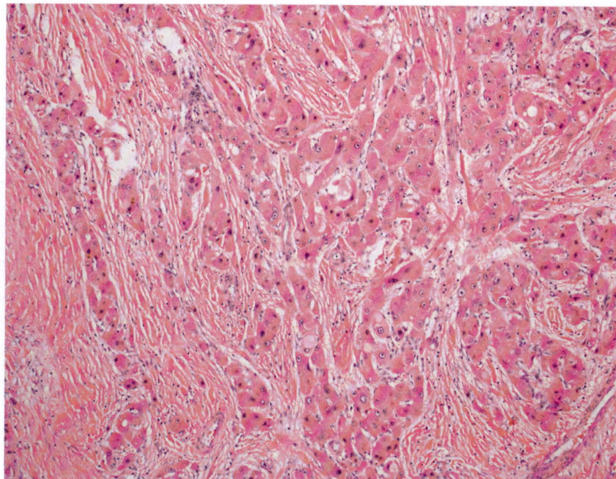

Figure 15.53. **Fibrolamellar carcinoma, intratumoral fibrosis.** The amount of fibrosis can vary, but this tumor had marked fibrosis.

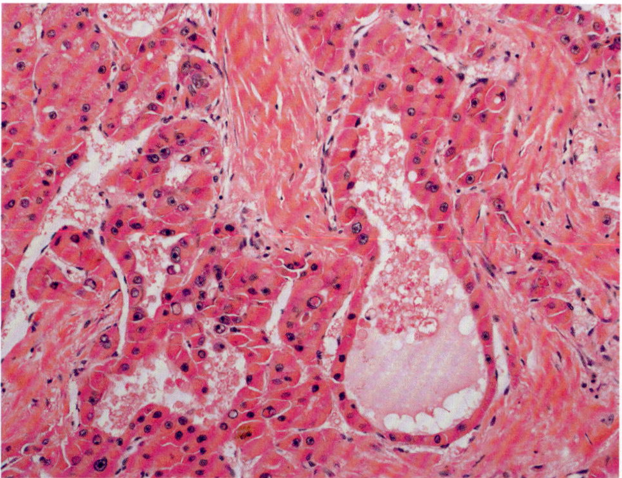

Figure 15.54. **Fibrolamellar carcinoma, psuedoglands.** Prominent psuedoglands are seen in this case.

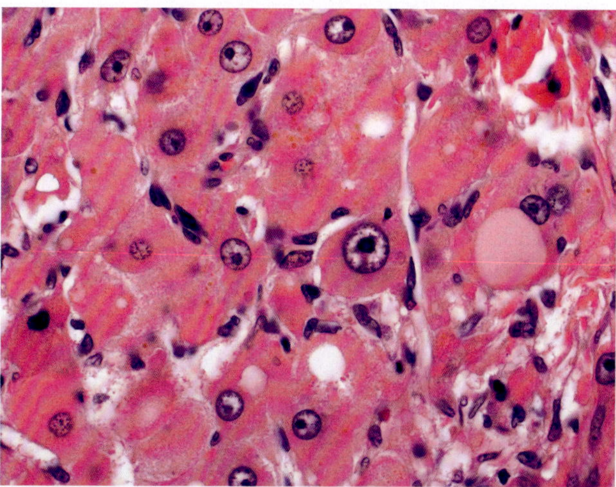

Figure 15.55. **Fibrolamellar carcinoma, pale bodies.** A pale body is present in the right side of this image.

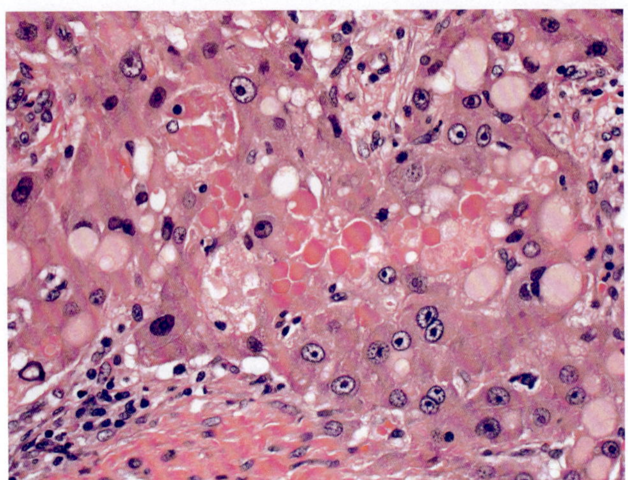

Figure 15.56. **Fibrolamellar carcinoma, hyaline bodies.** Prominent hyaline bodies are seen. Pale bodies are also present.

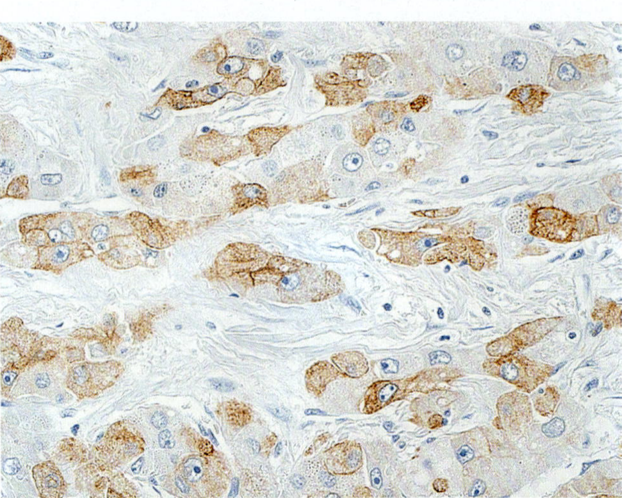

Figure 15.57. **Fibrolamellar carcinoma, CK7.** The CK7 is diffusely positive, although its not uncommon to have a mosaic staining pattern with clearly negative tumor cells admixed with the positive ones.

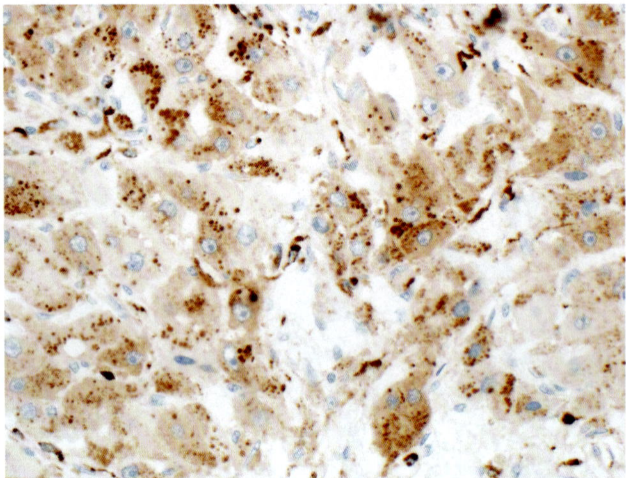

Figure 15.58. **Fibrolamellar carcinoma, CD68.** The CD68 show granular cytoplasmic staining.

KEY POINTS: Granulocyte Colony-Stimulating Factor–Producing Hepatocellular Carcinoma (Fig. 15.59)

- Frequency: <1%.
- Prognosis: worse.
- Serologies: elevated peripheral white blood cell counts, serum IL-6 levels,[43,60–62] and serum CRP levels.[43,60–63]
- Molecular correlates: the tumor secretes granulocyte colony-stimulating factor.
- Morphology: usually poorly differentiated tumors with numerous tumor-infiltrating neutrophils.
  - Focal areas of sarcomatoid morphology are common.
- Common pitfall: treated hepatocellular carcinomas can show areas of necrosis and sometimes focally intense neutrophil infiltrates.
- Differential diagnosis: rare cholangiocarcinomas[64] and metastatic carcinomas[65] can also produce granulocyte colony-stimulating factor, so there needs to be convincing evidence of hepatic differentiation.

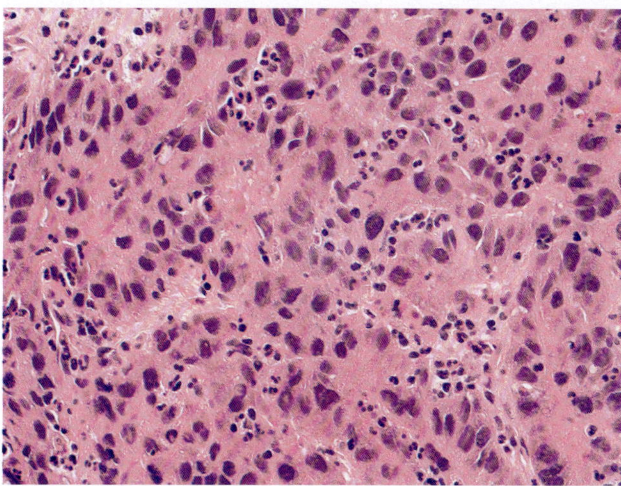

Figure 15.59. **Granulocyte colony-stimulating factor–producing hepatocellular carcinoma.** This poorly differentiated hepatocellular carcinoma has numerous infiltrating neutrophils.

KEY POINTS: Lymphocyte-Rich Hepatocellular Carcinoma (Figs. 15.60 and 15.61)

- Frequency: <1%.
- Prognosis: better.
- Molecular correlates: no consistent findings to date.
- Morphology: numerous tumor-infiltrating lymphocytes; there should be more lymphocytes than tumor cells in most fields.
  - Most tumors are well to moderately differentiated.
  - If the hepatocellular carcinoma is poorly differentiated, then the term lymphoepithelioma-like hepatocellular carcinoma is used (Fig. 15.61); in this setting hepatic differentiation should be proven with immunostains.
- Other findings: essentially all bona fide lymphocyte-rich hepatocellular carcinomas are EBV negative, in contrast to lymphocyte-rich cholangiocarcinomas, which are frequently EBV positive.
- Common pitfall: overcalling conventional hepatocellular carcinomas with mild diffuse patchy lymphocytosis, or dense but focal lymphocytosis, as lymphocyte-rich hepatocellular carcinoma.

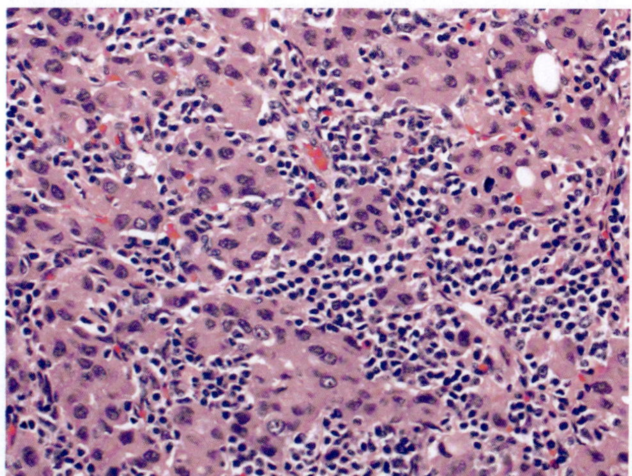

Figure 15.60. **Lymphocyte-rich hepatocellular carcinoma.** In this case, the lymphocytes outnumbered the tumor cells in essentially every field.

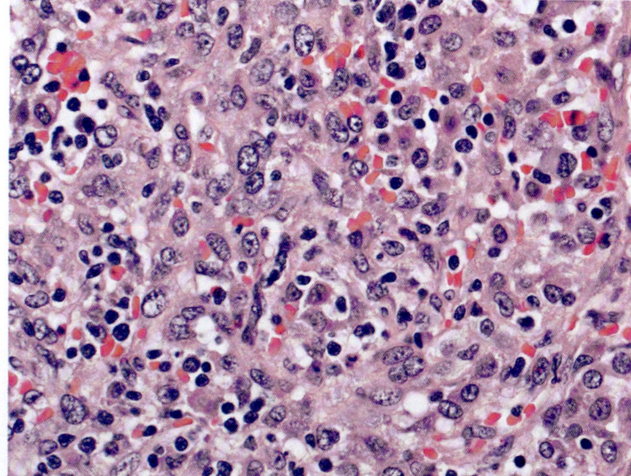

Figure 15.61. **Lymphoepithelial hepatocellar carcinoma.** The epithelial component is hard to see on H&E, but the tumor was keratin positive and showed patchy hepatic differentiation.

KEY POINTS: Macrotrabecular Hepatocellular Carcinoma (Fig. 15.62)

- Frequency: 5%.
- Prognosis: worse.
- Molecular correlates: P53 mutations, FGF19 amplifications.[66]
- Clinical correlates: elevated serum AFP, enriched for chronic hepatitis B.
- Morphology: macrotrabecular growth pattern with tumor cells generally showing basophilic and often scant cytoplasm.
    - Abundant vascular invasion.
    - Poor prognosis.
- Historical note: all of the key clinical and histological findings of this entity were originally described at the Laennec Liver Society meeting, 2013.

KEY POINTS: Sarcomatoid Hepatocellular Carcinoma (Fig. 15.63)

- Frequency: <1%.
- Prognosis: worse.
- Molecular correlates: no consistent findings to date.
- Morphology: moderately to poorly differentiated hepatocellular carcinoma with areas of spindle cell growth. A definite component of hepatocellular carcinoma is required.
    - Spindle cell pattern positive for keratin expression.
    - Spindle cell pattern occasionally retains expression of markers of hepatic differentiation.
    - Spindle cell component is often a minor component, but in some cases, most of the tumor shows a spindle cell growth pattern.
- Differential: carcinosarcoma. In contrast to carcinosarcomas, the sarcomatoid component of sarcomatoid hepatocellular carcinomas does not show specific mesenchymal differentiation by morphology or by immunostains.

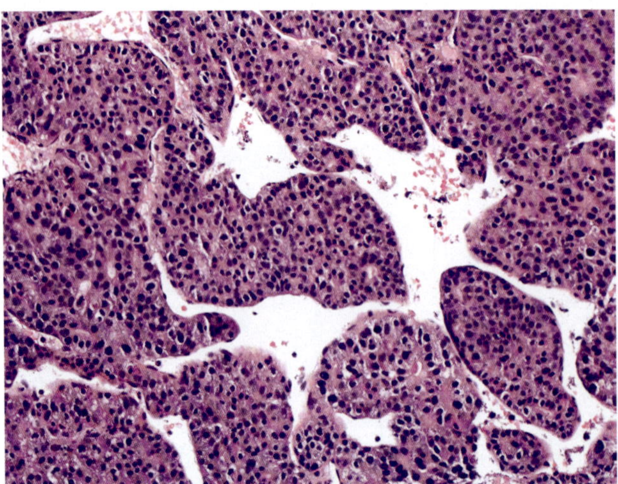

Figure 15.62. **Macrotrabecular hepatocellular carcinoma.** This variant is composed of basophilic tumor cells with a high N:C ratio. The tumor is essentially always positive for AFP on immunostain. Note that there also is a macrotrabecular growth pattern that is not the same as the macrotrabecular subtype and can be seen in conventional hepatocellular carcinomas as well as a variety of other subtypes.

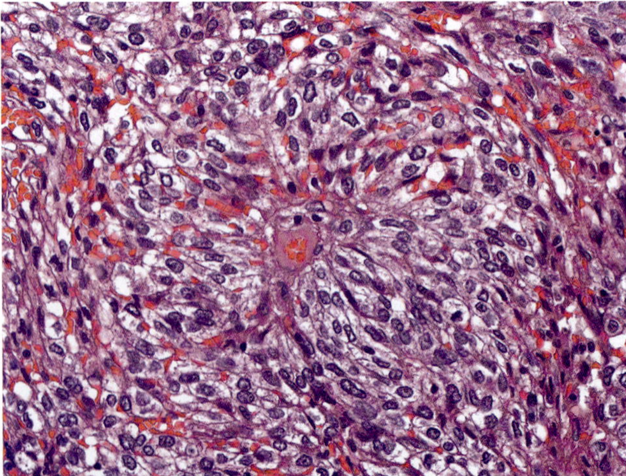

Figure 15.63. **Sarcomatoid hepatocellular carcinoma.** This hepatocellular carcinoma had an area of spindle cell growth, which still retained keratin and focal heppar1 expression.

KEY POINTS: Scirrhous Hepatocellular Carcinoma (Fig. 15.64)

- Frequency: 5%.
- Prognosis: similar to better.
- Molecular correlates: enriched for TSC1/TSC2 mutations.[66]
- Morphology: tumor defined by striking intratumoral fibrosis.
  - Hepatocellular carcinoma is well to moderately differentiated in most cases.
  - At least 50% of tumor should be made up of intratumoral fibrosis.
  - Grossly, the tumor is often composed of clusters of adjacent small subnodules.
  - Hyaline bodies and pale bodies are not uncommon.
- Special stains:
  - Reticulin loss is not always evident on biopsy specimens.
  - HepPar1 negative in about 50% of biopsy specimens, so arginase and glypican 3 should be part of immunostain evaluation.[67]
- Differential: fibrolamellar carcinoma, cholangiocarcinoma, and metastatic disease.
  - There should be positive immunostains for hepatic differentiation, and studies should rule out fibrolamellar carcinoma when needed, using immunostains for CK7 and CD68 or molecular testing to identify the DNAJB1-PRKACA genetic changes.

KEY POINTS: Steatohepatitic Hepatocellular Carcinoma (Figs. 15.65 and 15.66)

- Frequency: 20%.
- Clinical correlates: steatosis/steatohepatitis in the background liver from either the metabolic syndrome or ETOH.[68–70]
- Prognosis: similar.
- Molecular correlates: IL-6/JAK/STAT activation as well as a lower frequency of mutations in CTNNB1, TERT, and TP53.
- Morphology: tumor defined by steatohepatitis.

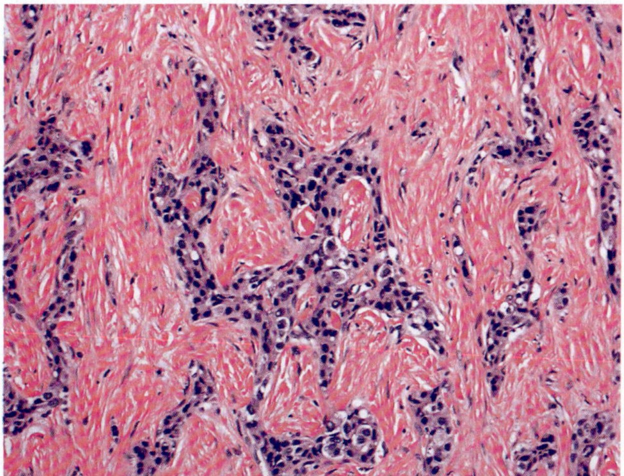

Figure 15.64. **Scirrhous hepatocellular carcinoma.** The hepatocellular carcinoma is growing as thin cords in a dense fibrotic background and can mimic cholangiocarcinoma or fibrolamellar carcinoma.

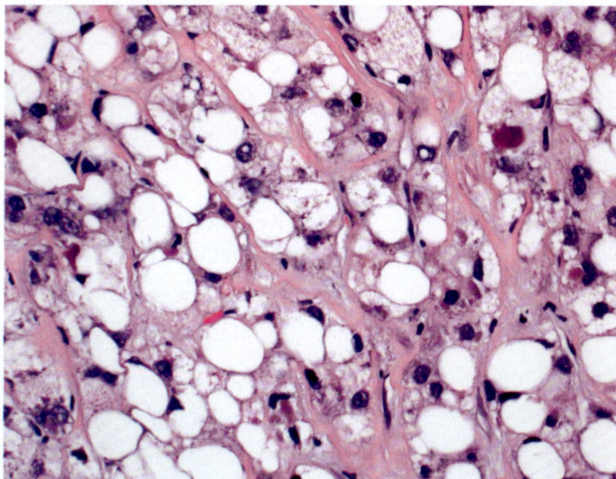

Figure 15.65. **Steatohepatitic hepatocellular carcinoma.** The carcinoma shows marked fat, lots of inflammation, and irregular areas of fibrosis.

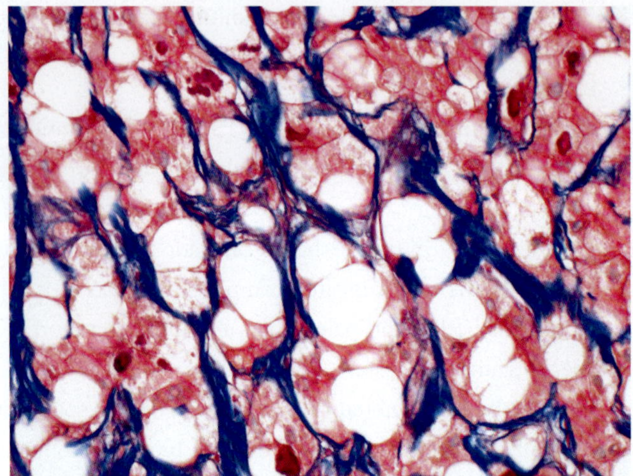

Figure 15.66. **Steatohepatitic hepatocellular carcinoma, trichrome.** The pericellular fibrosis is more apparent with the trichrome stain.

  - Macrovesicular steatosis (at least 5%; some studies have proposed at least 33%)
  - Balloon cells
  - Inflammation
  - Fibrosis
- Mechanism: there are two apparent mechanisms.[71]
  - The most common mechanism (>95% of cases) is that the entire liver shows fatty liver disease, and the tumor responds to the metabolic syndrome the same way as the background liver, by developing fatty liver disease.
  - A second, unknown mechanism leads to a steatohepatitic morphology in rare hepatocellular carcinomas in individuals who do not have the metabolic syndrome or ETOH use, and the background liver does not show steatosis. In these cases, the steatohepatitic morphology tends to be even more striking and is almost always diffuse.
- Common pitfall: hepatocellular carcinomas with mild macrovesicular steatosis alone do not qualify.
- Differential: tumor can be mistaken for nonneoplastic steatohepatitis. Focal nodular hyperplasia and inflammatory adenomas can also show steatosis but only very rarely steatohepatitis.

KEY POINTS: Chromophobe Hepatocellular Carcinoma (Figs. 15.67–15.69)

- Frequency: 1% to 5%.
- Prognosis: unclear.
- Molecular correlates: positive for alternating lengthening of telomeres (ALT).[41]
- Morphology: each component is present to varying degrees.
  - Abundant chromophobic to eosinophilic cytoplasm.
  - Background of low-grade tumor nuclei but then with patches of more distinct high-grade nuclear cytology (sudden anaplasia).
  - Irregular cystlike structure filled with pink flocculent material. Can also have intracystic hemorrhage.

PROVISIONAL SUBTYPES OF HEPATOCELLULAR CARCINOMA

The following subtypes are categorized as provisional because published data are limited to a few papers or because the best way to define them is not clear.

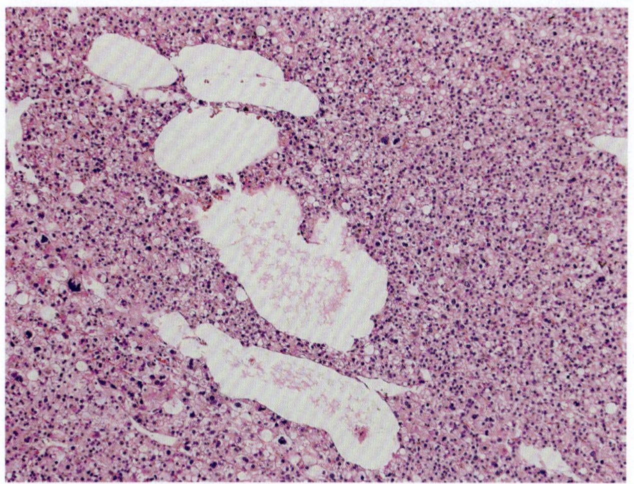

Figure 15.67. **Chromophobe hepatocellular carcinoma.** Scattered pseudocysts are seen at low power.

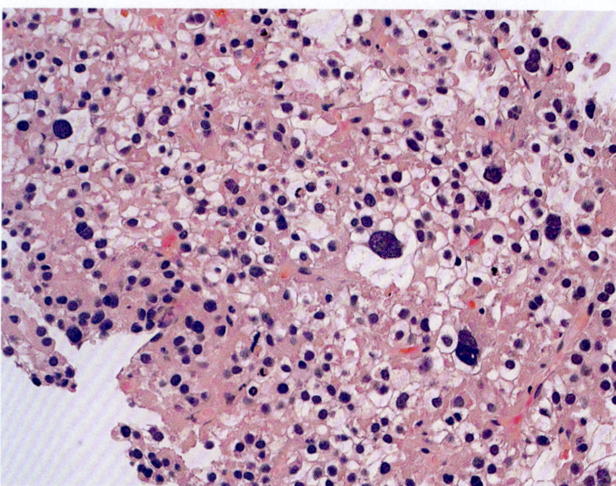

Figure 15.68. **Chromophobe hepatocellular carcinoma.** The tumor cells have almost a clear cell appearance, with generally bland nuclear cytology interrupted by sudden areas of more striking nuclear atypia.

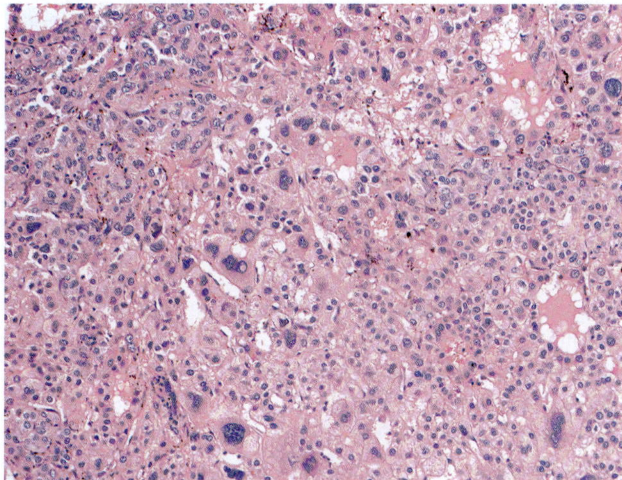

Figure 15.69. **Chromophobe hepatocellular carcinoma.** Another example with more eosinophilic cytoplasm.

KEY POINTS (Provisional Subtype): Combined Hepatocellular Carcinoma–Cholangiocarcinoma With Stem Cell Features

As originally conceived, this category was designed to capture cases that had conventional combined hepatocellular carcinoma–cholangiocarcinomas morphology but also had additional morphological findings or immunostain findings that suggested "stem-cellness." This original definition did not stick very well and has drifted considerably in the literature, so you have to read papers carefully to know what is being studied.

- Frequency: <1%.
- Prognosis: unclear.
- Clinical correlates: no consistent findings to date.
- Molecular correlates: no consistent findings to date.
- Morphology: three subtypes as follows.
  - **Typical subtype** (Fig. 15.70)**:** The edges of the hepatocellular carcinoma component have areas with a peripheral rim of smaller cells with a high nuclear to cytoplasmic ratio and hyperchromatic nuclei. The peripheral cells can be positive for CK7, CK19, and often CD56, c-Kit, and EpCAM. The center tumor cells are positive for the usual markers of hepatocellular differentiation.

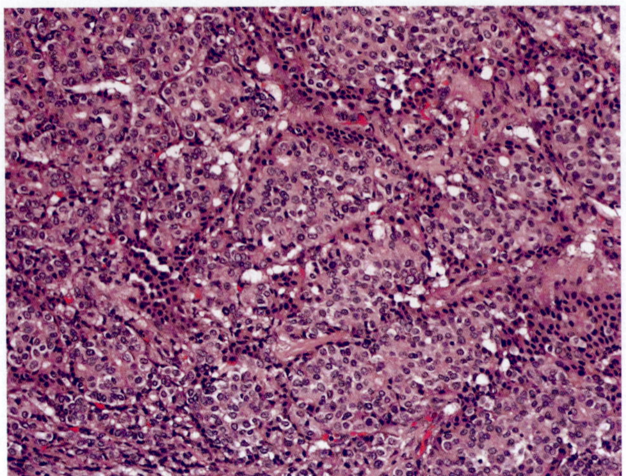

Figure 15.70. **Combined hepatocellular carcinoma–cholangiocarcinoma with stem cell features, subtype 1.** The hepatocellular carcinoma has islands of tumor cells surrounded by a rim or more primitive–looking tumor cells.

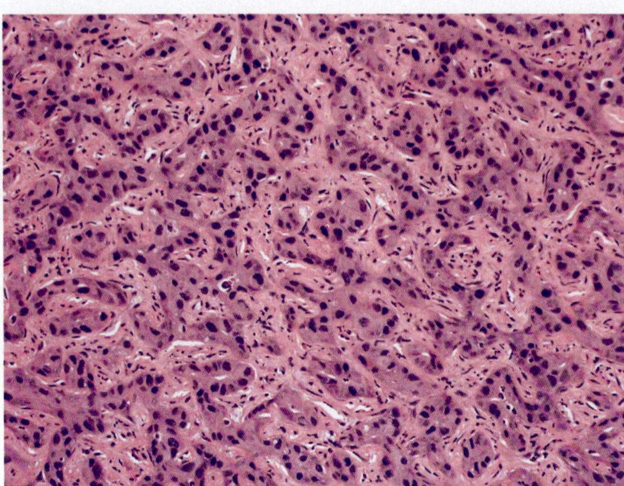

Figure 15.71. **Combined hepatocellular carcinoma–cholangiocarcinoma with stem cell features, subtype 3.** The growth pattern, cytology, and immunostains all support a cholangiocarcinoma. The tumor was also CD56 and CKIT positive.

- **Intermediate cell subtype:** The tumor cells are small- to medium-sized, plump-to-oval cells with mild to focally moderate cytological atypia. The tumor cells are hard to confidently classify as hepatic or biliary on morphology, and they can coexpress markers of hepatocellular and biliary differentiation. For example, a tumor could be positive for HepPar1, CK19, and CEA. Mucicarmine is negative, while CKIT expression is common.
- **Cholangiolocellular subtype** (Fig. 15.71)**:** This pattern is often associated with areas of conventional cholangiocarcinoma, and mostly it looks and stains like a cholangiocarcinoma. This subtype is often classified as cholangiocarcinoma and not a tumor with stem cell features. The tumor cells are small and show only mild cytological atypia. They have a branching, anastomosing cordlike pattern of growth, often with small tubular structures. The tumor stains like an ordinary cholangiocarcinoma. It was classified with other stem cell tumors because of positivity for the putative stem cell markers CD56, CKIT, and EpCAM.

KEY POINTS (Provisional Subtype): Lipid-Rich Hepatocellular Carcinoma (Fig. 15.72)

- Frequency: <1%.
- Prognosis: unclear.
- Molecular correlates: no consistent findings to date.
- Morphology: tumor cells have abundant cytoplasm filled with small lipid droplets, resembling microvesicular steatosis.[72]
  - This should be the predominant pattern.
  - Occasional foci of macrovesicular steatosis is acceptable.
- Differential: tumor can be mistaken for clear cell carcinoma at low power. On high power, the distinctive small lipid droplets indicate the proper diagnosis.

KEY POINTS (Provisional Subtype): Myxoid Hepatocellular Carcinoma[73]

- Frequency: <1%.
- Prognosis: unclear.
- Molecular correlates: no consistent findings to date.

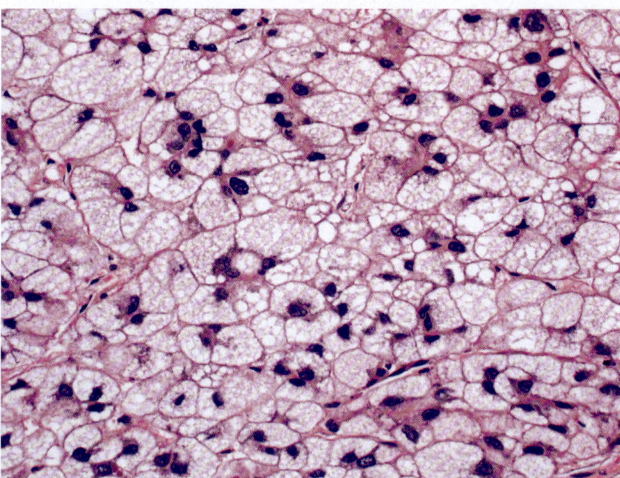

Figure 15.72. **Lipid-rich hepatocellular carcinoma.** At first examination, these tumors resemble clear cell hepatocellular carcinoma. Instead of glycogen, however, the cytoplasm is filled with small fat vacuoles.

- Morphology: tumor cells have distinctive extracellular myxoid material dissecting through the sinusoids.
- Adenomas can show similar morphology, so need to distinguish from myxoid hepatic adenoma.
- Distinct imaging findings have been reported.[74]

KEY POINTS (Provisional Subtype): Hepatocellular Carcinoma With Syncytial Giant Cells (Fig. 15.73)

- Frequency: <1%.
- Prognosis: unclear.
- Molecular correlates: no consistent findings to date.
- Morphology: tumor cells have distinctive syncytial giant cells.[75]
    - The giant cell transformation in the tumor cells resembles that of giant cell hepatitis, in contrast to the very atypical multinucleated giant cells in poorly differentiated hepatocellular carcinomas.

KEY POINTS (Provisional Subtype): Transitional Liver Cell Tumor (Fig. 15.74)

- Frequency: <1%.
- Prognosis: unclear.
- Clinical correlates: older children and adolescents.[76]
- Molecular correlates: no consistent findings to date.
- Morphology: tumor cells are well to moderately differentiated but have some areas that appear more primitive, resembling that of hepatoblastomas.
- Mechanism: unclear, but one possibility is that the tumor is a conventional hepatocellular carcinomas with more primitive areas that are more noticeable because of the patient's young age, which led the pathologist to consider the possibility of a hepatoblastoma. Another possibility that is sometimes proposed is that there may have been a hepatoblastoma that underwent "maturation"—a possibility that seems less likely based on current morphological and molecular findings.
- Note: this tumor has been renamed by some groups as hepatocellular malignant neoplasm, NOS.

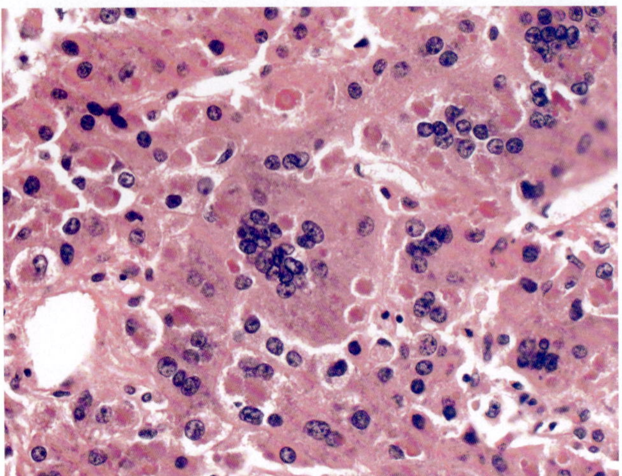

Figure 15.73. **Hepatocellular carcinoma with syncytial giant cells.** The tumor cells have abundant eosinophilic cytoplasm, and the nuclei show only mild cytological atypia, but there are scattered syncytial giant tumor cells.

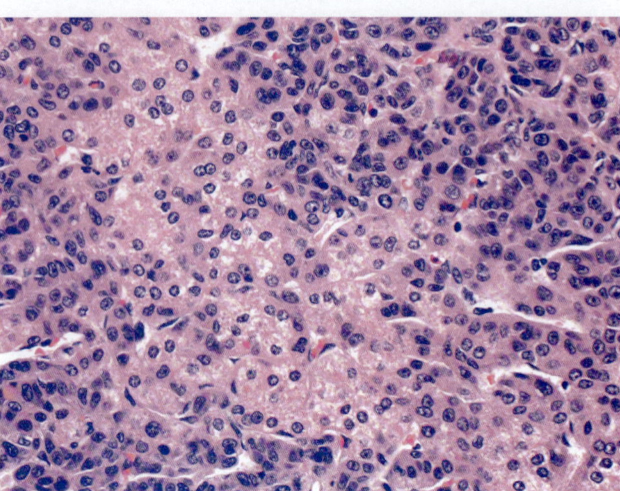

Figure 15.74. **Transitional liver cell tumor.** Most of this tumor looked like a conventional hepatocellular carcinoma, but there were areas with more primitive–looking tumor cells.

NEAR MISSES

CASE 1. A 57-year-old man had the metabolic syndrome and known fatty liver disease. A workup for fatigue showed a 5 cm liver mass. A biopsy was obtained and was initially interpreted as showing markedly active steatohepatitis with no evidence for tumor (Fig. 15.75). However, on review, it was noted that biopsy was lacking normal structures such as portal tracts and appeared to be all tumor. Further evaluation confirmed the steatohepatitic variant of hepatocellular carcinoma.

The steatohepatitic variant of hepatocellular carcinoma shows macrovesicular steatosis, intratumoral inflammation, ballooned tumor cells, and intratumoral pericellular fibrosis, all of which can mimic steatohepatitis in the background liver.

CASE 2. A 62-year-old woman with cirrhosis from hemochromatosis underwent liver transplantation. The explant showed a 6 cm hepatocellular carcinoma with patchy areas of necrosis. The case was received as consultation to rule out fibrolamellar carcinoma because there was intratumoral fibrosis that in some areas ran in parallel bands (Fig. 15.76). In addition, the tumor cells had abundant cytoplasm and vesiculated chromatin.

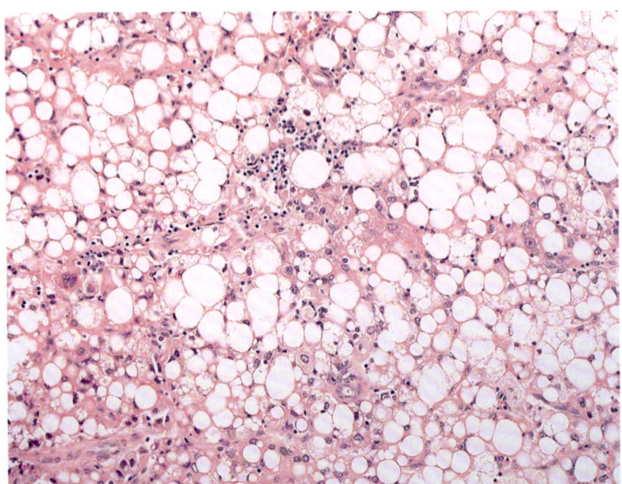

Figure 15.75. **Near miss case 1, steatohepatitic variant of hepatocellular carcinoma.** The diagnosis was initially missed in this case because of the well-differentiated morphology and the findings of steatohepatitis.

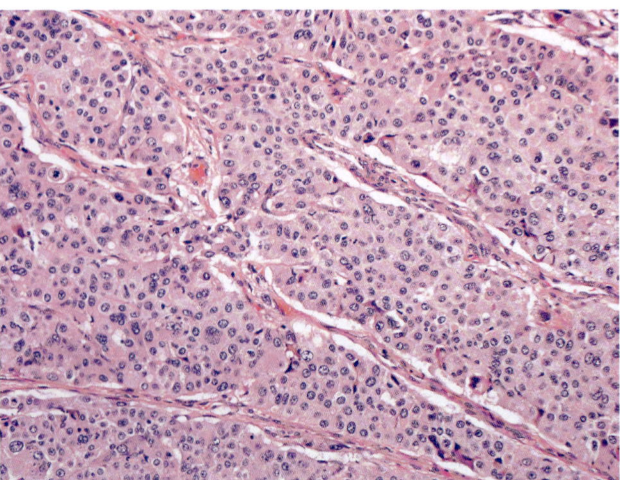

Figure 15.76. **Near miss case 2, hepatocellular carcinoma with intratumoral fibrosis.** The intratumoral fibrosis in this conventional hepatocellular carcinoma mimicked one aspect of the morphology of fibrolamellar carcinoma

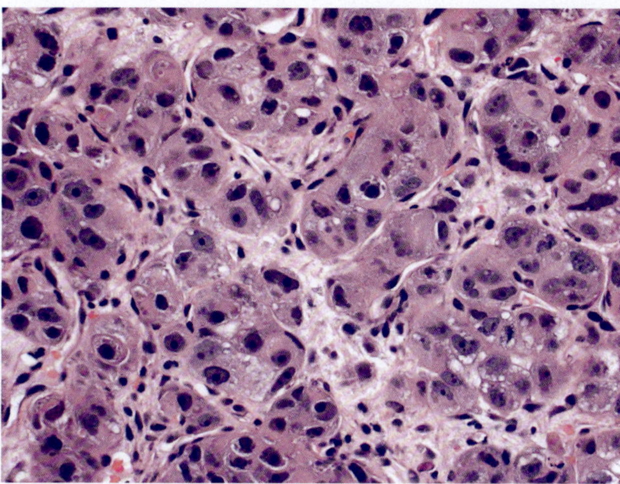

Figure 15.77. **Near miss case 3, renal carcinoma mimicking well-differentiated hepatocellular carcinoma.** The tumor has abundant cytoplasm and a trabecular growth pattern, mimicking hepatocellular carcinoma.

Fibrolamellar carcinoma was very unlikely because of the patient's age and the background of cirrhosis, but to more fully rule out fibrolamellar carcinoma, additional studies were performed. Immunostains confirmed hepatic differentiation, but immunostains (CD68, CK7) and molecular testing (FISH for the chromosome 19 deletion leading to the PRKACA-DNAJBA fusion) were both negative for fibrolamellar carcinoma.

This case illustrates the point that fibrolamellar carcinomas have a fairly narrow and well-defined clinical association (younger age, no background liver disease). Some hepatocellular carcinomas outside of this clinical range can resemble fibrolamellar carcinoma on H&E, as the morphology seen with fibrolamellar carcinoma is not entirely specific. Confirmatory tests, as used in this case, can help clarify the proper diagnosis.

CASE 3. A 41-year-old man had an incidentally discovered liver mass that was biopsied. The biopsy showed a tumor with a trabecular growth pattern composed of cells that resembled hepatocytes, suggesting hepatocellular carcinoma (Fig. 15.77). However, markers of hepatic differentiation were negative, including hepPar1 and arginase. Further workup found the tumor was positive for pax8, consistent with renal origin.

Well- and moderately differentiated hepatocellular carcinomas have several important mimics, the most common being metastatic renal carcinomas and metastatic neuroendocrine tumors. Immunostains to confirm hepatic differentiation are important, even when the morphology suggests hepatocellular carcinoma, as seen in this case.

References

1. Kim H, Park YN. Massive hepatic necrosis with large regenerative nodules. *Korean J Hepatol.* 2010;16:334-337.
2. Furuya K, Nakamura M, Yamamoto Y, Togei K, Otsuka H. Macroregenerative nodule of the liver. A clinicopathologic study of 345 autopsy cases of chronic liver disease. *Cancer.* 1988;61:99-105.
3. Hytiroglou P, Theise ND, Schwartz M, Mor E, Miller C, Thung SN. Macroregenerative nodules in a series of adult cirrhotic liver explants: issues of classification and nomenclature. *Hepatology.* 1995;21:703-708.
4. Seki S, Sakaguchi H, Kitada T, et al. Outcomes of dysplastic nodules in human cirrhotic liver: a clinicopathological study. *Clin Cancer Res.* 2000;6:3469-3473.
5. Iavarone M, Manini MA, Sangiovanni A, et al. Contrast-enhanced computed tomography and ultrasound-guided liver biopsy to diagnose dysplastic liver nodules in cirrhosis. *Dig Liver Dis.* 2013;45:43-49.
6. Sato T, Kondo F, Ebara M, et al. Natural history of large regenerative nodules and dysplastic nodules in liver cirrhosis: 28-year follow-up study. *Hepatol Int.* 2015;9:330-336.
7. Nakano M, Saito A, Yamamoto M, Doi M, Takasaki K. Stromal and blood vessel wall invasion in well-differentiated hepatocellular carcinoma. *Liver.* 1997;17:41-46.

8. Kojiro M, Roskams T. Early hepatocellular carcinoma and dysplastic nodules. *Semin Liver Dis*. 2005;25:133-142.

9. Kondo F. Assessment of stromal invasion for correct histological diagnosis of early hepatocellular carcinoma. *Int J Hepatol*. 2011;2011:241652.

10. Park YN, Kojiro M, Di Tommaso L, et al. Ductular reaction is helpful in defining early stromal invasion, small hepatocellular carcinomas, and dysplastic nodules. *Cancer*. 2007;109:915-923.

11. Seymour K, Charnley RM. Evidence that metastasis is less common in cirrhotic than normal liver: a systematic review of post-mortem case-control studies. *Br J Surg*. 1999;86:1237-1242.

12. Wang Q, Luan W, Villanueva GA, et al. Clinical prognostic variables in young patients (under 40 years) with hepatitis B virus-associated hepatocellular carcinoma. *J Dig Dis*. 2012;13:214-218.

13. Yeh MM, Daniel HD, Torbenson M. Hepatitis C-associated hepatocellular carcinomas in non-cirrhotic livers. *Mod Pathol*. 2010;23:276-283.

14. Baffy G, Brunt EM, Caldwell SH. Hepatocellular carcinoma in non-alcoholic fatty liver disease: an emerging menace. *J Hepatol*. 2012;56:1384-1391.

15. Alexander J, Torbenson M, Wu TT, Yeh MM. Nonalcoholic fatty liver disease contributes to hepatocellular carcinoma in non-cirrhotic liver: a clinical and pathological study. *J Gastroenterol Hepatol*. 2013.

16. Clark I, Shah SS, Moreira R, et al. A subset of well-differentiated hepatocellular carcinomas are Arginase-1 negative. *Hum Pathol*. 2017;69:90-95.

17. Singhi AD, Jain D, Kakar S, Wu TT, Yeh MM, Torbenson M. Reticulin loss in benign fatty liver: an important diagnostic pitfall when considering a diagnosis of hepatocellular carcinoma. *Am J Surg Pathol*. 2012;36:710-715.

18. Aigelsreiter A, Neumann J, Pichler M, et al. Hepatocellular carcinomas with intracellular hyaline bodies have a poor prognosis. *Liver Int*. 2017;37:600-610.

19. Nishihara Y, Aishima S, Kuroda Y, et al. Biliary phenotype of hepatocellular carcinoma after preoperative transcatheter arterial chemoembolization. *J Gastroenterol Hepatol*. 2008;23:1860-1868.

20. Rodriguez-Peralvarez M, Luong TV, Andreana L, Meyer T, Dhillon AP, Burroughs AK. A systematic review of microvascular invasion in hepatocellular carcinoma: diagnostic and prognostic variability. *Ann Surg Oncol*. 2013;20:325-339.

21. Ohashi M, Wakai T, Korita PV, Ajioka Y, Shirai Y, Hatakeyama K. Histological evaluation of intracapsular venous invasion for discrimination between portal and hepatic venous invasion in hepatocellular carcinoma. *J Gastroenterol Hepatol*. 2010;25:143-149.

22. Benckert C, Jonas S, Thelen A, et al. Liver transplantation for hepatocellular carcinoma in cirrhosis: prognostic parameters. *Transpl Proc*. 2005;37:1693-1694.

23. Zhou L, Rui JA, Wang SB, et al. Outcomes and prognostic factors of cirrhotic patients with hepatocellular carcinoma after radical major hepatectomy. *World J Surg*. 2007;31:1782-1787.

24. Lang H, Sotiropoulos GC, Brokalaki EI, et al. Survival and recurrence rates after resection for hepatocellular carcinoma in noncirrhotic livers. *J Am Coll Surg*. 2007;205:27-36.

25. Jonas S, Bechstein WO, Steinmuller T, et al. Vascular invasion and histopathologic grading determine outcome after liver transplantation for hepatocellular carcinoma in cirrhosis. *Hepatology*. 2001;33:1080-1086.

26. Nzeako UC, Goodman ZD, Ishak KG. Comparison of tumor pathology with duration of survival of North American patients with hepatocellular carcinoma. *Cancer*. 1995;76:579-588.

27. Durnez A, Verslype C, Nevens F, et al. The clinicopathological and prognostic relevance of cytokeratin 7 and 19 expression in hepatocellular carcinoma. A possible progenitor cell origin. *Histopathology*. 2006;49:138-151.

28. Uenishi T, Kubo S, Yamamoto T, et al. Cytokeratin 19 expression in hepatocellular carcinoma predicts early postoperative recurrence. *Cancer Sci*. 2003;94:851-857.

29. Christensen WN, Boitnott JK, Kuhajda FP. Immunoperoxidase staining as a diagnostic aid for hepatocellular carcinoma. *Mod Pathol*. 1989;2:8-12.

30. Kim H, Choi GH, Na DC, Ahn EY, et al. Human hepatocellular carcinomas with "Stemness"-related marker expression: keratin 19 expression and a poor prognosis. *Hepatology*. 2011;54:1707-1717.

31. Vlasoff DM, Baschinsky DY, Frankel WL. Cytokeratin 5/6 immunostaining in hepatobiliary and pancreatic neoplasms. *Appl Immunohistochem Mol Morphol*. 2002;10:147-151.

32. Shah SS, Wu TT, Torbenson MS, Chandan VS. Aberrant CDX2 expression in hepatocellular carcinomas: an important diagnostic pitfall. *Hum Pathol*. 2017;64:13-18.

33. Ferrone CR, Ting DT, Shahid M, et al. The ability to diagnose intrahepatic holangiocarcinoma definitively using novel branched DNA-enhanced albumin RNA in situ hybridization technology. *Ann Surg Oncol*. 2016;23:290-296.

34. Cotoi CG, Khorsandi SE, Plesea IE, Quaglia A. Histological aspects of post-TACE hepatocellular carcinoma. *Rom J Morphol Embryol*. 2012;53:677-682.

35. Herber S, Biesterfeld S, Franz U, et al. Correlation of multislice CT and histomorphology in HCC following TACE: predictors of outcome. *Cardiovasc Intervent Radiol*. 2008;31:768-777.

36. Vasuri F, Malvi D, Rosini F, et al. Revisiting the role of pathological analysis in transarterial chemoembolization-treated hepatocellular carcinoma after transplantation. *World J Gastroenterol*. 2014;20:13538-13545.

37. Sciarra A, Ronot M, Di Tommaso L, et al. TRIP: a pathological score for transarterial chemoembolization resistance individualized prediction in hepatocellular carcinoma. *Liver Int*. 2015;35:2466-2473.

38. Lai JP, Conley A, Knudsen BS, Guindi M. Hypoxia after transarterial chemoembolization may trigger a progenitor cell phenotype in hepatocellular carcinoma. *Histopathology*. 2015;67:442-450.

39. Zen C, Zen Y, Mitry RR, et al. Mixed phenotype hepatocellular carcinoma after transarterial chemoembolization and liver transplantation. *Liver Transpl*. 2011;17:943-954.

40. Kallini JR, Gabr A, Thorlund K, et al. Comparison of the adverse event profile of theraSphere((R)) with SIR-spheres((R)) for the treatment of unresectable hepatocellular carcinoma: a systematic review. *Cardiovasc Intervent Radiol*. 2017;40:1033-1043.

41. Wood LD, Heaphy CM, Daniel HD, et al. Chromophobe hepatocellular carcinoma with abrupt anaplasia: a proposal for a new subtype of hepatocellular carcinoma with unique morphological and molecular features. *Mod Pathol*. 2013;26:1586-1593.

42. Lao XM, Chen DY, Zhang YQ, et al. Primary carcinosarcoma of the liver: clinicopathologic features of 5 cases and a review of the literature. *Am J Surg Pathol*. 2007;31:817-826.

43. Aita K, Seki K. Carcinosarcoma of the liver producing granulocyte-colony stimulating factor. *Pathol Int*. 2006;56:413-419.

44. Xiang S, Chen YF, Guan Y, Chen XP. Primary combined hepatocellular-cholangiocellular sarcoma: an unusual case. *World J Gastroenterol*. 2015;21:7335-7342.

45. Lee KB. Sarcomatoid hepatocellular carcinoma with mixed osteoclast-like giant cells and chondroid differentiation. *Clin Mol Hepatol*. 2014;20:313-316.

46. Kuwano H, Sonoda T, Hashimoto H, Enjoji M. Hepatocellular carcinoma with osteoclast-like giant cells. *Cancer*. 1984;54:837-842.

47. Hood DL, Bauer TW, Leibel SA, McMahon JT. Hepatic giant cell carcinoma. An ultrastructural and immunohistochemical study. *Am J Clin Pathol*. 1990;93:111-116.

48. Sasaki A, Yokoyama S, Nakayama I, Nakashima K, Kim YI, Kitano S. Sarcomatoid hepatocellular carcinoma with osteoclast-like giant cells: case report and immunohistochemical observations. *Pathol Int*. 1997;47:318-324.

49. Tanahashi C, Nagae H, Nukaya T, Hasegawa M, Yatabe Y. Combined hepatocellular carcinoma and osteoclast-like giant cell tumor of the liver: possible clue to histogenesis. *Pathol Int*. 2009;59:813-816.

50. Dioscoridi L, Bisogni D, Freschi G. Hepatocellular carcinoma with osteoclast-like giant cells: report of the seventh case in the literature. *Case Rep Surg*. 2015;2015:836105.

51. Fan Z, van de Rijn M, Montgomery K, Rouse RV. Hep par 1 antibody stain for the differential diagnosis of hepatocellular carcinoma: 676 tumors tested using tissue microarrays and conventional tissue sections. *Mod Pathol*. 2003;16:137-144.

52. Murakata LA, Ishak KG, Nzeako UC. Clear cell carcinoma of the liver: a comparative immunohistochemical study with renal clear cell carcinoma. *Mod Pathol*. 2000;13:874-881.

53. Li R, Yang D, Tang CL, et al. Combined hepatocellular carcinoma and cholangiocarcinoma (biphenotypic) tumors: clinical characteristics, imaging features of contrast-enhanced ultrasound and computed tomography. *BMC Cancer*. 2016;16:158.

54. Torbenson M. Fibrolamellar carcinoma: 2012 update. *Scientifica*. 2012;2012:15.

55. Kakar S, Burgart LJ, Batts KP, Garcia J, Jain D, Ferrell LD. Clinicopathologic features and survival in fibrolamellar carcinoma: comparison with conventional hepatocellular carcinoma with and without cirrhosis. *Mod Pathol*. 2005;18:1417-1423.

56. Njei B, Konjeti VR, Ditah I. Prognosis of patients with fibrolamellar hepatocellular carcinoma versus conventional hepatocellular carcinoma: a systematic review and meta-analysis. *Gastrointest Cancer Res*. 2014;7:49-54.

57. Rondell PG, Lackner K, Terracciano L, et al. Fibrolamellar carcinoma in the Carney complex: PRKAR1A loss instead of the classic DNAJB1-PRKACA fusion. *Hepatology*. 2018;68:1441-1447.

58. Graham RP, Jin L, Knutson DL, et al. DNAJB1-PRKACA is specific for fibrolamellar carcinoma. *Mod Pathol*. 2015;28.

59. Ross HM, Daniel HD, Vivekanandan P, et al. Fibrolamellar carcinomas are positive for CD68. *Mod Pathol*. 2011;24:390-395.

60. Kohno M, Shirabe K, Mano Y, et al. Granulocyte colony-stimulating-factor-producing hepatocellular carcinoma with extensive sarcomatous changes: report of a case. *Surg Today*. 2012.

61. Amano H, Itamoto T, Emoto K, Hino H, Asahara T, Shimamoto F. Granulocyte colony-stimulating factor-producing combined hepatocellular/cholangiocellular carcinoma with sarcomatous change. *J Gastroenterol*. 2005;40:1158-1159.

62. Araki K, Kishihara F, Takahashi K, et al. Hepatocellular carcinoma producing a granulocyte colony-stimulating factor: report of a resected case with a literature review. *Liver Int*. 2007;27:716-721.

63. Joshita S, Nakazawa K, Koike S, et al. A case of granulocyte-colony stimulating factor-producing hepatocellular carcinoma confirmed by immunohistochemistry. *J Korean Med Sci*. 2010;25:476-480.

64. Takenaka M, Akiba J, Kawaguchi T, et al. Intrahepatic cholangiocarcinoma with sarcomatous change producing granulocyte-colony stimulating factor. *Pathol Int*. 2013;63:233-235.

65. Shimakawa T, Asaka S, Usuda A, et al. Granulocyte-colony stimulating factor (G-CSF)-producing esophageal squamous cell carcinoma: a case report. *Int Surg*. 2014;99:280-285.

66. Calderaro J, Couchy G, Imbeaud S, et al. Histological subtypes of hepatocellular carcinoma are related to gene mutations and molecular tumour classification. *J Hepatol*. 2017;67:727-738.

67. Krings G, Ramachandran R, Jain D, et al. Immunohistochemical pitfalls and the importance of glypican 3 and arginase in the diagnosis of scirrhous hepatocellular carcinoma. *Mod Pathol*. 2013;26:782-791.

68. Salomao M, Remotti H, Vaughan R, Siegel AB, Lefkowitch JH, Moreira RK. The steatohepatitic variant of hepatocellular carcinoma and its association with underlying steatohepatitis. *Hum Pathol*. 2012;43:737-746.

69. Shibahara J, Ando S, Sakamoto Y, Kokudo N, Fukayama M. Hepatocellular carcinoma with steatohepatitic features: a clinicopathological study of Japanese patients. *Histopathology*. 2014;64:951-962.

70. Jain D, Nayak NC, Kumaran V, Saigal S. Steatohepatitic hepatocellular carcinoma, a morphologic indicator of associated metabolic risk factors: a study from India. *Arch Pathol Lab Med*. 2013;137:961-966.

71. Yeh MM, Liu Y, Torbenson M. Steatohepatitic variant of hepatocellular carcinoma in the absence of metabolic syndrome or background steatosis: a clinical, pathological, and genetic study. *Hum Pathol*. 2015;46:1769-1775.

72. Orikasa H, Ohyama R, Tsuka N, Eyden BP, Yamazaki K. Lipid-rich clear-cell hepatocellular carcinoma arising in non-alcoholic steatohepatitis in a patient with diabetes mellitus. *J Submicrosc Cytol Pathol*. 2001;33:195-200.

73. Salaria SN, Graham RP, Aishima S, Mounajjed T, Yeh MM, Torbenson MS. Primary hepatic tumors with myxoid change: morphologically unique hepatic adenomas and hepatocellular carcinomas. *Am J Surg Pathol*. 2015;39:318-324.

74. Young JT, Kurup AN, Graham RP, Torbenson MS, Venkatesh SK. Myxoid hepatocellular neoplasms: imaging appearance of a unique mucinous tumor variant. *Abdom Radiol (NY)*. 2016.41.

75. Atra A, Al-Asiri R, Wali S, Al-Husseini H, Al-Bassas A, Zimmermann A. Hepatocellular carcinoma, syncytial giant cell: a novel variant in children: a case report. *Ann Diagn Pathol*. 2007;11:61-63.

76. Prokurat A, Kluge P, Kosciesza A, Perek D, Kappeler A, Zimmermann A. Transitional liver cell tumors (TLCT) in older children and adolescents: a novel group of aggressive hepatic tumors expressing beta-catenin. *Med Pediatr Oncol*. 2002;39:510-518.

16 BILIARY TUMORS

CHAPTER OUTLINE

BENIGN BILIARY LESIONS

CHECKLIST: Benign Biliary Lesions

- ☐ Benign reactive bile ductular proliferations in an area of parenchymal collapse
- ☐ Bile duct hamartoma (also called Von Meyenburg complex)
- ☐ Bile duct adenoma
  - ○ Clear cell bile duct adenoma
- ☐ Biliary adenofibroma

REACTIVE BILE DUCTULAR PROLIFERATIONS

Reactive biliary proliferations can present as mass lesions when there has been a focal injury, usually ischemic, to a segment or subsegment of the liver. Many of these lesions fall into the category of segmental atrophy/nodular elastosis. These reaction lesions have abundant mixed inflammation and a brisk bile ductular proliferation associated with parenchymal collapse. The parenchymal collapse typically leaves behind intact portal tracts that become closely approximated, with the lobules replaced by ductular proliferation and inflammatory cells.

BILE DUCT HAMARTOMA

Bile duct hamartomas are usually small lesions that can be located throughout the liver. Subcapsular lesions can be visible grossly as small white spots on the capsule and often lead to frozen sections to rule out metastatic disease during resections for abdominal tumors. Bile duct hamartomas can be found in noncirrhotic livers and cirrhotic livers but overall are more common in cirrhotic livers, especially cirrhosis resulting from chronic hepatitis C or alcohol-related liver disease. Bile duct hamartomas are also found in adult polycystic liver disease, with numerous lesions scattered diffusely throughout the liver parenchyma. In contrast, sporadic lesions are typically single or few in number.

Bile duct hamartomas are composed of interanastomosing biliary structures lined by bland biliary epithelium (Figs. 16.1 and 16.2). The lumens are typically dilated and commonly contain small bile plugs (Fig. 16.3). The intervening fibrous stroma can be loose or hyalinized and often shows mild inflammation (Fig. 16.3). The hamartomas are commonly found adjacent to or involving a portal tract.

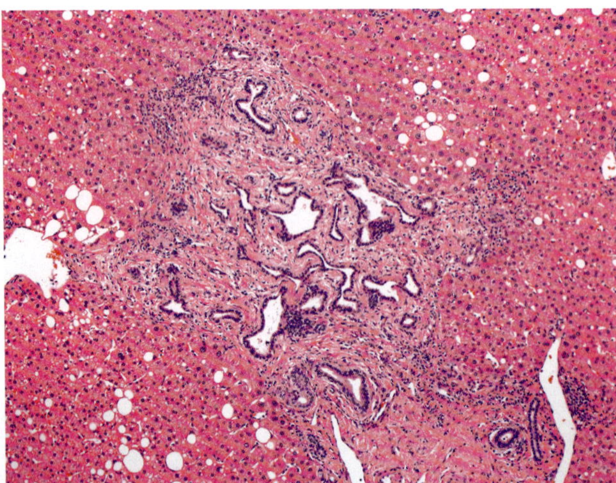

Figure 16.1. **Von Meyenburg complex/bile duct hamartoma.** At low power, the lesion is composed of interanastomosing bile duct–like structures with open lumens. A normal portal tract is present at the edge of the Von Meyenburg complex, in the lower right of the image.

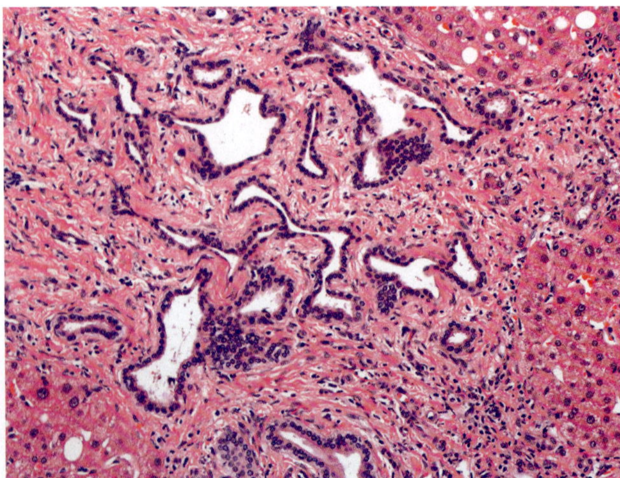

Figure 16.2. **Von Meyenburg complex/bile duct hamartoma.** At higher power, there is no cytological atypia and no mitotic figures. The background stroma is dense and fibrotic and shows mild patchy lymphocytic inflammation.

Most bile duct hamartomas are less than 10 mm, but occasional cases can be larger, with rare reports of lesions up to 20 cm. These larger lesions have been called *giant cystic bile duct hamartomas*[1,2] and show typical areas of bile duct hamartoma admixed with large dilated biliary cysts. Many of these (perhaps all) would now be classified as adenofibromas.

BILE DUCT ADENOMA

Bile duct adenomas are benign acquired lesions that are more common in cirrhotic livers than noncirrhotic livers. An older term in the literature is *peribiliary gland hamartoma*,[3] but the tumors are now known to be clonal proliferations and not hamartomas, so the term *bile duct adenoma* is preferred.

Bile duct adenomas are generally single and usually less than 10 mm, but they can be larger, up to several cm, and are multiple in about 10% of cases. Bile duct adenomas are composed of small round tubules with a variably dense fibrotic background (Figs. 16.4 and 16.5). The tubules have either no or very modest lumens and are lined by benign biliary epithelial cells. In contrast to hamartomas, the lumens do not contain bile. The biliary cells tend to be plumper than in bile duct hamartomas but are without cytological atypia. Occasionally, the adenomas can have an oncocytic appearance[4] or a clear cell appearance (Fig. 16.6).[5] Some bile duct adenomas are associated with dense

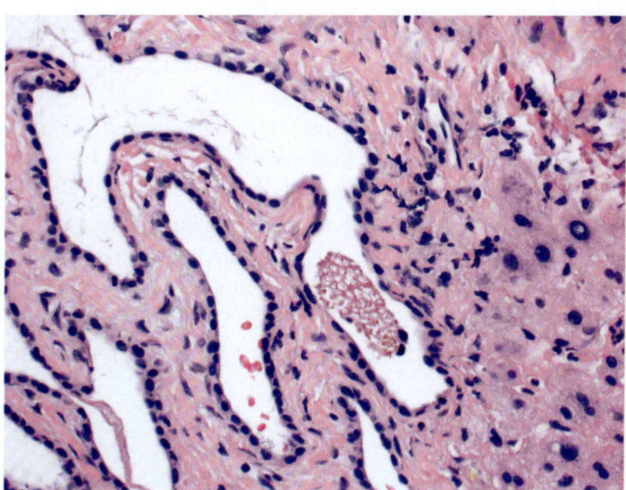

Figure 16.3. **Von Meyenburg complex/bile duct hamartoma.** Bile can be seen within the dilated lumens of the duct-like structures.

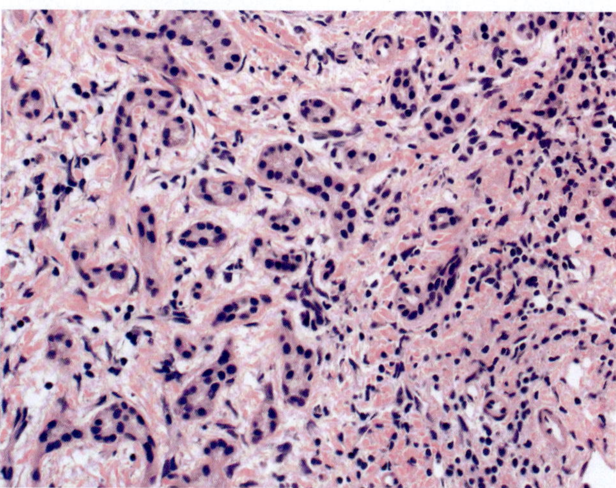

Figure 16.4. **Bile duct adenoma.** The bile duct adenoma is composed of smaller glands with lumens that are inconspicuous and lack bile.

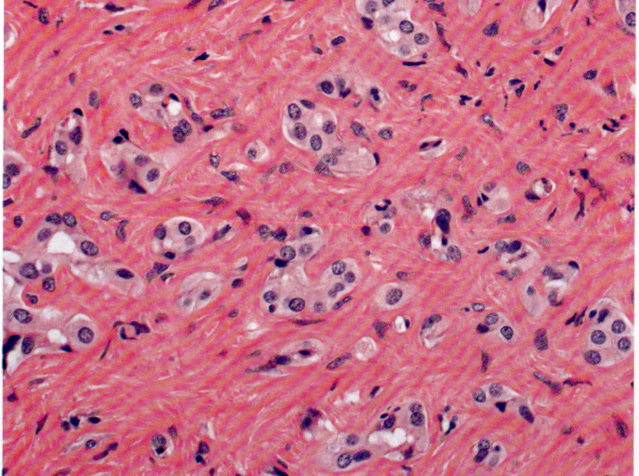

Figure 16.5. **Bile duct adenoma.** There is no cytological atypia and no mitotic figures.

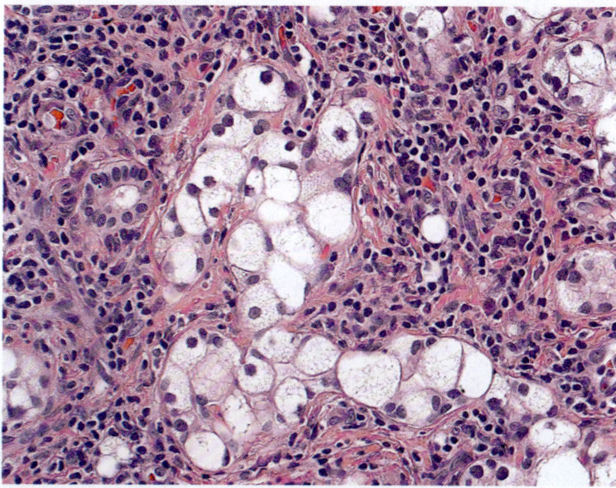

Figure 16.6. **Bile duct adenoma, clear cell type.** Clear cell bile duct adenomas have distinctive clear cytoplasm. They also tend to have significantly more chronic inflammation in the fibrotic stroma. Patchy, mild nuclear atypia can also be seen.

sclerosis, and the glands appear small and atrophic. In individuals with alpha1-antitrypsin deficiency, the adenomas can show eosinophilic cytoplasmic inclusions, even if inclusions are minimal in the background liver.[6,7] Rare bile duct adenomas have also been reported to have small clusters of endocrine cells surrounding the ducts in the adenoma.[8]

BILIARY ADENOFIBROMA

Biliary adenofibromas are larger tumors that range in size from 2 to 20 cm.[9–11] Most cases are single lesions, but rare examples with multiple tumors have been reported.[11] The tumors can recur if incompletely resected.[11]

Biliary adenofibromas are composed of dilated tubulocystic structures that often show areas of interanastomosing growth that resembles Von Meyenburg complexes (Fig. 16.7). The biliary structures are dilated and filled with varying amounts of bile, blood, and proteinaceous material. Cystic change is invariably present and can be either microcystic or macrocystic (cysts greater than 1 cm). The lining epithelium looks (Fig. 16.7) and stains like biliary cells. An oncocytic or apocrine type change can be seen in some cases. In other cases, there can be areas where the epithelium is more flattened (Fig. 16.8). Atypia is absent to equivocal. Sometimes, the lining biliary epithelium can have a micropapillary architecture.

The biliary structures are embedded in dense fibrotic stroma that shows mild chronic inflammation and frequently has entrapped islands of bland hepatocytes. Stromal calcifications are occasionally present.

The tumor is often over diagnosed when an ordinary bile duct hamartoma gets a bit large, which makes sense because small adenofibromas look pretty much like a large bile duct hamartomas. There are no well-established size criteria, but here is a useful general guideline: smaller lesions, 1 cm or less, are almost always hamartomas, while lesions greater than 2 cm are almost always biliary adenofibromas. Likewise, there are no firm histological criteria that will sharply separate these two lesions, but a prominent component of microcysts or macrocysts favors a biliary adenofibroma, while the presence of other typical bile duct hamartomas in the background liver favors the lesion being a larger but typical bile duct hamartoma.

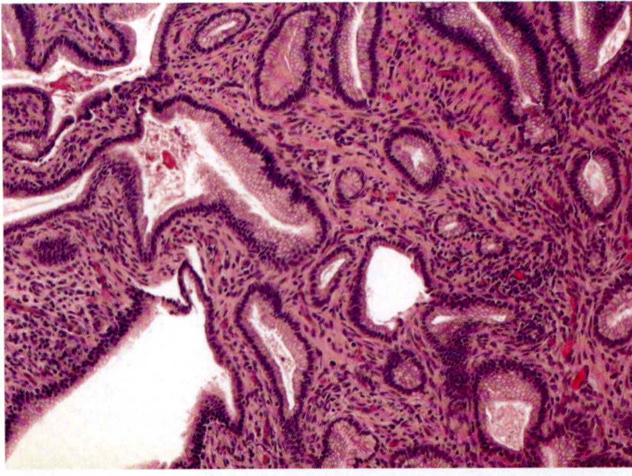

Figure 16.7. Biliary adenofibroma. The dilated interanastomosing glands can resemble those seen in a bile duct hamartoma. The lining cells look and stain like biliary epithelium.

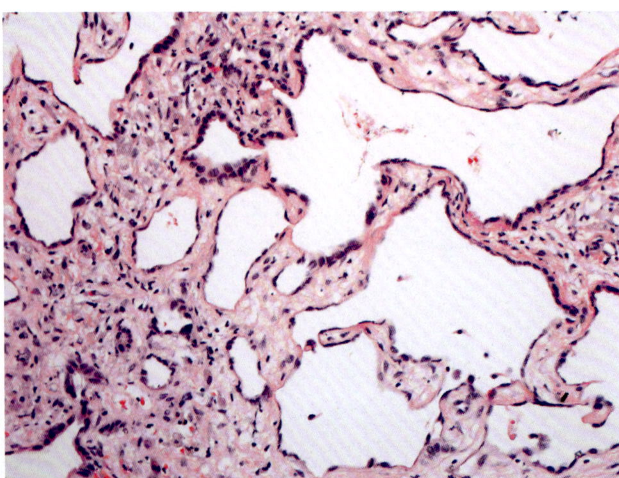

Figure 16.8. Biliary adenofibroma. In this example, the biliary epithelium was more attenuated.

IMMUNOSTAINS

Most benign biliary lesions are readily classified on H&E stains and immunostains are usually not necessary. They all stain with broad-spectrum cytokeratin stains and are always CK7 positive. CK20 is negative in bile duct hamartomas and in most bile duct adenomas, though one study did report CK20 positivity in 40% of bile duct adenomas.[12] Bile duct hamartomas, adenomas, and biliary adenofibromas all have a very low (~1%) to absent Ki-67 proliferate rate, which can be very helpful in cases if you are worried about malignancy.[13] About 50% of bile duct adenomas have BRAF V600E mutations,[14] and these can be detected by immunostains.[15] Bile duct hamartomas are negative for BRAF mutations.[15]

RISK FOR MALIGNANT TRANSFORMATION

Malignant transformation of bile duct hamartomas[16,17] and bile duct adenomas[18,19] has been reported, but is very rare. Malignant transformation of biliary adenofibromas is much more common.[20] Although there are insufficient data to determine their overall risk, currently about 30% of reported biliary adenofibromas had areas interpreted as malignancy.

For all three of these benign biliary lesions, the morphological findings that suggest malignancy are generally the same. Overall, the benign lesions tend to be well circumscribed, but some degree of infiltration is common at the edges, often leading to entrapped hepatocytes. However, a destructive pattern of infiltration should not be present. There should be no cytological atypia, including a lack of prominent nucleoli and no significant variation in nuclear size. There should be no glandular complexity and no luminal necrotic debris. Although there can be luminal hemorrhage in the larger cysts of adenofibromas, the luminal dirty necrosis that can be seen in some cholangiocarcinomas (Fig. 16.9) is absent in these benign lesions. In addition, there should be no population of "incomplete glands," where a tumor gland is not lined by epithelial cells around its entire circumference. Mitotic figures are usually absent and are never atypical.

The Ki-67 rate should be absent or low (~1% or less). Immunostains for p53 can show weak patchy staining in benign lesions,[13] but will not have the strong diffuse staining that can be seen in some cholangiocarcinomas and metastatic adenocarcinomas. All of the biliary lesions (benign and malignant) are typically positive for albumin in situ hybridization, which can be useful if your differential includes metastatic adenocarcinomas.[21]

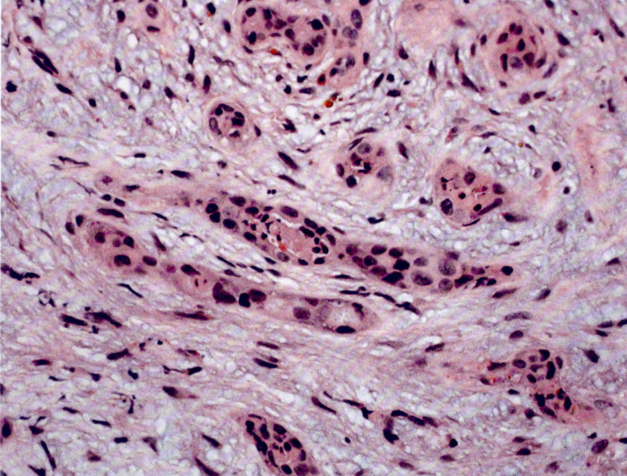

Figure 16.9. **Cholangiocarcinoma, dirty luminal necrosis.** This picture might look like a bile duct adenoma at first, but note the dirty necrosis within the gland lumens.

SIMPLE CYSTS INCLUDING BILIARY, MESOTHELIAL, AND FOREGUT

CHECKLIST: Benign Simple Cysts

- ☐ Simple biliary cyst (also called solitary biliary cyst)
  - ○ Lined by biliary epithelium
  - ○ Lacks ovarian stroma
- ☐ Mesothelial cysts
  - ○ Lined by mesothelial cells
  - ○ Always subcapsular in location, usually hilar in location
- ☐ Ciliated hepatic foregut cyst
  - ○ Lined by ciliated columnar epithelium. Not every cell will be ciliated, but cilia should be clearly present
  - ○ Cyst wall contains smooth muscle

The most common cyst in this group is the simple biliary cyst, which has a strong female predominance (8:1) and an average presentation in the sixth decade. Mesothelial cysts are usually hilar in location and are always subcapsular. They are lined by mesothelial cells and are positive for keratins, calretinin, and WT1. The ciliated hepatic foregut cyst is the least common, but they also tend to be subscapular and so are visible to surgeons and, when present, are often biopsied during intraabdominal surgeries. Ciliated hepatic foregut cysts lack the strong female predominance of simple biliary cysts. On average, they are 4 cm in size and are unilocular in 90% of cases.[22]

As a group, these cysts are lined by cytologically bland epithelium that can either be biliary (simple cyst, Fig. 16.10), mesothelial (mesothelial cyst, Figs. 16.11 and 16.12), or columnar with cilia (foregut cysts, Fig. 16.13). Other changes can include areas of metaplasia (intestinal, pyloric, squamous) and occasionally foci of dysplasia.

The cyst walls are usually fibrotic and can be densely hyalinized. Small atrophic portal tracts and/or islands of hepatocyte may be present. The cyst wall often has mild nonspecific inflammation and, if there has been cyst rupture, numerous pigment laden macrophages. Smooth muscle bundles are often seen in the walls of the ciliated hepatic foregut cyst. By definition, all of these cysts lack ovarian stroma.

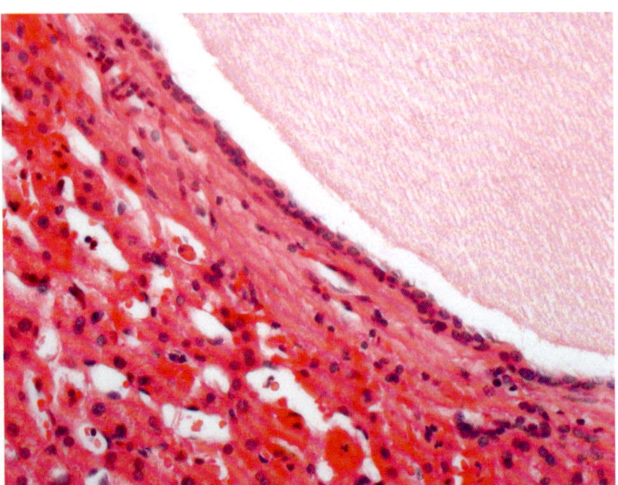

Figure 16.10. **Simple biliary cyst.** The cyst is lined by biliary epithelium.

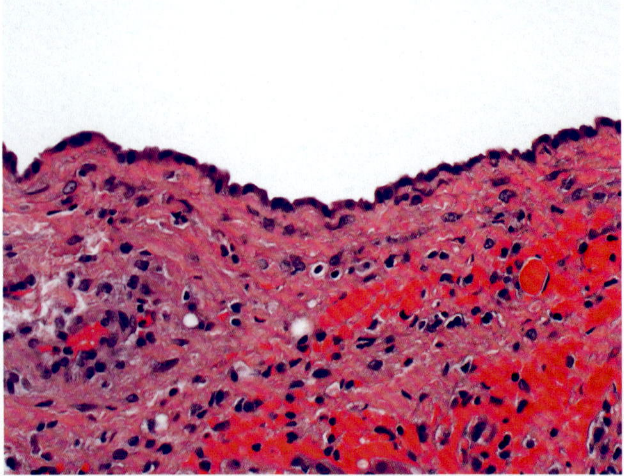

Figure 16.11. **Mesothelial cyst.** This small cyst was located in the hilum and is lined by mesothelial cells.

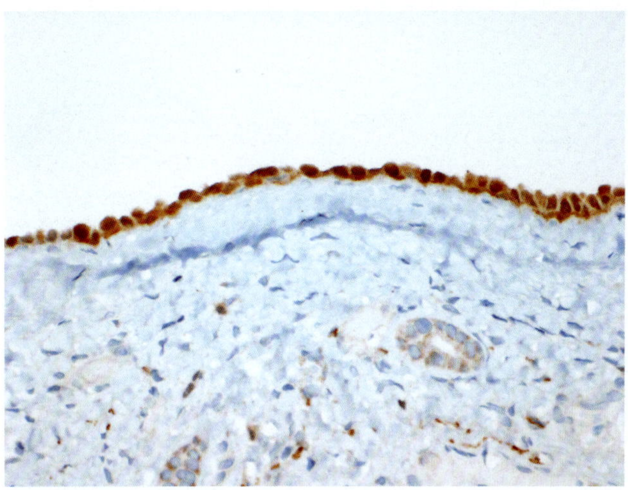

Figure 16.12. **Mesothelial cyst, calretinin immunonstain.** The cells are strongly positive.

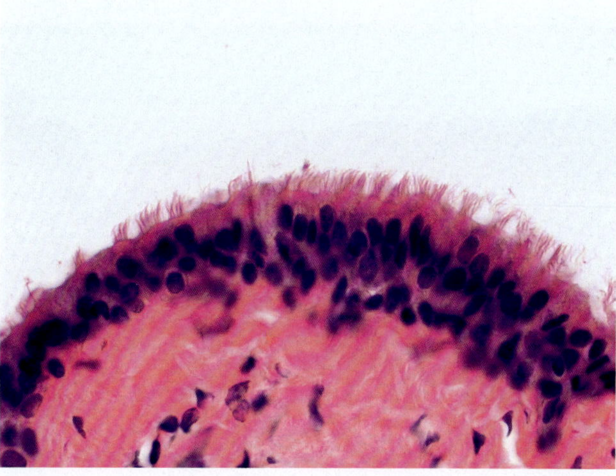

Figure 16.13. **Ciliated hepatic foregut cyst.** The cyst lining shows numerous ciliated cells.

MUCINOUS CYSTIC NEOPLASM

CHECKLIST: Mucinous Cystic Neoplasm

- ☐ Mucinous epithelium frequently admixed with biliary type epithelium
- ☐ Does not communicate with bile ducts
- ☐ Ovarian stroma

Histologically, mucinous cystic neoplasms are essentially the same as their counterpart in the pancreas. They have a strong female predominance (20:1), and most occur in the fourth and fifth decade of life. They used to be called biliary cystadenomas, hepatobiliary cystadenomas, or cystadenocarcinomas (when malignant), but the nomenclature was scrubbed up by the 2010 edition of the World Health Organization on tumors of the digestive system. The proposed nomenclature has been quickly adopted, and they are now classified as mucinous cystic neoplasms. Mucinous cystic neoplasms are further subtyped by their degree of dysplasia (low-grade vs. high-grade dysplasia) and by whether they have an invasive carcinoma.

Mucinous cystic neoplasms are solitary and multilocular and do not communicate with the bile ducts. They are defined by the presence of ovarian stroma (Fig. 16.14). These two observations, ovarian stroma and lack of communication with bile ducts, allow proper classification of essentially all cases. The ovarian stroma is positive for estrogen (Fig. 16.15), progesterone, and alpha-inhibin.[23] The epithelial cells forming the cyst lining are usually columnar with basally oriented nuclei and apical mucin. However, in most cases, the epithelium also includes nonmucinous cells that have a more classic biliary appearance.[24] Mucicarmine will highlight the mucinous nature of the epithelium, but the mucin can be reduced or absent in areas that show cuboidal or flattened epithelium. The epithelium can also show areas of intestinal metaplasia, pyloric gland metaplasia, and occasionally squamous metaplasia. The epithelium is positive for CK7, CK19, CK8, and CK18, while CK20 is typically negative, except in areas of dysplasia.[25] Synaptophysin or chromogranin stains often show occasional scattered endocrine cells in the epithelial lining.

Epithelial dysplasia, if present, is classified as low grade or high grade. The dysplasia can be cytological or architectural, with architectural changes including micropapillary projections into the cyst lumen, cryptlike invaginations into the cyst wall, or areas of epithelial multilayering. High-grade dysplasia typically has complex tubulopapillary projections into the lumen. Mitotic figures are easily found, and there is easily identified nuclear pleomorphism.

Mucinous cystic neoplasms tumor should be sectioned extensively for invasive adenocarcinoma. Sectioning should focus on any nodules within the cyst wall or areas of increased wall thickening.

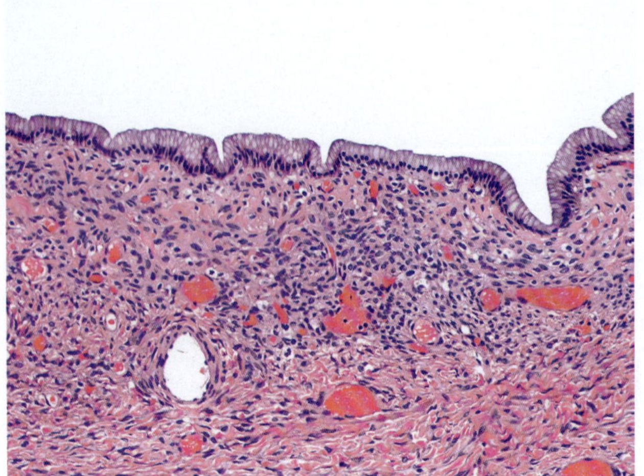

Figure 16.14. **Mucinous cystic neoplasm with ovarian stroma.** The cyst wall shows a dense spindle cell proliferation. The epithelium shows a mucinous morphology.

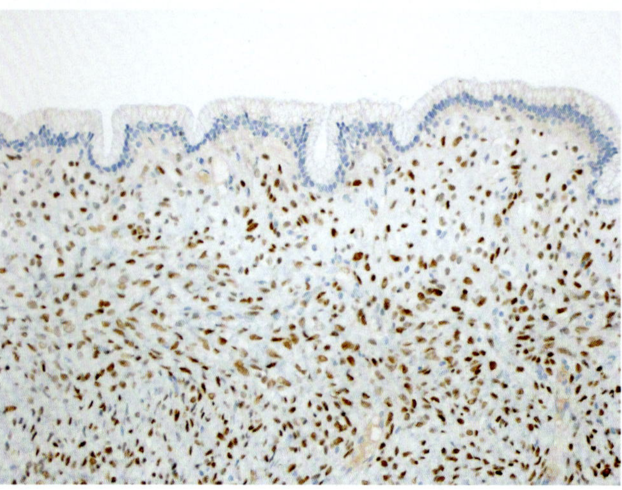

Figure 16.15. **Mucinous cystic neoplasm with ovarian stroma.** The stroma, but not the epithelium, is positive for estrogen receptor. The epithelium is ER positive in endometriosis.

The differential includes endometriosis. In cases of endometriosis, there often is iron-positive, pigment-laden macrophages in the stroma surrounding the cyst. Most helpful are immunostains for ER, which are positive in both the stroma and the epithelial cells in endometriosis, but only in the stroma of mucinous cystic neoplasms.

MUCINOUS CYSTIC NEOPLASM WITHOUT OVARIAN STROMA

Rare biliary tumors are challenging to classify[26,27] because they lack ovarian stroma (which is by definition found in a conventional mucinous cystic neoplasms), but they do not connect to the biliary tree (as would be found in an intraductal papillary biliary neoplasm), and they are lined by mucinous epithelium rather than biliary epithelium (so not a simple biliary cyst). These tumors defy the current classification schema, but a reasonable approach is to call them mucinous cystic neoplasm without ovarian stroma. Adenocarcinoma can also develop in these tumors.[28]

PEARLS & PITFALLS

Sometimes endometrioses of the liver can be mistaken for a mucinous cystic neoplasm. In general, the stroma in mucinous cystic neoplasms is more dense and cellular ("ovarian type stroma") while the stroma is less cellular in endometriosis ("endometrial stroma") and can contain iron-laden macrophages. The stroma in both tumors is positive for ER and PR. However, the epithelium is negative for ER and PR in mucinous cystic neoplasms but positive in endometriosis. In addition, the stroma is CD10 positive in endometriosis but negative in mucinous cystic neoplasms. In contrast, the stroma is inhibin positive in mucinous cystic neoplasms but negative in endometriosis.[29]

INTRADUCTAL PAPILLARY BILIARY NEOPLASM

CHECKLIST: Intraductal Papillary Biliary Neoplasm

- ☐ Papillary biliary neoplasm growing in bile ducts
- ☐ Cystic dilatation of involved bile duct
- ☐ Lack of ovarian stroma

This papillary tumor grows within the bile ducts, leading to areas of marked cystic change (Fig. 16.16). This tumor was previously known as biliary papillomatosis and biliary papilloma.

Intraductal papillary biliary neoplasms form large cysts with multiple subdivisions made of thin fibrous walls. They always connect to the rest of the biliary tree, but you may have to section carefully and correlate with imaging findings to document the connection. The tumor is composed of micropapillary or complex tubulovillous architecture and extends along the bile duct lumen (Figs. 16.17 and 16.18). The tumor leads to marked dilatation of the bile duct and so can mimic a mucinous cystic neoplasm but always lacks ovarian stroma. The epithelium in intraductal papillary biliary neoplasms can be biliary (most common), mucinous, intestinal with goblet cells, or oncocytic. Intraductal papillary biliary neoplasms have a high risk of invasive carcinoma and so should be sectioned extensively. The most common morphology is that of a typical cholangiocarcinoma, but adenocarcinomas associated with the intestinal epithelium tend to show a mucinous or colloid morphology.

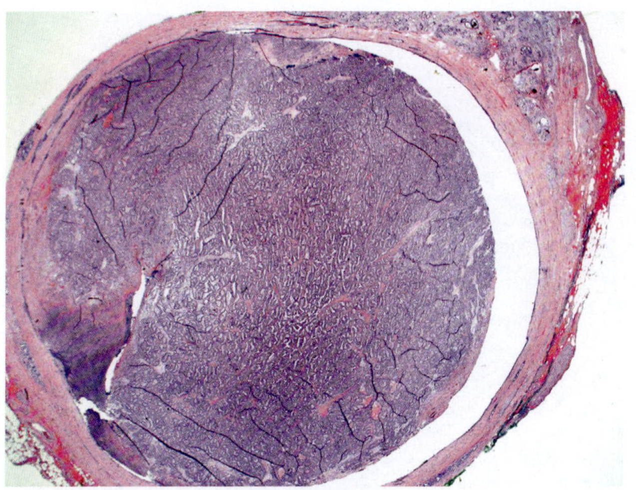

Figure 16.16. Intraductal papillary biliary neoplasm. A tumor expands and obstructs a bile duct.

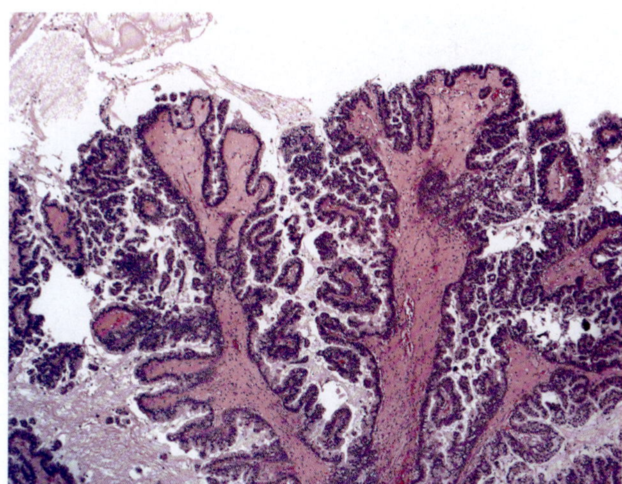

Figure 16.17. Intraductal papillary biliary neoplasm. This tumor shows a complex micropapillary architecture.

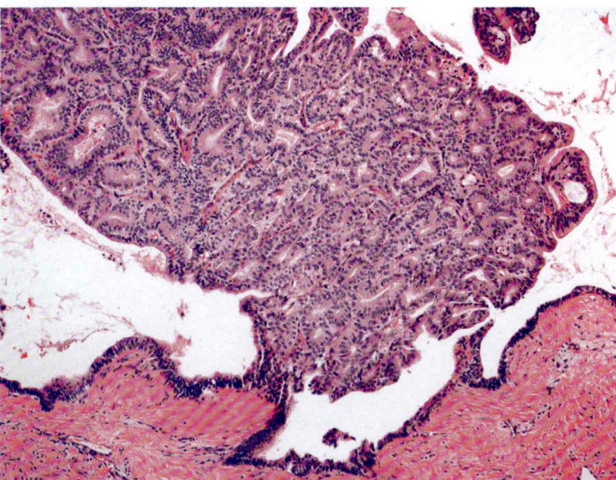

Figure 16.18. Intraductal papillary biliary neoplasm. This tumor shows a tubulovillous architecture.

FAQ: What is the difference between intraductal papillary biliary neoplasms and biliary intraepithelial neoplasm (BilIN)?

Answer: Both lesions are dysplastic biliary lesions that are precursors to cholangiocarcinoma, and both can have a papillary growth pattern. Biliary intraepithelial neoplasm (BilIN), however, is a microscopic lesion (Fig. 16.19) that is most commonly seen in cirrhotic livers with chronic hepatitis C, alcohol, or primary sclerosing cholangitis as the underlying risk factor.[30,31] Hepatolithiasis is also an important risk factor.[32] Most BilIN lesions are found in medium- or larger sized bile ducts.

BilIN is further divided into low-grade (Fig. 16.19) or high-grade dysplasia (Fig. 16.20) or sometimes into three grades called BilIN 1, 2 or 3. The images of BilIN 1 in many studies look more reactive than dysplastic, so BilIN 1 is probably not a very robust lesion. For that reason, BilIN low-grade dysplasia and BilIN high-grade dysplasia are more practical for clinical care.

Rarely, metastatic carcinoma can colonize the bile ducts, mimicking BilIN (Fig. 16.21).

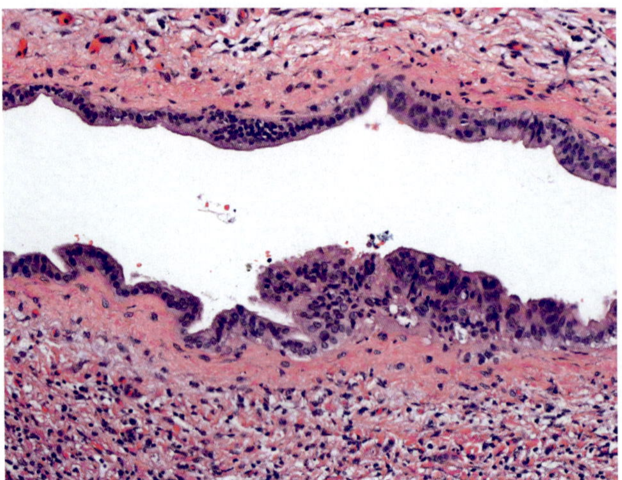

Figure 16.19. **Biliary intraepithelial neoplasm (BilIN).** A bile duct shows an area of low-grade dysplasia (BilIN) in the right side of the image.

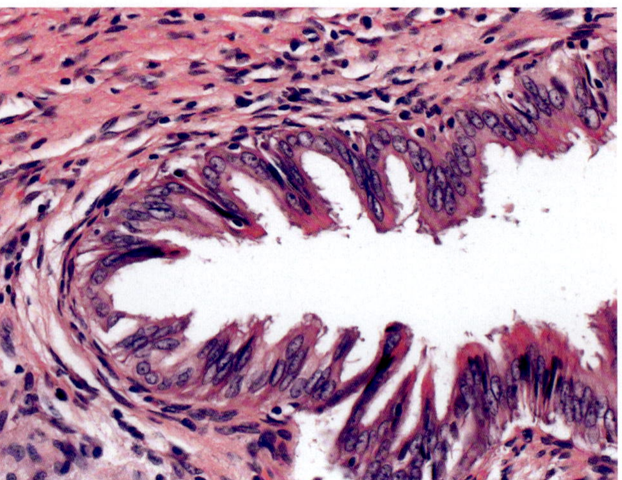

Figure 16.20. **Biliary intraepithelial neoplasm (BilIN).** This BilIN shows high-grade dysplasia.

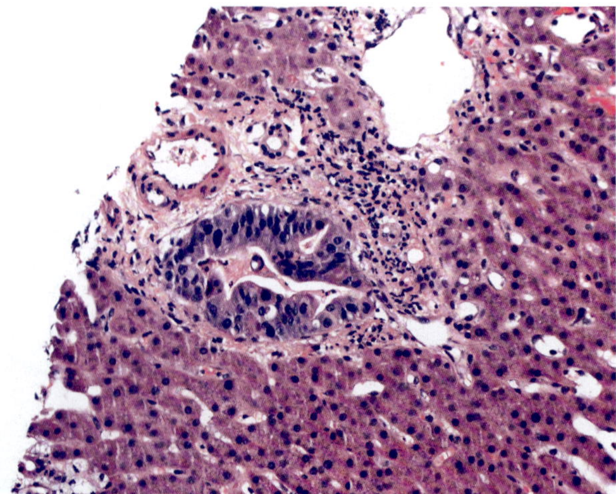

Figure 16.21. **Metastatic colon adenocarcinoma, colonizing bile ducts.** Colon and pancreas adenocarcinoma are the most common to show this growth pattern. Sometimes, this finding can mimic high-grade BilIN.

CHOLANGIOCARCINOMA

CHECKLIST: Cholangiocarcinomas

Locations

- □ Extrahepatic
- □ Perihilar ("Klatskin tumor")
- □ Intrahepatic

Patterns (have different names, but these are the basic patterns).

- □ Gland forming, with well-defined glands
  - ○ Clear cell
  - ○ Colloid
  - ○ Signet ring cell
  - ○ Lymphocyte rich (usually EBV positive)
- □ Solid growth
  - ○ Can be trabecular or solid nests
- □ Cholangiolocellular, with an anastomosing ductular reaction–like growth pattern

Cholangiocarcinomas are divided for clinical purposes, including surgical pathology, into extrahepatic, intrahepatic, and hilar. In many cases, the location of the tumor is clearly evident, but sometimes it can be challenging to decide if a tumor is best classified as perihilar or intrahepatic in location. Cholangiocarcinomas are classified as perihilar when they arise from the common hepatic duct (i.e., proximal to the cystic duct), or from the main right or left hepatic duct, or from the main bile duct branches in the liver hilum prior to their division into segmental branches. Perhilar cholangiocarcinomas can extend into the hepatic parenchyma, so the tumor is classified by where the bulk of the tumor is located.

Risk factors for cholangiocarcinoma depend on the tumor location. Hilar cholangiocarcinomas are most commonly associated with primary sclerosing cholangitis, while peripheral tumors are strongly linked to cirrhosis. The cirrhosis can be from any cause, but alcohol and chronic viral hepatitis appear to have the strongest increased risk.

Cholangiocarcinomas have a variety of growth patterns but most fall into one of the following patterns. The most common pattern is a gland-forming carcinoma composed of irregular, infiltrating glands (Figs. 16.22 and 16.23). The glands can be either large or small and are lined by columnar to cuboidal mucin-producing cells (Fig. 16.24). This pattern is sometimes called the bile duct pattern.[33] The large gland pattern tends to have the least desmoplastic stroma, while desmoplasia can be striking with the small gland pattern

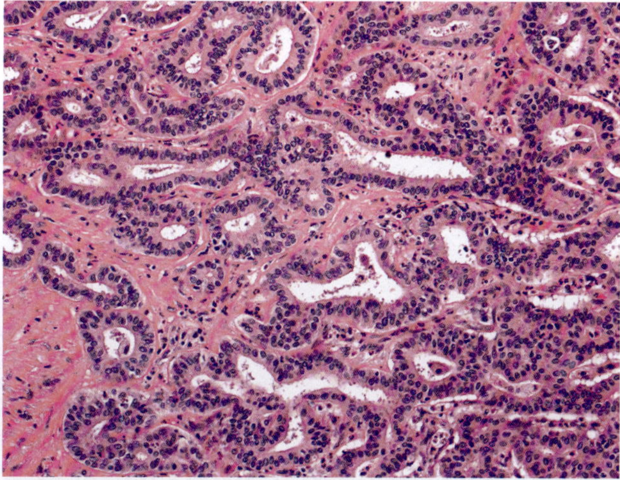

Figure 16.22. **Cholangiocarcinoma, gland forming.** A typical well-differentiated gland-forming cholangiocarcinoma.

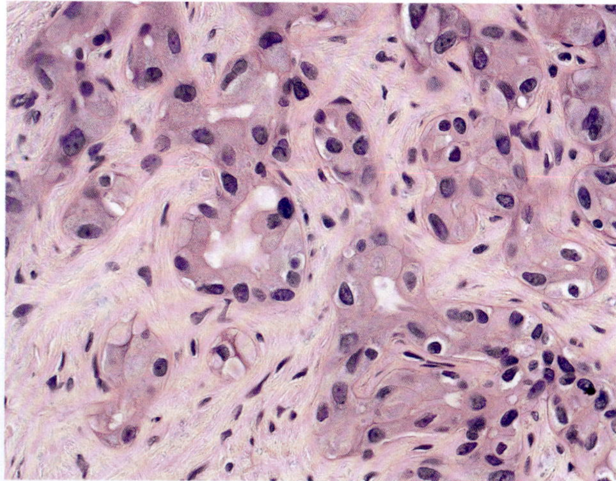

Figure 16.23. **Cholangiocarcinoma, gland forming.** Another example of a well-differentiated gland-forming cholangiocarcinoma.

(Figs. 16.25 and 16.26), with desmoplastic stroma making up most of the tumor in many cases. The second major pattern is colloid carcinoma, with tumor cells floating in abundant extracellular mucin. The third major pattern is tumor cells growing in solid trabeculae (Fig. 16.27) or solid nests (Fig. 16.28). This pattern also tends to have a dense desmoplastic response and can mimic the sclerotic variant of hepatocellular carcinoma. These solid patterns do not produce mucin, and hepatocellular carcinoma should be carefully excluded. Of note, many cases will have a mixture of more than one of these patterns, but one pattern tends to dominate. Other changes can be seen with any of these growth patterns, including clear cell morphology (Fig. 16.29) or areas of sarcomatoid growth (Fig. 16.30).

FAQ: How are solid cholangiocarcinomas distinguished from hepatocellular carcinoma?

Answer: They are distinguished by morphology and by immunostains. Morphological findings that would indicate hepatic differentiation are usually absent but would include bile production and steatosis. Pale bodies also favor hepatocellular carcinoma.

Immunostain panels are most useful than single or a few stains, as panel approaches are significantly more sensitive and specific compared with a single or a few stains. Cytokeratin stains are often not particularly helpful, but there are some patterns that can favor one diagnosis over another. Overall, immunostain stains for hepatic differentiation versus glandular differentiation are the most useful. Albumin in situ hybridization is not informative, being positive in both (Fig. 16.31). However, if albumin in situ hybridization is negative, then metastatic disease needs to be excluded.

Cytokeratin stains. Cytokeratin stains show significant overlap in hepatocellular carcinomas and solid cholangiocarcinomas, but they can be useful when they are negative. For example, the lack of CK7 or CK19 would somewhat favor hepatocellular carcinoma. The lack of CAM5.2 would somewhat favor cholangiocarcinoma.

The following strongly favor hepatocellular carcinoma.

- AFP
- Arginase
- Heppar1 (when more than focal).
- Glypican 3 (when strong and diffuse).

The following strongly favor cholangiocarcinoma.

- MOC31 (when strong and diffuse).
- CA19-9 (when strong and diffuse).

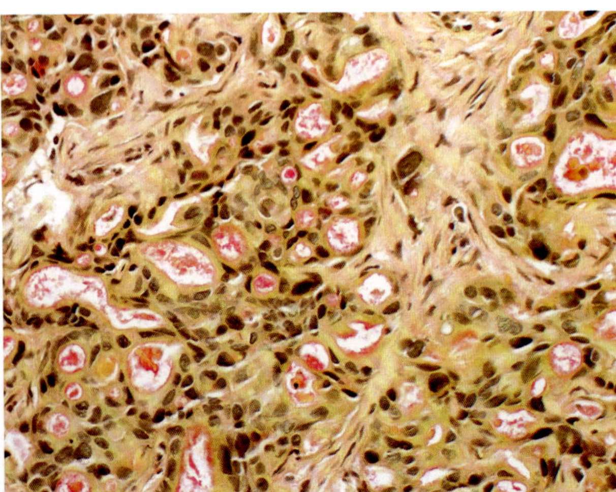

Figure 16.24. **Cholangiocarcinoma, mucicarmine.** A mucicarmine stain is strongly positive. Not all cholangiocarcinomas are mucicarmine positive.

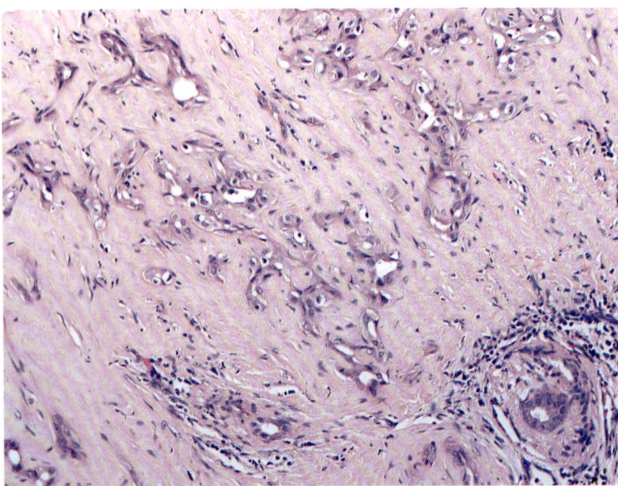

Figure 16.25. **Cholangiocarcinoma, dense fibrosis.** This moderately differentiated cholangiocarcinoma shows small glands and a densely fibrotic background.

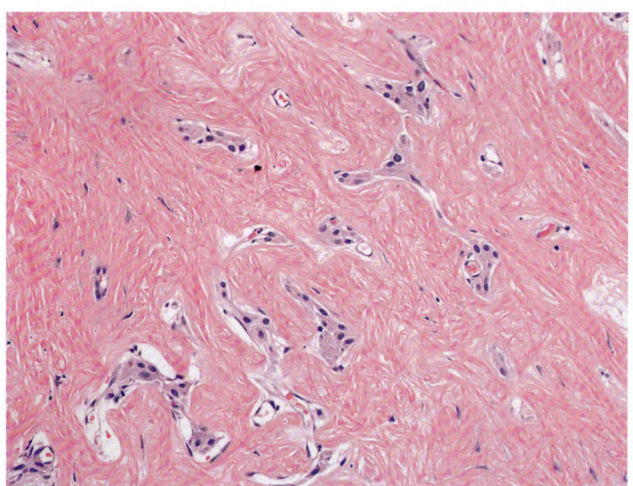

Figure 16.26. **Cholangiocarcinoma, dense fibrosis.** In this case, gland lumens are inconspicuous, and the image is dominated by fibrosis.

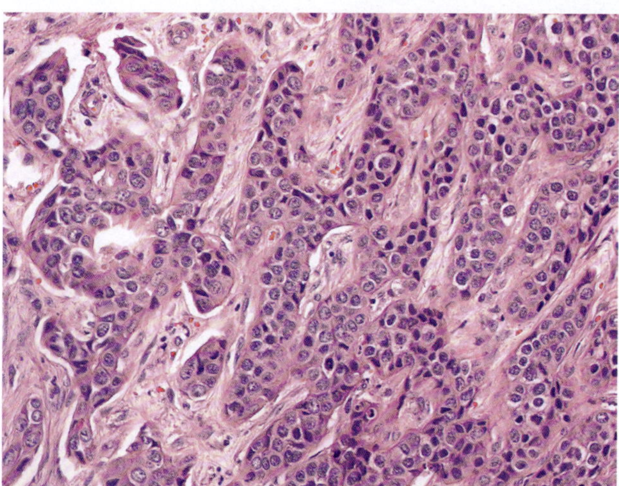

Figure 16.27. **Cholangiocarcinoma, trabecular growth pattern.** This cholangiocarcinoma has a trabecular growth pattern.

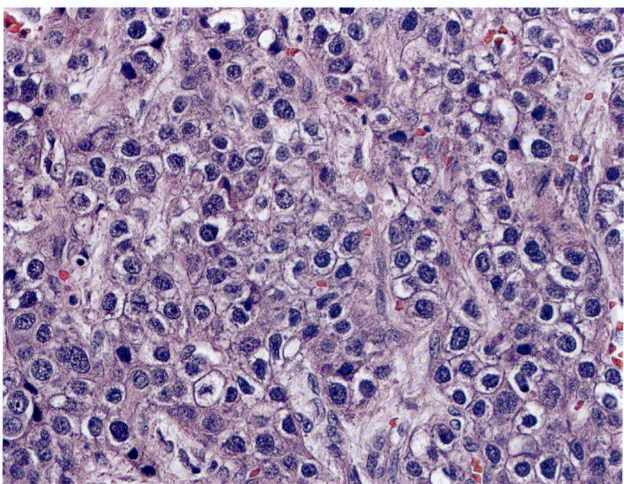

Figure 16.28. **Cholangiocarcinoma, solid nests.** This cholangiocarcinoma grew in solid nodules.

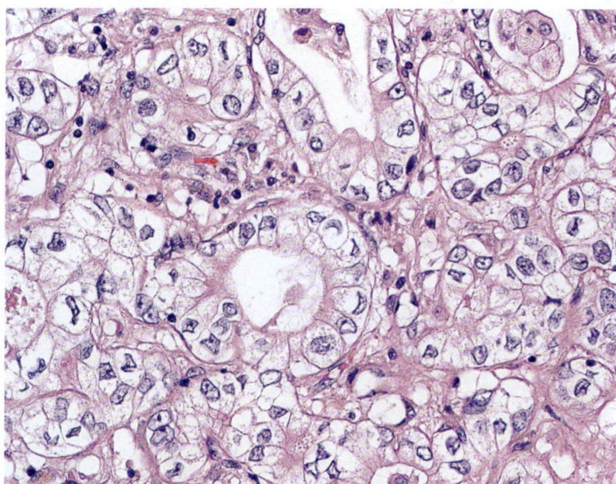

Figure 16.29. **Cholangiocarcinoma, clear cell.** The cholangiocarcinoma has a distinctive clear cell morphology.

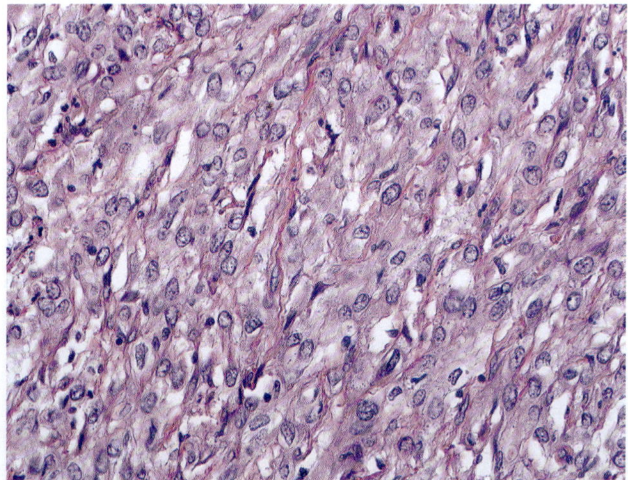

Figure 16.30. **Cholangiocarcinoma, sarcomatoid.** In some areas of this poorly differentiated cholangiocarcinoma, the tumor showed a spindle cell morphology

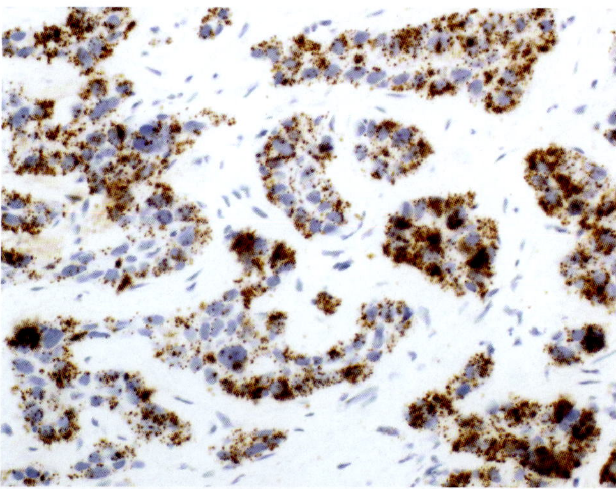

Figure 16.31. **Cholangiocarcinoma, albumin in situ hybridization.** The cholangiocarcinoma is strongly positive.

In the end, the final diagnosis often requires relative weighting of the morphology and immunostain results. This requires using some common sense, but still works well overall, with stains that are diffusely and strongly positive given more weight than those that are focally positive. For example, a tumor that is strongly and diffusely positive for HepPar, with focal patchy staining for MOC31, and negative for CK7 and CK19 is best classified as hepatocellular carcinoma. As another example, a tumor that shows focal Arginase and glypican 3 staining, with strong diffuse staining for CK19 and MOC31, would favor a cholangiocarcinoma.

Overall, there is a rough correlation between the major growth pattern and the location of the cholangiocarcinoma. Cholangiocarcinomas that are perihilar or are located in the large ducts near the hilum more commonly have well-formed glands and produce mucin. In contrast, cholangiocarcinomas developing in the periphery of the liver are more likely to grow as irregular trabecular or tubular structures without lumens. Sometimes these peripheral cholangiocarcinomas have a morphology that resembles proliferating bile ductules and have been called a *cholangiolocellular* pattern (Fig. 16.32).[33]

A small subset of cholangiocarcinomas has a dense lymphocytic inflammatory response including numerous intraepithelial lymphocytes.[34,35] These tumors usually show at least some degree of gland formation (Fig. 16.33), but much of the tumor can be dominated by a lymphoepithelioma morphology with irregular sheets of poorly defined epithelial cells embedded in an intense lymphocytic infiltrate (Fig. 16.34). They are more common in Asia and are strongly positive for EBV by in situ hybridization (Fig. 16.35) and/or EBV LMP. Some but not all studies have reported a better prognosis.

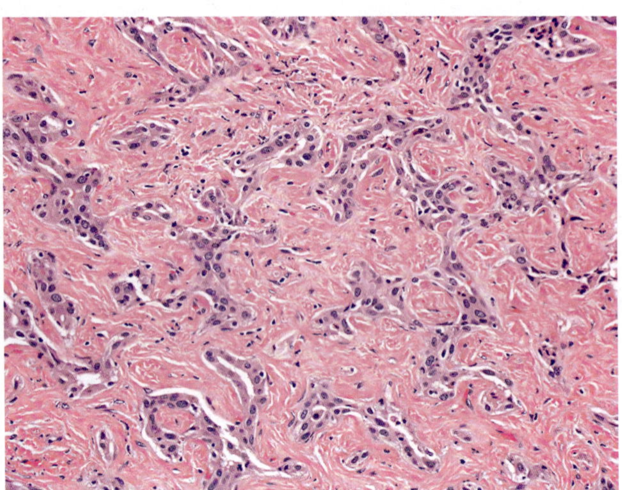

Figure 16.32. **Cholangiocarcinoma, cholangiolocellular.** The growth pattern somewhat resemble benign bile ductular proliferation.

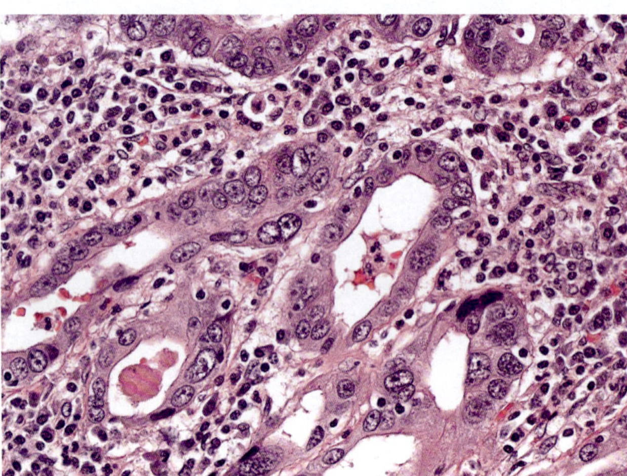

Figure 16.33. **Cholangiocarcinoma, lymphocyte rich.** The cholangiocarcinoma has numerous lymphocytes within the tumor stroma as well as within the epithelium.

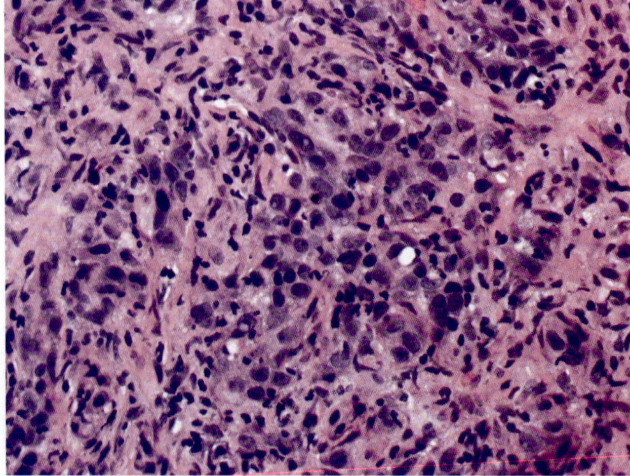

Figure 16.34. **Cholangiocarcinoma, lymphocyte rich.** This poorly differentiated cholangiocarcinoma has numerous and ill-defined tumor trabeculae and glands.

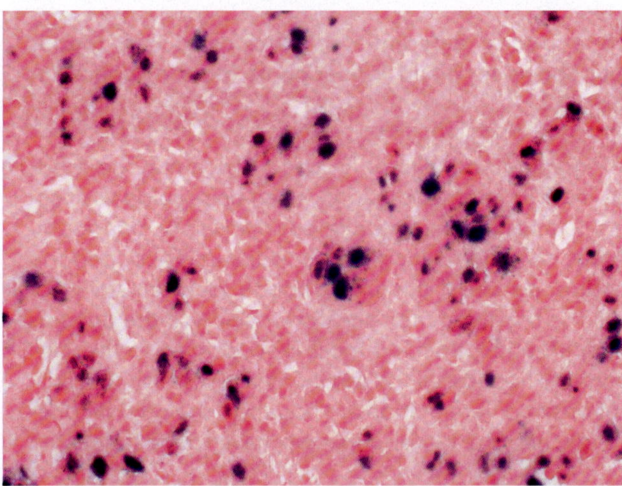

Figure 16.35. **Cholangiocarcinoma, lymphocyte rich, EBV in situ hybridization.** The tumor is strongly positive (same case as preceding image).

GRADING CHOLANGIOCARCINOMAS

CHECKLIST: Grading Cholangiocarcinomas a la CAP

- ☐ Grade 1. Well differentiated. Glands are seen in >95% of tumor.
- ☐ Grade 2. Moderately differentiated. Glands are seen 50% to 95% of tumor.
- ☐ Grade 3. Poorly differentiated. Glands are seen 5% to 49% of tumor.
- ☐ Grade 4. Undifferentiated. Glands are seen in <5% of tumor.

The CAP provides guidelines for grading cholangiocarcinoma based on the percent gland formation. This system makes sense for cholangiocarcinomas with a classic gland-forming morphology and less sense for those peripheral cholangiocarcinomas with trabecular, solid, or cholangiocellular growth patterns, as they all end up being classified as poorly differentiated, which is not necessarily the case. In these latter cases, the overall nuclear cytology can also be used to classify them as well, moderately, or poorly differentiated.

IMMUNOSTAINS

The diagnosis of cholangiocarcinoma is made using morphology, immunostains, and available imaging studies. Cholangiocarcinomas are positive for CK7 (~90%) and CK19 (80% to 90%), while centrally but not peripherally located cholangiocarcinomas can be positive for CK20.[36] The CK20 staining tends to be patchier in cholangiocarcinoma than it does in metastatic colon adenocarcinoma. Most cholangiocarcinomas are also positive for MOC31[37] and often show cytoplasmic staining for polyclonal CEA (~80%), though the staining can be weak and patchy. Albumin in situ hybridization (Fig. 16.31) is positive in most cholangiocarcinomas (~80%) but does not differentiate them from hepatocellular carcinoma. Rare metastatic tumors can also be positive for albumin in situ hybridization, so correlation with morphology and imaging findings is still important. As another potential diagnostic pitfall, CDX2 is positive in 40% of cholangiocarcinomas, especially hilar tumors.[38,39]

Makers of hepatic differentiation (Heppar1, arginase) are generally negative, though both stains can show patchy staining, more commonly in peripherally located tumors. Overall, glypican 3 is positive in about 5% of cholangiocarcinomas[40] and HepPar in 10%.[41,42] These tumors should not be called biophenotypic hepatocellular carcinoma–cholangiocarcinoma unless there are two distinctive morphologies on the H&E. Hilar cholangiocarcinomas can also be positive for both TTF1 and Napsin, an important diagnostic pitfall.[43]

FAQ: How do I approach a poorly differentiated carcinoma, one that is definitely keratin positive but shows no gland formation or other evidence for differentiation on H&E findings?

Answer: First correlate with imaging and clinical findings. There may be a history of prior malignancy or a mass in another organ that can help guide workup. Second, make sure the tumor is a carcinoma and rule out mimics. As one example, occasionally angiosarcomas can show patchy keratin staining. Third, perform CK7/CK20 to allow broad categorization of the tumor. Fourth, perform stains for organ-specific differentiation. The most common are shown below. If the tumor is positive for albumin in situ hybridization, then it is most likely primary to the liver, but this stain does not differentiate hepatocellular carcinoma from cholangiocarcinoma. Finally, if all markers of organ differentiation are negative, then the diagnosis is undifferentiated carcinoma, and the tumor origin will have to be suggested based on imaging findings.

The following are markers of organ differentiation (not exhaustive, but some of the most commonly used).

- Neuroendocrine: chromogranin, synaptophysin, keratin (keratin negative cases suggest a paraganglioma.
- Lung: Napsin, TTF1.
- Gastrointestinal (GI) tract: CDX2.
- Hepatic: HepPar1, Arginase, Glypican 3.
- Renal, mullerian: PAX8.
- Breast: GATA3, ER, mammaglobin GCDFP15.
- Squamous: p40, CK5/6.
- Urothelial: GATA3, p40, p63.
- Adrenal: MelA, inhibin.
- Mesothelial: WT1, calretinin, D240.
- Pancreatic acinar cell carcinoma: Trypsin.

NEAR MISSES

CASE 1. A biopsy was directed at an 8-cm tumor in a 69-year-old man who had no underlying liver disease. The case had been signed out as a bile duct adenoma, but a second review was requested by the clinical team.

The lesion was biliary in origin, with large dilated glands with an interanastomosing pattern (Fig. 16.36). The glands were embedded in a background of dense fibrosis. There was no significant cytological atypia and no mitotic figures, so the findings were consistent with a benign biliary lesion. However, the pattern of the glands (large, dilated, interanastomosing) is not that of a bile duct adenoma. The large size would also be unusual for a bile duct adenoma. Instead, the findings are that of biliary adenofibroma. The distinction is important. Although both are benign, biliary adenofibroma should be resected because they have a high risk for malignant transformation.

CASE 2. An 80-year-old man presented with unexplained weight loss and imaging showed an 8-cm liver mass. A biopsy showed a moderately differentiated adenocarcinoma (Fig. 16.37). There was no other primary site by imaging, so the presumptive clinical diagnosis was that of an intrahepatic cholangiocarcinoma. However, the pathologist was uncertain because the adenocarcinoma was CK7 negative, so submitted the case for consultation because they had limited in-house stains to complete a full evaluation.

The adenocarcinoma was moderately differentiated and was positive for pankeratin but negative for CK7, CK20, CK19, and for organ-specific markers including TTF1, CDX2, Pax8, PSA, and PACP. Albumin in situ hybridization was positive. The combination of imaging findings, morphology, and immunohistochemical findings was classified as most consistent with an intrahepatic cholangiocarcinoma.

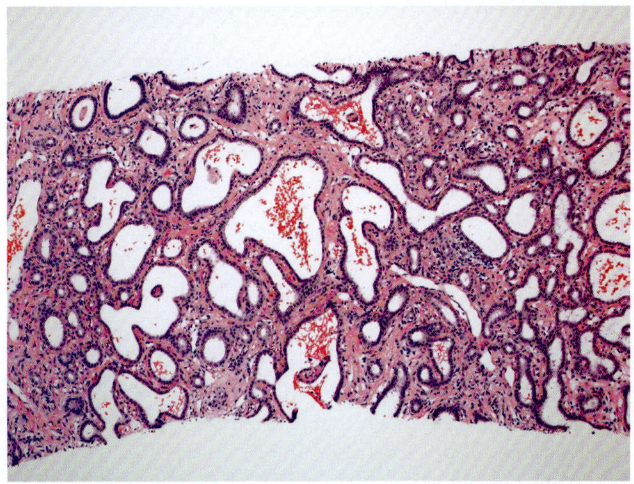

Figure 16.36. **Near miss, Adenofibroma.** Large dilated glands are seen, with a fibrotic background.

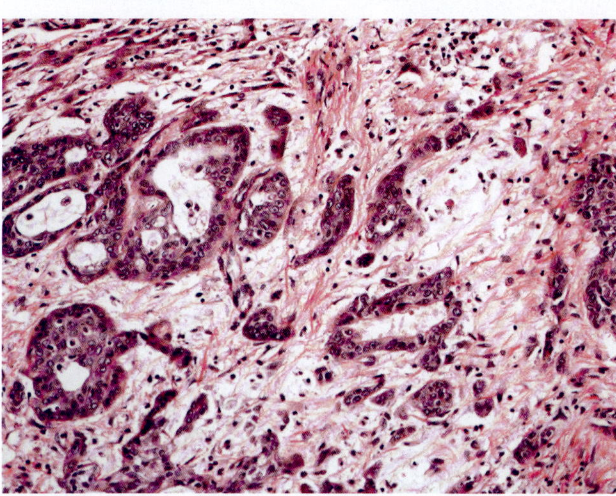

Figure 16.37. **Near miss, CK7 negative cholangiocarcinoma.**

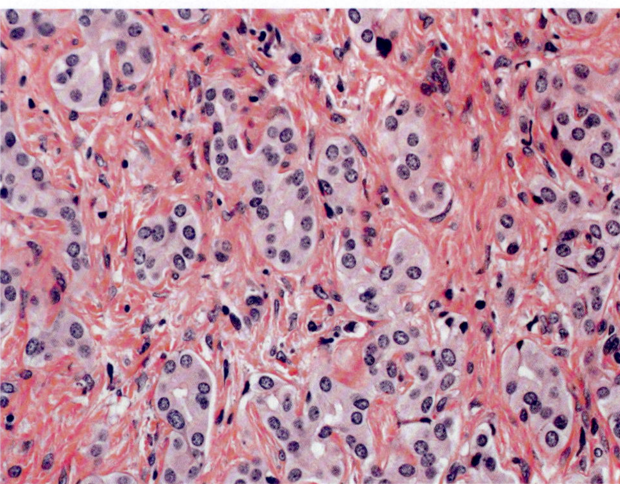

Figure 16.38. **Near miss, bile duct adenoma.**

The referring pathologist was correct that the majority of cholangiocarcinomas are CK7 positive. Most are also CK19 positive. However, cholangiocarcinomas can rarely be CK7 negative (10%) or CK19 negative (10% to 15%).

In this case, the morphology was clearly that of an adenocarcinoma, so hepatocellular carcinoma was not in the histological differential. In this setting, where hepatocellular carcinoma is not in the differential, the strong albumin in situ hybridization also supported the diagnosis of intrahepatic cholangiocarcinoma.

CASE 3. A 56-year-old woman underwent resection for a cecal colon carcinoma. During surgery, a subcapsular white lesion was noted and was submitted for frozen section. The lesion was interpreted as benign and most consistent with a bile duct adenoma. During evaluation of the permanent sections, the pathologist was less certain on the classification of the lesion. Immunostains were performed and showed the lesion to be CK7 positive, CK20 negative, and CDX2 negative, with a low ki-67 proliferative rate. So far so good, as these findings were consistent with a bile duct adenoma. The pathologist also performed an immunostain for mutant BRAF V600E, as the primary colon carcinoma was known to be positive. The liver lesion was also positive, leading to the uncertainty on how to classify the liver lesion, as the pathologist had learned during training that bile duct adenomas were actually hamartomas (biliary hamartomas) and not true neoplasms, implying they should not have BRAF V600E mutations.

On review, the pathologist's diagnosis on the liver lesion was correct (Fig. 16.38), as was his reasoning. However, in the past several years, bile duct adenomas have been proven to be neoplasms and not hamartomas, with about 50% having BRAF V600E mutations.

References

1. Martin DR, Kalb B, Sarmiento JM, Heffron TG, Coban I, Adsay NV. Giant and complicated variants of cystic bile duct hamartomas of the liver: MRI findings and pathological correlations. *J Magn Reson Imaging*. 2010;31:903911.
2. Singh Y, Cawich SO, Ramjit C, Naraynsingh V. Rare liver tumor: symptomatic giant von Meyenburg complex. *J Surg Case Rep*. 2017:2016.
3. Bhathal PS, Hughes NR, Goodman ZD. The so-called bile duct adenoma is a peribiliary gland hamartoma. *Am J Surg Pathol*. 1996;20:858-864.
4. Arena V, Arena E, Stigliano E, Capelli A. Bile duct adenoma with oncocytic features. *Histopathology*. 2006;49:318-320.
5. Albores-Saavedra J, Hoang MP, Murakata LA, Sinkre P, Yaziji H. Atypical bile duct adenoma, clear cell type: a previously undescribed tumor of the liver. *Am J Surg Pathol*. 2001;25:956-960.
6. Scheele PM, Bonar MJ, Zumwalt R, Ray MB. Bile duct adenomas in heterozygous (MZ) deficiency of alpha 1-protease inhibitor. *Arch Pathol Lab Med*. 1988;112:945-947.
7. Gambarotti M, Medicina D, Baronchelli C, Bercich L, Bonetti F, Facchetti F. Alpha-1-antitrypsin-positive "signet-ring" bile duct adenoma in a patient with M(MALTON) mutation. *Int J Surg Pathol*. 2008;16:218-221.
8. O'Hara BJ, McCue PA, Miettinen M. Bile duct adenomas with endocrine component. Immunohistochemical study and comparison with conventional bile duct adenomas. *Am J Surg Pathol*. 1992;16:21-25.
9. Tsui WM, Loo KT, Chow LT, Tse CC. Biliary adenofibroma. A heretofore unrecognized benign biliary tumor of the liver. *Am J Surg Pathol*. 1993;17:186-192.
10. Gurrera A, Alaggio R, Leone G, Aprile G, Magro G. Biliary adenofibroma of the liver: report of a case and review of the literature. *Patholog Res Int*. 2010;2010:504584.
11. Arnason T, Borger DR, Corless C, et al. Biliary denofibroma of liver: morphology, tumor genetics, and outcomes in 6 cases. *Am J Surg Pathol*. 2017;41:499-505.
12. Hornick JL, Lauwers GY, Odze RD. Immunohistochemistry can help distinguish metastatic pancreatic adenocarcinomas from bile duct adenomas and hamartomas of the liver. *Am J Surg Pathol*. 2005;29:381-389.
13. Tsokos CG, Krings G, Yilmaz F, Ferrell LD, Gill RM. Proliferative index facilitates distinction between benign biliary lesions and intrahepatic cholangiocarcinoma. *Hum Pathol*. 2016.
14. Pujals A, Amaddeo G, Castain C, et al. BRAF V600E mutations in bile duct adenomas. *Hepatology*. 2015;61:403-405.
15. Pujals A, Bioulac-Sage P, Castain C, Charpy C, Zafrani ES, Calderaro J. BRAF V600E mutational status in bile duct adenomas and hamartomas. *Histopathology*. 2015;67:562-567.
16. Song JS, Lee YJ, Kim KW, Huh J, Jang SJ, Yu E. Cholangiocarcinoma arising in Von Meyenburg complexes: report of four cases. *Pathol Int*. 2008;58:503-512.
17. Bhalla A, Mann SA, Chen S, Cummings OW, Lin J. Histopathological evidence of neoplastic progression of Von Meyenburg complex to intrahepatic cholangiocarcinoma. *Hum Pathol*. 2017;67:217-224.
18. Pinho AC, Melo RB, Oliveira M, et al. Adenoma-carcinoma sequence in intrahepatic cholangiocarcinoma. *Int J Surg Case Rep*. 2012;3:131-133.
19. Hasebe T, Sakamoto M, Mukai K, et al. Cholangiocarcinoma arising in bile duct adenoma with focal area of bile duct hamartoma. *Virchows Arch*. 1995;426:209-213.
20. Thompson SM, Zendejas-Mummert B, Hartgers ML, et al. Malignant transformation of biliary adenofibroma: a rare biliary cystic tumor. *J Gastrointest Oncol*. 2016;7:E107-E112.
21. Moy AP, Arora K, Deshpande V. Albumin expression distinguishes bile duct adenomas from metastatic adenocarcinoma. *Histopathology*. 2016;69:423-430.
22. Sharma S, Dean AG, Corn A, et al. Ciliated hepatic foregut cyst: an increasingly diagnosed condition. *Hepatobiliary Pancreat Dis Int*. 2008;7:581-589.
23. Lam MM, Swanson PE, Upton MP, Yeh MM. Ovarian-type stroma in hepatobiliary cystadenomas and pancreatic mucinous cystic neoplasms: an immunohistochemical study. *Am J Clin Pathol*. 2008;129:211-218.
24. Zhelnin K, Xue Y, Quigley B, et al. Nonmucinous biliary epithelium is a frequent finding and is often the predominant epithelial type in mucinous cystic neoplasms of the pancreas and liver. *Am J Surg Pathol*. 2017;41:116-120.

25. Zen Y, Pedica F, Patcha VR, et al. Mucinous cystic neoplasms of the liver: a clinicopathological study and comparison with intraductal papillary neoplasms of the bile duct. *Mod Pathol.* 2011;24:1079-1089.

26. Mano Y, Aishima S, Fujita N, et al. Cystic tumors of the liver: on the problems of diagnostic criteria. *Pathol Res Pract.* 2011;207:659-663.

27. Kishida N, Shinoda M, Masugi Y, et al. Cystic tumor of the liver without ovarian-like stroma or bile duct communication: two case reports and a review of the literature. *World J Surg Oncol.* 2014;12:229.

28. Ishibashi Y, Ojima H, Hiraoka N, Sano T, Kosuge T, Kanai Y. Invasive biliary cystic tumor without ovarian-like stroma. *Pathol Int.* 2007;57:794-798.

29. Hsu M, Terris B, Wu TT, et al. Endometrial cysts within the liver: a rare entity and its differential diagnosis with mucinous cystic neoplasms of the liver. *Hum Pathol.* 2014;45:761-767.

30. Torbenson M, Yeh MM, Abraham SC. Bile duct dysplasia in the setting of chronic hepatitis C and alcohol cirrhosis. *Am J Surg Pathol.* 2007;31:1410-1413.

31. Zen Y, Quaglia A, Heaton N, Rela M, Portmann B. Two distinct pathways of carcinogenesis in primary sclerosing cholangitis. *Histopathology*. 2011;59:1100-1110.

32. Zen Y, Adsay NV, Bardadin K, et al. Biliary intraepithelial neoplasia: an international interobserver agreement study and proposal for diagnostic criteria. *Mod Pathol.* 2007;20:701-709.

33. Liau JY, Tsai JH, Yuan RH, Chang CN, Lee HJ, Jeng YM. Morphological subclassification of intrahepatic cholangiocarcinoma: etiological, clinicopathological, and molecular features. *Mod Pathol.* 2014;27:1163-1173.

34. Sun K, Xu S, Wei J, et al. Clinicopathological features of 11 Epstein-Barr virus-associated intrahepatic cholangiocarcinoma at a single center in China. *Medicine (Baltimore).* 2016;95:e5069.

35. Jeng YM, Chen CL, Hsu HC. Lymphoepithelioma-like cholangiocarcinoma: an Epstein-Barr virus-associated tumor. *Am J Surg Pathol.* 2001;25:516-520.

36. Rullier A, Le Bail B, Fawaz R, Blanc JF, Saric J, Bioulac-Sage P. Cytokeratin 7 and 20 expression in cholangiocarcinomas varies along the biliary tract but still differs from that in colorectal carcinoma metastasis. *Am J Surg Pathol.* 2000;24:870-876.

37. Chan ES, Yeh MM. The use of immunohistochemistry in liver tumors. *Clin Liver Dis.* 2010;14:687-703.

38. Jinawath A, Akiyama Y, Yuasa Y, Pairojkul C. Expression of phosphorylated ERK1/2 and homeodomain protein CDX2 in cholangiocarcinoma. *J Cancer Res Clin Oncol.* 2006;132:805-810.

39. Chu PG, Schwarz RE, Lau SK, Yen Y, Weiss LM. Immunohistochemical staining in the diagnosis of pancreatobiliary and ampulla of Vater adenocarcinoma: application of CDX2, CK17, MUC1, and MUC2. *Am J Surg Pathol.* 2005;29:359-367.

40. Ryu HS, Lee K, Shin E, et al. Comparative analysis of immunohistochemical markers for differential diagnosis of hepatocelluar carcinoma and cholangiocarcinoma. *Tumori.* 2012;98:478-484.

41. Radwan NA, Ahmed NS. The diagnostic value of arginase-1 immunostaining in differentiating hepatocellular carcinoma from metastatic carcinoma and cholangiocarcinoma as compared to HepPar-1. *Diagn Pathol.* 2012;7:149.

42. Fan Z, van de Rijn M, Montgomery K, Rouse RV. Hep par 1 antibody stain for the differential diagnosis of hepatocellular carcinoma: 676 tumors tested using tissue microarrays and conventional tissue sections. *Mod Pathol.* 2003;16:137-144.

43. Surrey LF, Frank R, Zhang PJ, Furth EE. TTF-1 and Napsin-A are expressed in a subset of cholangiocarcinomas arising from the gallbladder and hepatic ducts: continued caveats for utilization of immunohistochemistry panels. *Am J Surg Pathol.* 2014;38:224-227.

ADULT BENIGN AND MALIGNANT MESENCHYMAL TUMORS 17

CHAPTER OUTLINE

SEGMENTAL ATROPHY AND NODULAR ELASTOSIS

CHECKLIST: Segmental Atrophy and Nodular Elastosis

- ☐ Benign pseudotumor
- ☐ Usually subscapular
- ☐ Morphology varies as the lesion progresses over time, starting with parenchymal collapse, followed by increasing elastosis, and finally with fibrosis

This benign pseudotumor results from a vascular insult that affects a segment or subsegment of the liver, leading first to parenchymal loss and then to gradual replacement by elastosis and fibrosis. They form mass lesions that are usually subcapsular and are either incidental findings during abdominal surgery for other reasons or, when large, can lead to mild nonspecific right upper quadrant abdominal pain and fullness. Imaging studies often suggest metastatic disease.[1]

The histological findings are discussed in more detail in chapter 9 on vascular-related tumors. In brief, the histology varies depending on the relative age of the lesion.[2] The earliest changes are parenchymal collapse, with the normal lobules replaced by inflamed and edematous stroma with an abundant bile ductular proliferation. Portal tracts are still evident, although in closer than normal proximity. Small islands of ordinary-looking hepatocytes are common. In some cases with early elastosis changes, the entrapped and normal bile ducts can dilate and form secondary biliary cysts. Additional common findings include thrombosed and fibrotic vessels.[2,3]

In time the inflammation and ductular proliferation diminishes and is replaced by increasingly dense deposits of elastic fibers. The original reticulin fibers of the lobules seem to be retained, so there ends up being a dense gray matrix composed of mixed elastic and reticulin fibers. Residual ghost portal tracts and small islands of ordinary-looking hepatocytes are common. This stage is called nodular elastosis and is quite distinctive (Fig. 17.1). Some cases can progress on to a fibrous scar.

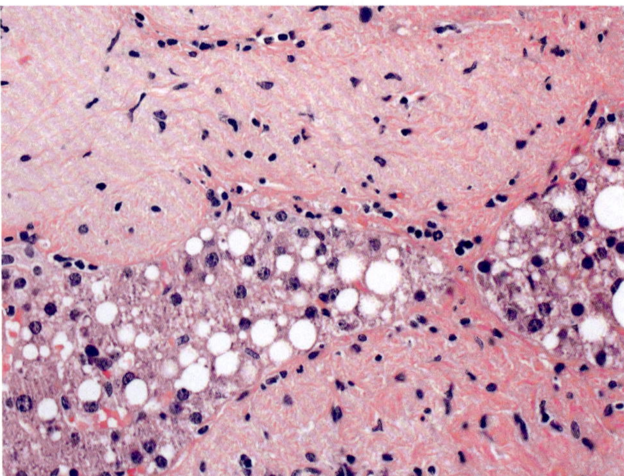

Figure 17.1. **Nodular elastosis.** A bland island of hepatocytes shows fatty change and is surrounded by dense elastosis.

INFLAMMATORY PSEUDOTUMOR

CHECKLIST: Inflammatory Pseudotumor

- ☐ Benign
- ☐ Modest male predominance of 2:1
- ☐ Average age: 50 years[4]
- ☐ Serum CA19-9 levels can be elevated, usually mild[5]
- ☐ Lesions can be single (2/3 of cases) or multiple (1/3)[4]
- ☐ Clinical associations are wide ranging, but these are the strongest:
  - ○ Biliary tract obstructive disease
  - ○ Syphilis
  - ○ IgG4 disease
- ☐ Outcome: Most sporadic cases will regress spontaneously or with antibiotic therapy

Inflammatory pseudotumors are fibrotic mass-forming lesions with varying amounts of inflammation. Patients can present with abdominal pain, distension, weight loss, and fever.[6] The average age at presentation is about 50 years, and there is a modest male predominance.[6,7] They are generally believed to be infection related, with most cases resulting from healing of abscesses. Other cases can be IgG4 related.[8,9] They do not recur after surgical resection, and most will disappear or shrink in size after antibiotic therapy.[7]

Inflammatory pseudotumors can be unifocal or multifocal, with multifocal lesions more common in the setting of biliary tract disease. Inflammatory pseudotumors tend to be more common in noncirrhotic livers but can also be seen in the setting of cirrhosis.

Histologically, they are composed of fibroblasts, collagen, and inflammatory cells (Figs. 17.2 and 17.3). The fibrosis can also vary in density and the degree of collagenization, but most cases have a fair amount of fibrosis. The collagen can be whorled/storiformed in some cases. Earlier lesions tend to be more inflamed and less fibrotic, while later lesions show the opposite, being less inflamed and more fibrotic. The lymphocytic component of the inflammation is composed primarily of T cells, with B cells found in scattered lymphoid aggregates or germinal centers. The inflammation is also often plasma cell rich (Fig. 17.4), with a predominance of IgG-positive plasma cells. Rare IgG4-positive plasma cells are common. Phlebitis is found in most resected specimens and sometimes on biopsies. Phlebitis is more commonly identified in larger lesions and, when present, involves medium- to larger sized veins.

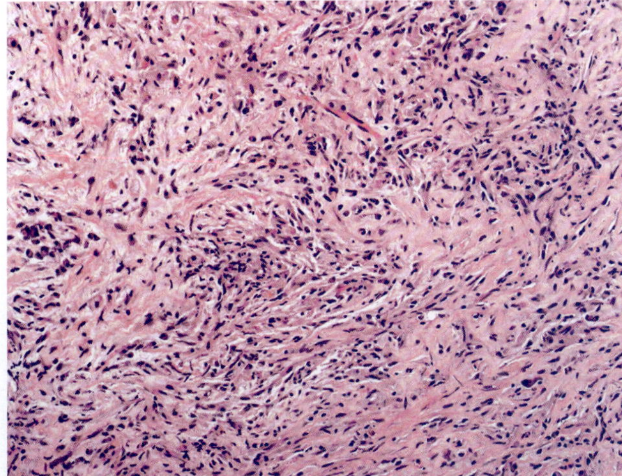

Figure 17.2. **Inflammatory pseudotumor.** At low power, the tumor is inflamed and fibrotic.

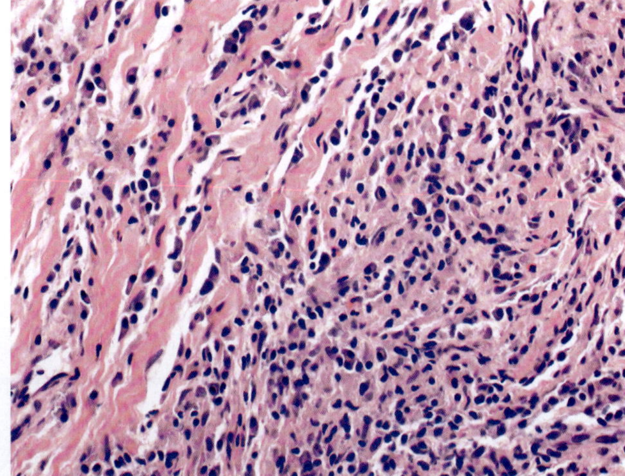

Figure 17.3. **Inflammatory pseudotumor.** The tumor is composed of fibroblasts, collagen, and inflammatory cells.

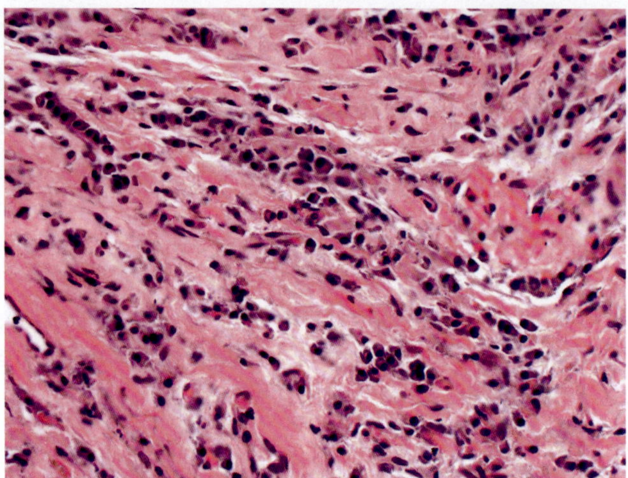

Figure 17.4. Inflammatory pseudotumor. At high power, the inflammatory cells are mostly lymphocytes but also show a mild prominence in plasma cells.

The diagnosis of an inflammatory pseudotumor is H&E based, with immunostains used mostly to exclude other diseases or to evaluate for etiology. The myofibroblasts are vimentin positive and often smooth muscle actin positive and can sometimes show patchy cytokeratin staining.[4] Syphilis is a rare but important infectious cause[10,11] and should be excluded by immunostains or be serological testing; a silver stain alone is insufficient in most cases owing to lack of sensitivity.

There are several diseases that can closely mimic inflammatory pseudotumors. These include Hodgkin lymphoma, especially on smaller biopsies, although Hodgkin lymphoma tends to have more eosinophils and, if you are lucky, occasional Reed Sternberg cells. Immunostains can also help to more fully exclude Hodgkin lymphoma. ALK staining is negative in hepatic inflammatory pseudotumors.[12] The rare "ALK-positive inflammatory pseudotumors" involving the liver that are sometimes presented at meetings or published in the literature essentially always represent systemic disease from an inflammatory myofibroblastic tumor, with liver involvement. Dendritic cell sarcomas are also in the differential and should be excluded by immunostains, such as CD21, CD35, or other markers.[13] Other tumors can sometimes have areas that closely mimic an inflammatory pseudotumor, including angiomyolipmas[14] and liposarcomas.[15]

HEMANGIOMA

CHECKLIST: Hemangioma

- ☐ Most common tumor of the liver
- ☐ More common in young adult women
- ☐ Single tumors in 90% of cases
- ☐ Histological patterns
  - ○ Cavernous (common)
  - ○ Capillary hemangioma (very rare)
  - ○ Anastomosing hemangioma (very rare)

CAVERNOUS HEMANGIOMA

Hemangiomas are found in approximately 5% of adult livers, usually in young adult women. They are usually unifocal and are mostly incidental findings. Symptoms can develop in larger tumors, typically those that are greater than 4 cm. Hemangiomas are benign neoplastic proliferations of cytologically bland blood vessels. Sometimes the literature states that hemangiomas are reactive or hamartomatous and not neoplastic, but in the liver this is not true.

The most common pattern is called a cavernous hemangioma and is made of dilated large caliber blood vessels, with generally sparse fibrous background stroma (Fig. 17.5). In some cases, the fibrous stroma can be more prominent and show mild chronic inflammation. Hemangiomas are not encapsulated, but the interface with the liver is generally fairly well demarcated. However, there can be patchy areas of irregular infiltration by smaller sized vessels, especially with larger tumors. The endothelial cells show no atypia and no mitotic figures. The centers of the hemangiomas can be sclerotic, and there can be ghostly remnants of the old cavernous vascular architecture. In other cases, there can be more irregular fibrosis in the center (Fig. 17.6), often with numerous pigment-laden macrophages and sometimes with scattered calcifications. In time, some hemangiomas can become completely sclerotic (Fig. 17.7). Hemangiomas have no malignant potential; they do not progress to angiosarcomas.

Larger cavernous hemangiomas, those greater than 8 cm in diameter, are called *giant cavernous hemangiomas*. This size cut off is not very strictly enforced, so there is wide variability in the use of this term. In general, they are histologically the same as ordinary hemangiomas, just bigger. The interface of the hemangioma and the background liver is also more likely to be fuzzy, with a fair amount of hemangioma infiltrating the adjacent liver (Fig. 17.8), leading to a cuff of admixed hepatocytes and hemangioma. This finding is called "hemangiomatosis" or "hemangioma-like vessels."[16,17]

CAPILLARY HEMANGIOMA

The capillary hemangioma, also called a lobular hemangioma, is rare variant in the liver.[18,19] The tumors are usually single but can be multiple. They have a modest female predominance, and most have been reported in adults, with a possible enrichment for Asian ethnicity.[19]

The capillary hemangioma is composed of blood vessels (Fig. 17.9) that are much smaller than the blood vessels in cavernous hemangiomas. In fact, sometimes the vessel lumens can be so small that the hemangioma can mimic a solid tumor, especially if there is substantial crush effect to the specimen. In uncrushed specimens, the vessels tend to be thin walled, round, and fairly uniform in size. Somewhat larger vessels can sometimes be found at the periphery or center of the tumor. The endothelial cells can be plump but lack cytological atypia and mitotic activity. A Ki-67 shows a low proliferative rate. In some cases, a lobular growth pattern can be observed at low power. The endothelial cells stain with ordinary markers of vascular differentiation.

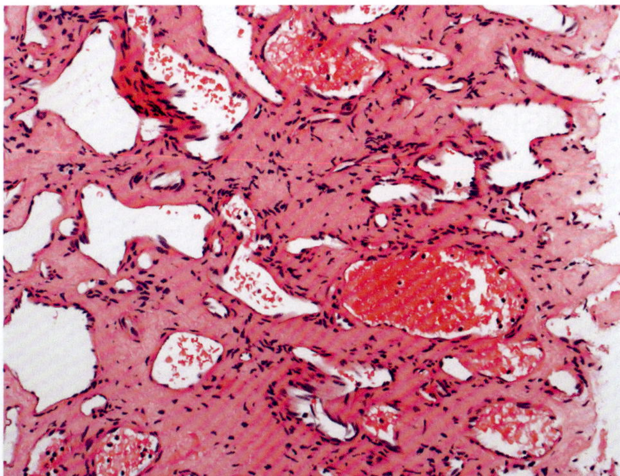

Figure 17.5. Hemangioma, cavernous. The tumor is composed of large caliber dilated vessels.

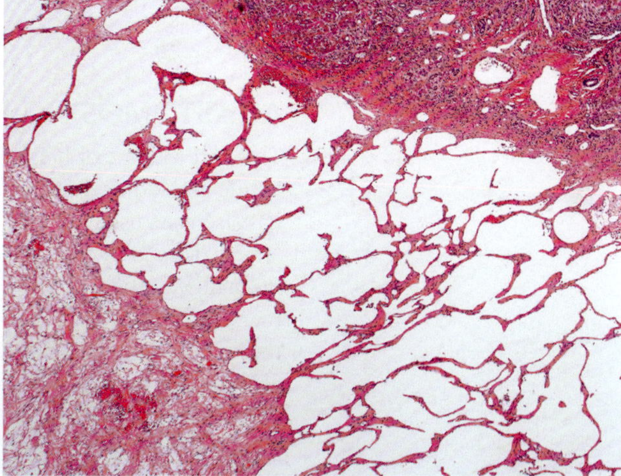

Figure 17.6. Hemangioma, cavernous. The center of the tumor (lower left of image) has become fibrotic.

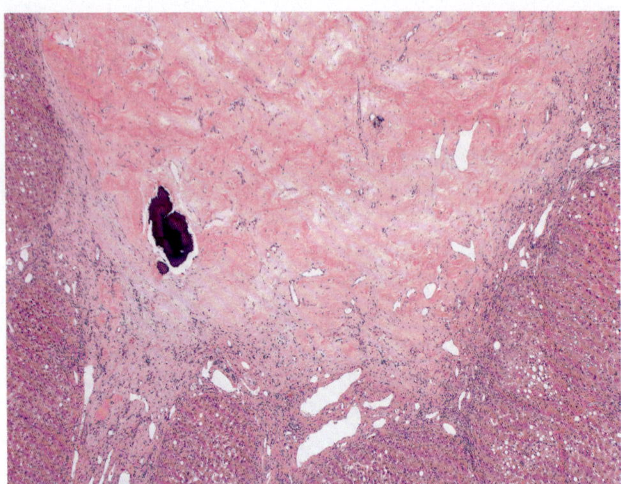

Figure 17.7. Hemangioma, sclerosed. This hemangioma shows almost total sclerosis, with focal calcifications.

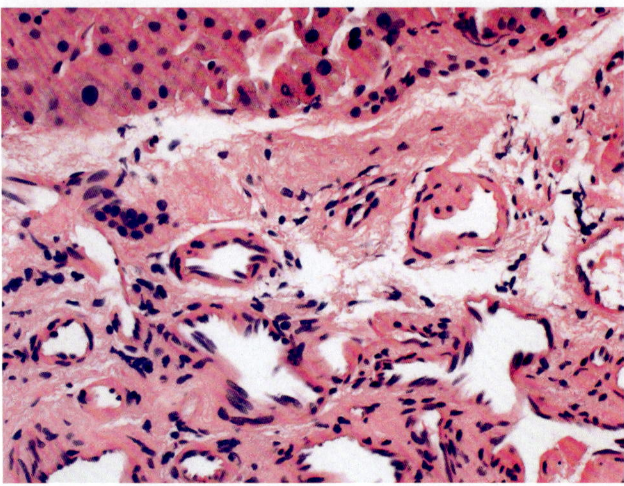

Figure 17.8. Hemangioma, infiltrative edges. This large hemangioma had irregular areas at the tumor edge that showed infiltration by the hemangioma.

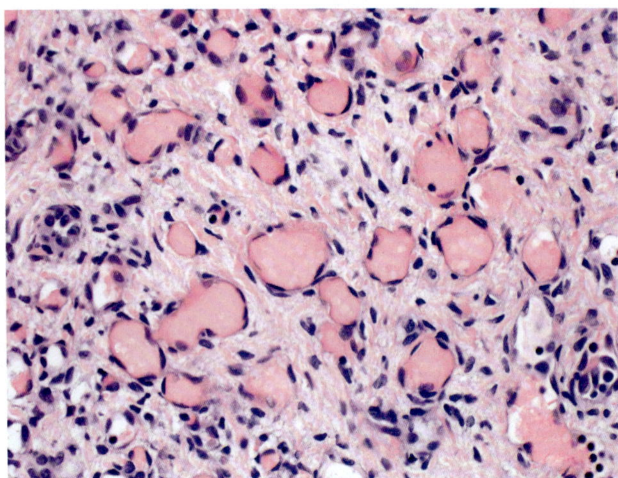

Figure 17.9. Hemangioma, capillary. This neoplasm has a lobular pattern at low power and is composed of small vessels with no atypia.

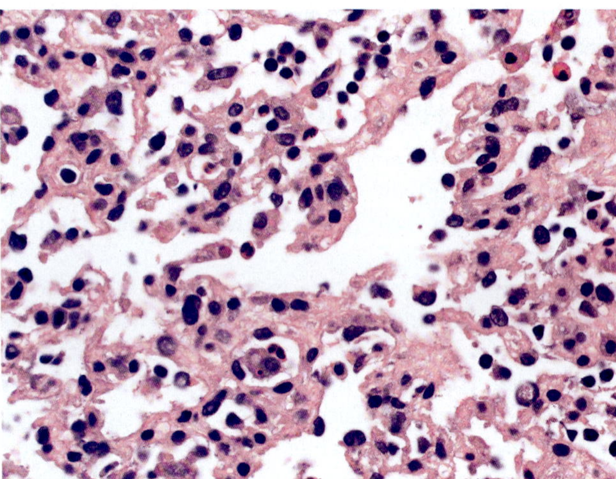

Figure 17.10. Hemangioma, anastomosing. This hemangioma shows tightly packed capillary-sized vessels with anastomosing channels lined by hobnail endothelial cells.

ANASTOMOSING HEMANGIOMA

This rare variant of hemangioma is more common in the male genital tract, retroperitoneum, and kidney but can also be found in the liver.[20,21] The term small vessel hemangioma has also been used for anastomosing hemangiomas when they are in the liver. This variant is largely defined by the cytology, which shows tightly packed capillary-sized vessels lined by hobnail endothelial cells (Fig. 17.10), with at least a focal anastomosing growth pattern of the vessels.[21] The vessels often have small thrombi. There can be mild cytological atypia, but there should be no mitotic figures and no necrosis. These lesions tend to be well circumscribed, but there can be admixed tumor cells and hepatocytes at the edges of the lesion, without parenchymal destruction.

EPITHELIOD HEMANGIOENDOTHELIOMA

CHECKLIST: Epithelioid Hemangioendotheliomas

- ☐ Malignant vascular tumor, less aggressive than typical angiosarcoma
- ☐ Does not have well-formed tumor vessels, instead tumor cells are epithelioid or dendritic in morphology, often with small intracellular lumina
- ☐ Tumor cells are embedded in abundant myxoid or hyalinized stroma
- ☐ Tumor cells can show keratin staining, so they are often misdiagnosed as metastatic adenocarcinoma

Epithelioid hemangioendothelioma is a rare malignant vascular tumor. Most patients present between the ages of 30 and 50 years, and there is a modest female predominance.[22] Clinical findings at presentation tend to be mild and nonspecific, such as vague abdominal pain or weight loss, with about 40% of cases identified as incidental findings during evaluation for other clinical problems.

The tumors arise in noncirrhotic livers and are almost always multifocal, in most cases involving both lobes of the liver. Histologically, the most striking finding at low power is the tumor matrix, which can be myxoid or hyalinized (Fig. 17.11). The tumor cells embedded within this matrix show scant to moderate cellularity, with the tumors typically more cellular at the periphery than in the center. In fact, the tumor center can be densely sclerotic and almost devoid of cells. Vessel formation is not a prominent feature in most cases, but occasionally can be seen.

Most of the tumor cells have an epithelioid morphology on H&E, with moderate amounts of pale eosinophilic to amphiphilic cytoplasm, often with intracellular lumina (Figs. 17.12 and 17.13). In some cases, red blood cells may be present within the lumina. A second population of tumor cells with a dendritic appearance is more challenging to see on H&E but is often brought out on immunostains. Mitotic figures tend to be rare or absent.

Epithelioid hemangioendotheliomas can be grossly well circumscribed but commonly have extensive parenchymal infiltration at the edges of the visible tumor masses. Microscopic tumor deposits can also be seen in sections considerably distant from the visible tumor mass. Epithelioid hemangioendotheliomas tend to spread along the sinusoids and the portal and central veins. As the tumor spreads, it often obliterates branches of the portal and central veins, leading to parenchymal atrophy (Fig. 17.14).

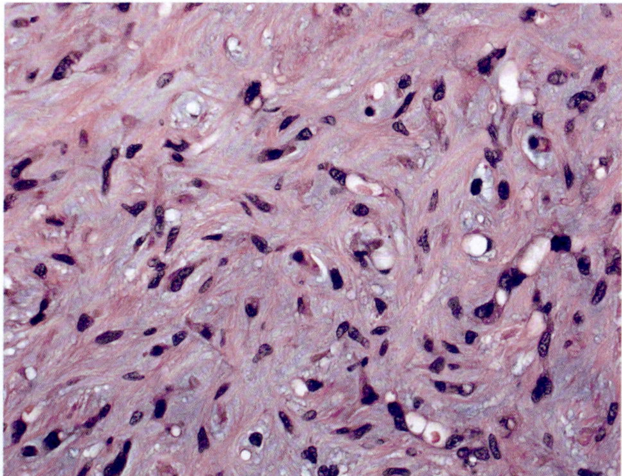

Figure 17.11. **Epithelioid hemangioendothelioma.** The tumor has a distinctive myxoid matrix, with atypical spindled and epithelioid cells.

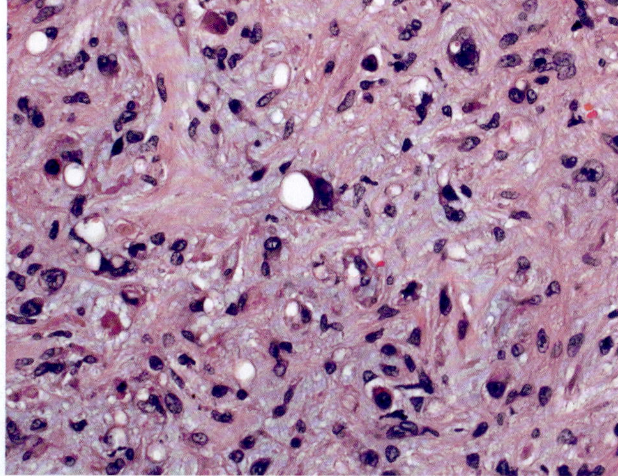

Figure 17.12. **Epithelioid hemangioendothelioma.** At higher power, some of the tumor cells have lumina.

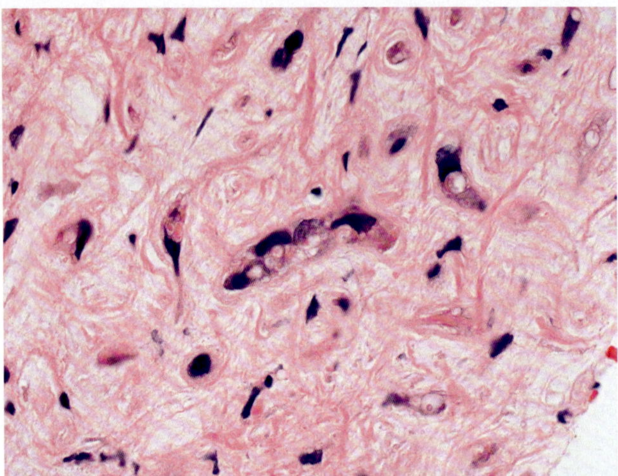

Figure 17.13. **Epithelioid hemangioendothelioma.** Another example showing the characteristic morphology. The background matrix is more collagenized in this case.

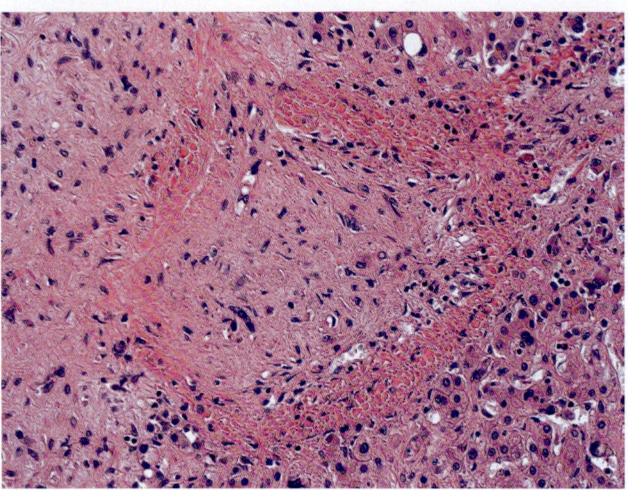

Figure 17.14. **Epithelioid hemangioendothelioma.** The tumor is growing along the central veins, leading to occlusion of the vein and collapse of the surrounding hepatic parenchyma.

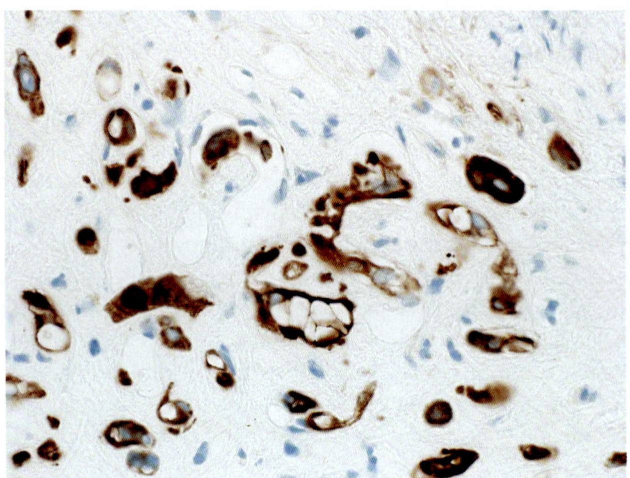

Figure 17.15. **Epithelioid hemangioendothelioma, CK7.** The tumor cells are strongly positive.

Epithelioid hemangioendotheliomas stain with the ordinary vascular markers, such as ERG, FLI-1, CD34, and CD31.[22–24] CD10 is also positive in most tumors,[25] D2-40 is positive in about 70% of cases,[24] while keratins can be positive in 10% to 30% of cases (Fig. 17.15).[24]

Angiosarcomas lack the distinctive matrix of epithelioid hemangioendotheliomas and tend to show more cytological atypia, readily identified mitotic figures, and more tissue destruction. Both are positive for markers of vascular differentiation.

At the molecular level, epithelioid hemangioendotheliomas have a WWTR1-CAMTA1 fusion gene[26] and less commonly other fusions including, YAP1-TFE3.[27,28] Some,[24] but not all, studies[29] have found that most epithelioid hemangioendotheliomas are TFE3 positive by immunostain, regardless of the type of fusion gene.

PEARLS & PITFALLS

- Always correlate the morphology with the immunostain results, as epithelioid hemangioendotheliomas can closely mimic other tumors.
- There should be compatible morphology plus immunostain confirmation of vascular differentiation.
  - Of the stains for vascular differentiation, CD34 is the least specific.
  - ERG is positive in all epithelioid hemangioendotheliomas but also positive in 30% to 50% of prostate cancers, some meningiomas, rare Ewing sarcomas, and rare mesotheliomas.[23,30]
  - FLI-1 is positive in all epithelioid hemangioendotheliomas.

ANGIOSARCOMA

Angiosarcomas of the liver are rare and aggressive malignancies, with few individuals alive >1 year after diagnosis.[31] Male gender is a general risk factor, but no specific etiological agent is identified in most cases. However, known risk factors include exogenous androgen use,[32] vinyl chloride exposure (an industrial chemical),[33] arsenic (found in the ground water in some parts of the world), and Thorotrast (a contrast agent previously used for imaging, no longer in use).[34] The latency between exposure to risk factors and the development of angiosarcoma can be very long. For example, the average latency in one study of vinyl chloride exposure was 37 years from exposure to clinical presentation with angiosarcoma, range 24 to 56 years.[35] In the pediatric population, most cases of angiosarcoma arise out of infantile hemangiomas.[36]

Angiosarcoma can be a metastatic or primary to the liver. They can be unifocal or multifocal. The background liver can show a range of nonspecific findings, including nonspecific chronic inflammation and fatty change. Most livers are noncirrhotic.

CHECKLIST: Morphological Patterns in Angiosarcoma

- ☐ Mass forming
  - ○ Vasoformative
  - ○ Solid/epithelioid
  - ○ Spindle cell
- ☐ Non-mass forming
  - ○ Sinusoidal infiltration
  - ○ Peliotic like

Morphologically, tumors can be mass forming or non-mass forming. The neoplastic cells in mass-forming lesions can be solid and epithelioid, mimicking a carcinoma (Fig. 17.16), or can be composed of spindled cells (Figs. 17.17 and 17.18). Some of the solid tumors will also be vasoformative (Fig. 17.19), with various sized vessels lined by malignant cells. In some cases, solid tumors undergo central cavitating necrosis, leaving behind a thin rim of malignant cells surrounding a cavity filled with blood and necrotic debris.

In addition to solid growth patterns, angiosarcomas can also show a very subtle sinusoidal infiltrative pattern (Figs. 17.19–17.22) or a sutle peliotic pattern, without forming a distinct mass either by imaging or by gross examination (Figs. 17.22–17.24). In these cases, imaging typically shows hepatomegaly and vascular perfusion changes. Histologically, the tumor cells extend along the sinusoids, replacing the normal endothelial cells, but leaving the hepatic plates relatively intact. There often is mild to moderate sinusoidal dilation, and this pattern is frequently mistaken for vascular outflow disease. This pattern is very subtle, and a large proportion of cases are initially misdiagnosed clinically, radiologically, and histologically. Important histological clues include subtle increased sinusoidal cellularity, cytological atypia, and mitotic figures.

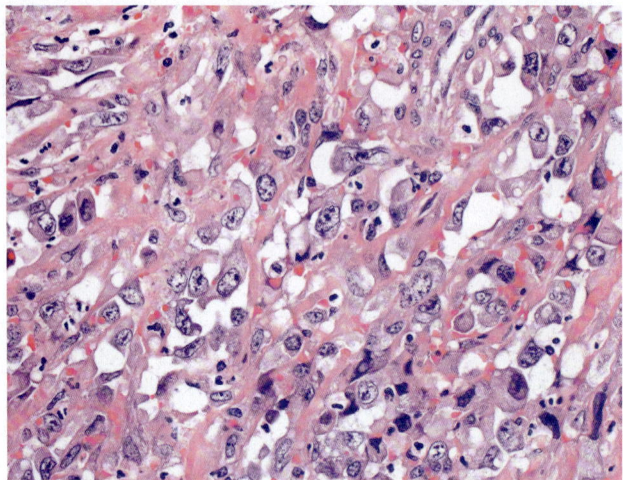

Figure 17.16. **Angiosarcoma, mass forming, epithelioid growth.** This mass-forming angiosarcoma at first suggested a carcinoma, but careful examination showed the tumor to be highly vascularized including tumor cells with intracytoplasmic red blood cells.

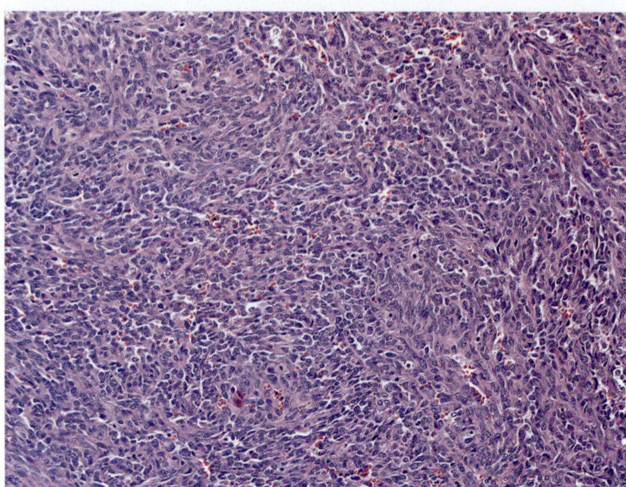

Figure 17.17. **Angiosarcoma, mass forming, spindle cell growth.** This mass-forming angiosarcoma has a spindle cell morphology.

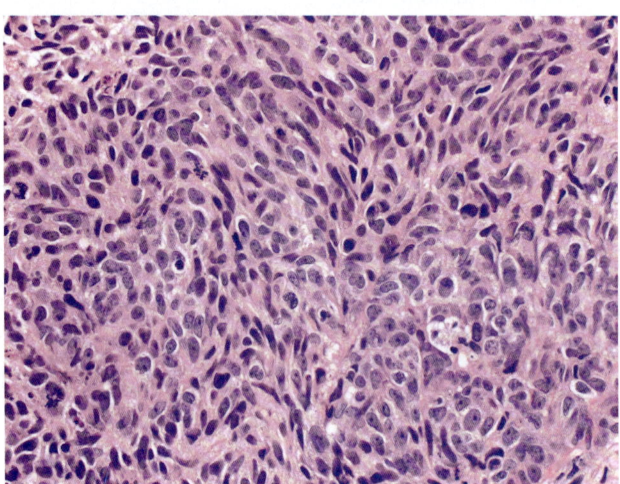

Figure 17.18. **Angiosarcoma, mass forming, spindle cell growth.** Another example of a mass-forming angiosarcoma with a spindled cell morphology.

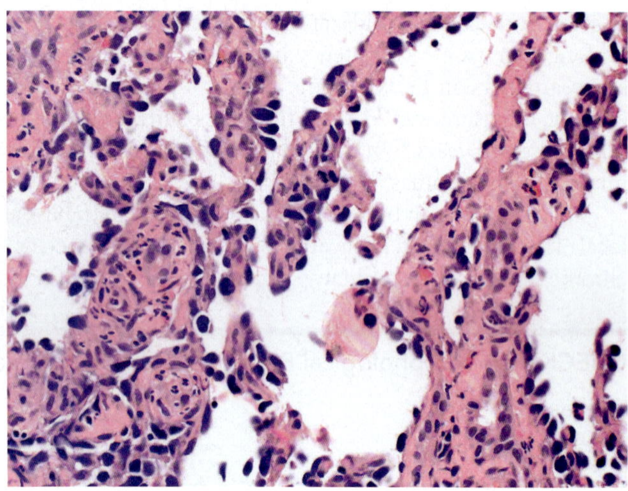

Figure 17.19. **Angiosarcoma, mass forming, vasoformative.** This angiosarcoma formed large, dilated vascular channels lined by very atypical cells.

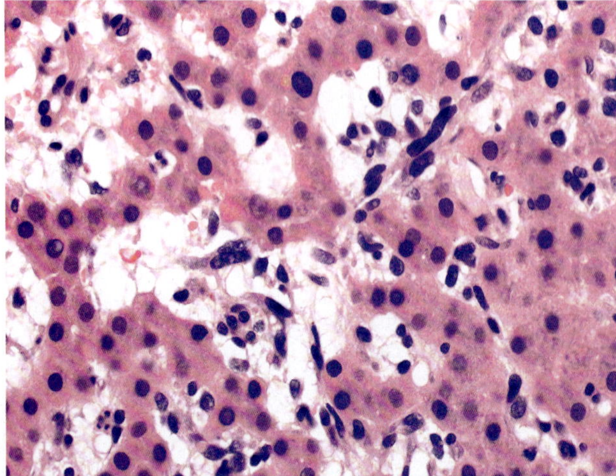

Figure 17.20. **Angiosarcoma, non-mass forming, sinusoidal growth pattern.** There were ill defined areas of vascular perfusion changes, but no mass lesion on imaging. The malignant cells are growing along the sinusoids, leaving intact hepatic trabeculae.

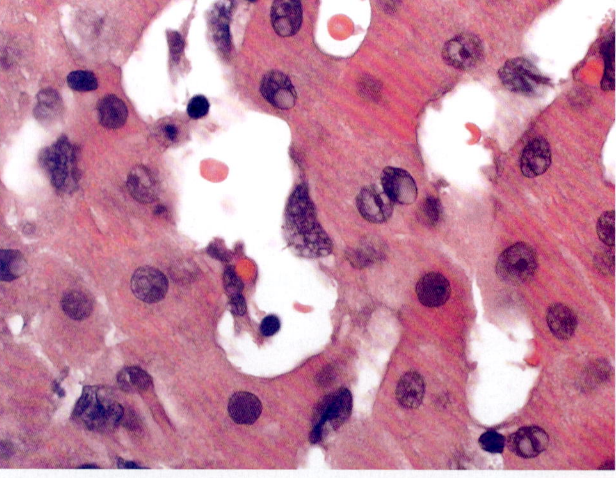

Figure 17.21. **Angiosarcoma, non-mass forming, sinusoidal growth pattern.** This case was very subtle and was initially misdiagnosed as congestive hepatopathy. Note the atypical endothelial cells. They had an increased proliferative rate (see below) and were p53 positive.

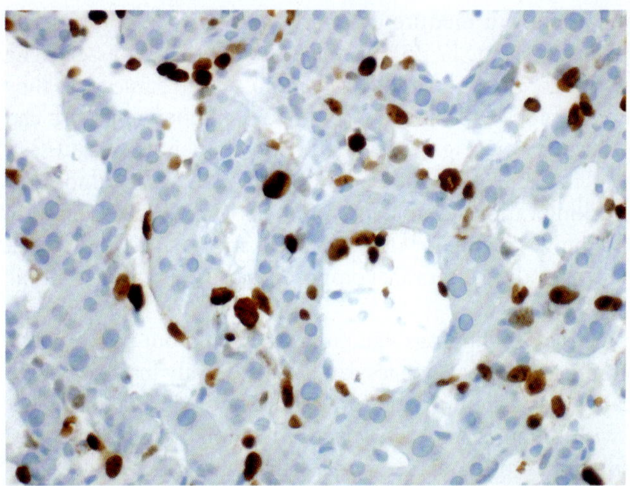

Figure 17.22. **Angiosarcoma, non-mass forming, sinusoidal growth pattern, Ki-67.** An immunostain for Ki-67 is strongly positive.

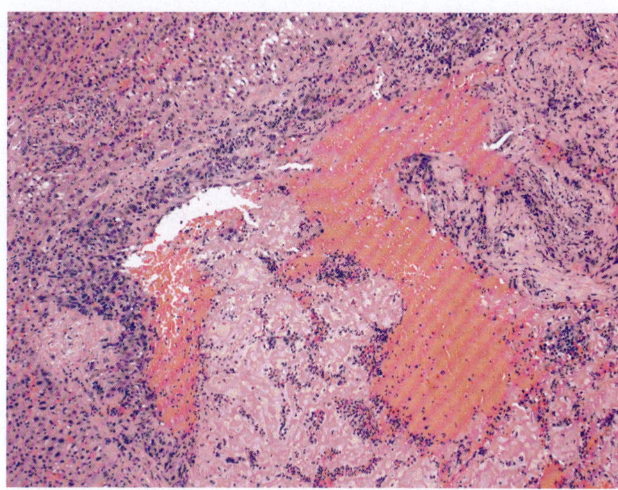

Figure 17.23. **Angiosarcoma, non-mass forming, peliosis hepatis pattern.** This case was originally interpreted as peliosis hepatis.

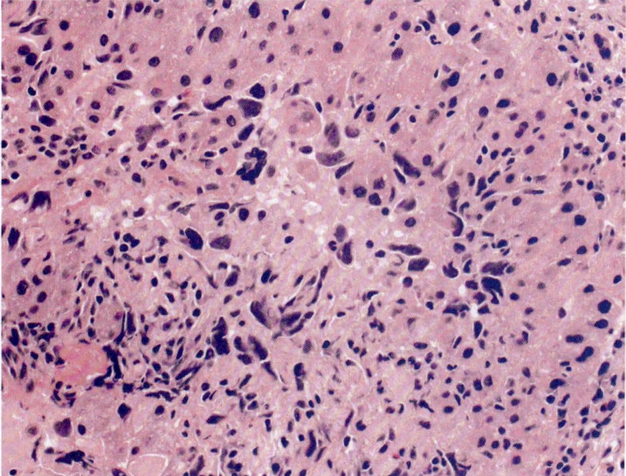

Figure 17.24. **Angiosarcoma, non-mass forming, peliosis hepatis pattern.** At higher power (same case as Fig. 17.23), atypical endothelial cells line the peliotic-like spaces.

Regardless of the growth pattern, the tumor cells show cytological atypia, a clearly increased Ki-67 proliferative rate, and often strong p53 expression. They are also positive for markers of vascular differentiation. ERG and FLI-1 are the most sensitive, but other markers can be positive: factor VIII (in 80% to 90% of cases), CD34 (75%), and CD31 (wide range of positive in the literature, 30% to 80%).[37] Also of note, aberrant expression of cytokeratin is common: AE1/3 (45% of cases) and CAM5.2 (30%).[37] Although the cytokeratin staining is usually patchy, it can be an important diagnostic pitfall.

ANGIOMYOLIPOMA

Angiomyolipomas are benign mesenchymal tumors composed of myoid cells, fat cells, and large irregular vessels. They are easy to recognize when all three components are present, but many hepatic angiomyolipomas are composed mostly of myoid cells, giving the tumors an epithelioid morphology that mimics carcinoma or a monomorphic spindle cell morphology that mimics smooth muscle tumors. In fact, half of the cases in some studies were initially misdiagnosed as other tumors.[38] Most hepatic angiomyolipomas are single tumors and are sporadic (not associated with the tuberous sclerosis complex). Angiomyolipomas have a strong female predominance, with an average at diagnosis of about 50 years.[38]

Histologically, angiomyolipomas show a mixture of tumor cells with smooth muscle or "myoid" differentiation, fatty change (Fig. 17.25), and large thick-walled vessels. The myoid cells can be spindled (Fig. 17.26) or epithelioid (Fig. 17.27), and in some cases they can be the only cell type evident in biopsy specimens. Epithelioid angiomyolipomas can sometimes show patchy pigment deposition (Fig. 17.28). The solid epithelioid variants can mimic hepatocellular carcinoma.[38] In some of the solid epithelioid variants, the tumor cells will show clear cell change, mimicking various clear cell carcinomas (Fig. 17.29). The solid spindle cell tumors can mimic leiomyosarcoma or other tumors, such as gastrointestinal stromal tumors (GIST).[39] In other cases, the tumors are composed mostly fat and can mimic a lipoma or liposarcoma.[38,40]

There are a number of other histological findings that are usually mild but rarely can be in sufficient quantity to cause confusion. Some changes can be seen focally in tumors with any morphology, including focal necrosis, hemorrhage, and cholesterol clefts, while other changes tend to be associated with different growth patterns. The following changes are seen most commonly in fat predominant tumors: (1) lipoblast-like cells (with multivacuolated cytoplasm and indented nuclei) and (2) extramedullary hematopoiesis. The following changes are seen most commonly with solid tumors: (3) striking peliotic changes, which is often accompanied by hemorrhage[38]; (4) spindle cell tumors with inflamed areas that mimic inflammatory pseudotumors; and (5) giant cell change in the epithelioid or spindle cell component,[41] with large, pleomorphic, and sometimes multinucleate cells (Fig. 17.30). The latter change does not indicate malignancy.

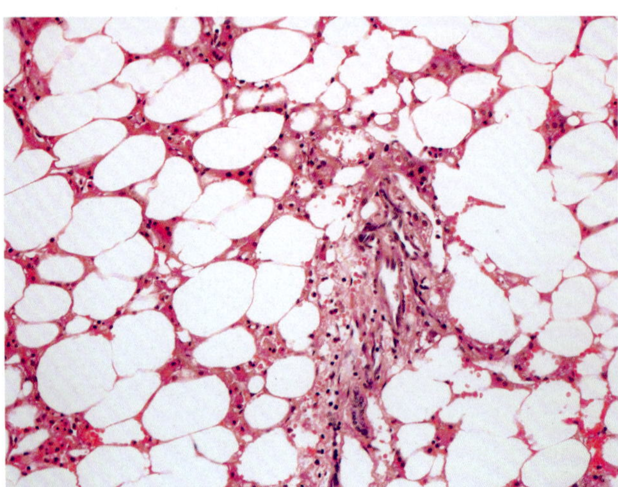

Figure 17.25. **Angiomyolipoma.** This tumor shows predominately a fatty pattern.

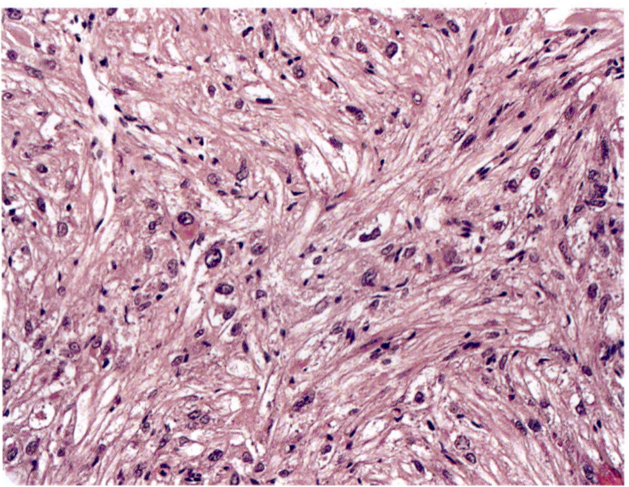

Figure 17.26. **Angiomyolipoma.** This case shows a spindle cell growth pattern.

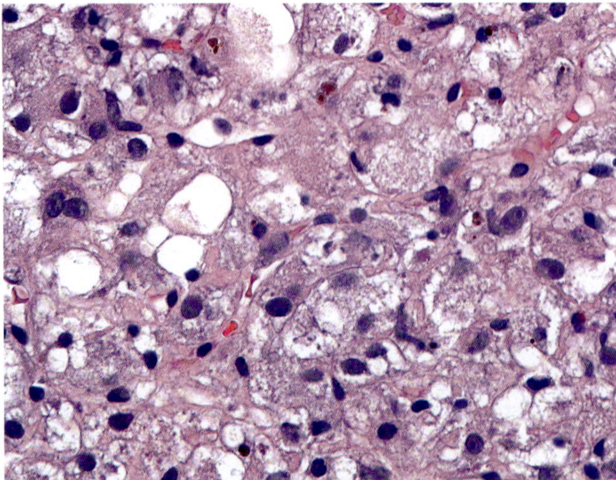

Figure 17.27. **Angiomyolipoma.** This case has case shows an epithelioid growth pattern.

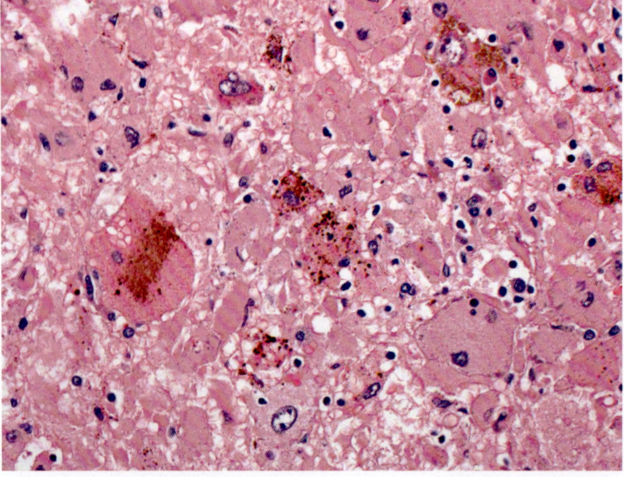

Figure 17.28. **Angiomyolipoma.** This case has an epithelioid growth pattern and shows patchy melanin pigment deposits.

Immunostains are important for confirming the H&E impression of an angiomyolipoma. Angiomyolipomas are negative for cytokeratins[38] and for HepPar1, arginase, and glypican 3. They are positive for HMB45 in essentially all cases (Fig. 17.31) and for MelA (>90% of cases), although the myoid component will have the strongest staining, and staining can be patchy or negative in fatty areas. CD68 is positive in nearly all cases with a myoid component (Fig. 17.32). CKIT (CD117) is also positive in nearly all cases[42] and can mimic a metastatic GIST. S100 is routinely positive in the fatty areas and often in the myoid areas.[38] Smooth muscle actin is positive, in more than half of cases, in particular in tumor cells with a spindle cell morphology.[38,42] Finally, TFE3 is frequently positive by immunohistochemistry, but there are no TFE3 gene rearrangements.[43]

Angiomyolipomas are benign tumors, but rarely, they become malignant. Because malignancy is a rare event in a rare tumor, the histological features that predict malignancy have not been well characterized. Cytological atypia alone does not indicate malignancy. In addition, rare cases of aggressive behavior in angiomyolipomas have been reported, despite the tumor showing ordinary histology with no worrisome features.[44] At this point, the best way to identify tumors that are at increased risk for aggressive behavior appears to be finding areas of tumor dedifferentiation, vascular invasion,[45] coagulative necrosis,[46] marked cytological atypia, or increased mitoses.[47] Immunostain findings are not characterized well enough to be helpful, but some studies have suggested an increased risk for malignancy if there is loss of CD117 staining[46] or strong P53 positivity.[47]

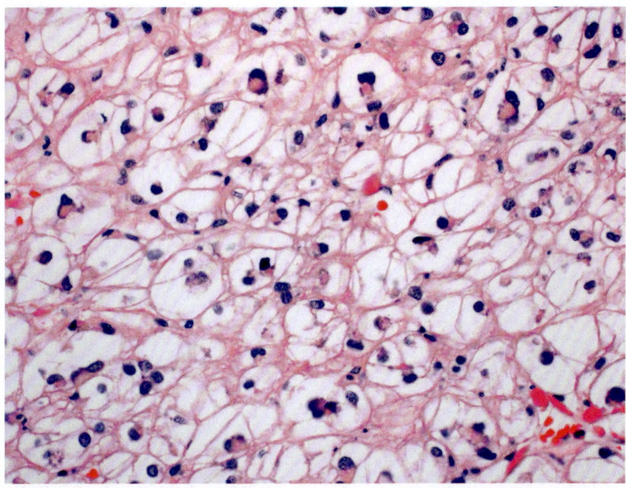

Figure 17.29. **Angiomyolipoma.** This epithelioid angiomyolipoma mimics a clear cell carcinoma.

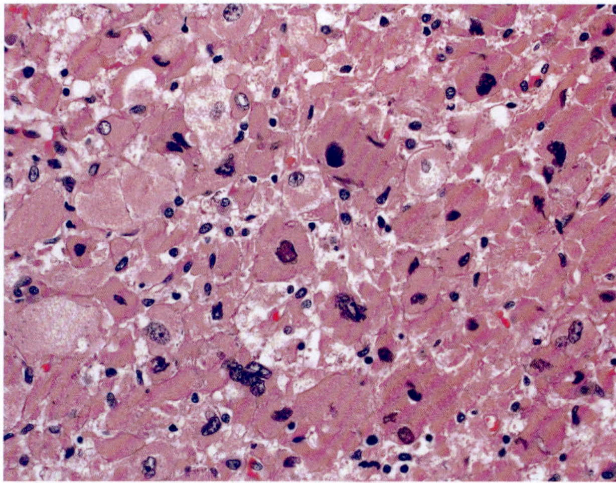

Figure 17.30. **Angiomyolipoma.** This epithelioid angiomyolipoma shows patchy but striking nuclear pleomorphism.

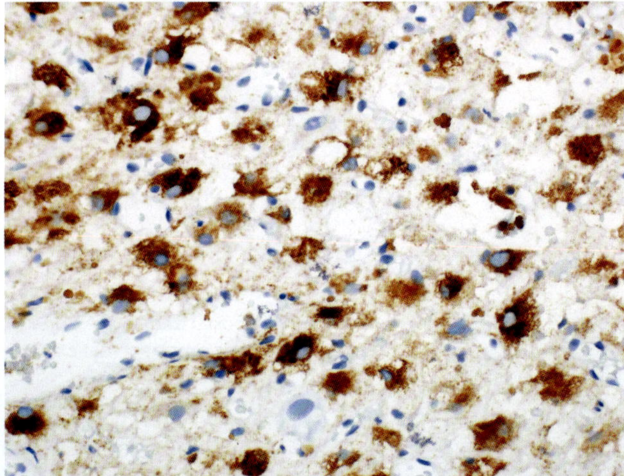

Figure 17.31. **Angiomyolipoma, HMB45.** The tumor cells are strongly positive, although not every cell stains.

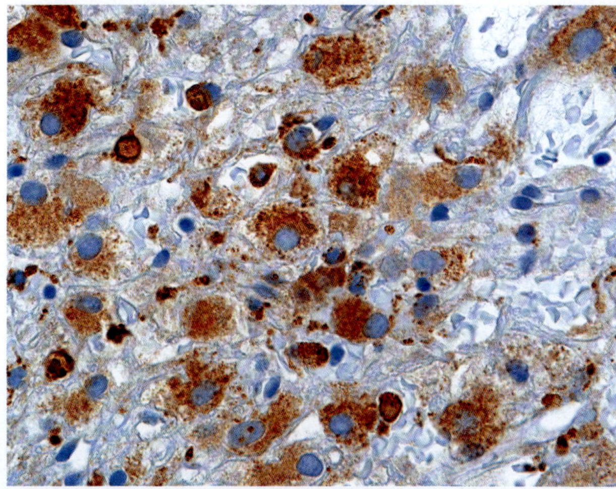

Figure 17.32. **Angiomyolipoma, CD68.** The tumor cells are strongly positive.

SOLITAR FIBROUS TUMOR

Solitary fibrous tumors are rare benign spindle cell tumors of uncertain etiology. They are thought to arise from fibroblast-like cells within Glisson capsule. However, most tumors are intraparenchymal, with only a small subset showing a direct connection to the liver capsule.[48] One possible explanation for this discordant finding is that Glisson capsule is thought to invaginate into the liver, surrounding at least some of the portal tracts with a sheath of connective tissue in the liver periphery.[49] While most solitary fibrous tumors are solitary, rare cases can be multifocal. At the molecular level, solitary fibrous tumors have a fusion gene, NAB2-STAT6,[50] but the diagnosis can be readily made in almost all cases by compatible morphology with immunostain confirmation. Because of the fusion gene, solitary fibrous tumors are STAT6 positive.

Most solitary fibrous tumors are identified in women over the age of 40 years with mild nonspecific clinical findings.[48] However, individuals can present with hypoglycemia if the tumor produces insulin-like growth factor-II.[51,52] Histologically, the tumors show low cellularity, with cytologically bland spindle cells embedded in a dense fibrous background. The spindled cells do not show any organizational patterns at low power, a finding called a "patternless pattern" (Fig. 17.33). Sometimes the stroma can appear more myxoid, while in other areas the stroma will become densely fibrotic and almost acellular. In rare cases, but more often when solitary fibrous tumors are multifocal, the tumors can entrap portal tracts, leading to additional benign changes in the portal tracts that include cystic dilatation of the bile duct, small clusters of proliferating bile ducts at the periphery (they look more like duct duplication than ductular proliferation), and pancreatic acinar cell metaplasia (Fig. 17.34) and/or hepatic metaplasia. Giant cell transformation alone is a benign change that does not indicate malignancy[53] (Fig. 17.35). The great majority of solitary fibrous tumors are benign, but about 10% of cases can have areas suggesting more aggressive biology, with foci of cytological atypia, increased mitoses, and necrosis.[54] Rarely, solitary fibrous tumors can show areas where the tumor has transformed into a high-grade fibrosarcoma.[52]

The diagnosis can be confirmed by immunostains, as tumors are positive for STAT6 (Fig. 17.36), BCL2, and CD34. Solitary fibrous tumors are negative for S100, desmin, smooth muscle actin, CKIT, and cytokeratins.

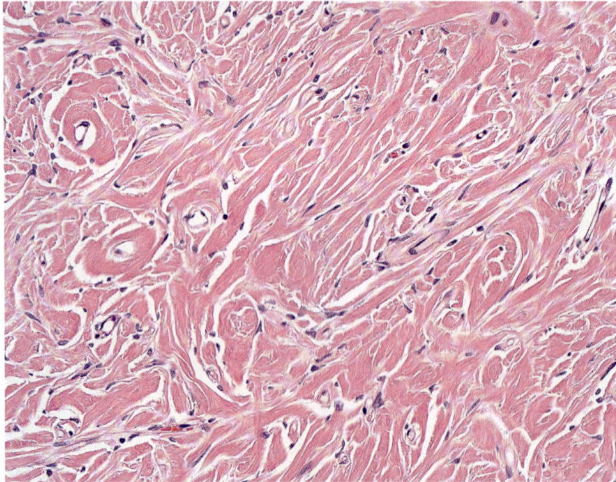

Figure 17.33. **Solitary fibrous tumor.** Small spindled cells are present in a densely collagenized background.

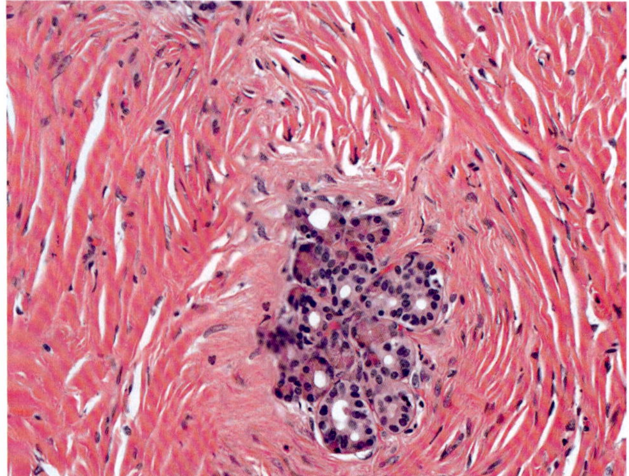

Figure 17.34. **Solitary fibrous tumor.** A portal tract at the edge of the lesion has become entrapped and underwent pancreatic acinar cell metaplasia.

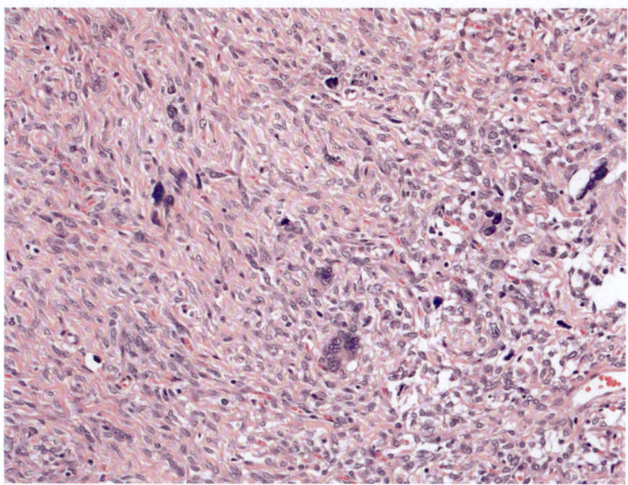

Figure 17.35. **Solitary fibrous tumor.** Focal areas of giant cell transformation and increased cellularity are seen. These changes alone do not indicate malignancy.

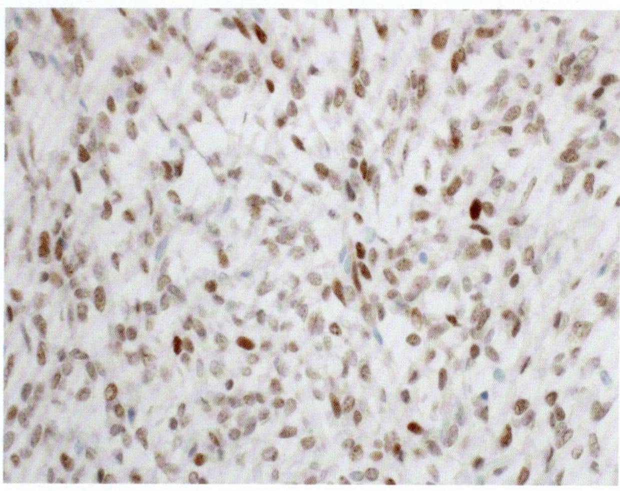

Figure 17.36. **Solitary fibrous tumor, STAT6.** The tumor shows strong diffuse nuclear staining.

NEAR MISSES

CASE 1. A biopsy was directed at a solitary 4-cm lesion in the liver of a 34-year-old woman. The lesion was clearly vascular on histology, and the initial interpretation was an angiosarcoma. However, the clinician noted that the clinical and imaging findings did not fit for angiosarcoma, and the biopsy was sent out for consultation.

The biopsy showed a well-differentiated vascular tumor composed of small interanastomosing vessels with plump endothelial cells but no atypia and no mitotic activity (Fig. 17.37). Mast cells were also mildly prominent in some areas. A diagnosis of anastomosing hemangioma was made.

Anastomosing hemangiomas have only been recently described, so many pathologists are less familiar with them. They often are initially classified as angiosarcomas, as seen in this case. The lack of cytological atypia, destructive growth, and mitotic figures helps exclude angiosarcoma. Also of note, many benign hemangiomas, including cavernous hemangiomas and anastomosing hemangiomas, can have an "infiltrative growth" at their edges, but these areas of infiltrative growth are not the same as a destructive growth pattern.

CASE 2. A 63-year-old man had weight loss and vague abdominal pain. Imaging showed parenchymal changes in the liver but no distinct mass lesions. A biopsy was performed and showed sinusoidal dilatation but no inflammation, fatty change, biliary tract disease, or fibrosis. The findings were initially interpreted as congestive hepatopathy, but further clinical evaluation showed no imaging evidence for vascular outflow disease. The biopsy was sent out for consultation, which also led to a diagnosis of findings most suggestive of congestive hepatopathy. Over the next 2 months, the patient deteriorated rapidly, and reimaging again showed diffuse liver parenchymal changes. The liver biopsy was sent a second time for consultation. This time, the sinusoidal cells were noted to be very atypical in some areas (Fig. 17.38), and a diagnosis of angiosarcoma, sinusoidal type, was made.

The sinusoidal pattern of angiosarcoma is particularly challenging to diagnose, and many cases are initially misdiagnosed as vascular outflow disease, as illustrated by this case. The clue is careful examination of the sinusoidal endothelial cells for atypia, inclusions (note the eosinophilic globes seen focally in Fig. 17.38), and mitotic figures. A p53 immunostain can sometimes be helpful if there is strong and diffuse positivity in the atypical cells, with no staining in the normal-appearing endothelial cells.

CASE 3. A 67-year-old woman had numerous liver tumors by imaging. Lesions were also present in the bones, lungs, and spleen. A biopsy of one of the large liver lesions showed a poorly differentiated epithelioid neoplasm (Fig. 17.39). The tumor showed strong patchy synaptophysin staining but was negative for chromogranin. Keratin markers were negative, other than focal weak CAM5.2 staining. Immunostains ruled out melanoma, lymphoma, GIST, neural malignancies, and leiomyosarcoma. There was temptation to sign out the case as a poorly differentiated malignancy, favor carcinoma with neuroendocrine differentiation, but one last round of stains revealed the correct diagnosis: angiosarcoma. The angiosarcoma was strongly positive for FLI-1, ERG (Fig. 17.40), and CD31.

Epithelioid angiosarcomas can be challenging to diagnose, mostly because it is easy to overlook angiosarcoma in the differential when evaluating a tumor with an epithelioid morphology. Aberrant keratin and synaptophysin staining can also contribute to confusion. However, once considered, the diagnosis can be confidently made using markers of vascular differentiation. None of the markers of vascular differentiation are perfectly sensitive or specific, so a panel approach works well in difficult cases.

CASE 4. A 47-year-old man had a 2-cm incidentally discovered liver mass while being evaluated for possible gallstones. A biopsy showed a vascular lesion with lymphoid aggregates (Fig. 17.41). The lesion was difficult to classify because it did not look like one of the typical hemangiomas (cavernous, capillary, anastomosing) and did not look like an angiosarcoma. The plan was to sign the case out descriptively but a final look before signing it out was helpful, as the correct diagnosis suddenly became clear: an ectopic spleen. An immunostain for CD8 confirmed the H&E impression (Fig. 17.42). Most patients with ectopic spleens in the liver have a history of blunt force trauma to the abdomen or prior splenectomy. In this case, no relevant history was evident in the medical charts.

Many times, a difficult case benefits from being set aside and reviewed a second (or third) time before punting with a descriptive diagnosis. In this case, the challenge was primarily to think of the possibility of an ectopic spleen. Once the possibility was in the differential, the subsequent work-up and diagnosis were clear.

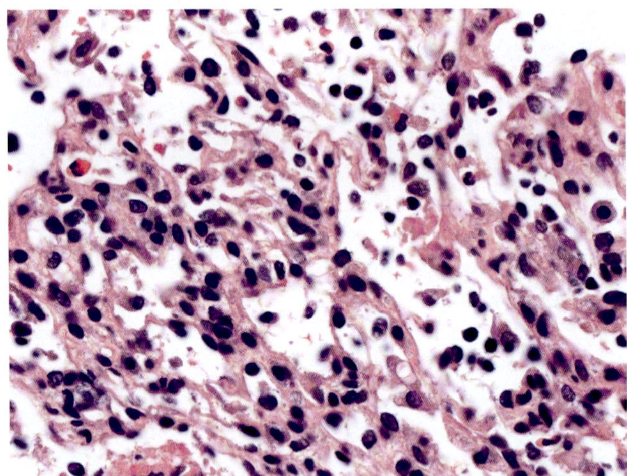

Figure 17.37. **Near miss case 1, anastomosing hemangioma.** This case was initially interpreted as an angiosarcoma. Note the lack of cytological atypia.

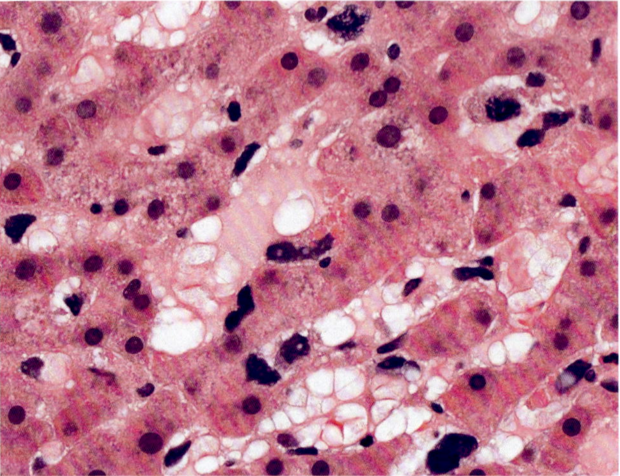

Figure 17.38. **Near miss case 2, angiosarcoma, sinusoidal growth pattern.** This angiosarcoma did not form a mass lesion, but instead showed diffuse sinusoidal growth. There is marked cytological atypia within the endothelial cells. One of the endothelial cells in the center of the image shows distinctive small eosinophilic globules.

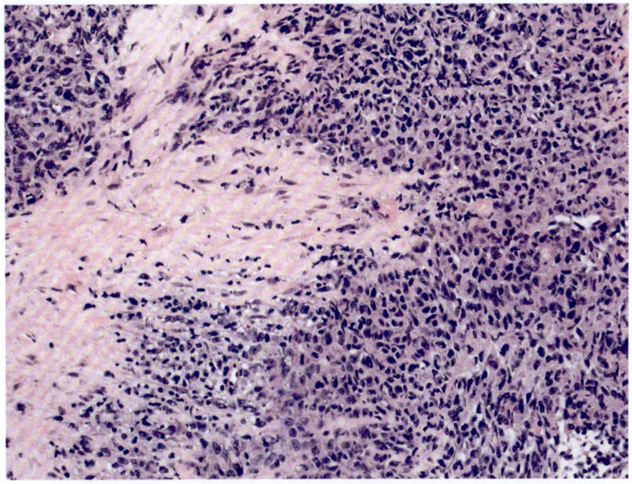

Figure 17.39. Near miss case 3, angiosarcoma, epithelioid growth pattern. The angiosarcoma has a solid growth pattern mimicking a poorly differentiated carcinoma or a lymphoma.

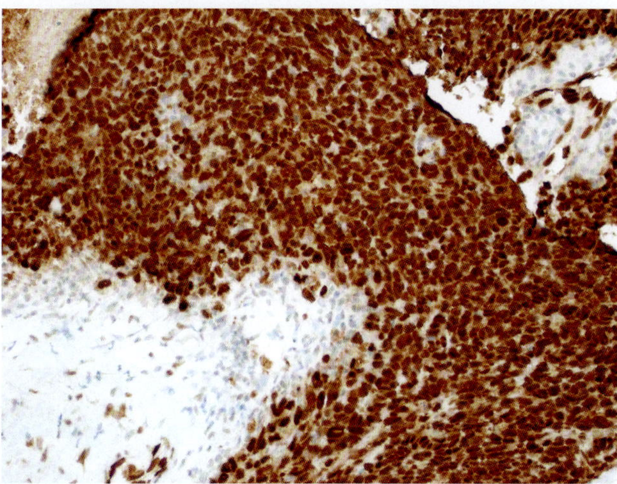

Figure 17.40. Near miss case 3, angiosarcoma, epithelioid growth pattern. An immunostain for ERG is strongly positive.

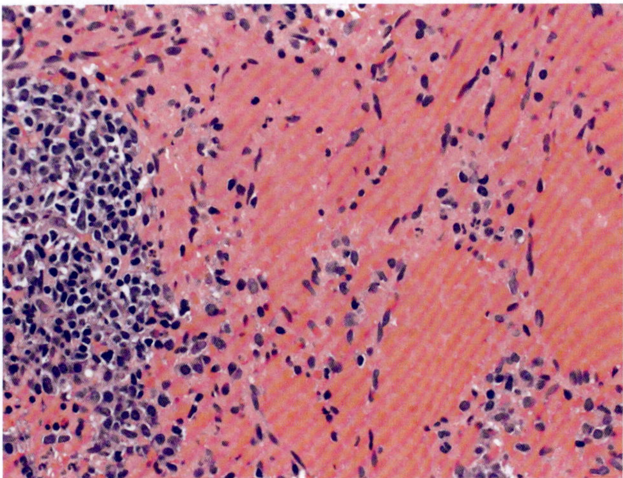

Figure 17.41. Near miss case 4, ectopic spleen. This case at first was thought to be a strange-looking hemangioma.

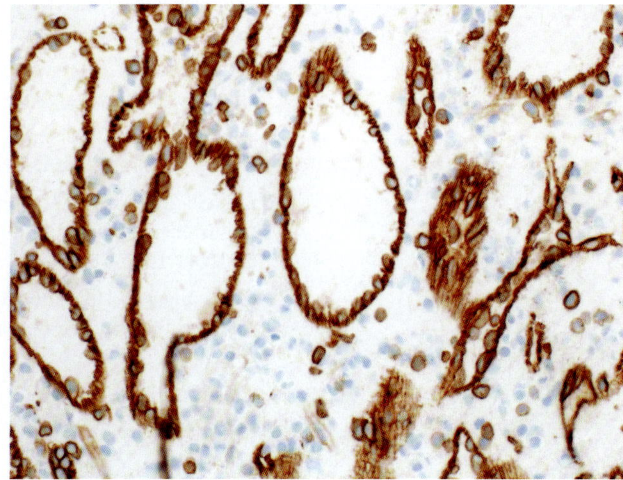

Figure 17.42. Near miss case 4, ectopic spleen. A CD8 immunostain highlights the endothelial cells.

References

1. Garg I, Graham RP, VanBuren WM, Goenka AH, Torbenson MS, Venkatesh SK. Hepatic segmental atrophy and nodular elastosis: imaging features. *Abdom Radiol (NY)*. 2017;42:2447-2453.
2. Singhi AD, Maklouf HR, Mehrotra AK, et al. Segmental atrophy of the liver: a distinctive pseudotumor of the liver with variable histologic appearances. *Am J Surg Pathol*. 2011;35:364-371.
3. Ishizaki Y, Mizuno T, Hara K, Kawasaki S. Advanced segmental atrophy of the liver with marked elastosis. *Surgery*. 2015;157:826-827.
4. Tang L, Lai EC, Cong WM, et al. Inflammatory myofibroblastic tumor of the liver: a cohort study. *World J Surg*. 2010;34:309-313.
5. Tsou YK, Lin CJ, Liu NJ, Lin CC, Lin CH, Lin SM. Inflammatory pseudotumor of the liver: report of eight cases, including three unusual cases, and a literature review. *J Gastroenterol Hepatol*. 2007;22:2143-2147.
6. Yang X, Zhu J, Biskup E, Cai F, Li A. Inflammatory pseudotumors of the liver: experience of 114 cases. *Tumour Biol*. 2015;36:5143-5148.
7. Park JY, Choi MS, Lim YS, et al. Clinical features, image findings, and prognosis of inflammatory pseudotumor of the liver: a multicenter experience of 45 cases. *Gut Liver*. 2014;8:58-63.
8. Mulki R, Garg S, Manatsathit W, Miick R. IgG4-related inflammatory pseudotumour mimicking a hepatic abscess impending rupture. *BMJ Case Rep*. 2015;2015.

9. Hastir D, Verset L, Lucidi V, Demetter P. IgG4 positive lymphoplasmacytic inflammatory pseudotumour mimicking hepatocellular carcinoma. *Liver Int.* 2014;34:961.
10. DeRoche TC, Huber AR. The great imitator: syphilis presenting as an inflammatory pseudotumor of liver. *Int J Surg Pathol.* 2017:1066896917745665.
11. Hagen CE, Kamionek M, McKinsey DS, Misdraji J. Syphilis presenting as inflammatory tumors of the liver in HIV-positive homosexual men. *Am J Surg Pathol.* 2014;38:1636-1643.
12. Chan JK, Cheuk W, Shimizu M. Anaplastic lymphoma kinase expression in inflammatory pseudotumors. *Am J Surg Pathol.* 2001;25:761-768.
13. Granados R, Aramburu JA, Rodriguez JM, Nieto MA. Cytopathology of a primary follicular dendritic cell sarcoma of the liver of the inflammatory pseudotumor-like type. *Diagn Cytopathol.* 2008;36:42-46.
14. Kojima M, Nakamura S, Ohno Y, Sugihara S, Sakata N, Masawa N. Hepatic angiomyolipoma resembling an inflammatory pseudotumor of the liver. A case report. *Pathol Res Pract.* 2004;200:713-716.
15. Argani P, Facchetti F, Inghirami G, Rosai J. Lymphocyte-rich well-differentiated liposarcoma: report of nine cases. *Am J Surg Pathol.* 1997;21:884-895.
16. Kim GE, Thung SN, Tsui WM, Ferrell LD. Hepatic cavernous hemangioma: underrecognized associated histologic features. *Liver Int.* 2006;26:334-338.
17. Jhaveri KS, Vlachou PA, Guindi M, et al. Association of hepatic hemangiomatosis with giant cavernous hemangioma in the adult population: prevalence, imaging appearance, and relevance. *Am J Roentgenol.* 2011;196:809-815.
18. Abaalkhail F, Castonguay M, Driman DK, Parfitt J, Marotta P. Lobular capillary hemangioma of the liver. *Hepatobiliary Pancreat Dis Int.* 2009;8:323-325.
19. Jhuang JY, Lin LW, Hsieh MS. Adult capillary hemangioma of the liver: case report and literature review. *Kaohsiung J Med Sci.* 2011;27:344-347.
20. O'Neill AC, Craig JW, Silverman SG, Alencar RO. Anastomosing hemangiomas: locations of occurrence, imaging features, and diagnosis with percutaneous biopsy. *Abdom Radiol (NY).* 2016;41:1325-1332.
21. Lin J, Bigge J, Ulbright TM, Montgomery E. Anastomosing hemangioma of the liver and gastrointestinal tract: an unusual variant histologically mimicking angiosarcoma. *Am J Surg Pathol.* 2013;37:1761-1765.
22. Makhlouf HR, Ishak KG, Goodman ZD. Epithelioid hemangioendothelioma of the liver: a clinicopathologic study of 137 cases. *Cancer.* 1999;85:562-582.
23. Miettinen M, Wang ZF, Paetau A, et al. ERG transcription factor as an immunohistochemical marker for vascular endothelial tumors and prostatic carcinoma. *Am J Surg Pathol.* 2011;35:432-441.
24. Flucke U, Vogels RJ, de Saint Aubain Somerhausen N, et al. Epithelioid hemangioendothelioma: clinicopathologic, immunhistochemical, and molecular genetic analysis of 39 cases. *Diagn Pathol.* 2014;9:131.
25. Weinreb I, Cunningham KS, Perez-Ordonez B, Hwang DM. CD10 is expressed in most epithelioid hemangioendotheliomas: a potential diagnostic pitfall. *Arch Pathol Lab Med.* 2009;133:1965-1968.
26. Errani C, Zhang L, Sung YS, et al. A novel WWTR1-CAMTA1 gene fusion is a consistent abnormality in epithelioid hemangioendothelioma of different anatomic sites. *Genes Chromosomes Cancer.* 2011;50:644-653.
27. Antonescu CR, Le Loarer F, Mosquera JM, et al. Novel YAP1-TFE3 fusion defines a distinct subset of epithelioid hemangioendothelioma. *Genes Chromosomes Cancer.* 2013;52:775-784.
28. Kuo FY, Huang HY, Chen CL, Eng HL, Huang CC. TFE3-rearranged hepatic epithelioid hemangioendothelioma-a case report with immunohistochemical and molecular study. *APMIS.* 2017;125:849-853.
29. Lee SJ, Yang WI, Chung WS, Kim SK. Epithelioid hemangioendotheliomas with TFE3 gene translocations are compossible with CAMTA1 gene rearrangements. *Oncotarget.* 2016;7:7480-7488.
30. Yaskiv O, Rubin BP, He H, Falzarano S, Magi-Galluzzi C, Zhou M. ERG protein expression in human tumors detected with a rabbit monoclonal antibody. *Am J Clin Pathol.* 2012;138:803-810.
31. Huang NC, Kuo YC, Chiang JC, et al. Hepatic angiosarcoma may have fair survival nowadays. *Medicine (Baltimore).* 2015;94:e816.
32. Falk H, Thomas LB, Popper H, Ishak KG. Hepatic angiosarcoma associated with androgenic-anabolic steroids. *Lancet.* 1979;2:1120-1123.

33. Guido M, Sarcognato S, Pelletti G, Fassan M, Murer B, Snenghi R. Sequential development of hepatocellular carcinoma and liver angiosarcoma in a vinyl chloride-exposed worker. *Hum Pathol.* 2016;57:193-196.

34. Yamamoto Y, Chikawa J, Uegaki Y, Usuda N, Kuwahara Y, Fukumoto M. Histological type of Thorotrast-induced liver tumors associated with the translocation of deposited radionuclides. *Cancer Sci.* 2010;101:336-340.

35. Collins JJ, Jammer B, Sladeczek FM, Bodnar CM, Salomon SS. Surveillance for angiosarcoma of the liver among vinyl chloride workers. *J Occup Environ Med.* 2014;56:1207-1209.

36. Grassia KL, Peterman CM, Iacobas I, et al. Clinical case series of pediatric hepatic angiosarcoma. *Pediatr Blood Cancer.* 2017;64.

37. Meis-Kindblom JM, Kindblom LG. Angiosarcoma of soft tissue: a study of 80 cases. *Am J Surg Pathol.* 1998;22:683-697.

38. Tsui WM, Colombari R, Portmann BC, et al. Hepatic angiomyolipoma: a clinicopathologic study of 30 cases and delineation of unusual morphologic variants. *Am J Surg Pathol.* 1999;23:34-48.

39. Nonomura A, Minato H, Kurumaya H. Angiomyolipoma predominantly composed of smooth muscle cells: problems in histological diagnosis. *Histopathology.* 1998;33:20-27.

40. Nonomura A, Mizukami Y, Shimizu K, Kadoya M, Matsui O. Angiomyolipoma mimicking true lipoma of the liver: report of two cases. *Pathol Int.* 1996;46:221-227.

41. Nonomura A, Mizukami Y, Takayanagi N, et al. Immunohistochemical study of hepatic angiomyolipoma. *Pathol Int.* 1996;46:24-32.

42. Makhlouf HR, Remotti HE, Ishak KG. Expression of KIT (CD117) in angiomyolipoma. *Am J Surg Pathol.* 2002;26:493-497.

43. Jimbo N, Nishigami T, Noguchi M, et al. Hepatic angiomyolipomas may overexpress TFE3, but have no relevant genetic alterations. *Hum Pathol.* 2017;61:41-48.

44. Parfitt JR, Bella AJ, Izawa JI, Wehrli BM. Malignant neoplasm of perivascular epithelioid cells of the liver. *Arch Pathol Lab Med.* 2006;130:1219-1222.

45. Dalle I, Sciot R, de Vos R, et al. Malignant angiomyolipoma of the liver: a hitherto unreported variant. *Histopathology.* 2000;36:443-450.

46. Nguyen TT, Gorman B, Shields D, Goodman Z. Malignant hepatic angiomyolipoma: report of a case and review of literature. *Am J Surg Pathol.* 2008;32:793-798.

47. Deng YF, Lin Q, Zhang SH, Ling YM, He JK, Chen XF. Malignant angiomyolipoma in the liver: a case report with pathological and molecular analysis. *Pathol Res Pract.* 2008;204:911-918.

48. Moran CA, Ishak KG, Goodman ZD. Solitary fibrous tumor of the liver: a clinicopathologic and immunohistochemical study of nine cases. *Ann Diagn Pathol.* 1998;2:19-24.

49. Launois B, Jamieson GG. The importance of Glisson's capsule and its sheaths in the intrahepatic approach to resection of the liver. *Surg Gynecol Obstet.* 1992;174:7-10.

50. Robinson DR, Wu YM, Kalyana-Sundaram S, et al. Identification of recurrent NAB2-STAT6 gene fusions in solitary fibrous tumor by integrative sequencing. *Nat Genet.* 2013;45:180-185.

51. Fama F, Le Bouc Y, Barrande G, et al. Solitary fibrous tumour of the liver with IGF-II-related hypoglycaemia. A case report. *Langenbecks Arch Surg.* 2008;393:611-616.

52. Chan G, Horton PJ, Thyssen S, et al. Malignant transformation of a solitary fibrous tumor of the liver and intractable hypoglycemia. *J Hepatobiliary Pancreat Surg.* 2007;14:595-599.

53. Trabelsi A, Hammedi F, Rammeh S, et al. Solitary fibrous tumor with giant multinucleated cells in the retroperitoneum - a case report. *N Am J Med Sci.* 2009;1:285-287.

54. Silvanto A, Karanjia ND, Bagwan IN. Primary hepatic solitary fibrous tumor with histologically benign and malignant areas. *Hepatobiliary Pancreat Dis Int.* 2015;14:665-668.

SELF-ASSESSMENT QUESTIONS

CHAPTER 1. BASIC PATTERNS IN LIVER PATHOLOGY

1-1. **What is acute-on-chronic hepatitis?**

a. A case of chronic hepatitis that has a superimposed acute injury
b. A case of acute hepatitis that transforms to chronic hepatitis
c. A case where the biopsy findings could be either acute hepatitis or chronic hepatitis
d. A case of chronic hepatitis that is undergoing acute fibrosis regression

1-2. **What is the best classification for a biopsy that shows mild lobular inflammation, mild portal inflammation, and no fibrosis?**

a. Acute hepatitis pattern of injury
b. Hepatitic pattern of injury
c. Chronic hepatitis pattern of injury
d. Paucisteatosis variant of steatohepatitis

1-3. **Which finding is NOT part of the injury pattern seen with chronic cholestatic liver disease?**

a. Ductopenia
b. Cholate stasis
c. Kupffer cell hyperplasia
d. Stellate cell hyperplasia

1-4. **Which finding is NOT part of the injury pattern seen with vascular outflow disease?**

a. Zone 3 sinusoidal congestion
b. Peliosis hepatis
c. Patchy bile ductular proliferation
d. Zone 3 hepatocyte dropout

1-5. **What is the best term to describe fat in the liver when hepatocytes diffusely show numerous tiny cytoplasmic droplets?**

a. Tiny droplet steatosis
b. Tiny round droplet steatosis
c. Microvacuolar steatosis
d. Microvesicular steatosis

1-6. **Which of the following statements is true regarding patterns of liver injury?**

a. Bland lobular cholestasis is often associated with drug effects
b. Zone 3 necrosis is always from acetaminophen toxicity
c. The pathologist should distinguish alcohol from nonalcohol causes of steatohepatitis
d. Fibro-obliterative duct lesions are specific for primary sclerosing cholangitis

CHAPTER 2. ACUTE AND CHRONIC VIRAL HEPATITIS

2-1. **Which of the following viral infections can cause punched out necrosis?**

a. Adenovirus
b. Hepatitis B
c. Hepatitis E
d. Epstein–Barr virus

2-2. **Which of the following viruses does not lead to chronic hepatitis?**

a. Hepatitis A
b. Hepatitis B
c. Hepatitis C
d. Hepatitis E

2-3. **What pattern is most likely to lead to chronic hepatitis D?**

a. Hepatitis D and B coinfection
b. Hepatitis D superinfection on chronic hepatitis B
c. Hepatitis D superinfection on chronic hepatitis C
d. Hepatitis D and E coinfection

2-4. **Which virus leads to ground glass inclusions?**

a. Hepatitis A
b. Hepatitis B
c. Hepatitis C
d. Hepatitis E

2-5. **Which injury pattern would be typical for a case of chronic viral hepatitis C?**

a. Marked portal inflammation with marked lobular activity
b. No portal inflammation and moderate diffuse lobular activity
c. Minimal portal inflammation with moderate lobular cholestasis
d. Mild portal chronic inflammation with mild patchy lobular inflammation

2-6. **Which clinical pattern is NOT seen with hepatitis A infection?**

a. Acute hepatitis A
b. Relapsing hepatitis A
c. Prolonged cholestatic hepatitis A
d. Fibrosing cholestatic hepatitis A

CHAPTER 3. NONVIRAL INFECTIONS OF THE LIVER

3-1. **Which is correct about inflammatory pseudotumors of the liver?**

a. Most are associated with bacterial infections of the liver
b. Most are associated with sarcoidosis of the liver
c. Most are associated with lymphomas of the liver
d. Most are associated with viral infections of the liver

3-2. **Malaria infection is associated with which finding in the liver?**

a. Lipofuschin
b. Hemozoin pigment
c. Hemosiderosis
d. Periportal copper deposition

CHAPTER 4. GRANULOMAS AND GRANULOMATOUS DISEASE

4-1. **Which of the following does NOT have a strong association with epithelioid granulomas?**

a. Primary biliary cirrhosis
b. Sarcoidosis
c. Common variable immunodeficiency
d. Steatohepatitis

4-2. **Necrotizing granulomas are strongly suggest with which of these diseases?**

a. Infection
b. Drug-induced liver injury (DILI)
c. Sarcoidosis
d. Primary biliary cirrhosis

4-3. **Granulomas can be associated with which of the following types of infections?**

a. Bacterial
b. Fungal
c. Viral
d. Parasitic
e. All of the above

4-4. **Which statement is true about lipogranulomas?**

a. Lipogranulomas are major risk factors for fibrosis
b. Lipogranulomas are associated with Q fever
c. Lipogranulomas are associated with steatosis
d. Lipogranulomas are associated with Zika virus

4-5. **Which statement is true about granulomas?**

a. Granulomas are generally ignored if they are not necrotizing
b. Granulomas are classified by their size: microgranulomas, small granulomas, medium granulomas, large granulomas, and jumbo granulomas
c. Polarizing granulomas can help identify foreign material
d. Granulomas are typically associated with a generalized Kupffer cell hyperplasia

4-6. **Which of the following pairing is incorrect?**

a. Granulomas with fibrosis—sarcoidosis
b. Lipogranuloma—fatty liver disease
c. Necrotizing granuloma—infection
d. Porlaizable material in a granuloma—fungal infection

CHAPTER 5. DRUG-INDUCED LIVER INJURY

5-1. **Which of the following is NOT a cause of ground glass type inclusions in hepatocytes?**

a. Drug reactions, usually in immunosuppressed individuals who are taking multiple medications
b. Chronic hepatitis B
c. Glycogen storage disease type IV
d. Alpha-1-antitrypsin deficiency

5-2. **Which of these causes a bland necrosis pattern of injury?**

a. Acute alcoholic hepatitis
b. Acetaminophen toxicity
c. Estrogen-related drug reactions
d. Poorly controlled diabetes mellitus

5-3. **Eosinophils are commonly prominent in which of the following patterns of DILI?**

a. Idiosyncratic drug reactions
b. Injury from direct toxins
c. Hypersensitivity type drug reactions
d. All of the above

5-4. **Which of the following is NOT a critical part of classifying a biopsy as a likely drug reaction?**

a. A compatible history of drug exposure
b. Compatible histological findings
c. Reasonable exclusion of other likely causes by clinical and laboratory testing
d. Positive serology to confirm a drug reaction

5-5. **Which of the following patterns of injury could be consistent with a drug reaction?**

a. Macrovesicular steatosis
b. Microvesicular steatosis
c. Bland lobular necrosis
d. Moderate lobular hepatitis
e. All of the above

CHAPTER 6. FATTY LIVER DISEASE

6-1. **What is used to distinguish steatosis from steatohepatitis?**

a. Pericellular fibrosis
b. The amount of fat (grade of steatosis)
c. Clinical findings, because histological criteria are arbitrary
d. Evidence of active injury, primarily balloon cells and or lobular inflammation

6-2. **Which finding is used to distinguish alcohol from non–alcohol-related liver disease?**

a. Mallory hyaline
b. Balloon cells
c. Neutrophilic inflammation in the lobules
d. None of the above

6-3. **Which of the causes below can lead to microvesicular steatosis pattern of injury?**

a. Autoimmune hepatitis
b. Drugs that cause mitochondrial injury
c. Sarcoidosis
d. Metabolic syndrome

6-4. **Which patterns of fibrosis can be seen with fatty liver disease?**

a. Portal fibrosis
b. Pericellular fibrosis
c. Perivenular fibrosis
d. Bridging fibrosis
e. All of the above

6-5. **What are the most common causes of steatohepatitis?**

a. Metabolic syndrome, celiac disease, Crohn disease
b. Metabolic syndrome, alcohol, and drug effects
c. Alcohol, tobacco, and drug effects
d. Metabolic syndrome, Carney syndrome, and Turner syndrome

6-6. **Steatohepatitis is NOT a risk factor for which of the following diseases?**

a. Cirrhosis
b. Focal nodular hyperplasia
c. Hepatic adenoma, inflammatory type
d. Hepatocellular carcinoma

6-7. **What is the best way to approach a lipogranuloma?**

a. Rule out infection
b. Rule out drug effect
c. Rule out primary biliary cirrhosis
d. Incidental finding

6-8. **What pattern is diagnosed as steatohepatitis?**

a. Fat plus balloon cells plus lobular inflammation
b. Fat plus cholestasis plus pericellular fibrosis
c. Fat plus lipogranulomas plus pericellular fibrosis
d. Fat plus portal chronic inflammation plus glycogenated nuclei

6-9. **Which features are characteristic of a ballooned hepatocyte?**

a. Microvesicular steatosis
b. Megamitochondria
c. Enlarged hepatocyte with rarified cytoplasm
d. Glycogenated nuclei

6-10. **Which one of the following activities does the pathologist NOT do?**

a. Identify the liver injury pattern as fatty liver disease
b. Grade the amount of active injury
c. Stage the amount of fibrosis
d. Differentiate alcohol from non–alcohol-related steatohepatitis

6-11. **Which fibrosis patterns are NOT consistent with a diagnosis of fatty liver disease?**

a. No fibrosis
b. Portal fibrosis
c. Pericellular fibrosis
d. Bridging fibrosis
e. None of the above

CHAPTER 7. AUTOIMMUNE HEPATITIS

7-1. **Which of the following findings are diagnostic for autoimmune hepatitis?**

a. Positive anti–smooth muscle antibodies
b. Plasma cell–rich inflammation
c. Interface activity
d. All of the above
e. None of the above

7-2. **Which pattern of autoimmune hepatitis is most likely to show mild non-specific inflammation without plasma cell–rich hepatitis?**

a. Fulminant hepatitis
b. Autoimmune hepatitis–primary biliary cirrhosis overlap syndrome
c. Autoimmune hepatitis with established cirrhosis
d. Autoimmune hepatitis in men

7-3. **The findings on a liver biopsy suggest autoimmune hepatitis. Which findings would be useful in evaluating for a possible autoimmune hepatitis–primary biliary cirrhosis overlap syndrome?**

a. Serology positive for AMA
b. Alkaline phosphatase levels 2X the ULN
c. GGT levels 5X the ULN
d. Florid duct lesion
e. All of the above

7-4. **Which of these patterns would be typical for a case of untreated autoimmune hepatitis?**

a. Plasma cell–rich hepatitis with moderate activity
b. Bland lobular cholestasis with abundant hepatic rosetting
c. Patchy moderate chronic inflammation mostly limited to the portal tracts, with bile duct lymphocytosis and injury
d. Moderate Kupffer cell hyperplasia with hemophagocytosis.

7-5. **Which of the following pairs of findings is incorrect?**

a. Autoimmune hepatitis–primary biliary cirrhosis overlap syndrome; moderately active plasma cell–rich hepatitis plus a florid duct lesion
b. Autoimmune hepatitis in a 15-year-old; imaging of the biliary tree shows findings that suggest early stricturing
c. Autoimmune hepatitis type 2; positive antinuclear antibodies (ANA) and anti–smooth muscle antibodies (ASMA)
d. Fulminant autoimmune hepatitis; massive live necrosis

7-6. **Which of the following potential diagnostic pitfall pairings is incorrect?**

a. Bridging necrosis—finding that can mimic bridging fibrosis
b. Plasma cell–rich hepatitis—pattern that can be seen with more than just autoimmune hepatitis, including acute viral hepatitis, Wilson disease, and drug effects
c. Lobular hepatitis with zone 3 accentuation—pattern that can be seen with more than just autoimmune hepatitis, including viral hepatitis and drug effects
d. None of the above

CHAPTER 8. CHOLESTATIC AND BILIARY TRACT DISEASE

8-1. **Which of the following would fit well for a diagnosis of primary biliary cirrhosis?**

a. Positive pANCA
b. Positive AMA
c. Positive ANA and/or ASMA
d. All of the above

8-2. **Which of the following diseases can have prominent plasma cells?**

a. Autoimmune hepatitis
b. Primary biliary cirrhosis
c. Drug effects
d. IgG4 disease
e. All of the above

8-3. **Which pediatric liver disease is characterized by a biliary obstruction pattern?**

a. Neonatal giant cell hepatitis
b. Paucity of intrahepatic bile ducts
c. Biliary atresia
d. All of the above

8-4. **Which type of bile salt deficiency disease is often associated with extrahepatic findings, such as hearing loss, diarrhea, or pancreatic disease?**

a. ATP8B1 (FIC) deficiency
b. ABCB11 (BSEP) deficiency
c. ABCB4 (MDR3) deficiency
d. All of the above

8-5. **Which pattern fits best for a diagnosis of ascending cholangitis?**

a. The portal tracts show a brisk bile ductular proliferation, one that is associated with numerous neutrophils
b. The bile ducts show lymphocytosis and injury, with a vague granulomatous response
c. The bile ducts are dilated, show attenuated epithelium, and have abundant neutrophils in the lumen
d. The portal tracts show fibro-obliterative duct lesions
e. All of the above

8-6. **Which of the following pairings is not correct?**

a. Primary biliary cirrhosis—florid duct lesion
b. Primary sclerosing cholangitis—fibro-obliterative duct lesion
c. IgG4 disease—plasma cell–rich fibroinflammatory nodule with storiform fibrosis and phlebitis
d. Segmental cholengiectasia—dilated and inflamed medium- to large-sized bile duct restricted to one segment of the liver
e. None of the above—all are correct

CHAPTER 9. VASCULAR DISEASE

9-1. **Which benign pseudotumor can result from a vascular insult?**

a. Focal nodular hyperplasia
b. Segmental atrophy and nodular elastosis
c. Hepatocellular pseudotumor
d. All of the above

9-2. **A person has chronic Budd–Chiari disease. Which types of tumor are they NOT at risk for?**

a. Hemangioma
b. Focal nodular hyperplasia
c. Hepatic adenoma
d. Hepatocellular carcinoma
e. All of the above

9-3. **A biopsy shows marked zone 3 sinusoidal congestion and zone 3 hepatocyte atrophy. Which is the most likely diagnosis?**

a. Hepatic artery thrombosis
b. Portal vein thrombosis
c. Sinusoidal obtrusive disease
d. Budd–Chiari syndrome
e. Any of the above

9-4. **Peliosis hepatis is associated with which of the following conditions?**

a. Medication effects
b. Debilitating illnesses
c. Malnutrition
d. All of the above

9-5. **Which of the following vascular diseases can show bile ductular proliferation in the portal tracts that can mimic biliary obstruction?**

a. Hepatoportal sclerosis
b. Peliosis hepatis
c. Budd–Chiari syndrome
d. Any of the above

9-6. **A biopsy shows portal vein atrophy, focal portal vein herniation, and nodular regenerative hyperplasia. Which is the most likely diagnosis?**

a. Hepatoportal sclerosis
b. Peliosis hepatis
c. Budd–Chiari syndrome
d. Any of the above

CHAPTER 10. SYSTEMIC DISEASES INVOLVING THE LIVER

10-1. **Which finding is not part of the glycogenic hepatopathy pattern of injury?**

a. Hepatomegaly
b. Increased AST and ALT
c. Advanced fibrosis
d. Pale swollen hepatocytes on H&E

10-2. **Which pairing of injury pattern and risk factor is the least correct?**

a. Mild nonspecific hepatitis: CVID
b. Arterial hyalinosis: hypertension and diabetes mellitus
c. Kupffer cell hemophagocytosis: viral infection
d. Glycogenic hepatopathy: pituitary disease, usually hypopituitary disease

10-3. **Which disease and possible injury pattern(s) pairing is the least correct?**

a. Cystic fibrosis: biliary obstruction; fatty liver disease
b. Celiac disease: necrotizing granulomas; biliary obstruction changes
c. Diabetes mellitus type 1: glycogenic hepatopathy; fatty liver disease
d. Crohn disease: nonspecific mild hepatitis; primary sclerosing cholangitis; fatty liver disease

10-4. **Which patterns of injury can be associated with sepsis?**

a. Nonspecific inflammatory changes
b. Bland lobular cholestasis
c. Cholangiolar cholestasis
d. Macrovesicular steatosis
e. All of the above

10-5. **Which of these entities does NOT have a propensity to mimic sclerosing cholangitis?**

a. Hemophagocytic syndrome
b. Cystic fibrosis
c. Mast cell disease
d. Langerhans histiocytosis
e. None of the above (all can mimic sclerosing cholangitis)

CHAPTER 11. TRANSPLANT PATHOLOGY

11-1. **Which of the following is NOT part of the typical acute cellular rejection pattern of injury?**

a. Portal lymphocytic inflammation
b. Endothelialitis
c. Granulomatous lobular inflammation
d. Lymphocytic bile duct injury

11-2. **Which of the following is NOT an accepted variant of acute cellular rejection?**

a. Hepatitic variant of rejection
b. Plasma cell–rich variant of rejection
c. Central venulitis variant of rejection
d. Steatohepatitic variant of rejection

11-3. **Which of the following statement are true regarding graft versus host disease (GVHD) of the liver?**

a. Liver GVHD is associated with a disproportionate elevation in serum alkaline phosphatase levels
b. Liver GVHD is often associated with skin GVHD
c. Liver GVHD is often associated with gut GVHD
d. The hepatitic variant of liver GVHD is associated with donor lymphocyte infusion
e. All of the above

11-4. **Which infection is most strongly associated with PTLD?**

a. EBV
b. Zika virus
c. Adenovirus
d. Herpes simplex virus
e. Cytomegalovirus

11-5. **Which of the following bile duct changes are typical for chronic rejection?**

a. Bile duct duplication
b. Bile duct loss
c. Florid duct lesions
d. Fibro-obliterative duct lesions

CHAPTER 12. GENETIC DISEASES

12-1. **Which of the following genetic diseases is autosomal dominant?**

a. Wilson disease
b. Alpha-1-antitrypsin deficiency
c. Ferroportin disease
d. HFE hemochromatosis

12-2. **Which alpha-1-antitrypsin alleles are not associated with hepatic globules?**

a. M
b. S
c. Z
d. Mmalton

12-3. **Which set of alpha-1-antitrypsin alleles is most strongly associated with clinical disease?**

a. MM
b. MS
c. MZ
d. ZZ

12-4. **Which of these patterns of injury should lead to further testing for genetic causes of hemochromatosis?**

a. Mild diffuse hepatocellular iron in a noncirrhotic liver with no other evidence for liver disease
b. Moderate diffuse hepatocellular iron in a noncirrhotic liver with fatty liver disease
c. Marked diffuse iron in a cirrhotic liver with a history of chronic hepatis C
d. All of the above

12-5. **Which of the following mutations is most likely to cause clinical disease?**

a. C282Y
b. H63D
c. S65Y
d. S6Y
e. None of the above.

12-6. **Which of these factors can lead to a negative copper stain in a person with Wilson disease?**

a. Staining a section cut at 4 or 5 microns instead of 10 microns
b. Early Wilson disease when the copper is in the cytoplasm and not the lysosomes
c. Patchy distribution of copper and a small liver biopsy
d. All of the above

CHAPTER 13. PEDIATRIC BENIGN AND MALIGNANT TUMORS

13-1. **Which hepatoblastoma subtype has the best prognosis?**

a. Small cell undifferentiated
b. Embryonal
c. Pure fetal with low mitotic activity
d. Macrotrabecular

13-2. **Which of these findings is highly specific for hepatoblastoma?**

a. High serum AFP levels
b. Age at presentation less than 5 years
c. Alternating light and dark swatches of epithelial cells seen on low power
d. Beta-catenin nuclear accumulation
e. None of the above

13-3. **Which of the following tumors typically develop in livers with chronic underlying disease?**

a. Hepatoblastoma
b. Infantile hemangioma
c. Mesenchymal hamartoma
d. Rhabdomyosarcoma
e. Calcified nested stromal epithelial tumor
f. None of the above

13-4. **Which of the following can have both neoplastic epithelial and neoplastic mesenchymal components?**

a. Hepatoblastoma
b. Infantile hemangioma
c. Mesenchymal hamartoma
d. Rhabdomyosarcoma
e. Calcified nested stromal epithelial tumor
f. All of the above

13-5. **Which of the following statement is most true?**

a. Increased mitoses in an infantile hemangioma = bad prognosis
b. Calcified nested stromal epithelial tumors can be associated with Cushing syndrome
c. AFP or glypican 3 expression in the entrapped hepatocytes of a mesenchymal hamartoma = early malignant degeneration to hepatocellular carcinoma
d. Embryonal sarcomas commonly arise from dedifferentiated hepatoblastomas

13-6. **Which of the following thumb nail sketches is most accurate for a typical tumor?**

a. Hepatoblastoma: Mixed epithelial and mesenchymal components. Epithelial component with hepatic differentiation and marked nuclear pleomorphism including multinucleated giant cells
b. Infantile hemangioma: Mildly atypical endothelial cells with disuse sinusoidal infiltration without forming a mass
c. Mesenchymal hamartoma: Spindle cell proliferation in a loose myxoid background with entrapped bile ducts and islands of hepatocytes
d. Rhabdomyosarcoma: Solid tumor with discohesive epithelioid cells showing INI-1 loss
e. Calcified nested stromal epithelial tumor: poorly differentiated subtype of hepatoblastoma with calcifications and an association with the Cushing syndrome

CHAPTER 14. HEPATOCELLULAR TUMORS

14-1. **Which of the following hepatic adenomas have an increased risk for malignant transformation?**

a. Inflammatory hepatic adenoma with beta-catenin activation
b. Myxoid hepatic adenoma
c. Androgen-related hepatic adenoma
d. Pigmented hepatic adenoma
e. All of the above

14-2. **Which of the following hepatic adenomas can show extensive reticulin loss?**

a. Inflammatory hepatic adenoma with beta-catenin activation
b. Myxoid hepatic adenoma
c. Androgen-related hepatic adenoma
d. Pigmented hepatic adenoma
e. None of the above

14-3. **A biopsy of a hepatic nodule shows well-differentiated hepatocytes. Maplike staining by glutamine synthetase supports a diagnosis of which of these tumors?**

a. Focal fatty nodule
b. Focal nodular hyperplasia
c. Hepatocellular adenoma
d. Hepatocellular carcinoma
e. None of the above

14-4. **Which statement is true?**

a. Copper staining in a benign liver tumor = focal nodular hyperplasia
b. Sinusoidal dilation in a benign liver tumor = inflammatory hepatic adenoma
c. Aberrant (naked) lobular arteries = hepatic adenoma
d. Ductal structures in a benign liver tumor = focal nodular hyperplasia
e. None of the above

14-5. **Which clinical association is NOT true?**

a. Female gender: Focal nodular hyperplasia
b. Female gender: Inflammatory hepatic adenoma
c. Fatty liver disease: Focal nodular hyperplasia
d. Fatty liver disease: Inflammatory hepatic adenoma
e. None of the above (all are true)

14-6. **Which interpretation of the staining pattern is correct?**

a. Strong diffuse sinusoidal CD34: hepatocellular carcinoma
b. Reticulin loss: hepatocellular carcinoma
c. Strong and diffuse glutamine synthetase staining: hepatocellular carcinoma
d. Beta catenin nuclear accumulation: hepatocellular carcinoma

CHAPTER 15. MALIGNANT HEPATOCELLULAR TUMORS AND PRECURSORS

15-1. **Which of the following findings are necessary to diagnosis combined hepatocellular carcinoma–cholangiocarcinoma?**

a. Two distinct morphologies
b. Immunostains of hepatic differentiation in a tumor that looks like a cholangiocarcinoma on H&E
c. Immunostains of biliary differentiation in a tumor that looks like a hepatocellular carcinoma on H&E
d. Molecular studies showing mutations common to both cholangiocarcinoma and hepatocellular carcinoma.

15-2. **Which tumor has a gene fusion of DNAJB1 and PRKACA?**

a. Steatohepatitic variant of hepatocellular carcinoma
b. Hepatocellular carcinomas that arise from hepatic adenomas
c. Fibrolamellar carcinoma
d. Combined hepatocellular carcinoma-cholangiocarcinoma

15-3. Which subtype of hepatocellular carcinoma is associated with fatty liver in the background liver?

a. Steatohepatitic variant of hepatocellular carcinoma
b. Clear cell variant of hepatocellular carcinoma
c. Lymphocyte rich hepatocellular carcinoma
d. Combined hepatocellular carcinoma–cholangiocarcinoma

15-4. Which subtype of hepatocellular carcinoma is associated with alternative lengthening of telomeres (ALT)?

a. Fibrolamellar carcinoma
b. Clear cell variant of hepatocellular carcinoma
c. Chromophobe variant of hepatocellular carcinoma
d. Combined hepatocellular carcinoma–cholangiocarcinoma

15-5. Which statement is true about hepatocellular carcinoma grade?

a. Tumor grade is prognostic for hepatocellular carcinomas in noncirrhotic livers
b. Tumor grade is prognostic for hepatocellular carcinomas in cirrhotic livers
c. Tumor grade is prognostic for hepatocellular carcinomas after resection of the tumor
d. Tumor grade is prognostic for hepatocellular carcinomas after liver transplantation
e. All of the above

CHAPTER 16. BILIARY TUMORS

16-1. What is different between biliary epithelial neoplasm (BilIN) and an intraductal papillary biliary neoplasm (IPBN)?

a. BilIN is microscopic and IPBN is not
b. IPBN is a precursor to cholangiocarcinoma, while BilIN is not
c. BilIN is seen mostly in noncirrhotic livers, while IPBN is primarily found in cirrhotic livers
d. Nothing, they are synonyms

16-2. Which of these lesions is composed of small glands with inconspicuous to absent lumens, embedded in a dense fibrous background?

a. Von Meyenburg Complex
b. Bile duct adenoma
c. Biliary adenofibroma
d. Intraductal papillary biliary neoplasm

16-3. The following stains have been matched up to their potential diagnostic pitfalls. Which is most correct?

a. CK20: can be positive in hilar cholangiocarcinomas, mimicking colon adenocarcinoma
b. TTF1: can be positive in hilar and extrahepatic cholangiocarcinomas, mimicking lung adenocarcinoma
c. Glypican 3: can be positive in 5% of cholangiocarcinomas, mimicking hepatocellular carcinoma
d. HepPar1: can be positive in 10% of cholangiocarcinomas, mimicking hepatocellular carcinoma
e. All of the above

16-4. **Which of the following tumors are associated with EBV?**

a. Cholangiocarcinoma with a lymphoepithelioma morphology
b. Adenofibroma with malignant transformation
c. Clear cell variant of cholangiocarcinoma
d. BilIN, when it occurs in noncirrhotic livers

16-5. **Which of the following has a high risk for malignant transformation?**

a. Von Meyenburg Complex
b. Bile duct adenoma
c. Biliary adenofibroma
d. None of above (risk is negligible for all of them)

CHAPTER 17. ADULT BENIGN AND MALIGNANT MESENCHYMAL TUMORS

11-1. **Which of the following tumors is STAT 6 positive on immunostain?**

a. Angiomyolipoma
b. Solitary fibrous tumor
c. Angiosarcoma
d. All of the above

17-2. **Which of the following stains are routinely positive in angiomyolipomas?**

a. HMB45
b. MELA
c. CKIT
d. CD68
e. All of the above

17-3. **Which of the following tumors is frequently positive for keratins?**

a. Solitary fibrous tumor
b. Angiomyolipoma
c. Hemangioma
d. Epithelioid hemangioma
e. None of the above

17-4. **Which of the following is the most common type of hemangioma in the liver?**

a. Anastomosing hemangioma
b. Capillary hemangioma
c. Cavernous hemangioma
d. Infantile hemangioma
e. Epithelioid hemangioendothelioma

17-5. **Which of the following morphological growth patterns can be seen with angiosarcoma?**

a. Spindle cell, mass forming
b. Epithelioid, mass forming
c. Sinusoidal growth, not mass forming
d. Peliotic growth pattern, not mass forming
e. All of the above

SELF-ASSESSMENT ANSWERS

CHAPTER 1. BASIC PATTERNS IN LIVER PATHOLOGY

1-1. Answer – a. Acute-on-chronic hepatitis indicates that a case of chronic hepatitis either has a new superimposed injury, for example, steatohepatitis with a superimposed biliary obstruction, or a case with a chronic underlying disease now has a flare of disease activity, which is most commonly seen with autoimmune hepatitis or chronic hepatitis B.

1-2. Answer – b. Acute and chronic hepatitis is largely defined by the duration of elevated liver enzymes (more than 6 months is chronic hepatitis). Histological findings can be informative on this point when there is definite fibrosis (indicates a chronic hepatitis) or when there is diffuse moderate or marked lobular inflammation (essentially always indicates either acute hepatitis or acute on chronic hepatitis).

1-3. Answer – d. Stellate cell hyperplasia is not part of the chronic cholestatic liver disease pattern, although sometimes Kupffer cell hyperplasia can be mistaken for stellate cell hyperplasia.

1-4. Answer – b. Peliosis hepatis is a vascular pattern of disease but is most often associated with debilitating chronic illness, chronic infection, or drug effects.

1-5. Answer – d. The correct term for this finding is microvesicular steatosis. The cytoplasmic changes are sometimes described as showing numerous tiny vacuoles, but the term *microvacuolar steatosis* is not used.

1-6. Answer – a. The bland lobular cholestasis pattern of injury most commonly results from a drug effect. There are many other causes of zone 3 necrosis beyond acetaminophen toxicity. Clinical findings, not the pathologist, distinguish alcohol from nonalcohol causes of steatohepatitis. Although some histological findings can suggest alcohol, the final determination is clinical. Most biopsies with fibro-obliterative duct lesions are in the setting of primary sclerosing cholangitis, but there are other causes.

CHAPTER 2. ACUTE AND CHRONIC VIRAL HEPATITIS

2-1. Answer – a. The punched out necrosis pattern is associated with adenoviral infection and herpes simplex viral infection but not the others.

2-2. Answer – a. Hepatitis A does not lead to chronic hepatitis, while all of the others can. Hepatitis E causes chronic hepatitis in immunosuppressed individuals.

2-3. Answer – b. Hepatitis D requires active infection with hepatitis B. Hepatitis D superinfection on chronic hepatitis B has a much higher risk of hepatitis D infection compared with Hepatitis D and B coinfection.

2-4. Answer – b. Chronic hepatitis B can lead to ground glass inclusions in hepatocytes. This finding is present only in livers with long-standing chronic hepatitis B infection, but even in this setting, they will not be evident in all biopsies.

2-5. Answer – d. The lobular inflammation in chronic viral hepatitis C is generally mild to patchy moderate in intensity, while the portal inflammation ranges from mild to moderate in most cases. None of the other patterns would be typical for chronic hepatitis C.

2-6. Answer – d. Hepatitis A can be acute or can show several other rare patterns. In relapsing hepatitis A, there is an initial clinical and biochemical recovery, followed weeks later by a hepatitis relapse, one that is associated with a spike in viral replication. In prolonged cholestatic hepatitis A, there is an extended clinical course characterized by cholestasis that lasts up to several months, despite viral clearance. Fibrosing cholestatic hepatitis occurs with hepatitis B and C, but not hepatitis A.

CHAPTER 3. NONVIRAL INFECTIONS OF THE LIVER

3-1. Answer – a. Most inflammatory pseudotumors of the liver are associated with bacterial infections of the liver and in most cases appear to represent healing abscesses.

3-2. Answer – b. Malaria infection can lead to hemozoin pigment, a black granular pigment seen in macrophages.

CHAPTER 4. GRANULOMAS AND GRANULOMATOUS DISEASE

4-1. Answer – d. Steatosis and steatohepatitis are strongly associated with lipogranulomas but not with epithelioid granulomas. Occasionally, incidental epithelioid granulomas can be found, but they are not a typical part of the disease pattern of fatty liver disease.

4-2. Answer – a. Necrotizing granulomas are almost always infectious in origin. All of the other diseases can have granulomas, but they should not be necrotizing. The so called necrotizing granulomas sometimes reported with sarcoidosis are, for the most part, large granulomas with central hyalinization, but without the typical dirty necrosis of infectious granulomas.

4-3. Answer – e. Granulomas can be seen with all major categories of infections including bacterial, fungal, viral, and parasitic infections.

4-4. Answer – c. Lipogranulomas are often associated with focal fibrosis but they are not a risk factor for generalized liver fibrosis. Lipogranulomas are associated with fatty liver disease but not with Q fever or Zika virus.

4-5. Answer – c. Sometimes foreign material in granulomas can be seen on H&E but other times only with polarization. Granulomas are frequently idiopathic, but they are not ignored. Microgranulomas are distinguished from true granulomas, but there is no other useful classification of granulomas based on their size. Granulomas can be associated with a generalized Kupffer cell hyperplasia in some cases, especially infection, but most granulomas in the liver are not associated with Kupffer cell hyperplasia.

4-6. Answer – d. Fungal infections can be epithelioid or necrotizing. The fungal organisms are identified with special stains, such as GMS, but not by polarization.

CHAPTER 5. DRUG-INDUCED LIVER INJURY

5-1. Answer – d. Ground glass type inclusions can be seen in drug reactions (usually in immunosuppressed individuals who are taking multiple medications), chronic hepatitis B, and glycogen storage disease type IV. The inclusions all look similar on H&E, but the clinical situations are distinct. In contrast to the large, gray, single inclusions in the hepatocyte cytoplasm that is seen with ground glass type inclusions, the hepatocyte globules in alpha-1-antitrypsin deficiency are smaller, often with numerous inclusions per cell, and are pink.

5-2. Answer – b. Acetaminophen toxicity leads to a bland pattern of necrosis, where the necrosis is not associated with significant inflammation. The necrosis first begins in zone 3 but can be panacinar in more severe cases. Acute alcoholic hepatitis shows a steatohepatitis pattern of injury, often with an additional component of cholestasis. Estrogen-related drug reactions can show a number of different patterns, including sinusoidal dilation and or peliosis, but is not associated with liver necrosis. Poorly controlled diabetes mellitus can be associated with glycogenic hepatopathy but does not show hepatocyte necrosis.

5-3. Answer – c. Eosinophils are commonly prominent in hypersensitivity type drug reactions but are usually inconspicuous to absent in idiosyncratic drug reactions or injury from direct toxins.

5-4. Answer – d. There are no serological tests that can be used to confirm a drug reaction. Serology is useful to rule out other potential causes such as autoimmune hepatitis and infection. All of the other listed items are critical steps in evaluating a liver biopsy for a possible drug reaction.

5-5. Answer – e. Drug reactions can have a wide range of patterns of injury. In fact, almost all patterns of injury have been associated with drug reactions.

CHAPTER 6. FATTY LIVER DISEASE

6-1. Answer – d. Steatosis and steatohepatitis are distinguished by the presence of active injury, which is defined primarily by the presence of balloon cells and/or lobular inflammation. Like any histological finding, reproducibility is not perfect, but the basic approach works well for clinical care. Pericellular fibrosis is not used to make the diagnosis of steatohepatitis and can be present in either steatosis or steatohepatitis. In general, at least 5% macrovesicular steatosis is needed before making a diagnosis of fatty liver disease, but the amount of fat does not otherwise influence the decision.

6-2. Answer – d. Clinical findings and not histology are used to distinguish alcohol from non–alcohol-related liver disease. It is generally true that cases with marked ballooning, abundant Mallory hyaline, and brisk lobular neutrophilic inflammation are more likely to be alcohol related than to be associated with the metabolic syndrome, but pathologists do not make an etiological assessment, as there is too much overlap between the pathology patterns for these diseases.

6-3. Answer – b. Drugs that cause mitochondrial injury can lead to a microvesicular steatosis pattern of injury. None of the other listed diseases are associated with microvesicular steatosis.

6-4. Answer – e. All of the above patterns of fibrosis can be seen with fatty liver disease.

6-5. Answer – b. There are many potential causes of fatty liver disease, but the most common are the metabolic syndrome, alcohol, and drug effects.

6-6. Answer – b. Steatohepatitis is an important risk factor for cirrhosis. Livers with steatohepatitis also have an increased risk for hepatocellular carcinoma, especially if the liver is cirrhotic. Fatty liver disease is also a known risk factor for inflammatory hepatic adenomas but not for focal nodular hyperplasia.

6-7. Answer – d. Lipogranulomas are incidental findings seen mostly with fatty liver disease and do not require any additional studies.

6-8. Answer – a. Steatohepatitis is defined as fat plus active injury, with active injury usually defined as some combination of balloon cells and/or lobular inflammation. Pericellular fibrosis is part of determining the fibrosis stage but is not used to determine whether there is steatosis or steatohepatitis. Lipogranulomas and glycogenated nuclei are incidental findings. Cholestasis is not part of the usual pattern of steatohepatitis and suggests an additional disease process, with one exception being acute alcoholic hepatitis, which can have a component of cholestasis.

6-9. Answer – c. Ballooned hepatocytes are enlarged and noticeably bigger than adjacent hepatocytes at low power. They have rarified cytoplasm with thin wisps of pink cytoplasm. Mallory hyaline can also be present.

6-10. Answer – d. Pathologists determine the pattern of injury, grade the amount of active injury, and stage the fibrosis. Although there can be some features that favor alcoholic hepatitis (marked ballooning, striking Mallory hyaline, abundant lobular neutrophilic inflammation, marked and diffuse pericellular fibrosis), the final determination of alcohol abuse is made by clinical findings.

6-11. Answer – e. All of these patterns can be seen with fatty liver disease. Fatty liver disease can be associated with pericellular fibrosis alone, with portal fibrosis alone, or with a combination of portal and pericellular fibrosis. Bridging fibrosis and cirrhosis can also be found.

CHAPTER 7. AUTOIMMUNE HEPATITIS

7-1. Answer – e. Histological findings compatible with autoimmune hepatitis include plasma cell–rich inflammation, interface activity, and lobular hepatitis, but none of these are diagnostic either in isolation or even when all are present. Instead, autoimmune hepatitis is diagnosed when there are compatible laboratory and histological findings and other causes have been excluded, such as drug effect and viral hepatitis.

7-2. Answer – c. The inflammation in autoimmune hepatitis can "burn out" when the liver becomes cirrhotic, leaving behind only mild nonspecific inflammation. Plasma cells can be less prominent in cases of autoimmune hepatitis in men, but plasma cells are still commonly enriched, and the overall degree of active inflammation is similar to that seen in women. The inflammation in fulminant hepatitis is never mild. Autoimmune hepatitis–primary biliary cirrhosis overlap syndrome shows features of both diseases, not a mild nonspecific pattern of inflammation.

7-3. Answer – e. All of these findings would be useful in considering a possible diagnosis of autoimmune hepatitis–primary biliary cirrhosis overlap syndrome.

7-4. Answer – a. The pattern of plasma cell–rich hepatitis with moderate lobular activity would be most consistent with autoimmune hepatitis. Bland lobular cholestasis with abundant hepatic rosetting would suggest a drug reaction. Patchy moderate chronic inflammation limited to the portal tracts, with bile duct lymphocytosis and injury, would suggest primary biliary cirrhosis. Moderate Kupffer cell hyperplasia with hemophagocytosis would suggest a hemophagocytic syndrome.

7-5. Answer – c. Type 1 autoimmune hepatitis shows positivity for ANA and/or ASMA. Type 2 autoimmune hepatitis shows positivity for liver kidney microsomal antibodies (LKM-1) and/or liver cytosol antibodies (LC-1).

7-6. Answer – d. All of these are important diagnostic pitfalls. Both of the patterns of plasma cell–rich hepatitis and of lobular hepatitis with zone 3 accentuation can be seen with autoimmune hepatitis, but they both have a wider differential that includes viral infection, drug effect, and Wilson disease. Bridging necrosis is an important mimic of bridging fibrosis.

CHAPTER 8. CHOLESTATIC AND BILIARY TRACT DISEASE

8-1. Answer – b. Primary biliary cirrhosis is strongly associated with a positive AMA. Autoimmune hepatitis is associated with positive ANA and/or ASMA, while primary sclerosing cholangitis is (weakly) associated with pANCA.

8-2. Answer – e. All of these conditions can have prominent plasma cells. Plasma cell–rich inflammation is an important histological observation, but the finding needs to be incorporated with other histological, laboratory, and clinical findings to arrive at the correct diagnosis.

8-3. Answer – c. The atretic portion of the biliary tree leads to a biliary obstruction pattern of injury in cases of biliary atresia.

8-4. Answer – a. The protein in ATP8B1 (FIC) deficiency is important for cellular function in organs outside the liver and mutations are also associated with hearing loss, diarrhea, and pancreatic disease in some patients.

8-5. Answer – c. The classic pattern for ascending cholangitis is that of dilated bile ducts that show attenuated epithelium and have abundant neutrophils in the lumen. Fibro-obliterative duct lesions are associated with chronic biliary obstruction and are seen most commonly in primary sclerosing cholangitis. Biliary obstruction typically shows a brisk bile ductular proliferation that is associated with neutrophils. A finding of bile duct lymphocytosis and injury with a vague granulomatous response would suggest primary biliary cirrhosis.

8-6. Answer – e. All of the pairings are correct.

CHAPTER 9. VASCULAR DISEASE

9-1. Answer – d. All of these three pseudotumors arise as a response to vascular injury. Focal nodular hyperplasia results from vascular shunting, while both hepatocellular pseudotumors and segmental atrophy and nodular elastosis are associated with vascular thrombi.

9-2. Answer – a. Chronic vascular outflow disease of the liver has an increased risk for focal nodular hyperplasias, hepatic adenomas, and hepatocellular carcinomas, but not for hemangiomas.

9-3. Answer – d. The pattern of marked zone 3 sinusoidal congestion and zone 3 hepatocyte atrophy is most consistent with vascular outflow disease such as Budd–Chiari syndrome.

9-4. Answer – d. Peliosis hepatis is defined by cyst-like spaces filled with blood in the hepatic lobules. The mechanism is unknown, but over the years several broad patterns have emerged, where peliosis hepatis is associated with debilitating illnesses including chronic infections, cancer, malnutrition, and medications effect.

9-5. Answer – c. Vascular outflow diseases from many different causes, including Budd–Chiari syndrome, can be associated with bile ductular proliferation in the portal tracts, which can closely mimic downstream biliary tract obstruction.

9-6. Answer – a. Portal vein atrophy, focal portal vein herniation, and nodular regenerative hyperplasia are all features of hepatoportal sclerosis. Peliosis hepatis is defined by cyst-like spaces filled with blood in the hepatic lobules. Budd–Chiari syndrome leads to vascular outflow disease, with zone 3 sinusoidal congestion, hepatic plate atrophy, and often hepatocyte dropout.

CHAPTER 10. SYSTEMIC DISEASES INVOLVING THE LIVER

10-1. Answer – c. Advanced fibrosis is not part of the glycogenic hepatopathy pattern of injury and, if present, indicates an additional disease process or that the diagnosis of glycogenic hepatopathy is incorrect.

10-2. Answer – d. Glycogenic hepatopathy is associated most strongly with type 1 diabetes mellitus and is not associated with pituitary disease.

10-3. Answer – b. The findings in celiac disease are typically that of a mild nonspecific hepatitis or fatty liver disease. Patients with celiac disease also have an increased risk for primary biliary cirrhosis and for autoimmune hepatitis. Necrotizing granulomas are not part of the celiac disease patterns of injury and instead suggests infection.

10-4. Answer – e. All of these patterns can be associated with sepsis. When there is severe hypotension, the liver can also show necrosis. None of these injury patterns are specific for sepsis, and the final diagnosis rests on clinicopathological correlation. The most common diagnostic error is to believe that cholangiolar cholestasis is either sensitive or specific for sepsis; it is neither. Instead, cholangiolar cholestasis tracks best with prolonged debilitating disease or prolonged cholestasis, which can be from many different causes.

10-5. Answer – a. Hemophagocytic syndrome is most commonly associated with viral infections or drug effects. The pattern of injury does not overlap with that of primary sclerosing cholangitis. In contrast, cystic fibrosis, mast cell disease, and Langerhans histiocytosis can all mimic primary sclerosing cholangitis.

CHAPTER 11. TRANSPLANT PATHOLOGY

11-1. Answer – c. Acute cellular rejection typically shows portal inflammation with lymphocytic bile duct injury. Endothelialitis can also be seen. Granulomatous inflammation is not part of the typical pattern of acute cellular rejection.

11-2. Answer – d. Steatohepatitis can occur after transplantation, usually as part of recurrent disease, but there is no steatohepatitic variant of acute cellular rejection.

11-3. Answer – e. All of the above statements are true. Liver GVHD is associated with a disproportionate elevation in serum alkaline phosphatase levels. Liver GVHD can rarely be an isolated finding, but most cases are associated with skin and or gut GVHD. The hepatitic variant of liver GVHD is a less common pattern that is associated with donor lymphocyte infusion.

11-4. Answer – a. Most cases of PTLD are associated with EBV infection.

11-5. Answer – b. Bile duct atrophy and loss are the key features of chronic rejection seen on peripheral needle biopsies. Resection specimens with chronic rejection can also show foam cell arteriopathy. Bile duct duplication and fibro-obliterative duct lesions are seen after long-standing biliary strictures but are not associated with chronic rejection. Florid duct lesions are part of the pathology of primary biliary cirrhosis or less commonly drug effects.

CHAPTER 12. GENETIC DISEASES

12-1. Answer – c. All of these conditions are autosomal recessive except for ferroportin disease.

12-2. Answer – a. M is the normal allele for the gene encoding alpha-1-antitrypsin protein.

12-3. Answer – d. The genotype ZZ is most likely to lead to clinical disease.

12-4. Answer – d. All of these setting would benefit from testing to rule out HFE mutations. There is no absolute cut off for when the findings on a Perls iron stain should trigger genetic testing. Instead the decision is based on the amount of iron, the iron location, the fibrosis stage, and relevant clinical findings.

12-5. Answer – a. The C282Y mutation in the HFE gene is most likely to cause clinical disease, either when there are homozygous mutations or compound heterozygote mutations, such as C282Y/H63D.

12-6. Answer – d. All of these conditions can lead to a negative copper stain, despite the patient having Wilson disease.

CHAPTER 13. PEDIATRIC BENIGN AND MALIGNANT TUMORS

13-1. Answer – c. The pure fetal with low mitotic activity subtype of hepatoblastoma has the best prognosis and is cured by complete surgical resection.

13-2. Answer – e. All of these are features of hepatoblastoma, but none are specific.

13-3. Answer – f. None of these tumors have been etiologically associated with a background of chronic liver disease.

13-4. Answer – a. Hepatoblastomas can be composed of neoplastic cells with both epithelial and mesenchymal differentiation. An epithelial component is required. Mesenchymal hamartomas can have entrapped bile ducts and hepatocytes, but the neoplasm is composed of mesenchymal cells. In calcified nested stromal epithelial tumors, the tumor is epithelial and the stromal component appears to be reactive based on current data.

13-5. Answer – b. About 20% of calcified nested stromal epithelial tumors are associated with Cushing syndrome. Increased mitoses in an infantile hemangioma are a common finding and do not indicate a worse prognosis. AFP or glypican 3 can be expressed in the entrapped hepatocytes of a mesenchymal hamartoma, but this does not indicate anything, other than being a diagnostic pitfall, mimicking hepatocellular carcinoma. Embryonal sarcomas commonly arise from dedifferentiated mesenchymal hamartomas, not hepatoblastomas.

13-6. Answer – c. Mesenchymal hamartomas are composed of a spindle cell proliferation in a loose myxoid background, often with cystic changes. Entrapped bile ducts and islands of hepatocytes are common, especially at the periphery of the lesion. Hepatoblastomas have mixed epithelial and mesenchymal components (about 40%), and the epithelial component shows hepatic differentiation, but the epithelial component does not show marked nuclear pleomorphism or multinucleated giant cells. Infantile hemangiomas form mass lesions that are visible both on imaging and gross examination. Rhabdoid tumors, not rhabdomyosarcomas, are composed of discohesive epithelioid cells with INI-1 loss. Calcified nested stromal epithelial tumors can be associated with the Cushing syndrome, but they are not a subtype of hepatoblastoma and typically are not poorly differentiated.

CHAPTER 14. HEPATOCELLULAR TUMORS

14-1. Answer – e. All of these subtypes of hepatic adenoma have an increased risk for malignant transformation.

14-2. Answer – e. Hepatic tumors with extensive reticulin loss are hepatocellular carcinomas. While all of the adenomas on this list have an increased risk for malignancy, none should have reticulin loss (unless they have undergone malignant transformation).

14-3. Answer – b. A maplike staining pattern on a glutamine synthetase stain supports a diagnosis of focal nodular hyperplasia in the setting of compatible morphology.

14-4. Answer – e. Copper staining is seen primarily in two benign liver tumors: focal nodular hyperplasia and inflammatory hepatic adenomas. Sinusoidal dilation can be prominent in inflammatory hepatic adenomas, but there can be dilation in other subtypes of adenomas and in focal nodular hyperplasia. Aberrant (naked) lobular arteries can be seen in a variety of tumors including focal nodular hyperplasia, hepatic adenoma, and hepatocellular carcinoma. Ductal structures can be present in both focal nodular hyperplasia and in inflammatory hepatic adenomas.

14-5. Answer – c. Female gender is associated with an increased risk for both focal nodular hyperplasia and for hepatic adenomas. Fatty liver disease is a known risk factor for inflammatory adenomas but not for focal nodular hyperplasia.

14-6. Answer – b. Of these findings, only reticulin loss indicates a diagnosis of hepatocellular carcinoma. All of the other findings can be seen in hepatocellular adenomas. Beta catenin nuclear accumulation and strong and diffuse glutamine synthetase staining indicate beta catenin activation, which has an increased risk for malignant transformation, but does not indicate malignancy itself.

CHAPTER 15. MALIGNANT HEPATOCELLULAR TUMORS AND PRECURSORS

15-1. Answer – a. The diagnosis of combined hepatocellular carcinoma–cholangiocarcinoma requires two distinct morphologies, with immunostains that support the morphology, e.g., biliary markers in the area that looks biliary and hepatic markers in the areas that look hepatic.

15-2. Answer – c. Fibrolamellar carcinomas have a DNAJB1–PRKACA gene fusion that leads to activation of protein kinase A. This fusion is unique to fibrolamellar carcinomas.

15-3. Answer – a. The steatohepatitic variant of hepatocellular carcinoma is strongly associated with fatty liver disease in the background liver, either from alcohol use or the metabolic syndrome.

15-4. Answer – c. The chromophobe variant of hepatocellular carcinoma is strongly associated with alternative lengthening of telomeres (ALT). ALT leads to telomere maintenance in neoplastic cells by homologous recombination, instead of by activation of telomerase. ALT is very common in some sarcomas, but rare in carcinomas in general.

15-5. Answer – e. The tumor grade for hepatocellular carcinoma provides prognostic information for all of these cases: hepatocellular carcinomas in cirrhotic livers, noncirrhotic livers, after partial hepatic resection, and after liver transplantation.

CHAPTER 16. BILIARY TUMORS

16-1. Answer – a. IPBN and BilIN are both precursors to cholangiocarcinoma, with BilIN found primarily in cirrhotic livers and IPBN in noncirrhotic livers. BilIN is a microscopic lesion, while IPBN forms grossly visible mass lesions.

16-2. Answer – b. The bile duct adenoma is composed of small glands with absent to inconspicuous (small) lumens. All of the rest of the lesions have prominent lumens.

16-3. Answer – e. All of the above are true and represent potential diagnostic pitfalls.

16-4. Answer – a. The tumor cells are EBV positive (by EBER or immunostains) in most cholangiocarcinomas with a lymphoepithelioma morphology.

16-5. Answer – c. The biliary adenofibroma has a high risk for malignant transformation. The risk for the other lesions is not zero but is negligible.

CHAPTER 17. ADULT BENIGN AND MALIGNANT MESENCHYMAL TUMORS

17-1. Answer – b. Solitary fibrous tumors are STAT 6 positive.

17-2. Answer – e. All of these stains are positive in angiomyolipomas. HMB45 is the most common stained used to confirm the diagnosis.

17-3. Answer – d. Epithelioid hemangiomas are frequently positive for keratins, which represents an important diagnostic pitfall.

17-4. Answer – c. By far, the most common hemangioma of the liver is the cavernous hemangioma. The remaining hemangiomas are all very rare. Epithelioid hemangioendotheliomas are malignant and are not hemangiomas.

17-5. Answer – e. Angiosarcomas can have many different growth patterns, including all of those listed here.

INDEX

Note: Page numbers followed by "f" indicate figures, "t" indicate tables and "b" indicate boxes.

H

I